Functional foods

Related titles:

Functional foods: principles and technology
(ISBN 978-1-84569-592-7)
Foods which have health-promoting properties over and beyond their nutritional value – products known as functional foods – have become a significant industry sector. *Functional foods: principles and technology* provides both students and professionals with an authoritative introduction to the key scientific aspects and major product categories in this area. The opening chapter introduces the principles of functional foods and explores industry and consumer roles in this evolving market. Subsequent chapters focus on the most significant product categories, reviewing ingredient sources, classification, properties, therapeutic effects and possible mechanisms of action, among other topics. Antioxidants, dietary fiber, prebiotics and probiotics, lipids and soy are among the foods and food constituents covered. The appendix contains laboratory exercises aimed at those using this book in a classroom situation.

Food for the ageing population
(ISBN 978-1-84569-193-6)
The world's ageing population is increasing. Food professionals will have to address the needs of older generations more closely in the future. This unique volume reviews the characteristics of the ageing population as food consumers, the role of nutrition in healthy ageing and the design of food products and services for the elderly. Chapters in Part 1 discuss aspects of the elderly's relationship with food, such as appetite and ageing and the social significance of meals. The second part reviews the role of nutrition in conditions such as Alzheimer's and eye-related disorders. Concluding chapters address issues such as food safety and the elderly and nutrition education programmes.

Food, diet and obesity
(ISBN 978-1-85573-958-1)
Obesity is a global epidemic, with large proportions of adults and children overweight or obese in many developed and developing countries. As a result, there is an unprecedented level of interest and research in the complex interactions between our genetic susceptibility, diet and lifestyle in determining individual risk of obesity. With its distinguished editor and international team of contributors, this collection sums up the key themes in weight control research, focusing on their implications and applications for food product development and consumers.

Details of these books and a complete list of Woodhead titles can be obtained by:

- visiting our web site at www.woodheadpublishing.com
- contacting Customer Services (e-mail: sales@woodheadpublishing.com; fax: +44 (0) 1223 832819; tel.: +44 (0) 1223 499140 ext. 130; address: Woodhead Publishing Limited, 80 High Street, Sawston, Cambridge CB22 3HJ, UK)

If you would like to receive information on forthcoming titles, please send your address details to: Francis Dodds (address, tel. and fax as above; e-mail: francis.dodds@woodheadpublishing.com). Please confirm which subject areas you are interested in.

Woodhead Publishing Series in Food Science, Technology and Nutrition: Number 205

Functional foods

Concept to product

Second edition

Edited by
Maria Saarela

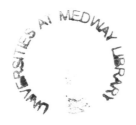

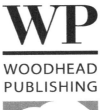

WP

WOODHEAD
PUBLISHING

Oxford   Cambridge   Philadelphia   New Delhi

Published by Woodhead Publishing Limited,
80 High Street, Sawston, Cambridge CB22 3HJ, UK
www.woodheadpublishing.com

Woodhead Publishing, 1518 Walnut Street, Suite 1100, Philadelphia, PA 19102-3406, USA

Woodhead Publishing India Private Limited, G-2, Vardaan House, 7/28 Ansari Road,
Daryaganj, New Delhi – 110002, India
www.woodheadpublishingindia.com

First edition 2000, Woodhead Publishing Limited and CRC Press LLC
Second edition 2011, Woodhead Publishing Limited
© Woodhead Publishing Limited, 2011
The authors have asserted their moral rights.

British Library Cataloguing in Publication Data
A catalogue record for this book is available from the British Library.

ISBN 978-1-84569-690-0 (print)
ISBN 978-0-85709-255-7 (online)
ISSN 2042-8049 Woodhead Publishing Series in Food Science, Technology and Nutrition (print)
ISSN 2042-8057 Woodhead Publishing Series in Food Science, Technology and Nutrition (online)

Typeset by RefineCatch Limited, Bungay, Suffolk

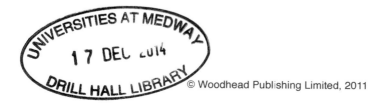

© Woodhead Publishing Limited, 2011

Contents

Part I General issues with functional foods

Contributor contact details

(* = main contact)

Editor and Chapter 18

Maria Saarela
VTT Technical Research Centre of
  Finland
PO Box 1000
02044 VTT
Finland

E-mail: maria.saarela@vtt.fi

Chapter 1

Marcel Roberfroid
Professor Emeritus
Faculty of Medicine
Catholic University of Louvain
7A rue du Rondia
B-1348 Louvain-La-Neuve
Belgium

E-mail: marcel@fefem.com

Chapter 2

Peter Berry Ottaway* and
  Sam Jennings
Berry Ottaway & Associates Ltd
Kivernoll
Much Dewchurch
Hereford
HR2 8DS
UK

E-mail: boa@berryottaway.co.uk;
  spj@berryottaway.co.uk

Chapter 3

Dr James E. Hoadley
EAS Consulting Group
PO Box 1816
Shepherdstown
West Virginia 25443
USA

E-mail: jhoadley@easconsultinggroup.
  com

Chapter 4

Dr Dilip Ghosh
Director, nutriConnect
23 Merrilong Street
Sydney
NSW 2154
Australia

E-mail: dilipghosh@nutriconnect.
  com.au

Chapter 5

Jerzy Zawistowski
Food, Nutrition and Health
Faculty of Land and Food Systems
University of British Columbia
2205 East Mall
Vancouver
British Columbia
Canada
V6T 1Z4

E-mail: jzawisto@interchange.ubc.ca

Chapter 6

Professor Liisa Lähteenmäki
Aarhus School of Business and Social
   Sciences
Aarhus University
Haslegaardsvej 10
DK-8210 Aarhus V
Denmark

E-mail: liisal@asb.dk

Chapter 7

Professor Hania Szajewska
Department of Paediatrics
The Medical University of Warsaw
01-184 Warsaw, Dzialdowska 1
Poland

E-mail: hania@ipgate.pl

Chapter 8

Professor Julie A. Lovegrove and
   Dr Kim G. Jackson
Hugh Sinclair Unit of Human
   Nutrition and the Institute for
   Cardiovascular and Metabolic
   Research (ICMR)
Department of Food and Nutritional
   Sciences
University of Reading
PO Box 226
Whiteknights
Reading
RG6 6AP
UK

Email: j.a.lovegrove@reading.ac.uk;
   k.g.jackson@reading.ac.uk

Chapter 9

Professor Ian T. Johnson
Institute of Food Research
Norwich Research Park
Colney
Norwich
NR4 7UA
UK

E-mail: ian.johnson@bbsrc.ac.uk

Chapter 10

Semone B. Myrie*
Richardson Centre for Functional
   Foods and Nutraceuticals
Department of Human Nutritional
   Sciences
University of Manitoba
Winnipeg, Manitoba
Canada
R3T 6C5

E-mail: myrie@cc.umanitoba.ca

Peter J. H. Jones
Richardson Centre for Functional
    Foods and Nutraceuticals
Departments of Food Science and
    Human Nutritional Sciences
University of Manitoba
Winnipeg, Manitoba
Canada
 R3T 6C5

E-mail: peter_jones@umanitoba.ca

Chapter 11

Jaana Lindström*
National Institute for Health and
    Welfare
Department of Chronic Disease
    Prevention
Diabetes Prevention Unit
PO Box 30
FI-00271 Helsinki
Finland

E-mail: jaana.lindstrom@thl.fi

Suvi M. Virtanen
National Institute for Health and
    Welfare
Department of Lifestyle and
    Participation
Nutrition Unit
PO Box 30
FI-00271 Helsinki
Finland

and

Tampere School of Public Health
FI-33014
University of Tampere and Tampere
    University Hospital
Research Unit
Finland

E-mail: suvi.virtanen@thl.fi

Chapter 12

Andrew Scholey*, David Camfield,
    Lauren Owen, Andrew Pipingas and
    Con Stough
NICM Collaborative Centre for
    Neurocognition
Brain Sciences Institute
Swinburne University
Melbourne
VIC 3122
Australia

E-mail: ascholey@swin.edu.au

Chapter 13

Susan J Whiting* and Hassanali
    Vatanparast
College of Pharmacy and Nutrition
University of Saskatchewan
Saskatoon SK
Canada
S7N 5C9

E-mail: Susan.whiting@usask.ca

Chapter 14

David G. Lindsay
Euroscience Perspectives
Apartado de Correos 353
Espinardo
MURCIA 30100
Spain

E-mail: eurofeda@yahoo.co.uk

Chapter 15

Professor Ann-Sofie Sandberg
Chalmers University of Technology
Food Science
SE 412 96 Gothenburg
Sweden

Email: ann-sofie.sandberg@chalmers.se

Chapter 16

Dr Anu Turpeinen* and Pirjo
   Merimaa
Valio Ltd
R&D
PO Box 30
00039 Valio
Finland

E-mail: anu.turpeinen@valio.fi

Chapter 17

Dr Charlotte Jacobsen
Division of Industrial Food Research
National Food Institute
Technical University of Denmark
B. 221, Søltofts Plads, DTU
DK-2800 Kgs. Lyngby
Denmark

E-mail: hja@food.dtu.dk

Chapter 19

Alexandra Drakoularakou, Bob Rastall
   and Glenn Gibson*
Department of Food and Nutritional
   Sciences
University of Reading
Whiteknights
Reading
RG6 6AP
UK

E-mail: g.r.gibson@reading.ac.uk

Chapter 20

Professor Hannu J. Korhonen
MTT Agrifood Research Finland
Biotechnology and Food Research
Myllytie 1
31600 Jokioinen
Finland

E-mail: hannu.j.korhonen@mtt.fi

Chapter 21

Keizo Arihara* and Motoko Ohata
Department of Animal Science
Kitasato University
Towada-shi
Aomori 034-8628
Japan

E-mail: arihara@vmas.kitasato-u.ac.jp

Chapter 22

Chao Wu Xiao
Nutrition Research Division
Food Directorate
Health Products and Food Branch
Health Canada
Ottawa
Ontario
Canada
K1A 0K9

and

Department of Cellular and
   Molecular Medicine
Faculty of Medicine
University of Ottawa
Ottawa
Ontario
Canada

E-mail: chaowu_xiao@hc-sc.gc.ca

Chapter 23

Professor Mercedes Careche* and
Professor Javier Borderías
Instituto de Ciencia y Tecnología de
   Alimentos y Nutrición (ICTAN)
CSIC
C/Jose Antonio Novais 10
28040 Madrid
Spain

E-mail: mcareche@ictan.csic.es

Isabel Sánchez-Alonso
Instituto de Estructura de la Materia
CSIC
C/Serrano 121
28006 Madrid
Spain

E-mail: isabel.sanchez@iem.cfmac.
    csic.es

Elisabeth K. Lund
Institute of Food Research (IFR)
Norwich Research Park
Colney
Norwich
NR4 7UA
UK

E-mail: liz.lund@BBSRC.AC.UK

Chapter 24

Professor Fabienne Guillon*,
    M. Champ, J.-F. Thibault and
    Luc Saulnier
INRA Research Centre
Rue de la Géraudière
44716 Nantes cedex 3
France

E-mail: guillon@nantes.inra.fr

Woodhead Publishing Series in Food Science, Technology and Nutrition

Preface

A healthy lifestyle (including a healthy diet), that would enable the onset of chronic conditions such as diabetes, elevated blood pressure or cholesterol either to be postponed or even prevented, has very much been a focus of public discussion for some time now. The alarmingly rapid increase in the incidence of obesity, already today called an 'epidemic', raises concerns and the trend of increasing obesity together with metabolic syndrome in children and young adults is especially worrying. Since the elderly populations of Western countries are increasing, we are in addition facing the threat that people will live longer, but that they will also be in less good health, which naturally reduces quality of life.

Diet – together with physical exercise – plays a major role when we try to prevent or postpone the onset of chronic conditions such as the metabolic syndrome. The food industry has already reacted to this challenge and a large number of products have been either reformulated or re-positioned to meet the current need for healthier foods. Thus a huge selection of various functional foods, i.e. foods that have a health-promoting or disease-preventing property beyond the basic function of supplying nutrients, is available for the consumer. However, healthiness is not enough – consumers, especially if they are still only at risk of developing a disease, are generally unwilling to compromise on the sensory qualities of food to gain the potential health benefits. A further obstacle in developing functional foods is that many consumers are suspicious of eating highly processed foods with a long list of ingredients and additives. Thus functional foods need to be at the same time healthy, tasty, convenient to use, and as 'natural' as possible (for a reference see Hardy 2009, *Future Innovations in Food and Drinks to 2015*, Business Insights Ltd).

Currently, those involved in the development and marketing of functional foods are facing new challenges in the European Union (EU) due to the recent changes in legislation. The Health and Nutrition Claims Regulation (Regulation (EC) No 1924/2006; see INFO-EUROPA no. 86 at http://www.europe.org.uk/

europa/view/-/id/747/) came into force in the EU on 1 July 2007. This regulation, which describes the criteria for health claims, applies to all human food and drink to be sold in the EU. The regulation describes the following claims:

- Reduction of disease risk claims and claims on children's development and health (Article 14);
- Function claims (Article 13.1): growth, development and functions of the body; psychological and behavioural functions; slimming and weight control; and
- New claims or claims for which protection of proprietary data is requested (Article 13.5).

The European Food Safety Authority (EFSA) has been given the mandate to evaluate health claims for the Commission. Since the majority of claims for functional foods fall into the category of Article 13.1 claims, these types of claim in particular have been the focus of interesting and exciting discussions. The European Commission will in time adopt a community list of permitted function claims (i.e. claims falling under Article 13.1), which are not product specific or proprietary. After a transitional phase only function health claims which are listed in the Community Register will be permitted to be used on food. The date when this community list can be adopted is currently not certain though, since the EFSA workload relating to claim evaluation has been very high. This is due to the vast number of claims submitted, which was much higher than initially expected. To date (July 2010) four Article 14(1)(a) health claims referring to the reduction of a risk factor in the development of a disease (on plant sterols/stanol esters and xylitol), six Article 14(1)(b) health claims referring to children's development and health (on a-linolenic acid/linoleic acid, essential fatty acids, calcium, vitamin D, phosphorus, and protein), and one Article 13(5) health claim based on newly developed scientific evidence and/or including a request for the protection of proprietary data (on water-soluble tomato concentrate) have been authorised by the Commission (see: DG health and consumers at http://ec.europa.eu/food/labellingnutrition/claims/community_register/authorised_health_claims_en.htm).

The outcome of the evaluation of Article 13.1 claims will potentially have a major impact on the functional foods market in Europe in the near future. So far a vast majority of these Article 13.1 claims have been rejected by EFSA due to a variety of reasons including, for example, poor characterisation of the product, incorrect target groups and insufficient or missing human intervention data on the health effect. Whether the food products that have so far failed to get a positive opinion will remain on the market or not remains to be seen. An important notion here is that even after negative evaluation these products can still be marketed, provided that this is without the health claims.

The recent debate relating to health claims regulation and evaluation has clearly indicated how complex the functional foods area is. Questions that arise include: Where do we draw the line between foods and medicines? How do we show a health benefit for a general (healthy) population? How strict should we be in the evaluation of claims if we on the one hand think that they are for foods and not medicines, but on the other need to ensure that they are scientifically substantiated and not misleading to the consumer? It will surely still take some time to solve all these complex issues.

This book provides the reader with an overview of current developments in the functional food area. It is divided into three parts: general issues (definitions, legislation, assessment of functional foods, and consumer issues related to functional foods); functional foods and health (including cardiovascular disease, diabetes and infectious diseases), and developing functional food products (e.g. plant-, dairy-, meat-based, pro- and prebiotics and fibres). The book should be of special interest to both scientists and industry professionals working in the area of functional foods as it covers a variety of related disciplines from medicine and jurisprudence (legislation) to microbiology, food technology and nutrition.

Maria Saarela

Part I

General issues with functional foods

1

Defining functional foods and associated claims

M. Roberfroid, Catholic University of Louvain, Belgium

Abstract: To understand functional foods it is first necessary to understand how the science of nutrition itself has changed. Nutrition has progressed from the prevention of dietary deficiency and the establishment of nutrition standards, dietary guidelines and food guides, to the promotion of a state of well-being and health, and the reduction of the risk of disease. This chapter reviews definitions of the concept of functional foods, followed by key aspects of functional food science, with emphasis on 'markers' for the development of functional foods. The communication issues associated with claims for functional foods are also addressed. The chapter then illustrates the concept of functional foods with case studies focusing on three major target functions for which relevance to the state of well-being and health as well as the reduction of risk of disease is established or very likely.

Key words: functional foods, health claims, FOSHU, FUFOSE, PASSCLAIM.

1.1   Introduction

To understand functional food it is first necessary to understand how the science of nutrition itself has changed. Nutrition has progressed from the prevention of dietary deficiency and the establishment of nutrition standards, dietary guidelines and food guides, to the promotion of a state of well-being and health and the reduction of the risk of disease.

1.1.1   Nutrition: a science of the twentieth century

Even though 'diet' and 'food' are very old terms, probably as old as human beings, the term 'nutrition' is rather modern, appearing for the first time in the nineteenth century. Nutrition is multidisciplinary as it integrates and applies broad and available knowledge (including basic science) about foods and/or nutrients and their effects on body physiology with the aim of maintaining/improving the state of well-being and health.[1]

During the twentieth century, essential nutrients have been discovered and nutrient standards, dietary guidelines and food guides established, mainly if not exclusively with the aim of preventing deficiencies and supporting body growth, maintenance and development. More recently, in the last 30 years, recommendations have also been made to avoid excessive consumption of some of these nutrients since their potential role in the aetiology of miscellaneous (mostly chronic) diseases has been recognised.[2] These advances are reflected in:

- Nutrient standards,[3] the recommended daily allowances (RDAs) or reference nutrition intakes (RNIs) which are the 'average daily amounts of essential nutrients estimated on the basis of available scientific knowledge to be sufficiently high to meet the physiological needs of nearly all healthy persons'.
- Dietary guidelines,[4] which are 'advice on consumption of foods or food components for which there is a related public health concern', mostly when RDAs or RNIs are not available. These are expressed in relation to total diet, often in qualitative terms (more/less/increased/reduced . . .), based on consensus research findings relating to diet and health.
- Food guides,[5] which are 'the translation of nutritional standards and dietary guidelines in terms of recommendations on daily food intake'. These form a conceptual framework for selecting the kinds and amounts of foods of various types that, together, provide a nutritionally satisfactory diet. They are based on nutrient standards, composition of foods, food intake patterns and factors influencing food choice.

Through these developments, one of the major contributions of nutritional science in the twentieth century has been the concept of the balanced diet, 'an appropriate mixture of food items that provides, at least, the minimum requirements of nutrients and a few other food components needed to support growth and maintain body weight, to prevent the development of deficiency diseases and to reduce the risk of diseases associated with deleterious excesses'.[6]

1.1.2   Nutrition: a science for the twenty-first century

At the turn of the twenty-first century, the society of abundance, which characterises most of the industrialised world, faced new challenges from an uncontrollable increase in the costs of health care, an increase in life expectancy, improved scientific knowledge and development of new technologies to major changes in lifestyles (Table 1.1), and nutrition had to adapt to these new challenges. As a consequence, nutrition as a science, in addition to keeping an emphasis on balanced diet, had to promote 'a 'preventive nutrition'[7] while, at the same time developing, the concept of 'optimum (optimised) nutrition'.[8]

Optimum (optimised) nutrition will aim at maximising the physiological functions of each individual, in order to ensure both maximum well-being and health but, at the same time, a minimum risk of disease throughout life. In other

Table 1.1   The challenges for nutrition in the twenty-first century

1. Application of new scientific knowledge in nutrition.
2. Improved scientific knowledge on diet–disease relationships.
3. Exponential increase of health-care costs.
4. Increase in life expectancy.
5. Consumer awareness of nutrition and health relationships.
6. Progress in food technology.

words, it will have to aim at maximising a healthy lifespan. At the same time, it will have to match an individual's unique biochemical needs and genetic make-up with a tailored selection of nutrient intakes for that individual. Such a selection will be based on a better understanding of the interactions between genes and nutrition.[8] These interactions include: genetic polymorphism and interindividual variations in response to diet, dietary alteration and modulation of gene expression, and dietary effects on disease risk. They play a role both in the modulation of specific physiological functions and/or pathophysiological processes by given food components, as well as in their metabolism by the body. They control the responsiveness of a particular individual to both the beneficial and deleterious effects of their diet.

Even though a balanced diet remains a key objective to prevent deficiencies and their associated diseases and to reduce the risk of the diseases associated with excess intake of some nutrients, optimum (optimised) nutrition will aim at establishing optimum (optimised) intake of as many food components as possible to support or promote well-being and health, and/or reduce the risk of diseases, mainly for those that are diet-related. At the beginning of the twenty-first century, the major challenge of the science of nutrition is thus to progress from improving life expectancy to improving life quality/wellness.

On the road to optimum (optimised) nutrition, which is an ambitious and long-term objective, functional food is, among others, a new, interesting and stimulating concept inasmuch as it is supported by sound and consensual scientific data generated by the recently developed functional food science aimed at improving dietary guidelines by integrating new knowledge on the interactions between food components and body functions and/or pathological processes.

1.2   Functional foods: defining the concept

Functional food cannot be a single well-defined/well-characterised entity. Indeed, a wide variety of food products are or will, in the future, be characterised as functional food with a variety of components, some of them classified as nutrients, affecting a variety of body functions relevant to either a state of well-being and health and/or to the reduction in risk of a disease. Thus no simple, universally accepted definition of functional food exists. Especially in Europe, where even defining the common term 'dietary fibre' took a very long time and required many meetings, it would be unrealistic to try to produce such a definition for something as new and diverse as functional food. Functional food has thus to be understood as a concept. Moreover, if it is function driven rather than product driven, the concept is likely to be more universal and not too much influenced by local characteristics or cultural traditions.[9]

1.2.1   Functional food: an international overview

Japan is the birthplace of the term 'functional food'.[10] Moreover, that country has been at the forefront of the development of functional foods since the early 1980s when systematic and large-scale research programmes were launched and funded by the Japanese government on systematic analysis and development of food functions, analysis of physiological regulation of function by food and analysis of functional foods and molecular design. As a result of a long decision-making process to establish a category of foods for potential enhancing benefits as part of a national effort to reduce the escalating cost of health care, the concept of foods for specified health use (FOSHU) was established in 1991. These foods, which are intended to be used to improve people's health and for which specific health effects (claims) are allowed to be displayed, are included as one of the categories of foods described in the Nutrition Improvement Law as foods for special dietary use. According to the Japanese Ministry of Health and Welfare, FOSHU are:

* foods that are expected to have a specific health effect due to relevant constituents, or foods from which allergens have been removed;
* foods where the effect of such an addition or removal has been scientifically evaluated, and permission has been granted to make claims regarding the specific beneficial effects on health expected from their consumption.

Foods identified as FOSHU are required to provide evidence that the final food product, but not isolated individual component(s), is likely to exert a health or physiological effect when consumed as part of an ordinary diet. Moreover, FOSHU products should be in the form of ordinary foods (i.e. not pills or capsules).

In the meantime, but mainly in the 1990s, a variety of terms, more or less related to the Japanese FOSHU, has appeared worldwide. In addition to functional foods, these include more exotic terms such as 'nutraceuticals', 'designer foods', 'f(ph)armafoods', 'medifoods', 'vitafoods', etc., but also the more traditional 'dietary supplements' and 'fortified foods'. According to Hillian[11] these terms intend to describe 'food substances that provide medical or health benefits including the prevention and treatment of disease'. As discussed in an editorial of the *Lancet*,[12] these are 'foods or food products marketed with the message of a benefit to health' and they 'sit in the murky territory between food and medicine'.[13] For the editors of two other books entitled *Functional Foods*, these terms cover 'foods that can prevent or treat disease'[14] or 'foods or isolated food ingredients that deliver specific non-nutritive physiological benefits that may enhance health'.[15] For these authors, these terms are interchangeable. But it appears that these terms either describe quite different entities that cannot be covered by a single heading or are formulated in such a general and broad sense that they lose specificity and become too vague to be really useful.

- Nutraceuticals have been described as 'any substance that is a food or part of a food that provides medical and/or health benefits, including the prevention and treatment of disease'[16] or 'a product produced from foods but sold in powders, pills and other medicinal forms not generally associated with food and demonstrated to have physiological benefits or provide protection against chronic disease'.[17]
- Vitafoods are defined by the Ministry of Agriculture, Fisheries and Food (MAFF) as 'foods and drinks to meet the needs of modern health conscious consumers which enhance the bodily or mental quality of life, enhance the capacity to endure or flourish or to recover from strenuous exercise or illness. They may also increase the healthy status of the consumer or act as potential deterrent to health hazard.'[18]
- Dietary supplements have, at least in the USA, a more elaborate definition which covers 'a product intended to supplement the diet and that bears or contains one or more of certain specified dietary ingredients (vitamins, minerals, herbs or other botanicals, amino acids, a dietary supplement) to supplement the diet by increasing total dietary intake, a concentrate, metabolite, constituent, extract or combination. It is a tablet, capsule, powder, softgel, gelcap or liquid droplet or some other form that can be a conventional food but is not represented as a conventional.'[19] However, in France the definition is more restrictive, being 'a product to be ingested to complement the usual diet in order to make good any real or anticipated deficiencies in daily intake'.[20]

Functional food has as many definitions as the number of authors referring to it. These definitions go from simple statements such as:

- foods that may provide health benefits beyond basic nutrition;[21]
- foods or food products marketed with the message of the benefit to health;[12] or
- everyday food transformed into a potential lifesaver by the addition of a magical ingredient;[13]

to very elaborate definitions such as:

- food and drink products derived from naturally occurring substances consumed as part of the daily diet and possessing particular physiological benefits when ingested;[11]
- food derived from naturally occurring substances that can and should be consumed as part of the daily diet and that serve to regulate or otherwise affect a particular body process when ingested;[22]
- food similar in appearance to conventional food, which is consumed as part of a usual diet and has demonstrated physiological benefit and/or reduces the risk of chronic disease beyond basic nutritional functions;[17]

- food that encompasses potentially helpful products including any modified food or food ingredient that may provide a health benefit beyond that of the traditional nutrient it contains;[23]
- food similar in appearance to conventional food that is intended to be consumed as part of a normal diet, but has been modified to subserve physiological roles beyond the provision of simple nutrient requirements.

Whatever definition is chosen, 'functional food' appears as a quite unique concept that deserves a category of its own, a category different from nutraceutical, f(ph)armafood, medifood, designer food or vitafood. . . . It is also a concept that belongs to nutrition and not to pharmacology. Functional foods are and must be foods, not drugs, as they have no therapeutic effects. Moreover their role regarding disease will, in most cases, be in reducing the risk of disease rather than preventing it.

1.2.2   Functional food: a European consensus[9,24,25]
The unique features of functional food are:

- being a conventional or everyday food;
- to be consumed as part of the normal/usual diet;
- composed of naturally occurring (as opposed to synthetic) components perhaps in unnatural concentration or present in foods that would not normally supply them;
- having a positive effect on target function(s) beyond nutritive value/basic nutrition,

and may enhance well-being and health and/or reduce the risk of disease or provide health benefits so as to improve the quality of life including physical, psychological and behavioural performances and have authorised and scientifically based claims.

It is in that general context that the European Commission's Concerted Action on Functional Food Science in Europe (FUFOSE), which actively involved a large number of the most prominent European experts in nutrition and related sciences, was initiated. It was coordinated by the International Life Science Institute – ILSI Europe. It developed in early 1996 and reached the European Consensus on 'Scientific Concepts of Functional Foods' in 1998.[9] To achieve that final objective, three major steps were undertaken:

1. Critical assessment of the science base required to provide evidence that specific nutrients and food components positively affect target functions in the body.
2. Examination of the available science from a function-driven perspective rather than a product-driven one.
3. Elaboration of a consensus on targeted modifications of food and food constituents, and options for their applications.[24]

In that context, 'target function' refers to genomic, biochemical, physiological, psychological or behavioural functions that are relevant to the maintenance of a state of well-being and health or to the reduction of the risk of a disease. Modulation of these functions should be quantitatively evaluated by measuring change in serum or other body fluids of the concentration of a metabolite, a specific protein or a hormone, change in the activity of enzymes, change in physiological parameters (e.g. blood pressure, gastrointestinal transit time, etc.), change in physical or intellectual performances, and so on.

The major deliverables of this concerted action are three publications:

Functional Food Science in Europe reviews the published literature to define the state of the art with respect to specific body systems, the methodologies to characterise and quantify specific related functions, the nutritional options modulating these functions, the safety implications related to these nutritional options, the role of food technology in nutritional and safety aspects and the science base required for providing evidence that specific nutrients positively affect function.[24]

Technological Aspects of Functional Food Science reviews the impact of processing, the importance of the source of materials to prepared food products, processing options to modulate functionality, safety implications of materials and processes, and process monitoring of functions.[25]

Scientific Concepts of Functional Foods in Europe: a consensus that proposes, for the first time, a consensual framework for the development of functional foods and for the elaboration of a scientific basis for claims.[9]

As already indicated above, because functional food is a concept rather than a well-defined group of food products, that consensus document proposes a working definition:

A food can be regarded as functional if it is satisfactorily demonstrated to affect beneficially one or more target functions in the body, beyond adequate nutritional effects, in a way that is relevant to either improved stage of health and well-being and/or reduction of risk of disease. A functional food must remain food and it must demonstrate its effects in amounts that can normally be expected to be consumed in the diet: it is not a pill or a capsule, but part of the normal food pattern.[9]

The main aspects of this working definition are:

- the food nature of functional food that is not a pill, a capsule or any form of dietary supplement;
- the demonstration of the effects to the satisfaction of the scientific community;
- the beneficial effects on body functions, beyond adequate nutritional effects, that are relevant to improved state of health and well-being and/or reduction of risk (not prevention) of disease;
- the consumption as part of a normal food pattern.

The definition encompasses all main features of functional foods identified above; it is aimed at stimulating research and development in the field of nutrition so as to contribute adequately to the scientific knowledge that will be required to define optimum (optimised) nutrition by elaborating new dietary guidelines. However, it should be emphasised that a functional food will not necessarily be functional for all members of the population, and that matching individual biochemical needs with selected food component intakes may become a key task as we progress in our understanding of the interactions between genes and diet.[8] From a practical point of view, a functional food can be:

- a natural food;
- a food to which a component has been added;
- a food from which a component has been removed;
- a food where the nature of one or more components has been modified;
- a food in which the bioavailability of one or more components has been modified, or any combination of these possibilities.

1.3   Functional food science

Being foods, functional foods need to be safe according to all criteria defined in current food regulations. But in many cases, new concepts and new procedures will need to be developed and validated to assess functional food risks. In Europe, some, but certainly not all, functional foods will be classified as 'novel foods' and consequently will require the decision tree assessment regarding safety that is described in the EU Novel Food Directive.[26]

However, it must be emphasised that this regulation does not concern the nutritional properties or the physiological effects of these novel foods. It is strictly a safety regulation. The requirement for safety is a prerequisite to any functional food development. Indeed, the risk versus benefit concept, which is familiar to pharmacologists developing new drugs, does not apply to functional foods except perhaps in very specific conditions for disease risk reduction when the scientific evidence is particularly strong. As described in the European consensus document:[9] 'The design and development of functional foods is a key issue, as well as a scientific challenge, which should rely on basic scientific knowledge relevant to target functions and their possible modulation by food components'. Functional foods themselves are not universal and a food-based approach would have to be influenced by local considerations. In contrast, a science-based approach to functional food is universal. The function-driven approach has the science base as its foundation – in order to gain a broader understanding of the interactions between diet and health. Emphasis is then put on the importance of the effects of food components on well-identified and well-characterised target functions in the body that are relevant to well-being and health issues, rather than, solely, on reduction of disease risk.

By reference to the new concepts in nutrition outlined above, it is the role of functional food science to stimulate research and development of functional foods (see Fig. 1.1).

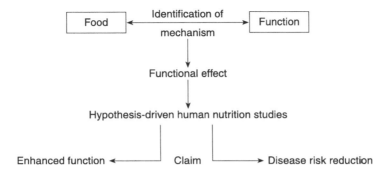

Fig. 1.1   The strategy for functional food development.

By reference to basic knowledge in nutrition and related biological sciences, such a development requires the identification and, at least partly, an understanding of the mechanism(s) by which a potential functional food or functional food component can modulate the target function(s) that is/are recognised or proven to be relevant to the state of well-being and health, and/or the reduction of a disease risk. Epidemiological data demonstrating a statistically validated and biologically relevant relationship between the intake of specific food components and a particular health benefit will, if available, be very useful. The conclusion of that first step will be the demonstration of a functional effect that should serve to formulate hypotheses to be tested in a new generation of human nutrition studies aimed to show that relevant (in terms of dose, frequency, duration, etc.) intake of the specified food will be associated with improvements in one or more target functions, either directly or indirectly in terms of a valid marker of an improved state of well-being and health and/or reduced disease risk. If well supported by strong scientific evidence, the conclusion could be a recommendation for improved or new dietary guidelines.

The new-generation human nutrition studies should be hypothesis driven but, in many cases, they will differ quite substantially from what is classically referred to as clinical studies. The main differences are that nutrition studies aim at testing the effect of a food as part of the ordinary diet; they may concern the general population or generally large, at-risk target groups; they are not diagnostic or symptom based; and they are not planned to evaluate a risk versus benefit approach. Most of these studies will rely on change(s) in validated/relevant markers to demonstrate a positive modulation of target functions after (long-term) consumption of the potential functional food. A (double) blind type of design based on parallel groups rather than crossing over will generally be appropriate. Data from these studies should be collected and handled according to good standards for data management, and data analysis should prove statistical as well as biological significance. Finally, the long-term consequences of interaction(s) between functional foods and body function(s) will have to be carefully monitored.

1.3.1   Markers: key to the development of functional foods

The development of functional foods will, in most cases, rely on measurements of 'markers'. These markers need to be identified and validated for their predictive value of potential benefits to a target function or the risk of a particular disease. Markers of correlated events are 'indicators' whereas markers representing an event directly involved in the process are 'factors'.[9] When related to the risk of disease, indicators and even factors might, in some instances, be equivalent to 'surrogate markers' defined as a biological observation, result or index that predicts the development of chronic disease.[27] The more that is known about the mechanisms leading to health outcomes, the more refined will be the identification of the markers and their appreciation. The markers should be feasible, valid, reproducible, sensitive and specific. They can be biochemical, physiological, behavioural or psychological in nature. However, dynamic responses might be as useful as, or more useful than, static or single point measurements. In many cases, a battery of markers might be needed in order to create a decision tree from multiple tests (see Fig. 1.2). These markers, most of which still need to be identified and validated, will relate to:

- Exposure to the food component under study by measuring serum, faecal, urine or tissue level of the food component itself or its metabolite(s), or the concentration of an endogenous molecule that is directly influenced by the consumption of the food component.
- Target function(s) or biological response such as change in serum or other body fluids of the concentration of a metabolite, a specific protein, an enzyme, a hormone, etc.

The following two markers are either indicators or factors.

An appropriate endpoint of an improved state of well-being and health and/or reduction of a disease risk. Such a marker is likely to be a factor rather than an indicator.

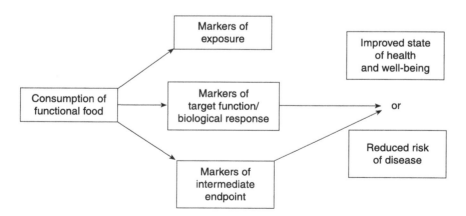

Fig. 1.2   Markers for functional food development.

Individual susceptibility or genetic polymorphism controlling the metabolism and/or the effect of the food component under study.[8]

To further develop these markers, a state-of-the-art literature review will be necessary to identify, define and characterise potential markers. Furthermore, the basic scientific knowledge underpinning these markers will be evaluated. The next step will include assessment of their relevance to physiological function, to well-being and health and eventually to disease risk. A validation will then be necessary both for the methodology and biological relevance. Finally, classification as indicator or factor will be made and potential dietary modulations demonstrated. New techniques such as those used by molecular and cellular biologists will be useful in identifying target groups who could benefit from the consumption of specific functional foods.

1.4   Communicating functional claims

1.4.1   A communication challenge

As stated in the European consensus on scientific concepts of functional foods:[9]

> As the relationship between nutrition and health gains public acceptance and as the market for functional foods grows, the question of how to communicate the specific advantages of such foods becomes increasingly important. Communication of health benefits to the public, through intermediates such as health professionals, educators, the media and the food industry, is an essential element in improving public health and in the development of functional foods. Its importance also lies in avoiding problems associated with consumer confusion about health messages. Of all the different forms of communication, those concerning claims – made either directly as a statement on the label or package of food products, or indirectly through secondary supporting information – remain an area of extensive discussion.

It is also the opinion of C. B. Hudson that 'the links between nutrition science and food product development will flow through to consumers only if the required communication vehicles are put in place'.[28] However, the communication of health benefits and other physiological effects of functional foods remains a major challenge because:

- science should remain the driving force;
- messages – claims – must be based on sound, objective and appropriate evidence;
- evidence must be consistent, able to meet established scientific standards and plausible.

Moreover, communication in nutrition generally comes from multiple sources that are sometimes contradictory, creating an impression of chaos. And chaotic information often generates ignorance and easily becomes misinformation (see Fig. 1.3).

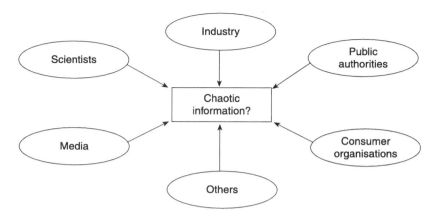

Fig. 1.3   The communication challenge for functional food development.

1.4.2   The scientific challenge: the claims

Regarding functional foods, claims associated with specific food products are the preferable means of communicating to consumers. In application of the fundamental principle, any claim must be true and not misleading; it must be scientifically valid, unambiguous and clear to the consumer. However, these basic principles should be safeguarded without becoming a disincentive to the production of functional foods or to their acceptance by consumers. Even though a general definition of 'claim' is widely accepted in the field of nutrition as 'any representation, which states, suggests or implies that a food has certain characteristics relating to its origin, nutritional properties . . . or any other quality',[29] one of the difficulties in communicating the benefits of functional foods is that distinct types of claims exist, and that in particular the term 'health claims', which is traditionally used to communicate the benefits of foods, is defined differently in different parts of the world.

Seeking clarity, *Codex Alimentarius*[29] has recently classified and defined four different categories of claims, but excluding the term 'health claim':

I.   Relate to dietary guidelines.
II. Relate to nutrient content.
III. Are comparative (reduced, less, more . . .).
IV. Describe nutrient function (contains . . ., that contributes to the development of . . .).

These claims refer to known nutrients and their role in growth, development and normal functions as well as to the concept of adequate nutrition. They are based on established, widely accepted knowledge but they do not refer to a particular effect over and above that expected from consuming a balanced diet. These claims are thus not really helpful to communicate the specific benefits of functional foods. Indeed, the claims for functional foods should be based on the scientific classification of markers (indicators and/or factors) for target functions and on the effects on these markers. If such an effect (which goes beyond what could be expected from the established role of diet in growth, development and other normal functions in the body) concerns a target function or a biological activity without direct reference to a particular disease or pathological process, claim will be made for an enhanced function. But, if the benefit is clearly a reduction of the risk of a disease or pathological process, claims will be made for disease risk reduction. These two types of claims, which are specific for functional foods, are the type A and type B claims, respectively, as they are described in the European consensus on scientific concepts of functional foods.[9] The type A claim is similar to the 'structure/function claim', whereas the type B claim can be regarded as equivalent to 'health claim' in the USA. The type B claim also corresponds to 'health claim' in Sweden.[30] In its last proposed draft recommendations for the use of health claims, *Codex Alimentarius* has included type A and type B claims and defined them as:[31]

> Type A or claims that concern specific beneficial effects of the consumption of foods and their constituents on physiological or psychological functions or biological activities but do not include nutrient function claims. Such claims relate to a positive contribution to health or a condition linked to health, to the improvement of a function or to modifying or preserving health.
>
> Type B or 'risk of disease reduction claims' that concern the reduction of a disease risk related to the consumption of a food or a food constituent in the context of the daily diet that might help reduce the risk of a specific disease or condition.

1.4.3   Scientific substantiation of claims

One of the major issues still to be resolved, especially with types A and B claims, concerns the biological level at which evidence can be accepted as 'satisfactorily demonstrating' an enhanced function or reduction of disease risk. This evidence should rely on all data available that can be grouped into three categories:

- biological observations;
- epidemiological data;
- intervention studies, mostly based on markers.

For any given specific food product, supporting evidence for enhanced function or reduction of disease risk might not be available or even not necessary from all three areas.[9] All supporting evidence should, however, be:

- consistent in itself;
- able to meet accepted scientific standards of statistical as well as biological significance, especially dose–effect relationship, if relevant;
- plausible in terms of the relationship between intervention and results, especially in terms of mechanism(s) of action;

- provided by a number of sources (including obligatory human studies) that give consistent findings able to generate scientific consensus.

To precisely define the requirements for the substantiation of functional food claims, two initiatives have been undertaken since the first edition of the present book. One was initiated, supported and published by the Council of Europe and, most importantly, the second (known as PASSCLAIM for 'Process for the Assessment of Scientific Support for Claims on Foods') was a research program funded by the EU and coordinated by ILSI Europe.[32–34] The main objective of PASSCLAIM was to produce a generic *corpus* for the evaluation of the quality of the scientific support of claims associated to foods or their components. As a starting point, the research has questioned the feasibility of the conceptual model developed in FUFOSE (see above). According to that model, consumption of a functional food component must be associated with functional/health effects scientifically substantiated by measuring either markers of target function(s) or intermediate endpoints between normal physiology and disease.

To reach these objectives, PASSCLAIM[32] has:

- identified seven physiological functions and reviewed all scientific data related to their modulation by foods and/or food components;
- defined scientific requirements concerning the quality of the data to justify potential claims;
- evaluated the relevance and value of the available markers.

Analysing the strengths and weaknesses of the available methodologies to evaluate the functional and health effects of foods and/or food components in different domains of the physiology allowed to identify general principles as well as criteria to be used in selecting and validating scientific data available to substantiate claims (Table 1.2). These general principles provide the context in which criteria can be operational (Table 1.3).

In summary, the criteria:

- underline the need for a direct relationship between the 'functional' benefice for humans in conditions that are compatible with the purported use;
- recognize the utility of the markers of intermediate endpoints when the 'ideal' target is not accessible to direct measurements;

Table 1.2   General principles applicable to substantiate a claim based on scientific evidence

PASSCLAIM

1. Food and food components for which a claim is made must conform to existing legislations and be compatible with a healthy nutrition.
2. Legislations must, in principle, reflect scientific progress by taking into consideration developments when appropriate.
3. A claim must reflect scientific justification and, at the same time, be understandable by the consumer while not misleading him.

Table 1.3   Criteria for the scientific substantiation of claims

PASSCLAIM

1. The food or food component for which a claim is made must be characterised.
2. The justification of a claim must be based on human data obtained, in priority, in intervention studies programmed as follows:

   2(a) Representative of the studied groups compared to the target group
   2(b) Relevant control group(s)
   2(c) Adequate duration of consumption and follow-up to demonstrate the searched effects
   2(d) Characterisation of the studied groups in terms of usual dietary habits and other ways of life
   2(e) Equality between the dose of food or food component in the study and the dose that will be recommended to the consumer
   2(f) Influence of the food matrix and of the dietetic context on the functional/health effect of the food or its component
   2(g) Control of the compliance of the food or its component during the study
   2(h) Statistical power of the study in relation to the tested hypothesis.

3. If the real target of the functional/health effect cannot be measured, markers including intermediate endpoints can be used in the studies.
4. These markers must be:

   • biologically relevant in the sense that they must have an established link with the final output and that their variability within the target population must be known;
   • methodologically validated from the point of view of their analytical characteristics.

5. In the study, changes in the target caused by the consumption of the functional food must be statistically and also biologically significant.
6. Scientific validation of a claim must take into account all the available data in evaluating the relative weight of each.

• underline the importance of using validated markers;
• claim for the necessity, for the importance and the nature of the demonstrated effect, to be not only statistically but also biologically significant.

In the conclusions of PASSCLAIM[32] it is underlined that the quality of the scientific data required to justify all claims (functional or health) is similar even if the nature of the data can vary. Claims concerning the usual roles of nutriments in maintaining health can be justified by the generally accepted scientific knowledge. For the claim on improvement of functions (type A) that are usually more precise, specific scientific studies will usually be required for their justification. Concerning the claims of disease risk reduction (type B), scientific substantiation will have to be found in a broad analysis of multiple data base and rely principally on studies demonstrating a reduction in a risk factor associated with a particular disease or pathology, e.g. measurement of markers of intermediate endpoints (Fig. 1.4).

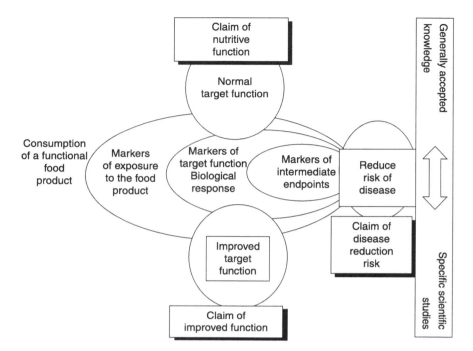

Fig. 1.4   Schematic representation of the process of scientific evaluation of the data required to justify claims (adapted from Asp *et al.*, 2004[34]).

1.5   Case studies

This section is aimed at illustrating the concepts of functional food by focusing on three major target functions for which relevance to the state of well-being and health as well as the reduction of risk of disease is established or very likely. It summarises the conclusions of expert groups that have recently reviewed the published literature to define the state of the art with respect to these specific body functions; they have identified and reviewed nutritional options modulating these functions and have critically assessed the science base required for providing evidence that specific nutrients positively affect target functions.[9,24]

1.5.1   Gastrointestinal functions[9,35]

The gastrointestinal target functions which are associated with a balanced microbiota together with an optimal gut-associated lymphoid tissue (GALT) are relevant to the state of well-being and health and to the reduction of the risk of diseases. The colonic microbiota is a complex ecosystem, the functions of which are a consequence of the combined action of the microbes that, besides interacting with the GALT, contribute to salvage of nutrient energy and produce end-metabolic products like short chain fatty acids (SCFAs) that play a role in cell differentiation, cell proliferation and metabolic regulatory processes. It is generally assumed that the group of potentially health-promoting bacteria includes, among others, bifidobacteria and lactobacilli which are and possibly should remain the most important genera in humans. Changes in the composition of the faecal microbiota, a recognised surrogate marker of the residual colonic microbiota, can be considered as a marker, indicator and factor of large bowel functions. They might play a role in gastrointestinal infections and diarrhoea, constipation, irritable bowel syndrome, inflammatory bowel diseases and colorectal cancer.

Probiotics (e.g. lactobacilli or bifidobacteria) and prebiotics (like inulin-type fructans) are recent concepts in nutrition that have already and will in the future be used to support the development of functional foods targeted towards gut function.[36] Their effects include:

• stimulation of the activity of the GALT (e.g. increased IgA response, production of cytokines);
• reduction in the duration of episodes of rotavirus infection;
• change in the composition of the faecal microbiota to reach/maintain a composition in which, for example, bifidobacteria and/or lactobacilli become predominant in number;
• increase in faecal mass (stool bulking) and stool frequency;
• increase in calcium bioavailability via colonic absorption (e.g. inulin);
• modulation of intestinal immunity;
• modulation of intestinal endocrine activities and control of satiety;
• strengthening of intestinal permeability, e.g. to lipopolysaccharides that cause metabolic endotoxemia and related diseases such as diabetes type II and obesity.

1.5.2 Defence against reactive oxidative species[9,37]

The generation of reactive oxidative species (ROS) is a general feature of any aerobic organism both during development and normal functions or pathological changes. These ROS can damage essential macromolecules like DNA, lipids and proteins by initiating or promoting oxidative processes. Many of these (bio) chemical reactions are thought to be involved in miscellaneous pathological processes such as cataracts, some cancers, cardiovascular diseases, rheumatoid arthritis and some neurodegenerative conditions. But it is becoming more and more evident that ROS also play an essential role in regulating gene expression and in participating in cell signalling. Maintaining a balance between production and destruction of ROS is thus a key element in well-being and health and it is likely to play a role in reducing the risk of disease. Examples of target functions for functional food development in relation to the maintenance of such a balance are:

• preservation of the structure and functional activity of DNA that can be evaluated by measuring DNA integrity (COMET assay), damaged DNA bases (e.g. 8 OH desoxyguanine) or specific gene expressions;

- preservation of structural and functional integrity of circulating lipoproteins by measuring either lipid hydroperoxides or their derivatives (e.g. malondialdehyde) or oxidised low-density lipoproteins in plasma;
- preservation of structural and functional integrity of proteins.

The major functional foods to rebalance oxidative processes are:

- vitamins (especially tocopherols, ascorbic acid and carotenoids);
- polyphenols such as flavonoids.

1.5.3   Psychological and behavioural functions[9,38]

Some foods or food components provide an important function by changing mood or mental state. They are involved in creating more a sense of 'feeling well' than 'being well'. Target functions for such foods and food components are:

- appetite, satiation and satiety, the most widely used markers of which are either visual analogue scales to evaluate subjectively sensations such as hunger, desire to eat and fullness or quantitative assessment of energy and/or nutrient intake;
- cognitive performance for which several markers are used like reaction to single stimulus test or complex interactive inputs;
- mood and vitality by focusing on behaviours such as sleep and activity, as well as feelings of tension, calmness, drowsiness and alertness, assessed either subjectively (e.g. with questionnaires) or objectively (e.g. with electro-physiological measurements);
- stress and distress management based on changes in physiological markers like heart rate, blood pressure, blood catecholamines, blood opioid levels.

The development of functional foods aimed at beneficially affecting behavioural and psychological functions has in the past and will in the future rely on:

- modulation of the intake of macronutrients especially by substitution (e.g. fat substitutes or intense sweeteners);
- use of components like caffeine with the aim of improving cognitive performance;
- use of specific amino acids like tryptophan or tyrosine to reduce sleep latency and promote feelings of drowsiness;
- activation of endogenous opioids (beta-endorphins) to reduce pain perception in the general population.

1.5.4   Food technology and its impact on functional food development[9,25]

From the point of view of food processing, the development of functional foods will often require an increased level of complexity and monitoring of food processing because the following will have to be considered carefully:

- new raw materials including those produced by biotechnologies;
- emerging thermal and non-thermal technologies;
- new safety issues;

- integration throughout the entire food chain especially to ensure preservation and/or enhancement of functionality.

The main areas for technological challenge that have been identified are as follows.

- The creation of new food components in traditional and novel raw materials that add or increase functionality. Examples of such challenges are: genetic modifications, use of under-utilised or unconventional natural sources (e.g. algae, seaweeds), and development of bioreactors based on immobilised enzymes or live micro-organisms.
- The optimisation of functional components in raw material and in foods to ensure maximal preservation of the component(s), to modify function, to increase their bioavailability. Examples of such challenges are: development of membrane-processing techniques, use of controlled and modified atmospheres, use of high hydrostatic pressure, high-intensity electric field pulse technology or ultrasound treatments.
- The effective monitoring, throughout the entire food chain, of the amount and functionality of the component(s) in raw materials and foods. Examples of such challenges are: monitoring of microbial viability and productivity for probiotic functions, development of sensitive markers to record changes in speciation and interactions with food components during processing, especially fermentation.

1.6   Conclusions and future trends

FUFOSE, the report of the council of Europe and PASSCLAIM have had a considerable impact not only within the EU but also the *Codex Alimentarius*. Criteria of PASSCLAIM provide a scientific background to facilitate the evaluation of health claims and to guarantee to the consumer that these claims are supported by well established scientific data. They also provide to the food industry a well defined and stable context for the development of new products likely to be beneficial for health and well-being. Consumers are assured that claims are substantiated and have been approved based on an evaluation that relies on the same criteria. Producers and distributors of food products who want to make claims know which data and which proofs are required. Government as well as European authorities who are responsible for laws and directives can have a clear understanding of the limits of the validity of each claim. Finally, those who want to develop new functional food or functional food component are guided by clear criteria defining the requirements to be fulfilled.

By reference to the conclusions of the FUFOSE concerted action,[9] future trends are as follows:

> Components in foods have the potential to modulate target functions in the body so as to enhance these functions and/or contribute towards reducing the risk of disease,

and functional food science will contribute to human health in the future provided that evidence is supported by sound scientific, mostly human, data.

Nutritionists and food scientists have the possibility through the development of functional foods to offer beneficial opportunities related to well-being and health and reduction of risk of disease. Such a new approach in nutrition is strongly dependent upon the identification, characterisation, measurement and validation of relevant markers as defined above. The design of such studies still needs to be carefully analysed and specifically developed by reference to, but differently from, classical clinical studies that have been elaborated to help in developing drugs, not food products.

Major target functions in the body that are or can be modulated by specific food products will have to be identified or characterised. The basic science to understand these functions and how they relate to well-being and health or a particular pathological process needs to be developed so as to give the necessary scientific base to develop new functional food products.

Progress in food regulation, which is the means to guarantee the validity of the claims as well as the safety of the food, have recently been giving the European Food Safety Agency (EFSA) the mission to evaluate the claims as defined in EU directive 1924/2006 (for more details see Chapter 2).

Optimised nutrition is a major challenge for nutritional science in the twenty-first century. The development of functional foods is part of this challenge but elaboration of claims should remain basically a scientific challenge, and not primarily a marketing one. The proper scientific validation of functional claims is critical to the success of functional foods, both for the benefit of human health and of the food industry.

1.7   References

1 Welsch, S. (1996) 'Nutrient standards, dietary guidelines and food guides'. In *Present Knowledge in Nutrition*, E.E. Ziegler and L.J. Filer eds, Washington DC, ILSI Press.
2 *Food and Nutrition Board Diet and Health, Implications for Reducing Chronic Diseases*, Washington DC, National Academy Press, 10th edn, 1989.
3 *Food and Nutrition Board Recommended Daily Allowances*, Washington DC, National Academy Press, 10th edn, 1989.
4 US Department of Agriculture/Department of Health and Human Services. *Nutrition and Your Health: Dietary Guidelines for Americans*, Home and Guide Bulletin No. 232, Washington DC, US Government Printing Office, 4th edn, 1990.
5 US Department of Agriculture/Department of Health and Human Services. *The Food Guide Pyramid*, Home and Guide Bulletin No. 252, Washington DC, US Government Printing Office, 1992.
6 James, W.P.T. (1998) *Healthy Nutrition: Preventing Nutrition-related Diseases in Europe*, WHO, Regional Publications European Series, **24**, 4–6.
7 Remesy, C. (2008) 'Bases d'une nutrition préventive.' In *Aliments Fonctionnels*, 2ème édition, Roberfroid, M.B., Coxam, V. and Delzenne, N. eds, Lavoisier, Paris, pp. 3–22.
8 Milner, J. (2000) 'Functional foods: the US perspective', 17th Ross Conference on Medical Issues, *Am J Clin Nutr*, **71**, 1654S–59S.

9 Diplock, A.T., Aggett, P.J., Ashwell, M., Bornet, F., Fern, F.B., Roberfroid, M.B. (1999) 'Scientific concepts of functional foods in Europe: consensus document', *Br J Nutr*, **81**(Supp. 1): S1–S28.

10 Kubomara, K. (1998) 'Japan redefines functional foods', *Prepared Foods*, **167**, 129–32.

11 Hillian, M. (1995) 'Functional foods: current and future market developments', *Food Technol Internat Europe*, 25–31.

12 Riemersma, R.A. (1996) 'A fat little earner', *Lancet*, **347**, 775–6.

13 Coghlan, A. (1996) 'A plateful of medicine', *New Scientist*, **2054**, 12–13.

14 Goldberg, I. (1994) *Functional Foods, Designer Foods, Pharmafoods, Nutraceuticals*, New York, Chapman & Hall.

15 Mazza, G. (1998) *Functional Foods: Biochemical and Processing Aspects*, Lancaster PA, Technomic.

16 Defelice, S.L. (1995) 'The nutraceutical revolution, its impact on food industry research and development', *Trends Food Sci Technol*, **6**, 59–61.

17 Health Canada (1997) *Policy Options Analysis: Nutraceuticals/Functional Foods*, Health Canada, Health Protection Branch, Therapeutic Products Programme and Food Directorate, Ottawa.

18 Ministry of Agriculture, Fisheries and Food Food Advisory Committee (1996) *Review of Functional Foods and Health Claims*, London.

19 Federal Register (1994) 'Diet Supplement Health Education Act (DSHEA)', Publ L, Washington DC, pp. 103–417.

20 Ministére de la Santé Publique, République Française Discret Définissant et Réglementat les Compléments Alimentaires, 14 October 1997, 97–964.

21 IFIC Foundation (1995) 'Functional foods: opening the door to better health', *Food Insight*, November/December.

22 Smith, B.L., Marcotte, M., Harman, G. (1996) *A Comparative Analysis of the Regulatory Framework Affecting Functional Food Development and Commercialization in Canada, Japan, the European Union and the United States of America*, Ottawa, Intersector Alliance Inc.

23 Food and Nutrition Board, Institute of Medicine, National Academy of Sciences (1994). In *Opportunities in the Nutrition and Food Sciences*, P.R. Thomas and R. Earl eds, Washington DC, National Academy Press, 1994.

24 Bellisle, F., Diplock, A.T., Hornstra, G., Koletzko, B., Roberfroid, M., *et al.* (1998) 'Functional food science in Europe', *Br J Nutr*, **80**(Supp. 1), S1–S193.

25 Knorr, D. (1998) 'Functional food science in Europe', *Trends in Food Sci Technol*, **9**, special issue, 295–340.

26 European Commission Novel Food Directive, 97/258/CEE.

27 Keystone (1997) 'The Keystone national policy dialogue on food nutrition and health: executive summary', *J Nutraceuticals, Functional and Medical Foods*, **1**, 11–32.

28 Hudson, C.B. (1994) 'The food industry's expectation', In *Health Claims: Substantiation and Research Needs*, ILSI–Australasia, 9–11.

29 Codex Alimentarius Codex General Guidelines on Claims, 1991, CAC/GL 1–1979, Revision 1.

30 *Swedish Nutrition Foundation Health Claims in the Labelling and Marketing of Food Products: The Food Industry's Rules (Self-Regulatory Programme)*, Lunc, 1996.

31 *Codex Alimentarius. Proposed Draft Recommendation for the Use of Health Claims*, Geneva, WHO, 1999.

32 Aggett, P.J., Antoine, J.-M., Asp, N.-G., Bellisle, F., Contor, L., *et al.* (2005) 'Process for the Assessment of Scientific Support for Claims on Foods (PASSCLAIM) – Consensus on Criteria'. *Eur J of Nutr* **44** (Suppl 1): S1–S27.

33 Asp, N.G., Cummings, J.H., Mensink, R.P., Prentice, A., Richardson, D.P (2003). 'Process for the Assessment of Scientific Support for Claims on Foods (PASSCLAIM) – Phase One: Preparing the Way'. *Eur J Nutr* **42** (Suppl 1): 1–119.

34 Asp, N.G., Cummings, J.H., Howlett, J., Rafter, J., Riccardi, G., Westenhoeffer, J. (2004). 'Process for the Assessment of Scientific Support for Claims on Foods (PASSCLAIM) – Phase Two: moving forward.' *Eur J Nutr* **43**(Suppl 2): 1–183.
35 Salminen, S., Bouley, C., Boutron-Ruault, M.C., Cummings, J.H., Franck, A., *et al.* (1998) 'Functional food science and gastrointestinal physiology and function', *Br J Nutr*, **80**(Supp. 1): S147–S171.
36 Gibson, G.R. and Roberfroid, M.B. eds, *Handbook of Prebiotics*, CRC Press, Boca Raton, 2008.
37 Diplock, A.T., Charleux, J.L., Crozier-Willy, G., Kok, F.J., Rice-Evans, C., *et al.* (1998) 'Functional food science and defense against reactive oxidative species', *Br J Nutr*, **80**(Supp. 1): S77–S112.
38 Bellisle, F., Blundell, J.E., Dye, L., Fantino, M., Fern, E., *et al.* (1998) 'Functional food science and behaviour and psychological functions', *Br J Nutr*, **80**(Supp. 1): S173–S193.

2

EU legislation and functional foods: a case study

P. Berry Ottaway and S. Jennings,
Berry Ottaway & Associates Ltd, UK

Abstract: Food legislation has always lagged behind innovation and product development, sometimes by more than a decade. The composition and proposed marketing of many functional foods, particularly those developed outside of the European Union (EU) can introduce a number of anomalies in the application of current EU food legislation. This chapter looks at the complexities associated with the development of functional foods within the EU, using a fortified beverage mix that had been successfully marketed outside of the EU as an example of the difficulties that may have to be surmounted in order to achieve compliance with the relevant European legislation.

Key words: European food legislation, functional foods, case study, product development.

2.1 Introduction

Food legislation has always lagged behind innovation and product development, sometimes by more than a decade. This was particularly true in Europe in the late 1990s, with advances in nutritional science and the general acceptance that some aspects of food could contribute to health in other ways than by providing an adequate supply of the classical nutrients. From a relatively slow start in the mid-1990s the concept of functional foods has been gaining ground world-wide, at the same time attracting the attention of the major multinational food companies. Through the first decade of the twenty-first century there has been an increasing recognition in Europe of the category of functional foods by the authorities, particularly in the area of health claims for the foods.

The composition and proposed marketing of many functional foods, particularly those developed outside of the European Union (EU), can introduce a number of anomalies in the application of current EU food legislation. There are also distinct differences in the approach to functional foods between legislators in Europe, the United States of America and Japan. This chapter looks at the complexities associated with the development of functional foods within the European Union, using a fortified beverage mix that had been successfully marketed outside of the EU as an example of the difficulties that may have to be surmounted in order to achieve compliance with the relevant European legislation.

2.2   Product description

The product, which was in an advanced state of development in a country outside the EU, was also being considered for the European market. The concept of the product was as a powdered beverage mix which could be made up with milk, water or fruit juice and which provided not only the essential macronutrients protein, carbohydrate and fat, but also a wide range of micronutrients, added fibre sources, fructo-oligosaccharides and a number of substances claimed to have '*in vivo*' antioxidant properties.

The micronutrients in the form of vitamins and minerals and trace elements were those listed in the amendment to the EU directive on nutrition labelling.[1,2] The vitamins C, E and betacarotene were present at levels above the recommended daily allowances (RDAs) for labelling purposes given in the directive. In addition, the formulators of the product wanted to add a number of other substances such as the carotenoids lycopene and lutein, and also some herbal extracts being marketed for their physiological properties.

The marketing objective in the country of origin of the product was that the product should be positioned not only as a nutritious beverage but also for athletes, convalescents and as a meal replacement for weight control purposes. It was intended that the product would be available in three flavours with appropriate colours.

2.3   Product positioning in the European market

The definition of the product from the marketing point of view was found to be critical. Some of the recommended uses fell into the definition of dietetic as given in the Directive on foods for particular nutritional uses (2009/39/EC) known as the PARNUTS Directive.[3] There is a specific Directive in force, 96/8/EC,[4] which controls both the composition and labelling of foods marketed as meal replacements for use in weight control diets. The composition of such meal replacements must comply with very detailed criteria with respect to the energy, protein, carbohydrate, fat and micronutrient content. The product as developed did not meet all the criteria so the decision had to be made to market it as a convenient healthy beverage applicable to a range of lifestyles.

2.4   Product composition

A detailed investigation had to be carried out on every component, whether ingredient or additive, to ensure compliance with the various European laws.

2.4.1   Protein

The protein contribution was made up of both isolated soya protein and casein (milk protein). The specifications and origins of both had to be checked. To comply with Commission Regulation (EC) No 1829/2003[5] on genetically modified food and feed and Regulation (EC) No 1830/2003[6] on the traceability and labelling of genetically modified organisms, the provenance of the soya had to be traced and certification obtained that it did not contain genetically modified protein or DNA. In addition, there is a European Directive 83/417/EEC[7] (as amended) laying down the specification and quality criteria for caseinates, and the ingredient specification had to be checked for compliance.

2.4.2   Fat

The fat contribution was supplied from a vegetable oil high in polyunsaturated fatty acids, a fish oil plus some lecithin. The specification and typical analyses of the oil were obtained to ensure that the permitted maximum level of erucic acid in the vegetable oil was not likely to be exceeded. Erucic acid is a normal constituent of seed oils which has been shown to have detrimental effects on health if consumed in large quantities. There is a limit for erucic acid from oils used in compounded foods where the overall fat content of the food exceeds 5%. The details are given in Directive 76/621/EEC[8] with the method of analysis in Directive 80/891/EEC.[9] Directive 76/621/EEC also gives derogation for member states to apply the provisions of the directive to foods where the total fat content is equal to or less than 5%.

Due to the high polyunsaturated content of the oil it was more susceptible to oxidation (rancidity) than many oils used in such products. The presence of a number of mineral salts in the product also increased the risk of rapid rancidity. Permitted antioxidants for fats and oils are given in Regulation (EC) No 1333/2008[10] on food additives, which points to the Annexes of Directive 95/2/EC[11] until such time as the ongoing review of food additives is completed. As the proposed source of the oil was North America, discussions had to be conducted with the suppliers to ensure that the oil was adequately protected using only the antioxidants and permitted levels given in the directive. As European law in this area differs from that in the United States of America, this caused considerable problems which were only resolved by changing to a different grade of oil to that originally preferred.

Legal complications were also encountered with the lecithin. Lecithins are approved additives and appear in Annex 1 to Directive 95/2/EC as being generally permitted in foodstuffs. According to the formulator of the product, the lecithin had been included for two reasons, the first was technological to improve the wetting-out characteristics when the powder was mixed into the liquid, and the second was nutritional to provide a source of phospholipids. This situation, where substances can have dual roles in foods as additives and nutrients, is not uncommon in European food law. The decision was made that the primary function of the lecithin was as an additive. However, while the decision was made to specify the lecithin as an additive, its contribution had to be added to the total fat content given in the nutrition information on the label. Directive 90/496/EEC (as amended)[2] on nutrition labelling specifically includes phospholipids in the definition of fat.

A further complication was that the lecithin had to be derived from a non-genetically modified (GM) source, otherwise the phrase 'This product contains genetically modified organisms' or 'This product contains genetically modified lecithin' would have to be added to the product label. As GM foods are not generally popular with European consumers, the decision was made to find a reputable supplier of non-GM lecithin, although this meant allowance had to be made in the product budget for an increase in the cost of this ingredient.

The addition of a fish oil high in omega-3 fatty acids was made with the intention of making a claim for the health benefits of the fatty acids. Within European legislation both a claim for omega-3 fatty acid content and a claim for a health benefit come under the Nutrition and Health Claims Regulation (EC) No 1924/2006 (as amended).[12] Both types of claim had a requirement for a minimum content of fatty acids (for more details see the later section on claims). At the time of formulation the European Commission had not agreed on the minimum level of the omega-3 fatty acids required to make the claim that the product contained the fatty acids. The health benefit claims for the fatty acids were still being assessed for scientific substantiation by the European Food Safety Authority (EFSA) and their opinions had not been released. The decision was made to retain the fish oil in the formulation but to defer the claims until further information became available.

As the source of the fish oil was from outside the EU it was necessary to ensure that the supplier was registered to the requirements of the Regulations on the hygiene on animal by-products (Regulations (EC) No 853/2004[13] and (EC) No 854/2004[14]). It was also necessary to ensure that the relevant documentation would be available from the suppliers of the fish oil and the manufacturers of the product.

2.4.3   Carbohydrate

The main carbohydrate component of the product consisted of a mixture of dextrose, fructose and maltodextrin. As these ingredients can be produced from maize the GM status of each had to be determined. The product was also found to contain relatively small amounts of sorbitol, principally as a component of some compounded ingredients. Under European law the definition of carbohydrates for labelling purposes includes the polyols, of which sorbitol is one, but requires the energy calculation for the contribution from sorbitol to be made with a different factor.[2] Carbohydrates (excluding polyols) must be calculated on the basis of 4 kcal/g, whereas polyols are at 2.4 kcal/g, Also, for the purposes of nutrition labelling, the statement of carbohydrate content had to be sub-divided into sugars, polyols and starch. The legal definition of sugars includes all monosaccharides and disaccharides in the foods, but excludes polyols.

2.4.4   Fibre

The added fibre and fructo-oligosaccharides presented a number of legal problems, particularly in the quantification of the fibre content. When Directive 90/496/EEC on nutrition labelling[2] was adopted, the definition of fibre was not given and the following statement appeared in the law:

> fibre means the material to be defined in accordance with the procedure laid down in Article 10 (of Directive 90/496/EEC) and measured by the method of analysis to be determined in accordance with that procedure.

This meant that there was no official definition of fibre and this situation prevailed for the next 18 years. During this period the United Kingdom was at odds with the rest of the EU on both the definition and determination of fibre, with the British authorities favouring the Englyst method and most of the other countries working to the American Association of Analytical Chemists (AOAC) method. For many foods the AOAC method gave higher values than the Englyst method for fibre as it was measuring some different substances.

Directive 2008/100/EC,[15] which amended Directive 90/496/EEC, brought in an EU definition of fibre as follows:

> For the purposes of this Directive 'fibre' means carbohydrate polymers with three or more monomeric units, which are neither digested nor absorbed in the human small intestine and belong to the following categories:
>
> - edible carbohydrate polymers naturally occurring in the food as consumed;
> - edible carbohydrate polymers which have been obtained from food raw material by physical, enzymatic or chemical means and which have a beneficial physiological effect demonstrated by generally accepted scientific evidence;
> - edible synthetic carbohydrate polymers which have a beneficial physiological effect demonstrated by generally accepted scientific evidence.

The amount of fibre needed to make a claim of a source of fibre, and any claim likely to have the same meaning for the consumer, may only be made where the product contains at least 3 g of fibre per 100 g or at least 1.5 g of fibre per 100 kcal. A claim that a food is high in fibre, and any claim likely to have the same meaning for the consumer, may only be made where the product contains at least 6 g of fibre per 100 g or at least 3 g of fibre per 100 kcal. This Directive only comes into force in October 2012 and, although there is now a chemical definition of the substances that can be considered as fibre, the analytical methodology was not agreed.

As the definition encompasses a large and heterogeneous group of substances there was no single method of analysis available which included all these substances. In mid-2009 the European Commission circulated an 'Issues Paper' outlining both the problem and the analytical options. As a consequence, the precise amount of fibre that could be declared was uncertain and it was decided that for the short term the AOAC method would be used and any discrepancies adjusted when the official EU method is finally agreed. Directive 2008/100/EC also required that for the total energy calculation of the product, the fibre content is calculated as 2 kcal/8 kJ per gram of fibre.

2.4.5 Micronutrients

The marketing proposal for the product relied on the presence of a range of vitamins and minerals. In 2006 the EU Regulation on the addition of vitamins, minerals and certain other substances to foods was adopted, Regulation (EC) No 1925/2006 (as amended).[16] This regulation specifies which vitamins and minerals are permitted in foods and also the permitted sources that can be used to supply the micronutrients. This law was brought in as, previously across Europe, there had been no consistent approach to the addition of micronutrients to foods, with some countries being considerably more liberal than others. Before 1996 many countries used the recommended daily allowance (RDA) values as a means of controlling the levels of vitamins and minerals in products with complex legislation. For example, Belgium controlled vitamins A and D at $1 \times$ RDA, the B vitamins and vitamins C and E at $3 \times$ RDA and the other micronutrients at $2 \times$ RDA. Germany prohibited the addition of vitamins A and D to most foods and permitted the other vitamins to be added up to $3 \times$ RDA. These complexities meant that a pan-European formula had to be reduced to the lowest common denominator from each country's requirements.

While Regulation 1925/2006 lists the permitted micronutrients and their sources, the permitted upper levels as required by the law have not yet been adopted and were still in discussion towards the end of 2010. Until maximum levels are adopted by the EU, national legislation will prevail, giving a wide range of approaches across the 27 countries of the EU. To ensure maximum coverage of the EU marketing opportunities it was decided that the vitamins and minerals would not be added at levels exceeding the RDAs for labelling purposes laid down in Directive 2008/100/EC.[1] Until this directive was adopted in October 2008 there were only 12 vitamins and 6 minerals which were officially recognised. The new directive increased this by assigning RDA values to all 13 vitamins and 14 minerals/trace elements permitted by the legislation.

The sources permitted for the supply of vitamins and minerals had to be checked against the amended list in Regulation 1925/2006. The final list is the result of an evaluation by EFSA of over 500 applications for additions. The list does not contain a number of sources, particularly mineral sources, commonly used in the USA at the present time.

In order to comply with the nutrition and health claims Regulation (EC) No 1924/2006,[12] any claim for 'source of' or 'high in' for the vitamins and minerals contained in the product had to comply with the levels specified in the Annex to the Regulation. This meant that each vitamin or mineral claimed had to be present at a level of at least 15% RDA in the product as consumed, for a claim of 'source of', or at least 30% RDA in the product as consumed for a 'high in' claim. As the majority of claims for the vitamin or mineral health benefits, which are also regulated by this legislation, required a minimum of 15% RDA for the vitamin/ mineral concerned, the product was formulated to ensure that the claimed amount of each vitamin/mineral was at least 15% of the RDA as laid down in Directive 2008/100/EC.

2.4.6   Novel foods and novel ingredients

The original proposal for the product included a number of substances, which were to be added for their *in vivo* antioxidant functions. The list of those to be considered consisted of a number of plant extracts including some with high levels of polyphenols. The first task was to check each proposed substance on the list for acceptability, both in terms of their status with regard to the Council Regulation (EC) No 258/97 on Novel Foods and Novel Ingredients,[17] and to the national situation in the countries of intended sale.

Although Regulation 258/97 had been in force for over 12 years at the time the review was carried out, the situation was found to be very confusing. The main criterion for classification as a novel food or ingredient is that the substance should not previously have been used for human consumption in the European Community *to a significant degree*. Unfortunately, no formal definition of the phrase 'to a significant degree' had been agreed between the European Commission and the original 15 Member States at the time the Regulation was adopted. Interpretations varied from that which accepted evidence that the substance had been on sale in a food product in one Member State before 15 May 1997 (the date the Regulation came into force), to evidence of a large distribution and sales in more than one Member State.

In 2005 the European Commission's Standing Committee on the Food Chain and Animal Health came to a decision that evidence of pre-1997 use that was entirely in food supplements, could not be used to claim exemption from the Regulation for foods in other categories

The main problem encountered was that, although evidence of prior sale in the United Kingdom and the Netherlands could be found for some of the substances, enquiries determined that they were not considered acceptable for use in food products in other countries such as Germany and France. The investigations highlighted a major weakness in the system. The intention of Regulation 258/97 is that novel foods and novel ingredients are reviewed and approved by the competent authority in the Member State of intended first sale. This is carried out with the knowledge of the other 26 Member States who are notified of the application by the European Commission. Once approved, the substance should be accepted throughout the EU. No provision was made in the Regulation or in any other European food legislation for mutual recognition of foods and ingredients which were introduced into one of the national markets a few years before the Regulation came into force. This left a number of ingredients, including some on the proposed list for the product, in a situation where approval for use still had to be obtained on a country by country basis.

A Regulation allowing for 'mutual recognition' (Regulation (EC) No 764/2008[18]) came into force in September 2008 and became applicable from May 2009. The principle of this Regulation is that a product lawfully marketed in one Member State and not subject to EU harmonisation should be allowed to be marketed in any other Member State, even when the product does not fully comply with the technical rules of the Member State of destination. The Regulation puts the onus of proof for denying entry of the product into their market on the destination Member State rather than on the company that is attempting to market the product across EU borders. However, early indications are that there are very few areas where there is a lack of EU harmonisation that enables this Regulation to be applied.

While lutein was found to be acceptable, the lycopene was an anomaly. The carotenoid had been approved for use as a food colouring in Europe, but with restricted levels of input. It appears in the legislation on colours for use in foodstuffs and its permitted use is restricted to specified categories of food and drink. It has also been used in food supplements. The introduction of the Standing Committee decision that supplement usage prior to 1997 did not give exemption for other foods, meant that the manufacturers of the lycopene had to submit an application under the Novel Foods Regulation for evaluation and approval for food use. Approval was finally granted in 2009,[19,20,21,22] but the only beverage categories in which it was permitted to be used were:

- fruit or vegetable juice-based drinks (including concentrates) to a maximum of 2.5 mg/100 g;
- drinks intended to meet the expenditure of intense muscular effort, especially for sportsmen, to a maximum of 2.5 mg/100 g.

These categories did not fit the concept of the product and it was reluctantly decided to remove the lycopene; however, the lutein was retained.

2.4.7   Plant extracts
The original formulation contained plant (herbal) extracts which claimed antioxidant properties. The use of plant extracts in foods and food supplements is one of the areas where there is a lack of harmonisation across the EU, with a number of different national laws in force across the Member States. As it was almost impossible to find plant extracts which were permitted for use in foods in all of the countries of the EU, it was decided to leave them out of the European formulation.

2.4.8   Colours and flavours
Both food colours and food flavourings are controlled by European legislation. The proposed colours and the levels of use had to comply with Regulation (EC)

No 1333/2008,[10] which refers to the Annexes of Directive 94/36/EC[23] until such time as the ongoing review of colours for use in foodstuffs is completed. As many of the proposed colours were carried on a base or were in the form of a lake, details of the pure dye content of each had to be obtained to enable the appropriate calculations to be made. Regulation (EC) No 1333/2008 includes the requirement, applicable from July 2010, that if certain azo (synthetic) colours were used in a product, the label of the product must carry a warning about sensitivity to these colours by certain children. The decision was made not to use azo-based colours for any versions of the product.

Legislation amending earlier EU laws on flavourings was adopted in 2008 as Regulation (EC) No 1334/2008.[24] This considerably changed the definitions of flavouring categories, with new criteria for the claims of 'natural flavourings'. There were also limits placed on the quantity of certain substances that can be naturally present in flavours derived from natural sources. As most food flavourings are compounded proprietary mixtures, certification had to be obtained from each of the proposed suppliers that their flavouring complied with the requirements of the Regulations.

2.5   Claims

One of the important aspects of the product concept was that both nutrition and health claims could be made for the product. This is a complicated area that was under discussion for over 26 years before the European Regulation (EC) No 1924/2006 on nutrition and health claims made on foods finally came into force.[12] Unfortunately, there are some areas of this relatively new regulation that have added to the complication of the issue and that are very dependent upon interpretation of the legislation.

The nutrition and health claims Regulation classifies claims into three categories:

- Nutrition claims, which are claims which state, suggest or imply that a food has particular nutritional properties due to the nutrients it contains or does not contain.
- Health claims, which are defined as any claim which states, suggests or implies that a relationship exists between a food category, a food or one of its constituents and health.
- Reduction of disease risk claims, which are health claims that state, suggest or imply that a food or one of its constituents significantly reduces a risk factor in the development of a human disease.

Claims which state, suggest or imply that a product can prevent, treat or cure a disease or condition are regarded as medicinal claims and are prohibited for foods.

The use of nutrition and health claims, whether stated, suggested or merely implied, are prohibited in the labelling, presentation and advertising of foods marketed in the EU, unless they comply with the legislation. Only those nutrition claims included in the Annex to the Regulation may be used, and any nutrition claim must comply with the terms and conditions which are detailed within the Annex. These terms are very specific with regard to the quantity of the nutrient or other substance that must/must not be present in the food if a claim is to be made and, most importantly, the terms relate to the food 'as consumed'. This means that the addition of liquids such as water, milk or fruit juice to a product must be taken into account when calculating the quantity of the specific nutrient or other substance per 100 g, 100 ml or 100 kcal in order to make a claim.

The only health claims that are permitted to be made are those which appear on lists held by the European Commission, known as the Community Register.[25] These lists, which are accessible from the Commission's website, not only give the wording that can be used but also specify the conditions (mainly compositional) that must be met before the claim is allowed. The claims that are currently held on the Community Register include the nutrition claims as per the amended Annex to the Regulation; health claims which fall under Article 13 but which have been submitted with newly developed scientific evidence or proprietary data (the 'Article 13(5)' claims); health claims which relate to children's development and health (Article 14(1)(a) claims); those which refer to the reduction of disease risk (Article 14(1)(b) claims); and a list of rejected health claims and the reasons for their rejection. Health claims authorised on the basis of proprietary data will appear in a separate Annex to the Community Register. There will also eventually be an additional generic list of health claims other than those referring to the reduction of disease risk and to children's development and health (the 'Article 13(1)' claims).

In order to appear on the Community Register, all the health claims, with their substantiating scientific literature, have to be submitted to the relevant Member States, who forward the claims to the European Commission. The claims are then sent to EFSA, who are tasked with assessing the scientific data that has been provided by the submitter for each claim and issuing an opinion on issues such as: the extent to which the claimed effect of the food is beneficial for human health; the extent to which a cause and effect relationship is established between consumption of the food and the claimed effect in humans; whether the quantity of the food and pattern of consumption required to obtain the claimed effect could reasonably be achieved as part of a balanced diet; and whether the specific study group(s) in which the evidence was obtained is representative of the target population for which the claim is intended. A simplified process of submission was put in place for the Article 13(1) claims, while comprehensive dossiers are required for Article 13(5) and Article 14 claims. However, although the submission process differs, the evaluation by EFSA is the same for all claims.

Following the issuance of an opinion from EFSA, the Commission have to present a draft decision to the Standing Committee on the Food Chain and Animal Health, taking into account the EFSA opinion, the relevant Community Law and other legitimate factors. The Commission proposal is then adopted by Comitology (Regulatory Committee) with the scrutiny right of the European Parliament.

By mid-2010, very few Article 14 claims and only one Article 13(5) claim had received a positive opinion from EFSA, and all those for which a negative opinion was received were added to the Community list of rejected claims. The date for the generic list of Article 13(1) claims to be published was stated in the legislation as the end of January 2010 but, as EFSA are issuing their opinions in batches, it is anticipated that the generic list will also be published in stages, with the last part not being finalised until possibly as late as 2011. Around 44 000 Article 13(1) claims covering all official languages of the EU were originally submitted to the Commission by the given deadline, but only around 4000 of these finally went to EFSA for assessment. Current expectations are that just a small proportion of the submitted claims will actually meet the stringent criteria to which EFSA are working and eventually make it on to the Community Register of approved generic health claims. Of the first 523 Article 13(1) health claims assessed by EFSA, relating to over 200 foods and food components, only about a third received positive opinions, the majority of these relating to functions of vitamins and minerals.

Until publication of the Community list of Article 13(1) health claims occurs, companies are having to work to the list of claims submitted to EFSA and make certain that their product complies with the stated conditions of use. However, until such time as the Community list is published, companies also have to ensure that the claims they wish to use are acceptable within the country of intended sale, and be aware that (i) the claim may receive a negative opinion from EFSA, which is likely to have an adverse effect on its placement in the Community Register; and (ii) if a positive opinion is given, the final conditions of use as prescribed by EFSA may differ to those on the originally submitted claim.

If the claim a company wishes to make is dependent on newly developed scientific evidence or proprietary data, or is a new claim relating to children's growth and development or disease risk reduction, then the company has to submit a comprehensive dossier for assessment, showing that substantiation of the claim is based on strong scientific data which is primarily obtained from methodologically sound human intervention studies. The proposed health claim cannot be used until it has been assessed by EFSA, accepted by the Commission and added to the Community Register. The company then has to ensure that the claim is compliant with national legislation in the member state of sale as, for example, certain claims may be permitted in one member state but may be considered to be medicinal claims in another.

These stringent requirements for health claims resulted in considerable discussion between the development and marketing teams of the company as it became apparent that further studies would be required to support the substantiation of some of the proposed claims. A cost–benefit appraisal had to be carried out by the marketing department to see if the cost of acquiring the extra data was likely to be returned from additional sales if the claims were made. The decision was taken to commence marketing using generic claims from the Article 13(1) list which had received a positive opinion from EFSA, in the expectation that these would be accepted by the Commission and added to the Community Register, while further research was carried out on the product in preparation for the compilation of a dossier of proprietary data to support a more specific claim at a later date.

2.6   Packaging

The proposed packaging had not only to be tested for its barrier properties in terms of product stability but also checked for compliance with a number of laws. The first group of legislation that had to be checked was that dealing with materials and articles in contact with food. Regulation (EC) No 1935/2004 (as amended)[26] is the framework Regulation which lays down a general requirement that all materials that come into contact with food should not transfer their constituents to food in quantities which could endanger human health or make the food unacceptable to the consumer.

Under the framework Regulation there is a large number of more specific directives and regulations, including Commission Directive 2002/72/EC (as amended)[27] on plastic materials and articles in contact with food, and Directive 82/711/EEC (as amended)[28] on the methods of testing the migration of the constituents of plastics to foods. As the inner surface of the packaging which came into contact with the product was a plastic, these directives were particularly relevant and certification of compliance to the directives had to be obtained from the supplier of the packaging.

Although not directly part of European food law, the requirements of the Directive on packaging and packaging waste (94/62/EC, as amended)[29] also had to be considered. Aspects of this Directive have a direct relevance to the packaging of the product. The main ones to be considered were the requirements that the packaging used must be the minimal subject to the safety, hygiene and acceptance for the packed product and for the consumer. The packaging used must be recoverable through at least one of the following:

- material recycling
- incineration with energy recovery
- composting or biodegradation.

The Directive also permits packaging to be reusable, but this was not appropriate for the product concept. Any noxious or hazardous substances in the packaging must be minimised in any emissions, ash or leachate from either incineration or landfill.

Within the packaging and packaging waste Directive there is also a very specific requirement for heavy metal limits in packaging or any of its components. These limits, which refer to the total concentration of cadmium (Cd), mercury (Hg), lead (Pb) and hexavalent chromium (Cr), refer to packaging in general and not just to that which comes into contact with food. The heavy metal limits for the total of all the elements (Cd, Hg, Pb and Cr) was 100 parts per million (ppm). Again, assurances had to be obtained from the manufacturers of all the components of the packaging that their products complied with the Directive, both in terms of recovery and the ability to meet the heavy metal limits. Instructions also had to be given to the packaging designers to ensure that the requirements for minimalisation of the packaging were taken into consideration. Within the United Kingdom the minimum fill of the container with product should not be less than 60% of the internal volume of the container.

2.7   Labelling

Once the pack design had been agreed it was important that all the legal requirements could appear on the label in the appropriate manner. The list of compulsory requirements is given in Directive 2000/13/EC (as amended)[30] and the main ones include the name of the product as a generic name, the list of ingredients, instructions for use, a statement of minimum durability, storage conditions and the name of the manufacturer, packer or seller established within the EU. The declaration of minimum durability, in this case a 'Best before end:' statement and the storage conditions, were based on the results of the product shelf life trials.

In the case of the declaration of ingredients, the marketing department had a preference to exercise the option of declaring the additives by their generic names as given in the directives instead of using the 'E' numbers for the additives.

As the original development of the product had taken place in North America, many of the values in the nutrition labelling had to be adjusted to the European requirements given in Directive 2008/100/EC,[1] which amended Directive 90/496/EEC on nutrition labelling.[2] Not only were the factors for calculating the energy content from the energy nutrients different between the two continents but there were also significant differences in the calculation of the activity of a number of vitamins. For example, the thiamin (vitamin B_1) level had been originally calculated on the basis of the input of the salt, whereas in Europe the declaration is as the amount of the thiamin cation present. There was also a major discrepancy in the calculation of vitamin A activity in beta carotene.

The formulation was checked to ensure that the composition did not trigger any statutory warnings or statements such as those required in Regulation (EC) No 1333/2008 on food additives,[10] where the presence in a product of the intense sweetener aspartame or polyols require prescribed warning statements. The national requirements in this area also had to be taken into consideration. For example, in the United Kingdom there is a voluntary agreement between the British Department of Health and the food industry that products containing added vitamin A (as retinol) should carry a warning for pregnant women if the vitamin A content of the recommended daily intake of the product exceeds 800 μg. The contribution of beta carotene to the vitamin A content is excluded from this requirement.

European food labelling law requires that all sub-components of a compounded ingredient are declared in the list of ingredients, regardless of the levels of the sub-components in the ingredient. The background to this requirement was the introduction of legislation requiring the identification of a number of potential allergens (soya, milk etc.). This caused considerable problems as a number of ingredients were considered to be proprietary blends by their suppliers who were very reluctant to give the details required.

2.8   Manufacture

The manufacture of the product was a dry-blending process followed by the spraying into the mix of oil and lecithin. While it was envisaged that the production for the launch of the product would be carried out in North America, there was a requirement to find a suitable production facility in Europe. As part of the evaluation of potential contract manufacturers, a technical, quality and hygiene audit was carried out on the main contenders. The hygiene part of the audit was designed to ensure that all the requirements of Regulation (EC) No 852/2004 on food hygiene were in compliance.[31] This included confirmation that a hazard analysis and critical control point assessment (HACCP) had been carried out by the company as required by the Regulation.

Regulation (EC) No 178/2002 on general food law[32] requires that there is full traceability of all materials and products on a supplier customer basis known as 'one up' (supplier) and 'one down' (customer). Detailed records of the traceability must be made and kept for a statutory period. As the production was likely to be outside of the EU, detailed operating procedures on compliance with the European traceability requirements had to be developed and arrangements made for them to be implemented and monitored in the production and packaging operations.

2.9   Conclusions

The complexities of developing a functional food to be in compliance with European Union food legislation are considerable. Much of the problem is due to advances in science and nutrition running ahead of the legislation. This case study has shown that a very detailed knowledge of the technology, function and compositional specification of every component of the formulation is essential. It has also shown that no great reliance can be placed on formulations developed for markets outside the European Union, as the disparity in the legislation between the EU and other countries such as the United States of America is substantial.

2.10   References

1. Commission Directive 2008/100/EC amending Council Directive 90/496/EEC on nutrition labelling for foodstuffs as regards recommended daily allowances, energy conversion factors and definitions. O.J. of E.U. L285/9 of 29 October 2008.

2. European Council Directive 90/496/EEC on nutrition labelling for foodstuffs. O.J. of E.C. L276/40 of 6 October 1990.
3. European Parliament and Council Directive 2009/39/EC on foodstuffs intended for particular nutritional uses (recast). O.J. of E.U. L124/21 of 20 May 2009.
4. Commission Directive 96/8/EC on foods intended for use in energy-restricted diets for weight control. O.J. of E.C. L55/22 of 6 March 1996.
5. European Parliament and Council Regulation (EC) No 1829/2003 on genetically modified food and feed. O.J. of E.U. L268/1 of 18 October 2003.
6. European Parliament and Council Regulation (EC) No 1830/2003 concerning the traceability and labelling of genetically modified organisms and the traceability of food and feed products produced from genetically modified organisms and amending Directive 2001/18/EC. O.J. of E.U. L268/24 of 18 October 2003.
7. European Council Directive 83/417/EEC relating to caseins and caseinates. O.J. of E.C. L237/25 of 26 August 1983.
8. European Council Directive 76/621/EEC on the maximum level of erucic acid in oils, fats and foodstuffs for human consumption. O.J. of E.C. L202/35 of 28 July 1976.
9. European Council Directive 80/891/EEC on method of analysis for determining the erucic acid content of fats and oils. O.J. of E.C. L254/35 of 27 September1980.
10. European Parliament and Council Regulation (EC) No 1333/2008 on food additives. O.J. of E.U. L354/16 of 31 December 2008.
11. European Parliament and Council Directive 95/2/EC on food additives other than colours and sweeteners. O.J. of E.C. L61/1 of 18 March 1995.
12. Corrigendum to European Parliament and Council Regulation (EC) No 1924/2006 on nutrition and health claims made on foods. O.J. of E.U. L12/3 of 18 January 2007.
13. European Parliament and Council Regulation (EC) No 853/2004 of the European Parliament and of the Council laying down specific hygiene rules for food of animal origin. O.J. of E.U. L226/22 of 25 June 2004.
14. Corrigendum to European Parliament and Council Regulation (EC) No 854/2004 laying down specific rules for the organisation of official controls on products of animal origin intended for human consumption. O.J. of E.U. L226/83 of 25 June 2004.
15. Commission Directive 2008/100/EC amending Council Directive 90/496/EEC on nutrition labelling for foodstuffs as regards recommended daily allowances, energy conversion factors and definitions. O.J. of E.U. L285/9 of 29 October 2008.
16. European Parliament and Council Regulation (EC) No 1925/2006 on the addition of vitamins and minerals and of certain other substances to foods. O.J. of E.U. L404/26 of 30 December 2006.
17. European Parliament and Council Regulation (EC) No 258/97 concerning novel foods and novel food ingredients. O.J. of E.C. L43/1 of 14 February 1997.
18. European Parliament and Council Regulation (EC) No 764/2008 laying down procedures relating to the application of certain national technical rules to products lawfully marketed in another Member State and repealing Decision No 3052/95/EC.
19. Commission Decision of 28 April 2009 authorising the placing on the market of lycopene oleoresin from tomatoes as novel food ingredient under Regulation (EC) No 258/97 of the European Parliament and of the Council. O.J. of E.U. L109/47 of 30 April 2009.
20. Commission Decision of 23 April 2009 authorising the placing on the market of lycopene as a novel food ingredient under Regulation (EC) No 258/97 of the European Parliament and of the Council. O.J. of E.U. L106/55 of 23 April 2009.
21. Commission Decision of 28 April 2009 authorising the placing on the market of lycopene from Blakeslea trispora as a novel food ingredient under Regulation (EC) No 258/97 of the European Parliament and of the Council. O.J. of E.U. L111/31 of 28 April 2009.

22. Commission Decision of 30 April 2009 authorising the placing on the market of lycopene as novel food ingredient under Regulation (EC) No 258/97 of the European Parliament and of the Council. O.J. of E.U. L110/54 of 30 April 2009.
23. European Parliament and European Council Directive 94/36/EC on colours for use in foodstuffs. O.J. of E.C. L237/13 of 10 September 1994.
24. European Parliament and Council Regulation (EC) No 1334/2008 on flavourings and certain food ingredients with flavouring properties for use in and on foods and amending Council Regulation (EEC) No 1601/91, Regulations (EC) No 2232/96 and (EC) No 110/2008 and Directive 2000/13/EC. O.J. of E.U. L354/34 of 31 December 2008.
25. The Community Register of nutrition and health claims made on food: http://ec.europa.eu/food/food/labellingnutrition/claims/community_register/index_en.htm
26. European Parliament and Council Regulation (EC) No 1935/2004 on materials and articles intended to come into contact with food and repealing Directives 80/590/EEC and 89/109/EEC. O.J. of E.U. L338/4 of 13 November 2004.
27. Commission Directive 2002/72/EC relating to plastic materials and articles intended to come into contact with foodstuffs. O.J. of E.U. L220/18 of 15 August 2002.
28. Council Directive 82/711/EEC laying down the basic rules necessary for testing migration of the constituents of plastic materials and articles intended to come into contact with foodstuffs. O.J. of E.C. 297/26 of 23 October 1982.
29. European Parliament and Council Directive 94/62/EC on packaging and packaging waste. O.J. of E.C. 365/10 of 31 December 1994.
30. European Parliament and Council Directive 2000/13/EC on the approximation of the laws of the Member States relating to the labelling, presentation and advertising of foodstuffs. O.J. of E.U. L109/29 of 6 May 2000.
31. Corrigendum to European Parliament and Council Regulation (EC) No 852/2004 of on the hygiene of foodstuffs. O.J. of E.U. L226/3 of 25 June 2004.
32. European Parliament and Council Regulation (EC) No 178/2002 laying down the general principles and requirements of food law, establishing the European Food Safety Authority and laying down procedures in matters of food safety. O.J. of E.U. L31/1 of 1 February 2002.

2.11   Appendix: note

This chapter is an illustration of some of the problems that could be encountered when developing a product for the European market, and the legislation detailed was up to date at the time of writing (mid-2010). It is important, if the reader is intending to use this chapter as a guide to the legislation, that the current status of the legislation is checked on the European Commission's website (http://ec.europa.eu/food/food/index_en.htm).

3

U.S. regulation of functional foods

J. E. Hoadley, EAS Consulting Group, USA

Abstract: Functional foods are regulated in the U.S. under the same regulatory framework as are conventional food and dietary supplements. The primary distinction between a functional food and food in general is in the claims made for benefits, other than nutritional, attributed to the functional food. As such, the aspect of U.S. food regulation of most relevance to functional food is the regulation of food label claims. In the U.S. there are three categories of regulated food label claims The U.S. regulatory framework makes a firm separation between products intended to be used as drugs and those intended for use as food. There are two subcategories of food in the U.S. regulatory framework (medical food and food for special dietary use) for foods intended to meet special dietary needs of people with existing disease.

Key words: U.S. food regulations, health claims, nutrient content claims, structure/function claims, medical food, food for special dietary use.

3.1 Introduction

The U.S. Food and Drug Administration (FDA) regulatory scheme does not recognize 'functional food' to be a distinct regulatory category. FDA believes existing food regulations are sufficient to provide for functional food.[1] Functional foods differ from food in general in being promoted for benefits in regards to enhancement of structures or functions of the body or in lowering health risks, rather than for traditional food attributes. The fundamental characteristic that sets functional food apart from other foods is the claims made about their intended function.

The U.S. regulatory framework for products intended for human consumption has a rigid separation between products intended to be used as food and products whose intended use is disease-related (drugs). The distinction between foods and drugs is based largely on intended use rather than on composition. The claims made for the functional effects of a food are one way in which the intended use for a product will be shown. A statement about the function of a food being related to a disease can cause the product to be regulated as a drug even when the product has an established use as a food. Because the food label is a primary vehicle for communicating information about the benefits attributable to a functional food, the food label has a major role in FDA's consideration of whether a functional food will be regulated as a food or a drug.

Although food and drugs are distinct regulatory categories, there are some areas of overlap. One such area is food label health claims in which a relationship between a nutrient and disease risk reduction may be communicated via food labels. Another overlap is the use of foods to affect structures or functions of the body not related to a disease condition. Both foods and drugs may be used to affect a structure or function of the body.

Functional foods are likely to be promoted with label claims about what beneficial effects are to be expected from consuming the functional food. Food label claims regulated by FDA fall into three categories: health claims, structure/ function claims and nutrient content claims. There also are two food subcategories (medical foods and foods for special dietary use) that have been considered by some parties as a route for promoting functional foods in the U.S., but neither is a viable option for functional foods.

The FDA is the U.S. agency primarily responsible for the regulation of food and drugs. FDA is responsible for ensuring that all food (except for meat and poultry which are regulated by the U.S. Department of Agriculture) (USDA)) are safe, sanitary, wholesome, and properly labeled. FDA regulates both the labeling and advertizing of drugs. But for foods, the regulation of advertising comes under Federal Trade Commission (FTC) jurisdiction.

The primary compilation of laws that prescribe FDA's regulation of foods and drugs is the Federal Food, Drug, and Cosmetic Act (FD&C Act). The regulations FDA issues to implement the provisions of the FD&C Act are compiled in Title 21 of the U.S. Code of Federal Regulations (21 CFR).

3.2   Food label health claims

Health claims describe an effect of a nutrient, food component, dietary ingredient, or specific food in reducing the risk of a disease or health-related condition. Health claims must be evaluated and authorized by FDA prior to their use in food labeling. There are three ways by which FDA exercises its oversight in determining which health claims will be authorized:

1   issuance of an authorizing regulation (the significant scientific agreement, or *SSA claims*);
2   notification from a third party of authoritative statements from a U.S. government scientific body other than FDA that ensues from that scientific body's deliberative review of scientific evidence on the substance/disease

relationship and that serves as the basis for a health claim (the *FDAMA claims*);

3 issuance of an 'enforcement discretion' letter permitting use of health claims where the quality and strength of the scientific evidence supporting the claim is less than that of the significant scientific agreement standard required for FDA to issue an authorizing regulation (the *qualified health claims*).

3.2.1 Significant Scientific Agreement (SSA) health claims

The FD&C Act requires that to issue a health claim-authorizing regulation, FDA must evaluate the supporting scientific evidence and reach a conclusion that

- scientific evidence from well-designed studies conducted in a manner consistent with generally recognized scientific procedures and principles supports the claims; and
- there is significant scientific agreement among qualified experts that the totality of publicly available scientific evidence supports the claim.

The SSA substantiation standard is intended to provide a high level of confidence in the validity of a substance/disease relationship. FDA explains how the SSA standard is applied in the evaluation of health claim substantiation in a document titled *Guidance for Industry: Evidence-based Review System for the Scientific Evaluation of Health Claims*, January 2009.[3]

The process for FDA to authorize a new SSA health claim begins with the submission, by the proponent of the claim, of a health claim petition. The requirements for submitting a health claim petition are explained in 21 CFR 101.70. Typically it takes FDA in excess of two years to evaluate the supporting evidence, make its SSA determination, and follow required rule-making steps to issue a regulation. Health claims authorized by regulations are listed in Table 3.1. A listing of authorized SSA health claims may also be found in the FDA document *A Food Labeling Guide*, Appendix C.[4]

3.2.2 Qualified health claims

FDA's authority to apply the SSA standard to health claims for dietary supplements was challenged in a lawsuit by dietary supplement distributors. In *Pearson v Shalala* (164 F.3d 650 (D.C. Cir. 1999)) the U.S. Court of Appeals for the District of Columbia ruled that FDA could not apply a blanket prohibition of all health claims that fail the SSA substantiation standard because although such claims are potentially misleading, they not necessarily inherently misleading. The Court concluded that the U.S. Constitution First Amendment protection of speech does not permit FDA to prohibit potentially misleading health claims unless the agency can also determine that adding a disclaimer to the claim would not eliminate the potential deception. The Court suggested that adding qualifying language

Table 3.1   Health claims authorized by regulation

Regulation no.*	Nutrient/disease relationship	Model health claim†
21 CFR 101.72	Calcium and osteoporosis	Regular exercise and a healthy diet with enough calcium helps teens and young adult white and Asian women maintain good bone health and may reduce their high risk of osteoporosis later in life.
21 CFR 101.73	Fat and cancer‡	Development of cancer depends on many factors. A diet low in total fat may reduce the risk of some cancers.
21 CFR 101.74	Sodium and hypertension	Diets low in sodium may reduce the risk of high blood pressure, a disease associated with many factors.
21 CFR 101.75	Saturated fat, cholesterol and cardiovascular disease‡	While many factors affect heart disease, diets low in saturated fat and cholesterol may reduce the risk of this disease.
21 CFR 101.76	Dietary fiber-containing grains, fruits, and vegetables, and cancer	Low fat diets rich in fiber-containing grain products, fruits, and vegetables may reduce the risk of some types of cancer, a disease associated with many factors.
21 CFR 101.77	Fruits, vegetables, and grains that contain fiber, particularly soluble fiber, and coronary heart disease	Diets low in saturated fat and cholesterol and rich in fruits, vegetables, and grain products that contain some types of dietary fiber, particularly soluble fiber, may reduce the risk of heart disease, a disease associated with many factors.
21 CFR 101.78	Fruits, vegetables, and cancer	Low fat diets rich in fruits and vegetables (foods that are low in fat and may contain dietary fiber, vitamin A, or vitamin C) may reduce the risk of some types of cancer, a disease associated with many factors. Broccoli is high in vitamin A and C, and it is a good source of dietary fiber.
21 CFR 101.79	Folate and neural tube birth defects	Healthful diets with adequate folate may reduce a woman's risk of having a child with a brain or spinal cord defect.
21 CFR 101.80	Dietary noncariogenic carbohydrate sweeteners and dental caries	Frequent between-meal consumption of foods high in sugars and starches promotes tooth decay. The sugar alcohols in [*name of food*] do not promote tooth decay.
21 CFR 101.81	Soluble fiber from certain foods and coronary heart disease [*eligible sources are oats, barley, and psyllium*]	Soluble fiber from foods such as [*name of soluble fiber source*], as part of a diet low in saturated fat and cholesterol, may reduce the risk of heart disease. A serving of [*name of food product*] supplies __ grams of the [*necessary daily dietary intake for the benefit*] soluble fiber from [*name of soluble fiber source*] necessary per day to have this effect.

| 21 CFR 101.82 | Soy protein and risk of coronary heart disease | 25 grams of soy protein a day, as part of a diet low in saturated fat and cholesterol, may reduce the risk of heart disease. A serving of [*name of food*] supplies __ grams of soy protein. |
| 21 CFR 101.83 | Phytosterols and coronary heart disease | Diets low in saturated fat and cholesterol that include two servings of foods that provide a daily total of 800 milligrams of phytosterols in two meals may reduce the risk of heart disease. A serving of [*name of food*] supplies __ milligrams of phytosterols.§ |

* Food labeling regulations are codified in Title 21 of the U.S. Code of Federal Regulations (CFR), Part 101. The regulation authorizing a health claim about the relationship of dietary calcium and osteoporosis risk is in section 72 of this part, i.e. 21 CFR 101.72.

† Authorizing regulations provide examples of model claims and prescribe elements that must be included within the claim statement (e.g. the claim must make it clear that inadequate calcium intake is not the only risk factor for this disease, the claim must identify the population at risk as white and Asian women in their bone forming years, etc.) but the actual wording of the claim can vary.

‡ The criteria for these health claims include meeting requirements of 'low' nutrient content claims for total fat, saturated fat and cholesterol. The 'low' nutrient content claims are not defined for most dietary supplements; therefore, these health claims are not available for use by dietary supplements.

§ FDA uses enforcement discretion to allow for greater flexibility in use of this claim than what is in the regulation. The variations from the regulatory criteria allowed are explained in a letter available at: http://www.fda.gov/Food/LabelingNutrition/LabelClaims/ HealthClaimsMeetingSignificantScientificAgreementSSA/ucm074779.htm.

to a claim to explain why the supporting evidence is inconclusive could correct the misleading character of a health claim that does not meet the SSA substantiation standard.

Because the FD&C Act does not permit FDA to issue a regulation authorizing a specific health claim without an SSA determination, the process for allowing qualified health claims involves issuing an enforcement discretion letter, instead of a regulation. Since the validity of the substance/disease relationship in a qualified health claim is not well established, the qualified health claim enforcement discretion letters are on an interim basis and note that the decisions to allow the claims will be re-evaluated by FDA as additional scientific evidence becomes available. A series of lawsuits by dietary supplement distributors pertaining to FDA's implementation of the *Pearson v Shalala* decision has contributed to a continuing evolution of FDA's processing of qualified health claim petitions. Under the more recent Court decisions FDA is compelled to allow most all requested qualified health claims when supported by any credible evidence. As a result there appears to have evolved a policy that the length of the required qualifying language is inversely proportional to the level of scientific support for a health claim. The qualifying language required of most qualified health claims allowed in recent years is too cumbersome for the claims to be of practical use in promoting a food product. There are close to 20 qualified health claims allowed by FDA. A listing of the currently allowed qualified health claims with the conditions under which the claims may be used can be found in

Appendix D to *A Food Labeling Guide*[5] (http://www.fda.gov/Food/Guidance ComplianceRegulatoryInformation/GuidanceDocuments/FoodLabelingNutrition/ FoodLabelingGuide/ucm064923.htm).

3.2.3   Food and Drug Administration Modernization Act (FDAMA) health claims

The 1997 FDA Modernization Act (FDAMA) amended the FD&C Act to provide an expedited process for authorizing new health claims. This expedited process is initiated by submission to FDA of a notification of a health claim about a substance/ disease relationship evaluated by U.S. government scientific bodies other than the FDA, or by the National Academies of Science. The health claim that is the subject of the notification becomes an authorized health claim at 120 days following FDA's receipt of the notification provided the notification was valid and FDA has taken no action within that time to prohibit or modify the claim with a regulation. The basis for a FDAMA health claim must be an 'authoritative statement' from either the National Academies of Science, or a U.S. government scientific body with official responsibility for public health protection or research directly relating to human nutrition [FD&C Act §403(r)(3)(C)]. The substantiation standard for a FDAMA health claim is the same as that for FDA-authorized SSA health claims; the two types of health claims differ only in the process leading to their authorization, and where within the U.S. government the evaluation of substantiating evidence is done. FDA provides more information on what constitutes an authoritative statement and how to submit a FDAMA health claim notification in the document *Guidance for Industry: Notification of a Health Claim or Nutrient Content Claim Based on an Authoritative Statement of a Scientific Body* (http://www.fda.gov/ Food/GuidanceComplianceRegulatoryInformation/GuidanceDocuments/ FoodLabelingNutrition/UCM056975).

Health claims authorized through the FDAMA authoritative statement-based claim notification process include claims for whole grains and heart disease/cancer, potassium and hypertension/stroke, fluoridated water and dental caries, and saturated fat, *trans* fat, and cholesterol and heart disease (Table 3.2). Authorized FDAMA health claims are listed in *A Food Labeling Guide*, Appendix C[4] (http://www.fda. gov/Food/GuidanceComplianceRegulatoryInformation/GuidanceDocuments/ FoodLabelingNutrition/FoodLabelingGuide/ucm064919.htm).

3.3   Food label structure/function claims

FDA uses the term *structure/function claim* collectively to refer to food label statements about the role of food substances in

- maintaining general well-being;
- maintaining normal structure and functions of the body;
- preventing essential nutrient deficiency diseases.

Table 3.2   Health claims based on authoritative statements (FDAMA Health Claims)

Notification docket no.*	Nutrient/disease relationship	Required claim statement
FDA-1999-P-4061	Whole grain foods and heart disease and certain cancers	Diets rich in whole grain foods and other plant foods and low in total fat, saturated fat, and cholesterol may reduce the risk of heart disease and some cancers.
FDA-2000-Q-0914	Potassium and high blood pressure and stroke	Diets containing foods that are a good source of potassium and that are low in sodium may reduce the risk of high blood pressure and stroke.
FDA-2006-Q-0034	Fluoridated water and dental caries	Drinking fluoridated water may reduce the risk of dental caries. Or Drinking fluoridated water may reduce the risk of tooth decay.
FDA-2006-Q-0509	Saturated fat, cholesterol, and *trans* fat, and heart disease	Diets low in saturated fat and cholesterol, and as low as possible in *trans* fat, may reduce the risk of heart disease.

* The notifications which serve as the basis for authorization of these claims are available at http://www.regulations.gov, filed under the Docket numbers indicated.

Structure/function claims cannot have any direct or implied connection to an effect on a disease or health-related condition leading to a disease. Label statements about a relationship of a substance and a disease (i.e. *disease claims*) are prohibited for foods unless the statement is in accordance with an authorized health claim. It is not always easy to draw the line between structure/function claims and disease claims. The consideration of whether a claim is a disease claim will take into account the meaning of the claim in context of other information on the label and labeling, and also implied meanings of the claim. As an aid to understanding FDA's thinking as to when a claim is or is not a disease claim, FDA has set ten criteria to clarify what types of claims may be made as structure/function claims. These criteria are listed in 21 CFR 101.93(g). FDA elaborates on the ten disease claim criteria in *Guidance for Industry: Structure/Function Claims Small Entity Compliance Guide*, January 2002 (http://www.fda.gov/Food/GuidanceComplianceRegulatoryInformation/GuidanceDocuments/DietarySupplements/ucm103340.htm).

Label statements will be considered disease claims when information presented on the label or in labeling:

- claims an effect on a disease or class of diseases;
- claims an effect on characteristic signs or symptoms of disease using scientific or lay terminology;

- claims an effect on an abnormal condition associated with a natural state or process;
- claims an effect on a disease through the product name, formulation, use of pictures, or other factors implies a disease claim;
- claims that a product belongs to a class of products that is intended to diagnose, mitigate, treat, cure, or prevent a disease;
- claims to be a substitute for a product that is a therapy for a disease;
- claims to augment a therapy or drug intended to diagnose, mitigate, treat, cure, or prevent a disease;
- claims to have a role in the body's response to a disease or to a vector of disease;
- claims to treat, prevent, or mitigate adverse events associated with a therapy for a disease;
- otherwise suggests an effect on a disease or diseases.

Although foods may be used to affect the structure or function of the body, unless the structure/function effect is derived from the 'food' attributes of the product (i.e. taste, aroma, or nutritive value), a structure/function claim will cause the product to be regulated as a drug. *Nutritive value* means a value in sustaining human existence by such processes as promoting growth, replacing loss of essential nutrients, or providing energy (21 CFR 101.14(a)(3)). Structure/function effects claimed for dietary supplements need not be derived from nutritive value.

3.3.1 Dietary Supplement Health and Education Act (DSHEA) and structure/function claims

The 1994 Dietary Supplement Health and Education Act (DSHEA) added to the FD&C Act structure/function claim provisions specific to dietary supplements. Included is an explicit listing of types of dietary supplement structure/function claims that are not subject to FDA review or approval [FD&C Act §403(r)(6)]. Also included is the requirement that dietary supplement structure/function claims must be accompanied by the statement:

> This statement has not been evaluated by the Food and Drug Administration. This product is not intended to diagnose, treat, cure, or prevent any disease.

The structure/function claim disclaimer statement must be placed prominently in bold type on every label or labeling panel where a structure/function claim appears. Dietary supplement manufacturers must submit a notification to FDA of all structure/function claims they use within 30 days of first marketing the dietary supplement with the claim. FDA reviews these submissions only to see that they are structure/function-type claims and not disease claims. FDA sends 'courtesy letters' to manufacturers when they find claims in a structure/function notice that are clearly disease claims. Not receiving an FDA reply to a

30-day structure/function claim notice does not constitute an FDA approval for use of the claim.

3.3.2   Substantiation of structure/function claims

FDA neither reviews nor approves the structure/function claims made on conventional foods and dietary supplements labels. All label statements, including structure/function claims, must be truthful and not misleading. Although the truthfulness of a structure/function claim must be substantiated by appropriate scientific evidence, FDA has no legal authority to request access to a manufacturer's substantiating evidence for structure/function claims. Some dietary supplement manufacturers have assumed that because of the lack of FDA oversight and sometimes vagueness of structure/function claim language, the substantiation standard for structure/function claims is lax. This is not true. Both the FDA and the Federal Trade Commission (FTC) have adopted a strong 'Competent and Reliable Scientific Evidence' substantiation standard for claims. Competent and reliable scientific evidence means:

> Tests, analyses, research, studies, or other evidence based on the expertise of professionals in the relevant area, that have been conducted and evaluated in an objective manner by persons qualified to do so, using procedures generally accepted in the profession to yield accurate and reliable results.

The key issues a manufacturer must consider in assessing whether the evidence to substantiate a claim meets the competent and reliable scientific evidence standard include:

- the meaning of the claim being made;
- the relationship of the evidence to the claim;
- the quality of the evidence;
- the totality of the evidence.

FDA has described the amount, type, and quality of evidence that it recommends manufacturers have to substantiate structure/function claims. This advice is available in *Guidance for Industry: Substantiation for Dietary Supplement Claims Made Under Section 403(r)(6) of the Federal Food, Drug, and Cosmetic Act*, December 2008 (http://www.fda.gov/Food/GuidanceComplianceRegulatoryInformation/GuidanceDocuments/DietarySupplements/ucm073200.htm).

Although FDA has little direct oversight authority over the use and substantiation of structure/function claims, there are potential consequences of using structure/function claims that are not adequately substantiated with credible scientific evidence. Companies that make inadequately substantiated structure/function claims are at risk of enforcement actions by the FTC and State Attorneys General, Better Business Bureau complaints, and class action lawsuits.

Curbing the use of deceptive and misleading dietary supplement advertizing claims is an enforcement priority for the FTC.[6] Unlike the FDA, the FTC has authority to review the evidence a manufacturer uses to substantiate that the claims used are truthful and not misleading. FDA food labeling regulations generally preempt state or local government authority in regulating food labels. However, state and local governments may take actions against misleading structure/function label claims. An example of such action is a 2009 charge by the Attorney General for the State of Oregon that the Kellogg's Company use of a 'helps support your child's immunity' claim on Rice Krispies breakfast cereal was misleading.[7] An example of class action lawsuits against manufacturers making structure/function claims is a suit alleging Dannon's claims for immune system-boosting benefits from the probiotic bacteria in Activia and DanActive branded yogurt were not truthful.[8]

The National Advertising Division (NAD) of the Council of Better Business Bureaus reviews national advertising for truthfulness and accuracy in response to competitors' complaints about potentially misleading national advertising claims. NAD investigates substantiation for performance claims, superiority claims against competitive products and all kinds of scientific and technical claims. If a company fails to follow NAD advice to remove or modify claims it has reviewed, NAD will refer the claims to the appropriate federal government regulatory agency.

3.4   Food label nutrient content claims

Nutrient content claims are food label statements that describe the level of a nutrient in a food using terms such as *free, high, and low*, or they compare the level of a nutrient in one food to another food using terms such as *more, reduced*, and *lite*. The descriptor terms are defined by regulation to ensure they are used consistently for all types of foods. For example, to characterize the amount of a nutrient in a food using the terms *high, rich in*, or *excellent source of* requires the food contains at least 20% of the Daily Value (guideline daily amount) for that nutrient per reference amount (the reference amount is a standardized serving size for a particular food category); and to characterize the amount of a nutrient as a *good source, contains*, or *provides* requires the food contain at least 10% of the Daily Value of the nutrient per reference amount (21 CFR 101.54). Nutrient content claims may only be used in accordance with an authorizing regulation, and generally the nutrient content claim regulations apply only to those nutrients permitted to be declared in the Nutrition Facts box. A summary of the rules for using nutrient content claims on food labels is in the FDA publication *A Food Labeling Guide*, Chapter VIII (http://www.fda.gov/Food/GuidanceComplianceRegulatoryInformation/Guidance Documents/FoodLabelingNutrition/FoodLabelingGuide/ucm064908.htm). Specific requirements of the authorized nutrient content claims are located in Appendices A and B of *A Food Labeling Guide* (http://www.fda.gov/Food/ GuidanceComplianceRegulatoryInformation/GuidanceDocuments/FoodLabeling Nutrition/FoodLabelingGuide/default.htm). Among the authorized nutrient content claims a few (e.g. healthy, antioxidants, and omega-3 fatty acids) are potentially of unique interest to the functional food industry.

3.4.1 Claims using the term 'healthy'

Use of the term *healthy* in association with a nutrient, e.g. healthy fats, is considered to be a nutrient content claim characterizing not only the nutrient named, but also implying that the levels of all other nutrients in the food are present at 'healthy' levels. The requirements for use of healthy claims on food labels are prescribed by regulation in 21 CFR 101.65(d). There are five criteria for a food to be labeled as healthy. For most packaged foods these criteria are:

1 low in total fat (≤3g total fat);
2 low in saturated fat (≤1 g saturated fat and ≤15% of calories from saturated fat);
3 cholesterol content ≤60 mg;
4 sodium content ≤480 mg;
5 contain at least 10% of the Daily Value for one or more of vitamin A, vitamin C, calcium, iron, protein, or dietary fiber.

The fifth criterion (the 'jelly bean rule') was included to preclude foods of little intrinsic nutritional value, such as candy, from being characterized as healthy. There are some variations in these criteria depending on whether the labeled food is a fruit/vegetable, a grain product, a seafood, or meal-type product. Further, there are a number of technical details in how the eligibility criteria are applied, so manufacturers interested in labeling a food as healthy should be familiar with 21 CFR 101.65(d).

3.4.2 Antioxidant nutrient content claims

Nutrient content claims that use the term *antioxidant* must be made in accordance with the requirements of 21 CFR 101.54(g). These requirements are:

1 the antioxidant nutrient has an established Daily Value for nutrition labeling;
2 the nutrient has recognized antioxidant activity in the body after it has been absorbed from the gastrointestinal tract;
3 the level of each nutrient that is the subject of the claim is sufficient to qualify for a *high* or *good source* claim;
4 the individual nutrients that are the subject of the claim are named in the claim;
5 the amount of the nutrients that are the subject of the claim be declared in the nutrition information.

The nutrients that meet both criteria 1 and 2 are vitamin C, vitamin E, and selenium. Beta-carotene may also be the subject of an antioxidant nutrient content claim when the amount of vitamin A activity in the food, present as beta-carotene, is sufficient to qualify for the claim. Vitamin A itself is not an antioxidant, and the bioavailability of beta-carotene's antioxidant potential is doubtful. However, beta-carotene was included in the antioxidant content claim regulation.

There are ways that information about antioxidant substances without established Daily Values can be presented other than as nutrient content claims. One alternative is to refer to antioxidant potential or function rather than content.

However, when a manufacturer has available information about *in vitro* antioxidant capacity (such as ORAC value) only and no evidence that the substance will function as an antioxidant within the body when consumed, then claims about antioxidant function are not substantiated. Another alternative is the use of truthful quantitative statements of the amount of an antioxidant. Quantitative statements of the amount of a nutrient, that do not 'characterize' the level (e.g. as high) are permitted. For example, the statement '30 mg of green tea antioxidants per serving' is a permissible quantitative statement.

3.4.3   Omega-3 fatty acid content claims

There are no Daily Values established for omega-3 fatty acids; and thus no omega-3 fatty acid content claims authorized by FDA regulation. However, FDAMA provides for authorization of nutrient content claims based on authoritative statements through a notification process. FDA has received three omega-3 fatty acid content claim FDAMA notifications and the claims in these notifications are, at this time, authorized claims. All three of the omega-3 fatty acid claim notifications were based on authoritative statements from the Institute of Medicine (IOM) Dietary Reference Intake (DRI) Report for macronutrients.[9] The IOM did not arrive at Recommended Dietary Allowances (RDAs) for omega-3 fatty acids in this DRI report, but did set an Adequate Intake for the essential omega-3 fatty acid alpha-linolenic acid (ALA) and an Acceptable Macronutrient Distribution Range (AMDR) for ALA of 0.6 to 1.2% of dietary energy. The IOM also commented that approximately 10% of the AMDR for ALA could be met by consuming long-chain omega-3 fatty acids (i.e. EPA and DHA). The three omega-3 content claim notifications each interpreted the IOM's intake recommendations differently resulting in different claim criteria for the same omega-3 content claims. These notifications provide for content claims for specific fatty acids (ALA, EPA, DHA, and EPA+DHA claims); there are no authorized claims for 'omega-3s' in general as the subject of the claim. As with all claims authorized through the FDAMA authoritative statement-based claim notification process, only the exact wording of the claim as stated in the notification may be used on food labels. For example, the required wording for a high DHA claim provided for in the Martek Bioscience Corporation notice is: *High in DHA. Contains __ mg of DHA per serving, which is __ % of the 160 mg Daily Value for DHA.* The only permitted variation from this text is that *Rich in* or *Excellent source of* may replace *High in*.

The inconsistent claim criteria situation resulting from the three omega-3 content claim notifications was unacceptable to FDA. As such, FDA has proposed a regulation[10] that would override the claims authorized under the FDAMA notifications. The regulation proposed by FDA will prohibit all EPA and DHA nutrient content claims, and authorize *good source, high,* and *more* nutrient content claims for ALA based on an ALA Daily Value of 1.6 g per day. The omega-3 fatty acid content claims that are to be authorized under the proposed regulation are summarized in Table 3.3. As of the time this chapter is being

Table 3.3 Omega-3 nutrient content claims to be authorized under the 2007 proposed regulation*

Omega-3 fatty acid	Good source†	High‡	More§	Daily Value	Comments
α-Linolenic acid (ALA)	≥160 mg ALA per RACC¶	≥320 mg ALA per RACC	≥160 mg (i.e. 10% DV) more ALA per RACC than an appropriate reference food	1.6 g	Because ALA is not listed in the Nutrition Facts, an ALA content claim must include: • the mg of ALA per serving; • the % Daily Value per serving; • state that the ALA Daily Value is 1.6 g.
Eicosapentaenoic acid (EPA)	*No claims will be authorized for EPA*				
Docosahexaenoic acid (DHA)	*No claims will be authorized for DHA*				

* Proposed Rulemaking. Food Labeling: Nutrient Content Claims; Alpha-Linolenic Acid, Eicosapentaenoic Acid, and Docosahexaenoic Acid Omega-3 Fatty Acids. November 27, 2007 (Ref. 10).
† *Contains* and *Provides* are allowed synonyms for *Good Source*.
‡ *Rich In* and *Excellent Source of* are allowed synonyms for *High*.
§ *Added, Extra, Plus,* and *Fortified* are allowed synonyms for *More*.
¶ Reference Amounts Customarily Consumed per Eating Occasion (RACC) are standardized serving sizes established for most food categories in 21 CFR 101.12. The RACC is used for uniformity in presenting nutrition information and nutrient content claims on food labels.

written, the FDA action remains only a proposed rule. The proposed rule becomes enforceable only after the rulemaking process progresses to the final rule stage and after a reasonable implementation period following publication of the final rule. Until that time, all omega-3 fatty acid content claims authorized through FDAMA claim notification process may continue to be used on food labels.

3.5 Medical food and food for special dietary use

As of around 1970 the FDA began a policy of regulating as foods dietary products specially formulated for use in the dietary management of diseases, rather than as drugs, even though they were specifically intended for use in disease conditions. The justification for this policy was that the included products did not require the level of regulatory oversight necessary for drugs because there was a very limited number of such products; they were produced by a small number of reputable manufacturers with high standards of quality control; the nutritional formulation requirements of these products were well established by the medical community; their usefulness was widely accepted by health care professionals; and their use was under close physician supervision.[11] These products were largely limited to formula for infants with rare metabolic disorders where the potential market was too limited for manufacturers to want to incur the expense of a new drug approval. FDA took this action to foster development of such products and to ensure they would be available at reasonable cost to people with rare genetic diseases whose survival depended on dietary therapy. Recognizing that such foods would not be appropriate, or necessarily safe, for consumption by the general population, FDA established a 'foods for special dietary use' regulatory subcategory to distinguish these products from foods for general use.

The 1988 Orphan Drug Act established, for the first time, a statutory definition of 'medical food.' The Orphan Drug Act provided economic incentives (such as drug application fee exemptions, and market exclusivity) for the development of new 'orphan drugs' for treatment of rare diseases. The sole purpose for 'medical food' to be defined within the Orphan Drug Act was to make such therapies, along with drugs, eligible for research grants to defray the costs of developing medical foods for rare diseases. A 'rare disease' within the context of medical foods means any disease or condition that occurs so infrequently in the U.S. that there is no reasonable expectation that a medical food for such disease or condition will be developed without assistance of the Orphan Drug Act incentives. Medical food was defined within the context of new drug development, not for regulating the use of such products. The Orphan Drug Act amended the FD&C Act to add the orphan drug development economic incentives to the drug sections of the FD&C Act, but the amendments did not add the medical food definition to the FD&C Act. If the U.S. Congress had intended to establish a regulatory subcategory for food formulated to meet distinctive nutritional requirements resulting from diseases or health conditions, the FD&C Act would have been amended to include the medical food definition.

The Orphan Drug Act definition of medical food is:

A food which is formulated to be consumed or administered enterally under the supervision of a physician and which is intended for the specific dietary management of a disease or condition for which distinctive nutritional requirements, based on recognized scientific principles, are established by medical evaluation.

Congress again amended the FD&C Act in 1990 with the Nutrition Labeling and Education Act (NLEA) which, in part, provided for mandatory nutrition labeling of most packaged food and provided for FDA regulation of label claims that characterized a relationship of a nutrient to any disease or health-related condition (i.e. health claims). FDA's pre-NLEA nutrition labeling regulations exempted foods for special dietary use that were intended for use solely under medical supervision in the dietary management of specific diseases and disorders, the rationale being that the nutrition labeling developed for foods intended for consumption by the general population was not well suited for these special use foods. NLEA followed suit and exempted 'medical foods,' as defined in the Orphan Drug Act, from mandatory nutrition labeling. NLEA also exempted medical foods from the new health claim regulation provisions. Another NLEA amendment revised the 'drug' definition to specify that a food would not be a drug solely because it made an FDA-authorized health claim. NLEA made no similar provision to ensure that 'medical foods' would not be regulated as drugs.

FDA's regulations to implement the NLEA nutrition labeling and health claim provisions (21 CFR 101.9 and 21 CFR 101.14) list 'medical food' among the exemptions in these regulations. The 1988 Orphan Drug Act 'medical food' definition was incorporated and expanded on in these regulations. Following the 1993 issuance of these regulations, awareness spread within the food industry that there is a subcategory of foods for which FDA regulations permitted manufacturers to make claims, not subject to FDA regulation, about effects on diseases.

FDA does not consider all foods that may be of some benefit to people who are sick, or all foods prescribed or recommended by a physician, to be medical foods. To clarify the statutory definition of a medical food, FDA set clarifying criteria in the nutrition labeling regulation (at 21 CFR 101.9(j)(8)). A food can be considered a medical food exempt from nutrition labeling only if:

- it has been specially formulated for feeding of a patient;
- it is intended for the dietary management of a patient who, because of therapeutic or chronic medical needs, has limited or impaired capacity to ingest, digest, absorb, or metabolize ordinary foodstuffs or certain nutrients, the dietary management of which cannot be achieved by the modification of the normal diet alone;
- it provides nutritional support specifically modified for the management of the unique nutrient needs that result from the specific disease or condition, as determined by medical evaluation;
- it is intended for use under medical supervision;
- it is intended only for a patient receiving active and ongoing medical supervision wherein the patient requires medical care on a recurring basis for, among other things, instructions on the use of the medical food.

FDA considers the statutory definition of medical foods to narrowly constrain the types of products that fit within the category. Outside of medical foods that have been developed for dietary management of rare diseases, FDA has considered most products marketed as medical foods, not to meet the definition of a medical food. In a number of situations where FDA has become aware of the marketing of products as medical foods, the agency has sent Warning Letters to the firms informing them that the products are illegal because (1) the product is mislabeled for not meeting the statutory definition of a 'medical food', and (2) the product is an unapproved new drug as it is intended to be used to treat or mitigate a disease. The types of products that have been the target of FDA medical food Warning Letters include products intended for the dietary management of allergies and asthma, lactose intolerance, psoriasis, constipation, irritable bowel syndrome, Crohn's disease, colitis, arthritis, failure-to-thrive, injury/trauma, pre/post surgery, and prenatal vitamins.

Under the FD&C Act a food is misbranded if it purports to be or is represented for special dietary uses, unless its label bears such information concerning its vitamin, mineral, and other dietary properties as FDA determines to be, and by regulation prescribes as, necessary in order fully to inform purchasers as to its value for such uses [FD&C Act §403(j)]. Prior to NLEA, FDA issued a number of 'food for special dietary use' (FSDU) regulations (21 CFR 105) that addressed conditions required (e.g. ingredients, labeling) to accommodate foods intended for use to supply the particular dietary needs of special populations (as opposed to the general healthy population). For example, there had been a FSDU regulation for low sodium foods intended for people with hypertension. The low sodium FSDU use regulation became obsolete following NLEA because the 'low sodium' properties of such foods now may be promoted by nutrient content claims, and the special dietary use may be promoted under the authorized health claim for sodium and hypertension (21 CFR 101.74). The only FSDU regulations that remain today are for hypoallergenic foods, infant foods (other than infant formula), and label statements relating to usefulness in reducing or maintaining body weight. Although functional foods are foods for special dietary uses, the likelihood of FDA creating new FSDU regulations to accommodate functional foods in nil because required FSDU labeling can be accommodated under the existing petition process for new health claims and nutrient content claims, or with use of structure/function claims.

3.6   Ingredient safety

U.S. food ingredient safety standards differ depending on whether a product is marketed as a dietary supplement or conventional food. A functional food ingredient acceptable as a dietary supplement ingredient may, when used as an ingredient of a conventional food, cause the product to be adulterated. The marketing of adulterated food in the U.S. is prohibited. A conventional food is adulterated unless all ingredients are (1) used in accordance with a food additive regulation, (2) are a GRAS use, or (3) were in the U.S. food supply prior to January 1, 1958. Dietary ingredients used in dietary supplements are presumed safe if marketed in the U.S. prior to October 14, 1994. Dietary ingredients not marketed in the U.S. prior to October 15, 1994 are 'new dietary ingredients' (NDI). To market a dietary supplement containing a NDI, the manufacturer must submit a notification to FDA, 75 days prior to marketing the product, that explains the NDI's history of use or other evidence of safety that establishes, when used under the conditions recommended in the labeling of the supplement, the use of the NDI-containing dietary supplement will reasonably be expected to be safe (21 CFR 190.6). NDIs that have been present in the food supply as an article used for food in a form in which the food has not been chemically altered are exempt from the premarket notification requirement [FD&C Act §413(a)]. FDA has concerns about the growth of conventional food products that contain added botanical ingredients that have not previously been used as food ingredients. Although the popular botanical ingredients used in dietary supplements are legal under DSHEA, most are not approved food additives or GRAS for use in conventional foods and thus their use may cause the food to be adulterated.[12]

The safety standard for conventional food ingredients requires that prior to use of the ingredient it be established that there is a reasonable certainty of no harm to consumers when the ingredient is used within the proposed conditions of use. The term 'reasonable certainty' is used in the standard as there cannot be 'absolute certainty' of no harm since safety determinations are based on extrapolation from experimental animal evidence. When FDA is satisfied that 'reasonable certainty of no harm' has been established, the agency issues a food additive regulation that specifies the types of foods in which the additive may be used, the maximum use levels, and how the additive is to be identified on the food label. The same safety standard applies to GRAS food ingredients, but the process for establishing the reasonable certainty of no harm differs from that of a food additive regulation.

The safety standard for dietary supplement ingredients requires that when used under the conditions recommended or suggested in the labeling of the dietary supplement, the dietary ingredient will reasonably be expected to be safe (FD&C Act §413(a)]. The 'reasonably expected' standard is a more lax standard than the 'reasonable certainty of no harm' required of conventional food ingredients. As such, many common dietary supplement ingredients cannot be used as conventional food ingredients.

The traditional rubric for food additive safety testing is to feed high levels of the substance to experimental animals to discover the adverse effects of high oral doses. Next, graded doses of the ingredient are fed to determine the 'no observable effect level' (NOEL) for the adverse effects. The third step is to apply safety factor to the NOEL (typically 100-fold) to derive an 'acceptable daily intake' (ADI) for the food ingredient. The food additive is considered safe when the 'expected daily intake' (EDI) is lower than the ADI. Functional food ingredients, intended for effects in the body, are typically added to foods in much greater amounts than are ingredients intended for effects in the food (e.g. flavors, emulsifiers, preservatives, etc). Such ingredients face difficulty in establishing a reasonable certainty of no harm because they are used in foods at levels too high to accommodate a 100-fold difference between the expected human intake and the amount that can be incorporated into diets of experimental animals.

3.7   Sources of further information and advice

The Federal Food, Drug, and Cosmetic Act, as Amended (FD&C Act): http://www.fda.gov/RegulatoryInformation/Legislation/FederalFoodDrugand CosmeticActFDCAct/default.htm

A Dietary Supplement Labeling Guide, U.S. Food and Drug Administration, April 2005: http://www.fda.gov/Food/GuidanceComplianceRegulatoryInformation/GuidanceDocuments/DietarySupplements/DietarySupplementlabelingguide/default.htm

A Food Labeling Guide, US Food and Drug Administration, April 2008: http://www.fda.gov/Food/GuidanceComplianceRegulatoryInformation/GuidanceDocuments/FoodLabelingNutrition/FoodLabelingGuide/default.htm

Conventional Foods Being Marketed as 'Functional Foods'; Public Hearing; Request for Comments. Notice of public hearing; request for comments. Docket No. 2002P-0122. The Food and Drug Administration. Federal Register. Vol 71, no. 206. Page 62400. October 25, 2006. http://edocket.access.gpo.gov/2006/pdf/06-8895.pdf

3.8   References

1. Food and Drug Administration. Notice of public hearing; request for comments. Conventional Food Being Marketed as 'Functional Foods.' Docket No. 2002P-0122. Federal Register Vol. 71(206). October 25, 2006. Available at: http://edocket.access.gpo.gov/2006/pdf/06-8895.pdf
2. Food and Drug Administration. Guidance for Industry: Factors that distinguish liquid dietary supplements from beverages, considerations regarding novel ingredients, and labeling for beverages and other conventional foods. December 2009. Available at: http://www.fda.gov/Food/GuidanceComplianceRegulatoryInformation/GuidanceDocuments/DietarySupplements/ucm196903.htm
3. Food and Drug Administration. Guidance for Industry: Evidence-based Review System for the Scientific Evaluation of Health Claims. January 2009. Available at: http://www.fda.gov/Food/GuidanceComplianceRegulatoryInformation/GuidanceDocuments/FoodLabelingNutrition/ucm073332.htm
4. Food and Drug Administration. A Food Labeling Guide, Appendix C. Health Claims. 2009. Available at: http://www.fda.gov/Food/GuidanceComplianceRegulatoryInformation/GuidanceDocuments/FoodLabelingNutrition/FoodLabelingGuide/ucm064919.htm
5. Food and Drug Administration. A Food Labeling Guide, Appendix D. Qualified Health Claims. October 2009. Available at: (http://www.fda.gov/Food/GuidanceComplianceRegulatoryInformation/GuidanceDocuments/FoodLabelingNutrition/FoodLabelingGuide/ucm064923.htm
6. David Vladeck, Director, Federal Trade Commission Bureau of Consumer Protection. Priorities for Dietary Supplement Advertising Enforcement. October 22, 2009. http://www.ftc.gov/speeches/vladeck/091022vladeckcrnspeech.pdf
7. Oregon Department of Justice Press Release. Kellogg Settlement Will Provide Nearly 500,000 Boxes of Cereal To The Hungry. December 17, 2009. http://www.doj.state.or.us/releases/2009/rel122209.shtml
8. Coughlin Stoia Geller Rudman & Robbins LLP. Dannon Activia and DanActive Settlement. January 27, 2010. http://www.dannonsettlement.com/
9. Institute of Medicine of the National Academies. Dietary reference intakes for energy, carbohydrate, fiber, fat, fatty acids, cholesterol, protein, and amino acids. 2005. National Academies Press. Washington, D.C.
10. Food and Drug Administration. Notice of Proposed Rulemaking. Food Labeling: Nutrient Content Claims; Alpha-Linolenic Acid, Eicosapentaenoic Acid, and

Docosahexaenoic Acid Omega-3 Fatty Acids. Federal Register. Volume 72, page 66103. November 27, 2007.

11. US Food and Drug Administration. Advanced Notice of Proposed Rulemaking. Regulation of Medical Foods. Federal Register Vol 61, No. 231, page 60661. November 29, 1996. At page 60662.

12. FDA. Letter to manufacturers regarding botanicals and other novel ingredients in conventional foods. http://www.fda.gov/Food/DietarySupplements/Guidance ComplianceRegulatoryInformation/ucm103443.htm

3.9   Appendix: definitions

Drug

The term *drug* is defined in the FD&C Act, in part, as (1) articles recognized in the official U.S. Pharmacopeia, official Homeopathic Pharmacopeia of the U.S., or official National Formulary, (2) articles intended for use in the diagnosis, cure, mitigation, treatment, or prevention of disease in man or other animals, and (3) articles other than food intended to affect the structure or any function of the body of man or other animals [FD&C Act §201(g)(1)].

A key aspect of this definition is that any article becomes a drug when it is intended to be used as a drug. For example, a *Cold and Flu Protection* statement made on an orange juice label would show the juice was intended to be used as a drug for the prevention of colds and flu. A second point is that both food and drugs may be intended to affect structure of function of the body provided the effects are not disease-related. Thus, *Calcium to build strong bones* is an acceptable type of statement for a food label about an affect on a body structure. *Calcium to reduce osteoporosis risk* however relates the effect to a disease and would not be an acceptable label claim for food (unless authorized as a health claim). The *drug* definition notes explicitly that a food label health claim made in accordance with FDA regulations does not cause the food to become a drug.

Food

Food is defined in the FD&C Act simply as: articles used for food or drink by man or other animals; articles used for components of food; and chewing gum [FD&C Act §201(f)].

The FD&C Act includes two food subcategories that have some unique regulatory requirements not common to food in general. These food subcategories are dietary supplements and Foods for Special Dietary Use. FDA uses the term conventional food to refer to any food that is not a dietary supplement. There is not a regulatory category for functional food, although the Foods for Special Dietary Use category is a similar concept. The original purpose for the Foods for Special Dietary Use regulatory category has largely been replaced by provisions for food label claims added to the FD&C Act by the 1990 Nutrition Labeling and Education Act (NLEA), and the provisions for dietary supplement structure/function claims added to the FD&C Act by the 1994 Dietary Supplement Health and Education Act (DSHEA). Although 'medical foods' are mentioned in NLEA, there is nothing within the FD&C Act that establishes medical foods as a regulatory subcategory of food.

Dietary supplement

The FD&C Act defines dietary supplements as:

> Products intended for ingestion (other than tobacco) to supplement the diet and that contain: a vitamin, a mineral, an herb or other botanical, an amino acid, a substance used by man to supplement the diet by increasing the total dietary intake, or a concentrate, metabolite, constituent, extract, or combination of any of the above substances.

Articles that are approved drugs cannot be used as dietary supplements unless the article had been marketed as a dietary supplement or food prior to the drug approval. The dietary supplement definition also notes that supplements must be in the form of a tablet, capsule, powder, softgel, gel cap, or liquid intended for ingestion in small quantities such as drops, or if not in such form they cannot be represented as a conventional food. Neither may dietary supplements be represented for use as the sole item of a meal. [FD&C Act §403(ff)].

Although the FD&C Act dietary supplement definition distinguishes between dietary supplements and conventional foods, the term 'conventional food' has not defined. FDA considers factors such as a product's name, packaging, serving size, recommended conditions of use, and other representations about the product, as determinants of whether a food product is represented as a conventional food.[2] For example FDA believes that the packaging of liquid products in bottles or cans similar to those in which single or multiple servings of beverages like soda, bottles water, fruit juices, and iced tea are sold, represent the product as a conventional food rather than as a dietary supplement. In addition, the name of a product can represent the product as a conventional food. Product or brand names that use conventional food terms such as beverage, drink, water, juice, or similar terms represent the product as a conventional food.

Dietary ingredient

FDA uses the term *dietary ingredient* to refer to the dietary supplement ingredients used to supplement the diet. Ingredients used for technical purposes such as colors, excipients, tablet coatings, etc. are food additives rather than dietary ingredients. The FD&C Act distinguishes between dietary ingredients marketed in the U.S. prior to October 15, 1994 (the date of enactment of the Dietary Supplement Health and Education Act (DSHEA)) and new dietary ingredients (NDI), i.e. dietary ingredients not marketed in the U.S. prior to October 15, 1994. Before marketing a dietary supplement containing a NDI, the manufacturer or distributor of the product must submit a NDI notification to FDA with details of the basis on which the manufacturer or distributor has concluded that a dietary supplement containing the NDI will reasonably be expected to be safe. Dietary ingredients marketed in the U.S. prior to enactment of DSHEA are presumed to be safe and are exempt from the premarket FDA notification requirement.

Food additive

The term *food additive* means any substance the intended use of which results, or may reasonably be expected to result, directly or indirectly, in its becoming a component or otherwise affecting the characteristics of any food [FD&C Act §201(s)]. Food additives require FDA premarket approval based on safety data submitted to FDA in a food additive petition. FDA issues food additive regulations specifying conditions of use (i.e. technical functions, categories of food, and maximum levels of use) under which a food additive has been demonstrated to be safe.

Dietary ingredients of dietary supplements are not food additives and not subject to the standard of safety required of food additives. Also excluded from the food additive definition are food ingredients whose use in foods is generally recognized as safe (GRAS) by qualified experts under the conditions of their intended use. The use of any substance in a food that is not an approved food additive or a GRAS use causes the food to be adulterated and it cannot be legally marketed in the U.S.

Food for special dietary use

The FD&C Act defines the phrase *food for special dietary use* (FSDU) to mean:

> A food represented to be used to supply (1) a special dietary need that exists by reason of a physical, physiological, pathological, or other condition, including but not limited to the condition of disease, convalescence, pregnancy, lactation, infancy, allergic hypersensitivity to food, underweight, overweight, or the need to control the intake of sodium; (2) a vitamin, mineral, or other ingredient used by man to supplement the diet; or (3) a special dietary need by reason of being a food for use as the sole item of the diet. [FD&C Act §412(c)]

The FSDU regulatory category was added to the FD&C Act long before the contemporary concept of functional foods. The purpose for creating the FSDU regulatory subcategory of food was to clarify that certain special uses of food could be regulated as food, not drugs, even though the special nutritional needs were disease or health condition related; e.g., a need to control dietary sodium intake due to hypertension. Dietary supplements were originally included within the FSDU category. However, when DSHEA amended the FD&C Act in 1994, a separate dietary supplement definition was created within FD&C Act §201(ff) in conjunction with establishing new regulatory requirements for dietary supplements.

Medical food

The term *medical food* was defined within the 1983 Orphan Drug Acts for the purpose of making medical foods eligible for federal government research grants for development of therapies for rare diseases. The Orphan Drug Act defined medical food as:

A food which is specially formulated to be consumed or administered enterally under the supervision of a physician and which is intended for the specific dietary management of a disease or condition for which distinctive nutritional requirements, based on recognized scientific principles, are established by medical evaluation.

The FD&C Act neither defines medical food nor provides for a medical food regulatory subcategory of foods.

Disease

For the purpose of distinguishing between claims made about effects of food on maintaining healthy structures or functions of the body and claims made about effects on diseases, the term *disease* has been defined as:

Damage to an organ, part, structure, or system of the body such that it does not function properly (*e.g.* cardiovascular disease), or a state of health leading to such dysfunction (*e.g.* hypertension); except that diseases resulting from essential nutrient deficiencies (e.g. scurvy, pellagra) are not included in this definition [21 CFR 101.93(g)]

In 21 CFR 101.93(g)(2) FDA expands on the disease definition by discussing 10 criteria that cause FDA to consider a claim to be a claim about effects on a disease.

Labels and labeling

The term *label* means a display of written, printed, or graphic material upon the immediate container of a food. The term *labeling* means all labels and other written, printed or graphic materials upon any food or any of its containers or wrappers, or accompanying the food [FD&C Act §201(k) and (m)]. While most mandatory label information (e.g. nutrition information, list of ingredients) requirements apply to labels only, the rules for using claims apply to both labels and labeling. Internet websites are considered to be labeling when (1) a customer can purchase the product from the website, or (2) the website is identified on the product label.

Health claim

The term *health claim* means a food label or labeling statement that characterizes the relationship of a nutrient to a disease or health-related condition [FD&C Act §403(r)(1)(B)]. FDA has expanded the FD&C Act definition a health claim by replacing 'nutrient' with 'substance' to be inclusive of nutrients, other food components, dietary supplement ingredients, and specific foods. The health claim definition in the FD&C Act does not alter the definition of a drug – the 'relationship' characterized in a food health claim cannot be that of a drug use, i.e. to cure, mitigate, treat, or prevent disease. Health claims are limited to characterizing disease risk reduction effects of foods and food components. The use of food health claims requires FDA premarket approval through a petition and regulation process. The FD&C Act also provides for health claims based on authoritative statements to be authorized through a notification process. The health claims authorized by FDA regulations are located in 21 CFR 101.14 and 21 CFR 101.72 through 101.83.

Structure/function claim

The FD&C Act drug definition acknowledges that foods are used to affect the structure or functions of the body. Inherent within the drug definition is recognition that food labels may contain information about intended effects on structure or functions. To make clear the parameters for acceptable claims about structure or function effects of dietary supplements, DSHEA amended the FD&C Act to add a definition of 'nutritional support' claims (in FDA's jargon, structure/function claims). Structure/function claims include:

1 statements about a benefit related to a classical nutrient deficiency disease, provided the claim discloses the prevalence of the disease in the U.S.;
2 statements about a role of a dietary ingredient to affect the structure or function in humans;
3 statements characterizing the documented mechanism by which a dietary ingredient acts to maintain the structure or function;
4 statements describing general well-being resulting from consumption of a dietary ingredient. [FD&C Act §403(r)(6)]

Structure/function claims are not subject to FDA review or approval. There is a notification requirement for dietary supplement structure/function claims.

Nutrient content claim

A nutrient content claim is a statement that characterizes the level of a nutrient in a food [FD&C Act §403(r)(1)(A)]. Nutrient content claims must be approved by FDA prior to their use and are permitted only for those nutrients permitted to be listed in the food label nutrition information. The use of a nutrient content claim that has not been authorized by an FDA regulation misbrands the product. The nutrient content claims authorized by FDA regulations are located in 21 CFR 101.13 and 21 CFR 101.54 through 101.67.

4

Australia and New Zealand regulations on nutrition, health and related claims made on foods*

D. Ghosh, nutriConnect, Sydney, Australia

Abstract: Consumers are increasingly health conscious and want to obtain more information about the food they buy. The health benefit evidence may then be used by companies to underpin marketing strategies regulated under a health claims framework. Regulation is important in food innovation because it governs the means by which health benefits can be translated into messages for consumers. This chapter describes the current regulatory framework in Australia and New Zealand, examines issues related to substantiation of health claims, and provides commentary on the proposed new regulations for nutrition, health and related claims that are currently in preparation by Food Standards Australia New Zealand (FSANZ).

Key words: Australia, functional foods, New Zealand, health, health claims, nutrition, regulation, substantiation.

4.1   Introduction

Foods and food components have an extensive history of use to prevent or ameliorate many diseases (Lupton, 2005; Heinrich and Prieto, 2008), but much more strategically designed research is required to provide scientific evidence of such potential effects. Companies are using this evidence to underpin marketing strategies regulated under a health claims framework. Since the advent of regulation governing the different health claims and public health, it is an important step in the whole food innovation process (Williams and Ghosh, 2008).

---

*With kind permission of The Dairy Industry Association of Australia, Inc. to reproduce some portions of Ghosh, D (2009) 'Functional food and health claims: regulations in Australia and New Zealand,' *Aust J Dairy Technol*, **64**, 152–155.

There is some variation in the way different countries regulate health claims on foods, but there is also international communication and efforts to consolidate and harmonise the activity. This article describes the current regulatory framework in Australia and New Zealand, examines issues related to substantiation of health claims, and provides commentary on the proposed new regulation for nutrition, health and related claims that are currently under revision by Food Standards Australia New Zealand (FSANZ).

4.2   Functional foods: current trends and market

The term 'functional foods' is a relatively new food category or concept, which first emerged in Japan, and has become more widely used over the past decade (Ghosh, 2009). Functional food is touted as a convenient means for consumers to promote optimal health, including the prevention of disease. The Food and Nutrition Board of the National Academy of Sciences, USA has suggested that a functional food is 'any modified food or food ingredient that may provide a health benefit beyond the traditional nutrients it contains' (http://www.iom.edu/). Others (Katan, 2004; Katan and de Roos, 2003) argue that a functional food is any food promoted or consumed for a specific health effect, regardless of whether the food has been modified in some fashion. The term 'functional foods' is not currently defined in food legislation and does not fall within either the general- or special-purpose categories under FSANZ jurisdiction. FSANZ defines it as a working option (Allen *et al.* 2005) as 'similar in appearance to conventional foods and are intended to be consumed as part of a usual diet, but have been modified to have physiological roles beyond the provision of simple nutrients requirements'. The National Centre of Excellence in Functional Foods (NCEFF), Australia, has defined functional foods broadly to include any food containing 'known bioactives', promoting 'general health and wellbeing' or promoted on a 'health platform', as long as these are underpinned by 'good scientific evidence' (NCEFF, 2005). Functional foods encompass a broad range of products, in one or more respects, including calcium-fortified orange juice, whole grains, fruits and vegetables (and components thereof, including lycopene, polyphenols, indoles, and other phytochemicals), soybeans, omega-3 fatty acids, phytosterols, and cocoa.

There is clearly a difference between the Western perspective on functional foods and the Eastern outlook. In the West, functional foods are viewed as a revolution and represent a fast growing segment of the food industry. In the Orient (East), in contrast, functional foods have been a part of the culture for centuries. In traditional Chinese medicine, foods that have medicinal effects have been documented since at least 1000 BC. From ancient times, the Chinese have believed that foods have both preventive and therapeutic effects and are an integral part of health, a view that is now being increasingly recognised around the world (Patwardhan *et al.*, 2005). *Ayurveda* is the traditional healing system of India and is more than 5000 years old and this system regards health as a normal state resulting from a suitable balance in mind, body, and emotions brought about by proper attention to diet, herbal supplements, and physical and meditative actions (Mitscher, 2007). In this sense Ayurveda has an emphasis on health rather than disease, cause rather than symptom, the individual rather than the symptom, and a relationship to Chinese traditional medicine and to Japanese Kempo is clear.

The world market for functional foods and beverages is highly dynamic. According to Euromonitor survey, Japan is the world's largest market at US$11.7 billion, then US is the second one market with around US$10.5 billion while the European market is less developed with an estimated market of US$7.5. The 'big four' European markets being UK (US$2.6 billion), Germany (US$2.4 billion), France (US$1.4 billion), and Italy (US$1.2 billion) (Bech-Larsen and Scholderer, 2007; Consumer Trends: Functional Foods, 2009).

4.3   Australia and New Zealand legislation and functional foods

Health claims are regulated in Australia and New Zealand through an integrated food regulatory system involving both governments, under the statuary agency Food Standards Australia New Zealand (FSANZ), established by the Food Standards Australia New Zealand Act 1991. Australia and New Zealand are regarded as one of the safest food supplies in the world. Australia is in the top five Organisations for Economic Cooperation and Development nations with the safest food supplies, according to a study conducted by Canadian academics. The 'Food Safety Performance World Ranking 2008' placed the UK first and Australia fourth, one ahead of Canada, but all the top five ranked as having 'superior' performance (Charlebois and Yost, 2008).

4.3.1   Current regulatory framework in Australia and New Zealand

Currently in Australia and New Zealand, claims on food labels (encompassing nutrition content and function claims) are regulated by various means. Some claims (for example, enhanced nutrient function claims, disease risk-reduction claim, etc) are not permitted under the Australia New Zealand Food Standards Code (the Code, http://www.foodstandards.gov.au/thecode/); others are permitted and regulated under the Code. At present, nutrient content claims are allowed (for example, those related to vitamins and minerals, fatty acids, lactose, gluten, and sodium), as are some general level health-maintenance claims (for example, calcium is needed for strong bones and teeth; iron helps carry oxygen around your body). Nutrient function claims are left to the general requirements of fair-trade laws (that is, that the information should not be false or misleading). However, there is a prohibition on other types of health claims such as enhanced nutrient function claims, disease risk-reduction claims or any other therapeutic claims, with the exception of claims about the benefit of maternal consumption of folate, to reduce the risk of foetal neural tube defects. It is important to distinguish between nutrient content claims, which are currently regulated and allowed, and health claims (general and high) relating to disease prevention, which are not currently allowed under the transitional Standard 1.1A.2 of the Australia New Zealand Food Standards Code.

4.3.2   New (proposed) regulatory framework in Australia and New Zealand

The development of new regulations for nutrition, health and related claims was initiated in December 2003 following the provision of the Policy Guideline by the Ministerial Council and has evolved through extensive risk analysis by FSANZ in consultation with all stakeholder groups. On the basis of this evaluation, FSANZ recommended a regulated approach with the introduction of the draft Standard for nutrition, health and related claims for the management and substantiation of nutrition content, general level and high level health claims   (http://www.foodstandards.gov.au/standardsdevelopment/proposals/ proposalp293nutritionhealthandrelatedclaims/index.cfm).

The objectives of this Proposal are to provide regulatory arrangements that:

- enable industry to innovate, and also giving consumers a wider range of healthy food choices;
- ensure the supply of adequate information of food labels bearing nutrition, health or related claims to enable consumers to make informed choices;
- prevent misleading or deceptive nutrition, health or related claims on food labels or in food advertising;
- develop strong substantiation framework that aligns levels of scientific evidence with the level of claims along the theoretical continuum of claims, and also draw on the best elements of international regulatory systems for nutrition, health and related claims.

The proposed Claims Classification Framework sets out criteria for two types of claims as nutrition content and health claims. There are two types of health claims: general-level health claims and high-level health claims. The level of a claim determines how the claim is regulated, including the evidence required for substantiation.

Nutrition content claims are statements regarding the amount of a nutrient, energy or a biologically active substance in the food. Manufacturers must have proof that the nutrient, substance, or property that is the subject of the claim is present at levels referred to in the claim. This category of claims is already in use and will now be regulated in the Code. For example, claims can be made about a food being a 'source' of a nutrient if it contains 10% of the Recommended Daily Intake (RDI) per serve, and a 'good source' if it contains 25% of the RDI per serve.

Health claims are of two types based on the state of health effects.

1 **General-level health claims** can refer to the presence of a nutrient or substance in a food and to its effect on a health function. A general-level health claim

cannot refer to a serious disease or condition or to an indicator of a serious disease (e.g. blood cholesterol). This claim will include qualifying criteria, the nutrient profiling scoring criteria (NPSC), scientific substantiation, and wording condition. The nutrient profiling scoring system is require to decide which foods will be able to carry claims and is based on the amount of energy, saturated fat, sodium, sugar, fibre, protein, fruits, vegetables, nuts and legumes in the food. One of the current areas of disagreement is whether this prerequisite system should be extended to nutrient content claims as well (Submission Summary – Preliminary Final Assessment Report, Proposal P293 – Nutrition, Health, and Related Claims). Specific conditions about weight management and weight loss, maternal folic acid consumption, biologically active substances and wholegrain will be the major criteria in the new Standard along with some specific exemptions for foods carrying health claims about lactose and gluten and for the special purpose foods (for example, amino acid modified food).

2   **High-level health claims** are those claims that make reference to a serious disease or biomarker and will need to be pre-approved by FSANZ through an application process.

Seven diet–disease relationships have undergone a review by external experts and of these, five have been substantiated. Claims about these will be allowed on food products, subject to certain conditions:

(i)   sodium (with or without potassium) AND hypertension;
(ii) fruit and vegetables AND coronary heart disease;
(iii) saturated fat and/or trans fat AND elevated serum cholesterol or heart disease;
(iv) calcium (with or without vitamin D) AND osteoporosis;
(v)   folate AND neural tube defects.

The following two diet–disease relationships were assessed but did not reach a sufficient level of evidence for high level health claims:

(i)   whole grains AND coronary heart disease;
(ii) omega-3 fatty acids AND cardiovascular disease.

4.4   Scientific substantiation of health claims

Currently, the increasing health concerns of non-communicable diseases have intensified the necessity for dietary interventions including the role of functional foods and how to communicate responsible health and wellness claims. Globally, different approaches have been taken to formalise the scientific substantiation of claims. In general, nutrition and health claims on food will have to be substantiated scientifically. FSANZ is developing a Substantiation Framework, which should be used by manufacturers before making a claim on a product. A range of approaches is taken towards substantiation of the general level health claims (structure/function claims). The new system will provide a guidance list of pre-substantiated nutrient-function statements. Alternatively, manufacturers may utilise the same process required for high-level health claims. Claims in the high-level category require the most rigorous substantiation evidence. The totality of the evidence must be convincing to support the food–disease relationship. The key elements include a consistent association between the property of food(s) and the claimed health effect; a number of well-designed experimental human studies; and ultimately a biologically plausible relationship between food and disease.

4.5 Australia and New Zealand regulatory framework in the light of global harmonisation

The draft Standard is broadly consistent with comparable arrangements overseas, particularly with US and European Commission (EC). A new regulation on nutrition and health claims made on foods came into force on 19 January 2007 by EC (Regulation (EC) No 1924/2006, http://www.fsai.ie/legislation/food/eu_docs/Labelling/Cor_Reg1924_2006.pdf.). The applications for authorisation of health claims (EC No 353/2008) was published on 18 April 2008 which adequately and sufficiently demonstrated that 'the health claim is based on and substantiated by generally accepted scientific evidence, by taking into account the totality of the available scientific data and by weighing the evidence'. In addition to the requirement of Article 15(3)(g) of Regulation (EC) No 1924/2006, the new regulation should emphasise on sound scientific substantiation. The important features of new proposed regulations are:

- relationship between the food and the claimed effect should be supported by the totality of human data;
- the pertinent non-human studies may help to support the relationship between the food and the claimed effect in humans;
- the totality of the data, including evidence in favour and not in favour and by weighing the evidence would be in consideration for final decision making process.

4.6 Implementation

Following approval of the draft variation to the Code by the FSANZ Board, the final Assessment Report was sent to the Ministerial Council for consideration, but the Council has asked for further review of the proposal, which will require more consumer research to be undertaken. It is likely that the revised standard will be submitted to the Council in the middle of 2010 so, if accepted, the earliest date of implementation is likely to be late 2010. In Australia, the proposed Standard will be enforced by state and territory government agencies and by the Australian Quarantine and Inspection Service (AQIS) for imported foods. In New Zealand, the New Zealand Food Safety Authority is responsible for enforcing the Standard. A health claims 'Watchdog' established by the governments of Australia and

New Zealand will monitor and record complaints received about food-related nutrition content and health claims.

4.7   Implications for the development and manufacture of functional foods

Most early developments of functional foods were those of fortified with vitamins and/or minerals such as vitamin C, vitamin E, folic acid, zinc, iron, and calcium (Sloan, 2000). Subsequently, the focus shifted to foods fortified with various micronutrients such as omega-3 fatty acid, phytosterol, and soluble fiber to promote good health or to prevent diseases such as cancers (Sloan, 2002). More recently, food companies have taken further steps to develop food products that offer multiple health benefits in a single food (Sloan, 2004).

Functional foods have been developed in virtually all food categories, but are not homogeneously scattered over all segments of the food and drink market and consumer health concerns and product preferences may vary between markets. From a product point of view, the functional property can be expressed in numerous different ways such as, 'add good to your life', e.g. improve the regular stomach and colon functions (pre- and probiotics) or 'improve children's life' by supporting their learning capability and behaviour. It is difficult, however to find good biomarkers for cognitive, behavioural and psychological functions. A second group of functional food is designed for reducing an existing health risk problem such as high cholesterol or high blood pressure. A third group consists of those products, which 'makes your life easier' (e.g. lactose-free, gluten-free products) (Siro et al., 2008). The value of the US and European natural (excluding organic) food and drinks market was worth $11.7bn in 2005 and it is expected to reach $19.2bn by 2010. The high consumer acceptance of the natural and exotic trend, as opposed to the functional trend which requires consumer education, indicates that this is a worthwhile area for manufacturer investment.

4.8   Future trends

Where are the challenges and future opportunities for functional foods? Historically, there has been an association between foods and health, but for functional foods to have a place in public health it will be necessary to optimise both the nutritional value and taste. With increasing knowledge of human genetics food may play a role for the individual needs and predispositions (nutrigenomics). Also, emerging food technologies (e.g. nanotechnologies) can potentially lead to increased safety, convenience, quality and nutritional value, but these new technologies will only be an asset if their application is transparent to the consumer. The future of functional foods will depend on continued advances in food science and developments of innovative technologies, facilitating regulatory milieu and improved consumer understanding of claims.

Despite new health claims regulations and vast regional differences in the uptake of functional food and drinks, there remain growth opportunities in the global health market as scientific studies uncover the benefits of emerging and existing ingredients. The discovery of the benefits of new natural ingredients is an important development in the market as consumers become increasingly conscious of what they are putting in and on their bodies.

4.9   Sources of further information and advice

The Institute of Medicine of the National Academies (http://www.iom.edu/).

The Australia New Zealand Food Standards Code (http://www.foodstandards. gov.au/foodstandards/foodstandardscode/).

Proposal P293 – Nutrition, Health and Related Claims (http://www. foodstandards.gov.au/standardsdevelopment/proposals/proposalp293 nutritionhealthandrelatedclaims/index.cfm).

Nutrient Reference Values for Australia and New Zealand Including Recommended Dietary Intakes (http://www.nhmrc.gov.au/publications/synopses/n35syn.htm).

The Australian Quarantine and Inspection Service (AQIS, http://www.daff.gov. au/aqis).

The New Zealand Food Safety Authority (NFSA, http://www.nzfsa.govt.nz/).

EC Regulation on Nutrition and Health Claims (http://www.fsai.ie/legislation/ food/eu_docs/Labelling/Cor_Reg1924_2006.pdf).

4.10   References

Allen J L, Abbott P J, Campion S.L, Lewis J L and Healy M J (2005), 'Functional foods: Australia/New Zealand. In Hasler C M (ed.), *Regulation of Functional Foods and Nutraceuticals: A Global Perspective*, Oxford: Blackwell, pp. 321–335.

Bech-Larsen T and Scholderer J (2007), 'Functional foods in Europe: Consumer research, market experiences and regulatory aspects', *Trends Food Sci Technol*, **18**, 231–234.

Charlebois S and Yost C (2008), The Food Safety Performance World Ranking 2008. Available from http://www.uregina.ca/news/releases/2008/may/21.shtml (accessed 2 February, 2010).

Consumer Trends: Functional Foods, Agriculture and Agri-Food Canada (2009). Available from http://www.gov.mb.ca/agriculture/statistics/pdf/marketanalysis%20 report_functionalfoods-en.pdf (accessed 2 February, 2010).

Ghosh D (2009), 'Functional food and health claims: regulations in Australia and New Zealand', *Aust J Dairy Technol*, **64**, 152–155.

Heinrich M. and Prieto J M (2008), 'Diet and healthy ageing 2100: will we globalise local knowledge systems?' *Ageing Res Rev*, **7**, 249–274.

Katan M B (2004) 'Health claims for functional foods', *BMJ*, **328**, 180–181.

Katan M B and de Roos N M (2003), 'Toward evidence-based health claims for foods', *Science*, **299**, 206–207.

Lupton J R (2005), 'Determining the strength of the relationship between a food, food component, or dietary supplement ingredient and reduced risk of a disease or health-related condition', *J Nutr*, **135**, 340–342.

Mitscher L A (2007), 'Traditional medicines', in *Comprehensive Medicinal Chemistry II*, Elsevier Ltd., 406–430.

National Centre of Excellence in Functional Foods (NCEFF) (2005), *Functional Foods for the Australian Industry: Definitions and Opportunities.* University of Wollongong, NCEFF, Australia.

Patwardhan B, Warude D, Pushpangadan P and Bhatt N (2005), 'Ayurveda and traditional chinese medicine: a comparative overview', *Evid Based Complement Alternat Med*, **2**, 465–473.

Siro I, Kápolna E, Kápolna B and Lugasi A (2008), 'Functional food. Product development, marketing and consumer acceptance–A review', *Appetite*, **51**, 456–467.

Sloan A E (2000), 'The top ten functional food trends'. *Food Technol*, **54**, 33–62.

Sloan A E (2002), 'The top 10 functional food trends. The next generation', *Food Technol*, **56**, 32–57.

Sloan A E (2004), 'The top ten functional food trends'. *Food Technol*, **58**, 28–51.

Williams P and Ghosh D (2008), 'Health claims and functional foods', *Nutr Diet*, **65**, S89–93.

5

Legislation of functional foods in Asia

J. Zawistowski, University of British Columbia, Canada

Abstract: The term 'functional foods' has various meanings in different Asian countries. These include health foods, functional health foods, foods that are fortified with minerals and vitamins, dietary supplements and even traditional Chinese medicine products. Regardless of what name functional foods fall under, their defining attribute is their health function. This concept was introduced over 20 years ago in Japan, and was followed by the implementation of a regulatory system to govern such foods. Since then, functional and health foods have shown sustainable growth on the Japanese and other Asian markets. The Japanese example prompted China, South Korea and many other Asian jurisdictions to develop and implement regulations for the production and sale of functional foods. Some countries chose to either utilize existing food and drug regulations or to develop their own systems. Others followed Codex Alimentarius guidelines or chose to adopt already established global regulations. This chapter reviews regulatory frameworks for functional foods in Asian countries. The definition and categories of functional foods, various function claims and disease risk reduction claims in Japan, China, South Korea, Taiwan and South-East Asia are also discussed.

Key words: Asia, functional foods, regulations, function claims, health claims.

5.1 Introduction: historical background

5.1.1 China and Japan: ancient versus modern era of functional foods

The health benefits of foods and natural health products have been recognized for a very long time in Asia. Herbs, nuts, sesame, tea and lilies were used in ancient China to protect from, and treat, various diseases in clinical practice. Shen Nong (Divine farmer), who is considered a legendary father of Chinese agriculture, tested hundreds of herbs in order to establish and record their medicinal value. According to legend, Shen Nong is attributed with discovering tea as a healthy drink about 5000 years ago. The medicinal value of tea connected to 'benefits of brain and improvement of sight' was first described in Shen Nong's *Material Medica* (Zeng and Liu, 2008). During the Tang Dynasty (618–907), the tea plant was cultivated in 42 China prefectures, and the consumption of tea was encouraged among people of all social ranks and classes. The blooming tea culture gave impetus to the research of tea health benefits. During this period, the very first ten health claims associated with tea drinking were established. Tea function claims such as: 'tea is beneficial to health, able to dredge body channels, relieve headaches, xerophthalmia and fatigue', 'tea can be used to eliminate toxins from the body', 'it is conducive to longevity', became well recognized (Wang, 2002). Although these claims are over a thousand years old, some of them are currently substantiated by science, and with some modification they are approved in countries like Canada, Japan and USA. For example, Health Canada's Natural Health Products Directorate health claim states: 'tea is accredited for the maintenance of good health and increasing alertness' (Canadian Food Inspection Agency, 2007).

In addition to herbs and teas, fruits and vegetables were part of traditional Chinese medical therapy. In some ancient medical books such as *Yellow Emperor's Internal Classic* and *Li Shizhen's Compendium of Material Medica*, the functional health values of fruits and vegetables are well represented. A systemic review of preventive and therapeutic properties of fruits and vegetables was published by Xiu (2002). The health functionality of foods is the important essence of Chinese culture. In addition to their nutritional value, foods were also used for their medicinal properties as per an assumption that 'food and medicine share the same roots' (Xiu, 2002). San Simiao of the Tang Dynasty prescribed a combination of almonds, dates and plums to 'prevent and treat pain in the heart' (Xiu, 2002). Physicians of the Ming Dynasty used haws (fruits of a hawthorn) in their medical practice to promote digestion. Fruits, vegetables, nuts, and other edible plants are extensively used in today's traditional Chinese medicine (TCM). Chinese physicians still prescribe haws to treat hypertension and coronary heart disease, and apples to treat colitis (Xiu, 2002).

Although one can argue that foods cannot be used to treat disease, for over thousands of years the use of foods in Chinese medical practice illustrates the point that functionality and health benefits of foods have been known in Asia for a very long time (Liu, 2004).

The modern term 'functional foods' was created in Japan in the late 1980s as a result of nine years of cooperation among government, academia and industry associations. In order to improve the health status of the Japanese population and to reduce health care costs, the Ministry of Education (presently Ministry of Education, Science and Culture) and the Ministry of Health and Welfare (presently Ministry of Health, Labour and Welfare, MHLW) initiated two research projects: 'Systematic analysis and development of functions of foods' (1984–1986) and 'Analysis of functions for adjusting physical conditions of human body with foods' (1988–1990). A group of Japanese scientists (Kinousei Shokuhin Konwakai) led by Professor T. Abe, has been studying the tertiary function of foods (Nakagawa, 2004). In the search of understanding and defining an effect of food constituents on function/structure of human body as well as risk reduction of chronic diseases, this group established the basis for the current TOKUHO system (short for *Toku*tei *Ho*ken-yo shokuhin): Food for Specified Health Uses (FOSHU). An interim report on functional foods was published in 1989 providing the background to institute a new approval system for functional foods in Japan. In 1991, Japanese MHLW established a legal system and implemented policies in order to permit selling and approving health claims on FOSHU functional foods (Arai, 2002; Ministerial Ordinance, 1991). Amelioration of Japanese food law has created a well-defined approval venue for marketing foods with health benefits. Furthermore, for the first time in World legislation, functional foods have been recognized as a unique and specific food category outside conventional foods and medicine. The approval of FOSHU foods was restricted to foods 'explicitly recognized as food' for ten years in order to avoid confusion between foods and drugs. However, in 2001, the Japanese government has again reformed the health food system and allowed the use tablets and pills under FOSHU regulations (Ohama et al., 2008). As of 2007, there are more than 700 FOSHU products labelled with different health claims being approved in Japan (Arai et al., 2008).

The Japanese success of regulatory reform and the marketing of FOSHU have a significant impact on food legislation in many countries and have generated tremendous interests in functional foods. This food category has gained popularity due to expectation that consumption of functional foods may increase life expectancy, improve life quality and reduce health care cost. Due to demographic changes, globalization, and improved economy, functional foods have also started to gain popularity in other Asian countries (Arvantitoyannis and Van Houwelingen-Koukaliaroglou, 2005; Arai et al. 2008). An increasing number of lifestyle-related diseases has encouraged food and nutritional scientists as well as health professionals to study and work on the bioactive components in functional foods that may carry potential physiological benefits (Doyon and Labrecque, 2005).

5.1.2   TOKUHO: a tertiary function for conventional foods

It is a common belief that unbalanced nutrition creates abnormal physiological conditions and leads to chronic diseases. The consumption of excess fat and cholesterol leads to hyperlipidaemia and hypercholesterolaemia, while the consumption of too much salt may cause hypertension. In addition, a shortage of iron or calcium in a diet may result in anaemia and osteoporosis, respectively. These conditions may be corrected by the consumption of a balanced diet and a healthy lifestyle. It could, however, take five to ten years to introduce such corrections. An adjustment of adverse physiological conditions to the normal state in a relatively short period of time constitutes the underlining principles of the physiological function of foods and the basis for TOKUHO. Such adjustment has to be proven by human clinical studies (Nakagawa, 2004).

The tertiary function of foods is, unlike conventional (primary – nutrition and secondary – taste) functions, directly involved in the modulation of human physiological systems such as the cardiovascular, immune and digestive systems (Arai, 1996). It has become clear that food can be designed not only to satisfy primary functions but also for adjusting conditions of the human body's function. For example, a significant number of clinical studies have demonstrated that consumption of phytosterol-containing foods (2–3 g/day) for three to four weeks leads to a decrease in serum low density lipoprotein (LDL)-cholesterol by 10–15% (Zawistowski and Kitts, 2004). Therefore, consumption of these kinds of functional foods may correct one of the causative factors of coronary heart disease (CHD) and reduce the risk of CHD by about 25% in a relatively short period of time (Law, 2004).

5.2   Regulatory challenges for marketing of functional foods

Asian countries such as China and India are leading suppliers of functional ingredients and raw materials for the formulation of food with health benefits. In addition, they have a long tradition of using food for treatment and protection against chronic diseases. However, Asian countries are facing challenges in developing and marketing functional foods for a number of reasons. One major reason is the costly requirement for the clinical support of functionality and health claims of foods that are destined for the global market, despite that some Asian foods already have a long history of health benefits (Williams *et al.*, 2006) based primarily on testimonials.

The cost associated with bringing a new product to the market is relatively high. In addition to the cost of clinical studies, it also includes costs of R&D, safety assessment, and food manufacturing under specific GMP standards as demanded by regulators in the most jurisdictions. For example, the cost of regulatory approval of a new FOSHU product with a health claim is estimated to be up to $US 1 500 000 (Patel *et al.*, 2008).

Outside of Japan, most consumers are still confused over the definition of functional foods. That is because most countries still lack a clear regulatory venue for functional foods, including production, import, approval and distribution of these products. In addition, health claims that can be used on a label as a way to communicate health benefits to consumers are lacking, prohibited or limited. Well-defined regulatory systems together with proper enforcement are critical factors in protecting as well as building confidence of consumers for functional foods (Williams *et al.*, 2006). A regulatory framework with adequate health claims is important for the food industry to encourage product innovation and promote fair competition. Another challenge faced by Asian countries is the harmonization of regulations within a region to avoid trade barriers, as well as understanding the regulatory demands of export countries.

5.3   Definition and categories of functional foods in various Asian countries

Generally, functional foods can be defined as any food product that is marketed or perceived to deliver a health benefit in addition to the basic nutritional value of a food product. Doyon and Labrecque (2005) have identified 28 definitions for functional foods based on the nature, health benefits, function and composition of the food. Worldwide diversity of the functional food concept is also reflected in Asian countries.

The definition of Japanese functional foods (FOSHU) captures the essence of what makes foods functional in a very specific way: 'A food derived from naturally occurring ingredients that can and should be consumed as part of the daily diet.' The definition (Furukawa, 1993) states that functional foods contain constituents that have science-based specific health benefits on physiological functions or biological activities of the body. This type of food has a particular function when ingested, serving to regulate particular body processes as such as:

- enhancement of the biological defence mechanisms;
- prevention of a specific disease;
- recovery from a specific disease;
- control of physical and mental conditions;
- slowing the aging process.

Since 2001, a category of FOSHU may not only include the food format that is 'explicitly recognized as food' but also a medicinal format that resembles US dietary supplements such as capsules, tablets and/or powder. Following the Japanese example, a number of Asian jurisdictions have succeeded to develop regulations and introduce a definition of functional foods.

Health properties are reflected in the Chinese definition of foods. The Food Hygiene Law of 1995 describes food as 'a product that has traditionally served as both food and medicament'. Subsequently, the amendment to the Food Hygiene Law defines functional foods as health foods with a specific effect on biological functions of the body and can be taken as a supplement. This definition includes herbs, botanicals, vitamins, minerals, dietary supplements, and some TCM. Health foods cannot be used for therapeutic purposes. This category excludes any conventional foods and TCM that are designated for mitigating and treating diseases (Reynolds, 1999).

Similar to Chinese regulations, Taiwanese regulations define food with health benefits under the category of health foods. Accordingly, 'health foods' are food products that possess 'special nutritious elements' (bioactive components) or 'specific health care abilities' to improve health, or/and reduce the risk of disease. This type of foods is not intended for use in mitigation, curing or/and treating human diseases. Any food products that are labelled or advertised as food matching this definition is specified and governed by the Health Food Control Law (HFCA), regardless whether they are named health foods or functional foods. This category includes food formats such as yogurt or fish oil as well as tablets, powders and capsules forms (HFCA, 2006).

In South Korea, the term 'Health Functional Foods' is used to describe functional foods and is defined as 'a processed food used with the intention to enhance and maintain human health by (consuming) physiologically functional ingredients and/or components in forms of tablets, capsules, powder granules, liquid and pills'. Health functional foods contain 37 generic categories of foods/ bioactive ingredients including vitamins, minerals, essential amino acids, proteins, dietary fibre, essential fatty acids and other nutrient supplements such as ginseng products, aloe, squalene, and chlorella (Chay, 2005). There is one critical element in this definition that makes it so different in comparison to the definition used in the Western regulatory jurisdictions such as Canada, the US and EU. Korean functional foods are doseable and can be used in medicinal formats. They resemble the form of dietary supplements that are regulated in the US under the Dietary Supplement Health and Education Act (DSHEA), rather than functional foods as they are defined by Canada and the EU.

Many Asian countries do not have a clear definition and regulatory venue for the approval of functional foods. In many cases regulators adopt existing law to define this category of foods. In Thailand, functional foods are grouped under the notification for foods for special dietary uses, and defined by the Thai Food and Drug Administration as foods which are similar in appearance to conventional foods, consumed as part of a normal diet and exhibit physiological benefits including the possibility of reducing the risk of chronic diseases.

However, sometimes these products cannot be classified as either foods or drugs. Since Thailand does not have a specific regulation for functional foods, most of these foods are now being confused with drugs. A clear-cut identification is necessary in the pre-marketing process in order to determine whether a product can be classified under the Drug Act or the Food Act. To classify a functional food as a drug or a food depends mainly on the type and concentration of active ingredients in the product and the claims it makes. If a product is classified as a food, three aspects need to be considered together: safety, quality and efficacy (Charoenpong and Nitithamyong, 2004).

In Indonesia, functional foods are defined as processed foods that contain one or more functional components (proven to be harmless) with a certain physiological function and proven by scientific studies to be beneficial for health (HK 00.05.52.0685, 2005). These types of products may be classified as dietary foods, and/or may be in line with the food fortification program that was launched in 1996 to improve the nutritional status of the community (Bogor Agricultural University, 2003). Dietary foods, and for the most part, traditional foods, contain natural bioactive components. These foods, which may provide health benefits to consumers, have been available in Indonesia for a long time and have the potential to be developed as functional and supplemental foods.

In Hong Kong, there is no universally accepted definition of health foods or functional foods. Alternative terms such as dietary supplements, nutraceuticals, designed foods, functional foods and natural health products are used on different occasions to refer to similar products.

The Philippines adapted the Codex Alimentarius definition of functional foods as being a 'food that satisfactorily demonstrates that it beneficially affects one or more target functions in the body beyond adequate nutritional effects, in a way which is relevant to either an improved state of health and well-being, or reduction of risk to disease'. The term 'functional foods' may include foods that are fortified with minerals and vitamins, and which are regulated under the Philippine Food Fortification Act of 2000. The government has implemented this act to make the fortification of certain staple foods mandatory in order to help combat the problem of malnutrition in the country. However, functional foods can also be promoted under this act to be an effective solution to the aforementioned problem. Dietary supplements in medicinal format may also be considered 'functional foods'.

Functional foods are not well defined and regulated in countries such as Singapore and Malaysia. Both countries are actively working to adapt international guidelines to provide a better regulatory control of this category of foods. It is worthwhile to notice that Malaysian regulations comprised dietary supplements as a category, which includes ingredients such as vitamins, minerals, amino acids, natural substances of plant/animal origin, enzymes, and substances with nutritional/ physiological functions in the form of pills, capsules and other medicinal types. However, in contrast to China, South Korea, Indonesia and other Asian countries, this category is not considered to represent a functional food and it is regulated as a drug by the National Pharmaceutical Control Bureau. Any product that is used to prevent and/or reduce risk of disease, control body weight, maintain and/or promote health and wellbeing is classified as a drug (Act 368 of 1989).

In India, until recently, functional foods, as a category, did not exist and comparable products were either regulated as foods or drugs. Nutritional foods were the closest category to functional foods. This category is defined by the Prevention of Food Adulteration Act (PFA) of 2004 as 'food[s] claimed to be enriched with nutrients such as minerals, proteins or vitamins'. Currently, Act no. 34 of 2006 (2009) dedicated a section for functional foods. Functional foods, foods for special dietary uses, nutraceuticals and health supplements share the same category and are defined as 'foods which are specially processed or formulated to satisfy particular dietary requirements which exist because of a particular physical or physiological condition; or specific disease or disorder which are presented as such, wherein the composition of these foodstuffs must differ significantly from the composition of ordinary foods of comparable nature'. This food category may include botanical and animal ingredients, minerals, vitamins, proteins, enzymes and dietary supplemental substances. In addition to the conventional food format, functional foods can exist in the form of powder, tablets, capsules, liquid and other dosage formats for oral administration. It is worthwhile to notice that there is a new food safety and standards regulations draft that was prepared in consultation with various stakeholders along with the Food Authority in India, and was published in December 2009. In this document, functional foods are not defined and the aforementioned definition relates only to foods for special dietary uses (FSSAI, 2009).

5.4 Food and drug interface: regulatory framework for functional foods

Functional foods share the properties of both foods and drugs as define in the regulations in many countries and for this reason such products present a classification and regulatory challenge. There is also a lot of consumer confusion how to discriminate functional foods from conventional foods. For the majority of consumers, orange juice is a conventional beverage. The same orange juice that

Table 5.1   Comparison of functional foods with drugs and their conventional counterparts

Items	Conventional food	Functional food	Drug
Function	To feel 'full' and to survive	Maintain health, improve health	Cures diseases or has curative functions
Property	Conventional properties	Conventional + drug properties	Drug properties
Dosage	No	Yes	Yes
Suitable for:	All groups of people	Certain groups of people	Certain groups of people

has been a subject of clinical studies, however, is considered a functional food. In fact, some clinical studies show that flavonoids present in orange juice may favourably change a human lipid profile upon consumption (Kurowska *et al.*, 2000). Functional foods can exist in many forms. For example, raw foods may be functional as long as they contain endogenous constituents with health benefits; e.g. tomatoes rich of lycopene, which may reduce the risk of cancer. Processed foods such as oat bran cereal may reduce serum cholesterol, and beverage-formatted foods, such as calcium-enriched orange juice, may reduce the risk of osteoporosis. Clearly, there is little demarcation between the health benefits of functional foods and drugs. Like drugs, this type of food should be taken in doses by a specific group of consumers (Table 5.1). In contrast to conventional foods, such products contain active ingredients that may act to prevent disease and enhance the health and wellness of consumers. Subsequently, these products may carry health claims on a label. In fact, International Life Sciences Institute (ILSI) defines functional foods as foods associated with health claims (Asp, 2005).

Generally there are four ways to regulate functional foods in Asia:

1   As food–drug interface products.
2   As foods.
3   As drugs.
4   As functional foods (health foods) using a specific regulatory venue, established for this particular category.

5.4.1   Malaysian food–drug interface products

In Malaysia, if a product is not clearly a food or a drug it is classified by the Committee for the Classification of Food–Drug Interface Products (Jawatankuasa Pengkelasan Keluaran Food–Drug Interphase) as a food–drug interface (FDI) based on its composition. Subsequently, the sale of FDIs, which resemble functional foods, is regulated either by the Drug Act or Food Act. If a product contains 80% or more food ingredients and 20% or less bioactive ingredient with pharmacological and/or therapeutic properties, such a product is regulated by the Food Safety and Quality Division (FSQD). However, if the product contains more than 20% bioactives and less than 80% food-based ingredients, it is regulated by the National

Pharmaceutical Control Bureau (NPCB). In addition, NPCB is responsible for approval of any products in 'pure' forms such as vitamins, minerals, amino acids, fatty acids, fibre, enzymes, etc, as well as products which are not traditionally used as foods or beverages with health benefits, such as alfalfa, spirulina, royal jelly, noni juice, rooibose tea and other herbal products (Ministry of Health Malaysia, 2007).

5.4.2   Adapting existing regulations

There are no specific regulations to govern functional foods in countries like Hong Kong and Thailand. In most cases the regulation of health (functional) food products is based on their ingredient content and falls under the classification of either foods or drugs. Depending on the composition, Hong Kongese health foods (functional foods) may be classified as drugs and regulated under the existing drug (Pharmacy and Poisons Ordinance, PPO; Cap. 138) or the Traditional Chinese Medicine regulations (Chinese Medicine Ordinance, CMO; Cap. 549) (Wu, 2001). Health food products, which do not contain any medicinal constituents, are regulated as general foods and are subjected to the regulation of the Public Health and Municipal Service Ordinance (PHMSO; Cap.132). These products are not allowed to carry a claim for the diagnosis, treatment, prevention, alleviation, or mitigation of disease or any symptoms of disease (Wu, 2001). Some Chinese medicines or foods containing Chinese medicines as active ingredients may be regarded as health foods, and they are subject to CMO regulations (Cap. 549). The latter products are allowed substantiated health claims but are prohibited to carry or advertise claims regarding curative or preventive effects against diseases (Undesirable Medical Advertisements Ordinance; Cap. 231) listed in the schedule to the Ordinance (the Government of Hong Kong, 2006).

Thailand also adapted the existing regulations for the marketing approval of functional foods based on the type and concentration of active ingredients. If a functional food is classified as a food, it must obey food regulations and must be manufactured according to food safety and quality standards (Charoenpong and Nitithamyong, 2004). However under existing food regulations, health claims are not permitted.

5.4.3   Developing new regulations

Traditionally, Asia has always been conscious of healthy eating habits. It is not surprising that a number of Asian countries – Japan, China, Taiwan and South Korea – have developed their own legislation systems to govern functional foods.

Japan was the first country which recognized the potential for the health benefits of functional foods and the need to regulate the use and marketing of these types of foods. The Japanese Ministry of Health, Labour and Welfare (MHLW) also recognized a need for approved health claims that can be used on a label to inform consumers about the functionality of foods. In 1991, Japan introduced FOSHU, which is currently grouped under Foods with Health Claims together with Foods with Nutrient Function Claims, and governed by the current Health Promotion

Law (Yamada *et al.*, 2008). The approval of FOSHU is a stand-alone system and products can only be approved on a one by one basis. To approve a new FOSHU product, MHLW requires a dossier containing information regarding product composition and specification, formulation, stability (shelf life), dosage, nutritional information, manufacturing procedure, and clinical as well as safety substantiation. Clinical and safety data are very crucial. FOSHU product effectiveness must be proven by well designed, randomized placebo-controlled double-blinded trials that are conducted for more than 12 weeks using a specific product (Ohama *et al.*, 2008). Safety must be confirmed by *in vivo* and *in vitro* toxicity tests as well as clinical studies (Ohama *et al.*, 2008). The evaluation process is stringent and is performed by the Council on Pharmaceutical Affairs and Food Sanitation, and the Food Safety Commission along with MHLW (Fig. 5.1). Once approved, FOSHU products are given specific health claims that can be displayed on a label along with a seal of approval (Fig. 5.2) (MHLW, 2006). For a decade, FOSHU products were allowed to only exist in food forms so as to encourage the consumption of FOSHU products as foods and as part of a regular diet (Bailey, 2004). However, in 2001, the FOSHU regulatory system was amended to accommodate the American Chamber of Commerce of Japan's request to remove a trade barrier in regards to dietary supplements, between the US and Japan (Ohama *et al.*, 2008). As a result of this amelioration, FOSHU products, when approved, can be marketed as food as well as in medicinal formats such as pills, tablets, capsules, powders, potions etc. In 2005, FOSHU was deregulated again to include new product categories and health claims. In addition to a regular FOSHU, MHLW created three new categories based on the efficacy substantiation (levels A, B, and C); qualified FOSHU (level C), standardized FOSHU (level B), and the disease risk reduction FOSHU (level A) (MHLW, 2006). This system is somewhat similar to USA qualified health claims on foods (Pearson claims) and was introduced to reduce the growth of non-FOSHU products on the Japanese market (Yamada *et al.*, 2008).

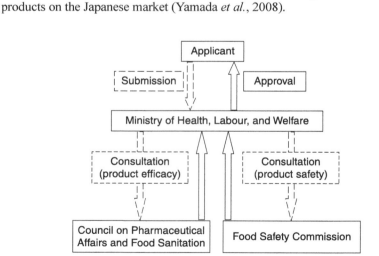

Fig. 5.1   FOSHU approval flow chart (modified from MHLW, 2006).

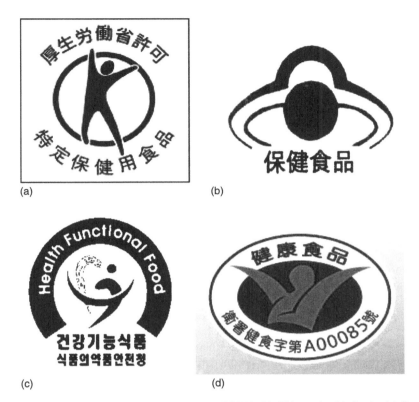

(a)   (b)

(c)   (d)

Fig. 5.2   Seals of approval for (a) Japanese FOSHU, (b) Chinese health foods, (c) South Korean health functional foods, and (d) Taiwanese health foods.

Products with health benefits that are not fully substantiated but suggestive or lacking elucidation of the mechanism of action are classified at level C and approved as qualified FOSHU. These products must bear the label statement that 'evidence has not necessarily been established' and use the word 'possible' in conjunction with a health claim (Patel *et al.*, 2008). Products that contain active ingredients, which were previously proven to meet requirements for specific health claims, are qulified as standardized FOSHU (level B) and do not require a rigorous review (Patel *et al.*, 2008). Regular and disease reduction FOSHU (level A) must be supported by statistically proven efficacy data generated from well established clinical trials and backing by the clear mechanism of action of a key ingredient (Ohama *et al.*, 2008). It is worthwhile to note that the Japanese market capitalized on the well established regulatory venue. The FOSHU products on the Japanese market reached a total number of 755 in 2007, representing the three largest categories; gut health, heart health and dental care (Datamonitor, 2008). Apparently, this number is slightly higher, and as of the end August 2008, 797 FOSHU products with health claims have been approved (Tee, 2009).

Following the Japanese example, China has introduced a series of laws and rulings to curb abundant health products in a previously under-regulated market. In 1996, the administrative policy of health food, law and policy regulating health foods was promulgated by legislature in China. This law was further revised by the newly formed State Food and Drug Administration (SFDA), and in 2005, it became Interim Administrative Measures for Health Food Registration. Chinese health foods include both categories: functional foods and dietary supplements. Botanicals, herbal bioactives, fungi, probiotics, amino acids, essential fatty acids, vitamins and minerals are classified as health foods. The Ministry of Health of the People's Republic of China issued and enforced a decree (Decree of State Food and Drug Administration No. 19) that specifies an administration procedure for health foods (Ford *et al.*, 2007). SFDA is a main regulatory authority to govern registration and approval of health foods for both domestically made and imported products. Patel and coworkers (2008) describe all details of the application and registration steps involved in the approval process. Health (functional) foods can be only approved by SFDA if they are supported by the proper safety data (toxicity testing), efficacy, quality assessment (hygiene, stability, and analytical tests), and full characterization of product. The Food Hygiene Law of 1995 describes sanitary standards for the manufacturing and import of health foods and health food additives (Law of the People 59 of 2005). If a product is approved, a Health Food Approval Certificate is issued which is valid for five years. During this time the product can be sold on the Chinese market; however, the product must be re-registered three months in advance of the expiry date of the certificate (Patel *et al.*, 2008).

Health foods are allowed to bear health (function) claims as per the 27 approved claims published by SFDA (Table 5.2). Depending on the type of claim, the level of evidence support must be substantiated by human clinical studies, animal studies or both. For example, a claim 'enhancing immune systems' requires only animal studies, a claim 'alleviating eye fatigue' must be supported by human studies, while a claim 'assisting blood lipids reduction' must be proven by animal and human studies (Patel *et al.*, 2008). Clinical studies must be conducted on Chinese subjects. Health foods must be manufactured and properly labelled according to the current GMP (Good Manufacturing Practice), with indication of functionality for a specific consumer group. SFDA is also responsible for the approval of health food advertisements under the Interim Rules on Reviewing Health Food Advertisements regulations. This ruling requires provincial-level approval for all health food advertisements before publications. Information on products must be true and not misleading to consumers. Any references to mitigating, treating or curing diseases are strictly prohibited. It is also required for products to carry the disclaimer 'this product is not a substitute for medicine' (Zhu, 2005).

Taiwan is another Asian country which has recently introduced specific regulations to govern functional foods. In 1999, the Executive Yuan, Department of Health (DOH), which is the highest Taiwanese authority on health, issued and implemented the Health Food Control Act (HFCA). The HFCA has been amended several times. The most recent of these amendments was made in May 2006

Table 5.2 Approved function health claims in People's Republic of China*

	Function		Function		Function
1	Enhance immunity[†]	10	Improve sleep[†]	19	Help to prevent against chemical liver damage[†]
2	Blood lipid regulation[§]	11	Stimulate milk secretion[§]	20	Remove acne[‡]
3	Blood sugar regulation[§]	12	Anti-fatigue[†]	21	Improve skin moisture[‡]
4	Anti-aging to improve memory[§]	13	Enhance anoxia endurance[†]	22	Improve skin oil content[‡]
5	Moisten and clear throat[§]	14	Radiation protection[†]	23	Remove skin chloasma[‡]
6	Blood pressure regulation[§]	15	Weight loss[§]	24	Improve gastrointestinal function[§]
7	Help to exclude lead[§]	16	Improvement of child growth and development[§]	25	Improve digestion[§]
8	Vision improvement[‡]	17	Improve bone density[†]	26	Help prevent gastric mucosa damage[§]
9	Anti-oxidative functions[§]	18	Improve nutritional anaemia[§]	27	Improve regularity[§]

* Modified from Ministry of Health China (2003), and Patel *et al.* (2008).
† Must be supported by animal studies.
‡ Must be supported by human studies.
§ Must be supported by animal and human studies.

(HFCA, 2006). The act governs all matters relating to health foods and dietary supplements, such as health food permits; manufacturing; importing; management of safety and sanitation; labelling and advertising; inspection of food facilities; manufacturers and vendors practices; and enforcement and sanction. Any products with health-care abilities, including health foods, must be registered within the Department of Health. In order to obtain an approval, products must be supported by safety and efficacy data with the clear indication of any bioactive(s) that exert a health benefit effect. If it is not possible to identify specific ingredient(s) that are contributing to the health effect, the beneficial effects should be listed and supporting literature should be provided to the central health authority for evaluation and verification. In addition, all methodology that is used to assess efficacy and safety of products must be also presented in the support of an application (HFCA, 2006). The approval process is well described by Wong (2001). Once all documents are submitted, DOH conducts an assessment of the dossier and if the review is successful, the manufacturer or importer is granted a permit valid for five years to sell the health product. The permit may be extended for another five years by applying for renewal within three months prior to the expiration of the issued permit. The DOH has the right to revoke the permit if scientific support of the product's efficacy is in doubt or when the bioactive ingredients, formulation, or method of manufacturing is changed, and when the safety of the product is in doubt during its validity period.

South Korea also recently has developed and implemented a new regulatory system for functional foods. The Korean term 'functional health foods' encompasses both functional foods and dietary supplements and is similar to the term health foods that is used in other regulatory jurisdictions mentioned in this section. In 2004, the Korean Food and Drug Agency (KFDA) introduced the Korea Health Functional Food Act (HFFA) to encourage the industry to produce and market health foods that are easy and convenient to use by average Korean consumers. This act is composed of four sets of regulations: standards and specifications for health functional foods (KFDA Notice #2004–11, January 31, 2004); regulations on recognition of raw materials or ingredients of health functional foods (KFDA Notice #2004–12, January 31, 2004); regulations on imported health functional food notification and inspection procedures (KFDA Notice #2004–8, January 31, 2004); and labelling standards for health functional foods (KFDA Notice #2004–6, January 31, 2004) (GAIN report, 2005).

The HFF Act refers to two types of foods: generic and product-specific health functional foods. If the functional ingredient is on the official HFF list of 37 health functional foods and bioactives, food containing this ingredient is classified as generic and the active ingredient does not require extensive characterization and specific proof of its efficacy in functional food products. However, many new physiologically active ingredients used in the formulation of functional foods are not listed in the HFF Code and require approval by KFDA (Kim, 2004).

In 2004, another set of regulations, the Functional Food Code (FFC) was developed, revised and promulgated. This code contains general standards and specifications governing functional food, individual standards and specifications for 37 functional food categories (Kim *et al.*, 2005). Functional foods can be in the form of tablets, pills, capsules, granules, powder, or liquid. A food product that meets the criteria for one of the 37 defined categories is permitted to carry a health efficacy claim. Anyone wishing to export a functional food that is not part of one of 37 categories specified in the Code can apply to KFDA for a separate approval to recognize the new category or raw materials that have specific health effects (GAIN report, 2005).

5.4.4   Influence of US and EU legislation on the functional foods regulations in Asia

A lack of regulation for functional foods in Indonesia and Singapore, prompts these countries to partially adapt the US and EU systems and implement them within their own legislation used to control conventional foods.

Functional foods in Indonesia are regulated under the same regulatory system that is applied for conventional foods, as long as this category of foods contains food-approved ingredients (PP 28, 2004). Functional foods can be classified as dietary foods, and/or food fortified with vitamins, minerals, essential fatty acids and botanicals such as ginseng and ginger (Bogor Agricultural University, 2003). Currently, the Indonesian National Agency for Drug & Food Control (NADFC) has adapted all eleven health claims from the US Nutrition Labeling and Education Act of 1990 (NLEA). Furthermore, the regulations promulgated on January 27, 2005 have approved 15 classes of functional food components that can be used in foods with health claims (HK 00.05.52.0685, 2005). These include: dietary fibre; prebiotics and probiotics; soy isoflavones; phytosterols and phytostanols; and tea polyphenols (Table 5.3). Some of the functional foods approved in the US have been granted approval for sale in Indonesia. For example, phytosterol-enriched milk powder for heart health was approved as a functional food by NADFC (Zawistowski, 2008). Approved functional foods must comply with safety, quality and nutritional standards as well as with food packaging and laboratory testing requirements, regardless of whether products are manufactured nationally or imported from outside of Indonesia. The production of functional foods must be conducted in facilities under the Hazard Analysis and Critical Control Points (HACCP) system. Food standards and rules are described in the governmental regulations on food safety, quality and nutrition (PP 28, 2004), regulations on food labelling and advertisement (PP 69, 1999), and the Food Act (UU 7, 1996).

Although Singapore does not have specific regulations regarding functional foods, the government does feature relevant standards that are applied internationally and have been adopted and/or modified to suit Singapore's conditions. In 2009, in order to control the marketing of functional foods (foods with health claims), the Agri-Food and Veterinary Authority (AVA) together with the Health Promotion Board (HPB) published five health claims for use on foods. These are all disease risk reduction claims that have been adopted from the US NLEA regulations. Food industries may now apply for the approval to AVA or HPB to market functional foods with the listed health claims. Eligible food products must first be pre-screened by HPB and qualified to carry the Healthier Choice Symbol before the health claim

Table 5.3 Classes of food components approved for use in functional foods in Indonesia*

Class	Food component	Class	Food component
I	Vitamin	IX	Probiotics
II	Mineral	X	Choline, lecithin, inositol
III	Sugar alcohols	XI	Carnitine, squalene
IV	Unsaturated fatty acids	XII	Isoflavones (soy)
V	Peptides and proteins	XIII	Phytosterols, phytostanols
VI	Amino acids	XIV	Polyphenols (tea)
VII	Dietary fibre	XV	Others to be determined later
VIII	Prebiotics		

* Modified from HK 00.05.52.0685 (2005).

approval is granted. All functional foods for the Singapore market are required to meet provisions, standards, and labelling specifications of the Singapore Food Regulations (1988). To continue evaluating new health claims, in August 2009, the government of Singapore established the Advisory Committee on the Evaluation of Health Claims. The committee is composed of scientific experts from the government, universities, consumer and industry associations. It is challenged by AVA to establish a framework for evaluation of other health claims based on Codex Alimentarius recommendations. By the end of 2009, the Committee approved the first claim that links consumption of plant sterol-containing foods with the reduction of blood cholesterol as a risk factor in the development of coronary heart disease. This claim can be used on selected functional foods such as vegetable fat spreads, salad dressing, mayonnaise and low fat dairy products (AVA, 2010). Food categories and labelling requirements are similar to the EU novel foods regulations (EC 333, 2004) while a health claim related to the effect of sterols on blood cholesterol, and health claim wording are in line with the EU approved claim (EC 983, 2009; EC 384, 2010). The regulatory authorities have already approved phytosterol-containing foods such as fat spreads and milk-type products for sale in Singapore (Zawistowski, 2008).

5.4.5   Role of Codex Alimentarius

Codex Alimentarius is neither a regulatory authority nor does it have any enforcement power to implement legislation within member countries. However, Codex standards, guidelines and definitions are used by many countries to create their own legislation. This is particularly true for Asian countries that can not financially afford to develop their own regulations. Another benefit of adopting codex food standards is the international uniformity that can lead to harmonization of regulations within Asian. This is in line with Codex objectives to establish internationally agreed upon food policies 'for national food control systems based on the criteria of consumer health protection and fair practices in trade and taking into account the needs and special concerns of all countries' (Codex, 2008). Since Codex play an important role in forming regulations in Asia, most countries of the region actively participate in Codex meeting and setting food standards which can be later adopted for they own benefits. Some Asian countries closely follow Codex development in the area of functional foods and health claims. The Philippines adopted the Codex definition of functional foods. Thailand has established nutrient content claims, comparative claims and nutrient function claims based on the Codex guidelines (Kongchuntuk, 2000). Malaysia, a member of Codex since 1971, is in the process of consolidating health claims and establishing conditions that require making these claims along with the Codex guidelines (Tee *et al.*, 2002). The newly instituted advisory committee to the Singapore AVA is examining scientific substantiation for health claims based on Codex recommendations. The committee is also making recommendations to the government for adopting function claims as defined by Codex (AVA, 2010). Some of the functional foods that have been approved for the Asian market such as sterol-containing foods must meet the specifications established by the Codex Joint Expert Committee on Food Additives (JECFA, 2008).

5.5   Nutrition and health claims

Functional foods have existed on the Asian market for over two decades. They are providing consumers with a potential means to improve their wellbeing and health benefits to reduce risk of some chronic diseases. Since these types of products are associated with health claims, the regulations of claims are important to consumers, manufacturers and governmental authorities. Moreover, the established regulatory frameworks, in respect to the approval of health claims, protect consumers from false labelling information. This system creates also fair competition within the food industry and encourages innovation in the marketing of new products with health benefits.

Most Asian countries use the term 'health claim' as defined by Codex Alimentarius: 'Health claim means any representation that states, suggests or implies that a relationship exists between a food or a constituent of that food and health' (Codex, 2004). The majority of countries allow nutrition content (nutrition) claims on foods; however, only a few such as Japan, China, Indonesia, Philippines, Singapore and Malaysia permit to use health claims. Nutrition content and health claims are governed by country's food labelling regulations and applied to selected prepackaged foods, either in labelling or in advertising. The regulations stipulate conditions of use and food categories that claims can be used on.

5.5.1   Nutrient content and comparative claims

Nutrient content and comparative claims are permitted on foods in most Asian countries (Table 5.4). Claim components such as energy, fat, saturated fat, cholesterol, sugars, sodium, dietary fibre, vitamins and minerals are generally based on the Codex's recommendations. There are basically two types of nutrient content claims; the first being a negative claim that allows a food to carry 'low', 'free' or 'non-addition' statements in respect to certain health-adverse food constituents, such as cholesterol, sodium, saturated fat or trans fat. An example of such a claim is the 'cholesterol free' statement listed on foods. The second type of claims are considered positive claims that allow label statements such as 'good/excellent source', 'high', 'enriched', 'fortified' in food constituents that are beneficial to health (Tee, 2000). Although descriptors are similar to those of the Codex (Codex, 2004), conditions for using those claims vary from country to country. For example, nutrient reference values (NRVs) for protein, vitamins and minerals are based on a country's specific recommendations (Tee, 2009). To make a claim 'a source of vitamin C' in Japan, Indonesia, and South Korea, solid food must contain not less than 15% of the NRV value. However, to make the same claim in Singapore, a product should contain at least one-sixth of the daily allowance as specified by the Singapore Food Regulations (AVA, 2010).

Table 5.4 Nutritient content and comparative claims in selected Asian countries*

Country	Nutrient content claims	Comparative claims	Format	Criteria
Japan	Yes	–	Codex	Different criteria
China	Yes	Yes	Codex	Codex
South Korea	Yes	Yes	Codex	Codex
Indonesia	Yes	Yes	Codex	Different criteria
Singapore	Yes	Yes	Codex	Different criteria
Thailand	Yes	Yes	Codex	Different criteria
Malaysia	Yes	Yes	Codex	Codex
Hong Kong	Yes	Yes	Codex	Different criteria
Philippines	Yes	Yes	Codex	Different criteria

* Adapted partially from Tee (2009).

5.5.2 Nutrient function claims

A nutrient function claim is a nutrition claim that describes the physiological role of the nutrient in growth, development and normal functions of the body (Codex, 2004). The claim refers specifically to the function of a nutrient. Some examples of nutrient function claims are 'calcium is an important component in the development of healthy bones and teeth', 'folate is an important component in red cell formation' and 'protein helps build and repair body tissues'. In order to make these types of claim, the specific nutrient must be present in foods in certain quantities. Claims related to protein, fat, essential fatty acids, energy, carbohydrates, vitamins and minerals are widely permitted on foods by Asian countries.

In China, there are currently 60 authorized nutrient function claims for macronutrients, minerals and vitamins (Tee, 2009). Since April 1, 2001, the Japanese Ministry of Health, Labour and Welfare have permitted 12 claims in this category for vitamins, β-carotene and five for minerals. The minimum and maximum daily doses for each nutrient were also established (Ohama et al., 2008).

In current Malaysian regulations, 23 claims are permitted (GAIN, 2006; Tee, 2009). These claims are similar to the Canadian biological role claim nutrients. However, in contrast to Canadian regulations, Malaysian claims are allowed for foods that already contain bioactives such as probiotics, prebiotics, and cholesterol-lowering ingredients (Zawistowski, 2008).

Thai regulations stipulate 29 claims and conditions for the use of protein, dietary fibre, vitamins and minerals (Tee, 2009). These claims and conditions are similar to those in the Codex guidelines.

Singapore authorities have published a list of acceptable nutrient function claims for foods. This list include 37 claims for protein, lactose, dietary fibre, vitamins, minerals and other food constituents such as collagen, probiotics and prebiotics. Interestingly, there is more than one claim for some nutrients. For example, there are four folate claims on foods for pregnant women. Singapore authorities have approved five nutrient function claims on foods for infants and children below six years old. These claims link the role of choline, docosahexaenoic (DHA) and arachidonic (ARA) acids, nucleotides, taurine and zinc to the mental and physical development of children (AVA, 2010).

The South Korean Health/Functional Food Act posted 13 vitamins and 11 minerals among 37 generic functional food products. Nutrient function claims can be made on foods containing these vitamins and minerals only if they have their own recommended daily allowance (RDA). Food products must contain at least 30% of RDA of eligible nutrients to qualify for claims (Kim *et al.*, 2005). Fifteen nutrient function claims are permitted in Indonesia (Tee, 2009). Claims such as 'fibre helps to improve digestion', 'iron is a factor in red blood cell formation' are acceptable, while claims such as 'omega 3 develops the brain cells and intelligence' or 'iron prevents anaemia' are not (GAIN, 2006). Although the Philippines do not have a specific list of approved claims, the country's regulatory body allows nutrient functional claims according to the Codex (Tee, 2009).

5.5.3   Enhanced function claims

In contrast to the nutrient function claims, where a claim refers to food nutrients, enhanced function claims (named by Codex as 'other function claims') link a food constituent to the maintenance and improvement of human health. According to the Codex Alimentarius, other function claims provide 'specific beneficial effects of the consumption of foods or their constituents, in the context of the total diet on normal functions or biological activities of the body. Such claims relate to a positive contribution to health or to the improvement of a function or to modifying or preserving health' (Codex, 2004). Enhanced function claims are used in Asia according to the Codex to differentiate a stronger category of claims than nutrient function claims, but softer than disease risk reduction claims. This definition is similar to a definition of structure/function claims that are used on foods in the US (FDA, 2003). The Chinese claim 'improves bone density', is in line with the US structure/function claim 'calcium helps build strong bones'.

In China, 27 function claims are approved by the Ministry of Health (2003) for use on health (functional) foods (Table 5.2). Claims only may be used on foods that are pre-approved by the State Food and Drug Administration (SFDA), not harmful for human health, and do not claim the 'therapeutic effect' (Reynolds, 1999). In order to obtain approval, health claims must be supported by human clinical studies, animal data or both (Table 5.2). Testing of the products must be conducted by SFDA qualified laboratories. Eligible products may only be certified for a maximum two functions. In the Chinese market one can find the approved products with health claims such as: 'clinical experiment shows that it [tea] has a special function in regulating human blood sugar'; 'it [health tea] is capable of regulating men's blood lipids and [it is] suitable for the middle-aged, the old and the people suffering from hyperlipidaemia and adiposity'. It is worthwhile to note that function claims such as weight loss, blood pressure, lipids, and sugar control are considered by some regulatory experts as disease risk reduction claims (Yang, 2008). However, other experts seem to argue the merits of this approach (Tee, 2009).

Japanese FOSHU are the only category of functional foods that are qualified to carry health function claims in this country. There are eight groups of function claims on FOSHU (Table 5.5). These include gastrointestinal conditions, blood

Table 5.5 Approved FOSHU products and examples of health function claims*

Specified health uses	Examples of health claims	Principal ingredients (ingredients exhibiting health functions)
Foods to modify gastrointestinal conditions	Helps maintain good gastrointestinal condition. Helps improve bowel movement.	Oligosaccharides, lactose, *Bifidobacterium, Lactobacillus*, dietary fibre, ingestible dextrin, polydextrol, guar gum, psyllium
Foods related to blood cholesterol level	Good for those who have higher serum cholesterol.	Chitosan, soybean protein, degraded sodium alginate, dietary fibre, plant sterols/stanols
Foods related to blood sugar levels	Good for those who have mildly higher blood glucose.	Indigestible dextrin, wheat albumin, guava tea polyphenols, L-arabinose
Foods related to blood pressure	Good for those with high blood pressure.	Lactotripeptide, casein dodecapeptide, tochu leaf glycoside (geniposidic acid), sardine peptide
Foods related to dental hygiene	Helps maintain strong and healthy teeth.	Xylitol, polyols, paratinose, erythrytol, Ca-phosphate, tea polyphenols
Foods related to mineral absorption	Helps improve absorption of calcium. Good for those who have mild anaemia.	Calcium citrated malate, casein phosphopeptide, hem iron, fructooligosaccharides, soya isoflavones, polyglutamin acid, CPP (casein phosphopeptide), CCM (calcium citrate malate)
Foods related to osteogenesis	This product is suitable for those who are concerned about their bone health. Helps maintain calcium in bone.	Soy, MBP (milk basic protein), vitamin K2, fructooligosaccharides
Foods related to triacylglycerol/body fat	Good for those who have higher serum triglycerides. Helps prevent accumulation of body fat.	Middle chain fatty acid, diacylglycerides, EPA/DHA (eicosapentaenoic acid/ docosahexaenoic acid), tea catechins

* Modified from MHLW (2006).

pressure, serum cholesterol, blood glucose, blood lipids, dental hygiene, bone health, and absorption of minerals (MHLW, 2006). Since 2001, these claims are also allowed on FOSHU dietary supplements in addition to foods (Yamada *et al.*, 2008). In spite of the fact that FOSHU health claims are relatively soft, regulators require a cumbersome dossier containing data from double-blind, placebo-control, randomized clinical studies. For instance, for cholesterol-related claims, clinical trials must be conducted for more than 12 weeks on Japanese subjects with mild hypercholesterolaemia using a specific food product. Health claims must also be supported by the mechanism of action (Ohama *et al.*, 2008). With the de-regulation of FOSHU in 2005, some products are allowed to carry a qualified health function claim, which is not substantiated by scientific evidence needed for the standardized FOSHU (MHLW, 2006).

South Korea's enhanced function claims are compatible with those by the Codex Alimentarius. Generic functional foods and ingredients approved by HFFA, such as dietary fibre, green tea extract, fructooligosaccharides (FOS), EPA/DHA and others (Table 5.6) are eligible for health claims. Examples of claims include

Table 5.6 Generic health/functional foods and ingredients eligible for health claims in South Korea*

Nutritional supplement	Grape seed oil
Ginseng	Fermented vegetable-extract
Red ginseng	Mucopolysaccharide
Eel oil	Chlorophyll-containing product
EPA/DHA-containing product	Mushroom
Royal jelly	Aloe
Yeast	Japanese apricot extract
Pollen	Soft-shelled turtle
Squalene-containing product	Beta-carotene
Yeast-containing product	Chitosan-containing product
Probiotics-containing product	Chitooligosccharide-containing product
Chlorella	Glucosamine-containing product
Spirulina	Propolis extract
Gamma-linolenic acid-containing product	Green tea extract
Embryo bud oil	Soy protein-containing product
Embryo bud	Phytosterol-containing product
Lecithin	Fructooligosaccharide-containing product
Octacosanol-containing product	Red yeast rice product
Alcoxy-glycerol-containing product	

* Modified from Kim *et al.* (2005).

Table 5.7   Examples of enhanced (other) function claims allowed on foods in Malaysia*

Bioactive ingredient	Acceptable claims
Inulin	Helps increase intestinal bifidobacteria and helps maintain good intestinal environment. Inulin is bifidogenic.
Fructooligosaccharides	Helps increase intestinal bifidobacteria and helps maintain a good intestinal environment. Oligofructose (fructooligosaccharide) is bifidogenic.
Bifidobacterium	Helps increase the growth of intestinal biobacteria.
Beta-glucan from oat	Helps lower or reduce cholesterol.
Plant sterols/stanols	Helps lower or reduce cholesterol.
Soy protein	Helps to reduce cholesterol.

* Modified from Zawistowski (2008).

'maintaining good gastrointestinal conditions' for food with FOS or with dietary fibre (Kim *et al.*, 2005).

Malaysia allows 21 function claims on foods with ingredients such as inulin, FOS, gluco-oligosaccharides (GOS), FOS and GOS mixture, polydextrose, resistant starch, plant sterols and stanols, β-glucan, soya protein and probiotics. Examples of function claims are listed in Table 5.7.

5.5.4   Disease risk reduction claims

Disease risk reduction claims are statements that link a food or a food ingredient to reducing the risk of a particular chronic disease or its condition in the context of a total diet. The claim, food containing dietary fibre may reduce risk of coronary heart disease (CHD), links a food constituent (dietary fibre) to chronic disease (CHD) and shows the claimed benefits (risk reduction). In contrast, the claim, dietary fibre may reduce the plasma cholesterol level, links fibre to a factor that is associated with the conditions of CHD. In the latter case, the reduction of cholesterol is the claimed benefit that may be associated with the risk reduction of CHD. These kinds of claims are on an edge with drug claims and prohibited in some countries (e.g. Malaysia, Thailand, and China). Currently, there are several disease risk reduction claims permitted on foods in Singapore, Philippines, Japan and South Korea. These claims must be supported by totality of scientific evidence.

Newly established regulations in Singapore allow six claims related to osteoporosis, CHD, and cancer (AVA, 2010). Table 5.8 shows health claims, principal ingredients and conditions of use on food products. Five claims are

Table 5.8   Approved disease risk reduction claims on functional foods in Singapore*

Principal ingredient/ disease	Health claim	Conditions of use
Calcium and vitamin D – osteoporosis	A healthy diet with adequate calcium and vitamin D, with regular exercise, helps to achieve strong bones and may reduce the risk of osteoporosis. (*Name of food*) is a good source of/high in/ enriched in/fortified with calcium.	– The reference quantity of the product must contain at least 50% of calcium RDA (800 mg) – The product should also either be low in fat (≤3 g fat per 100 g or ≤1.5 g fat per 100 ml) or fat free (≤0.15 g fat per 100 g or 100 ml)
Sodium – stroke and heart disease	A healthy diet low in sodium may reduce the risk of high blood pressure, a risk factor for stroke and heart disease. (*Name of food*) is sodium free/low in/very low in/ reduced in sodium.	– Salt/sodium free (≤5 mg sodium per 100 g) – Very low in salt/sodium (≤40 mg per 100 g) – Low in sodium (≤120 mg per 100 g) – Reduced sodium (≤15% of sodium RDA (2 g) – The product should contain no added salt
Saturated fat and trans fat – heart disease	A healthy diet low in saturated fat and trans fat, may reduce the risk of heart disease. (*Name of food*) is free of/low in saturated fats, trans fats.	– Low in saturated fat (≤1.5 g saturated fat per 100 g, and ≤10% of kilocalories from saturated fat) – Free of saturated fat (≤0.5 g saturated fat per 100 g, and ≤1% of the total fat is trans fat, and is free of trans fat (<0.5 g per 100 g) – Product must be at least low in sugar (≤5 g per 100 g or ≤2.5 g per 100 ml), unsweetened and has no added sugar – Contains ≤100 mg per 100 g cholesterol (1/3 of cholesterol daily allowance) – Contains ≤25% of sodium RDA (2 g)
Dietary fibre – heart disease	A healthy diet rich in whole grains, fruits and vegetables that contain dietary fibre, may reduce the risk of heart disease. (*Name of food*) is low/free of fat and high in dietary fibre.	– Eligible food groups: whole grains, fruit, vegetables or fibre fortified foods – Low in fat or fat free – High in dietary fibre (≥3 g per 100 kcal or ≥6 g per 100 g or 100 ml) – Soluble fibre ≥25% of dietary fibre

Continued

Table 5.8   Continued

Principal ingredient/ disease	Health claim	Conditions of use
Dietary fibre – cancer	A healthy diet rich in fibre-containing foods such as whole grains, fruits and vegetables may reduce the risk of some types of cancers. (*Name of food*) is free/low in fat and high in dietary fibre.	– Eligible food groups: whole grains, fruit, vegetables or fibre fortified foods – Low in fat or fat free – High in dietary fibre ($\geq$3 g per 100 kcal or $\geq$6 g per 100 g or 100 ml) – Soluble fibre $\geq$25% of dietary fibre
Plant sterols and stanols – heart disease	Plant sterols/stanols have been shown to lower/reduce blood cholesterol. High blood cholesterol is a risk factor in the development of coronary heart disease.	– Eligible food groups: margarine-type spreads, mayonnaise, salad dressing, low fat dairy products, or special dietary food products approved by AVA – Sterols/stanols should meet specifications established by JECFA (2008) – Intake of >3 g sterols/stanols should be avoided

* Modified from AVA (2010).

similar to the US Food and Drug Administration (FDA) approved claims under the Nutrition Labelling and Education Act (NLEA) (CFR, 2002), while the plant sterols/stanols claim resembles a recently approved claim by the European Commission (OJ, 2009).

Eleven disease risk reduction claims were adopted from the US NLEA regulations (CFR, 2002) by Indonesian authorities and now are allowed for use on foods (Tee, 2009). Permitted claims are listed in Table 5.9. In addition, marketing food products for weight reduction in Indonesia may be permitted if the caloric value of food is at least 25% lower than its conventional counterpart (GAIN, 2009).

Philippines does not have a positive list with health claims, however this country authorized disease risk reduction claims according to the Codex Alimentarius (Tee, 2009). Currently, only two health claims are allowed in the Philippines: 'calcium and osteoporosis risk of reduction', and 'food low in fat and some type of cancer risk reduction'.

Under the ameliorated FOSHU regulations, two disease risk reduction claims have been approved by Japanese MHLW. These claims are for calcium linked with osteoporosis and folic acid as related to neural tube defect. The permitted health claims are listed below (MHLW, 2006; Ohama *et al.*, 2008):

• Calcium and osteoporosis – 'Intake of proper amount of calcium contained in

Table 5.9   Disease risk reduction claims on foods permitted in Indonesia*

1 Calcium and osteoporosis
2 Dietary fat and cancer
3 Dietary saturated fat and cholesterol and coronary heart disease (CHD)
4 Fibre-containing grain products, fruits and vegetables and cancer
5 Fruits, vegetables and grain products that contain fibre, particularly soluble fibre and risk of CHD
6 Sodium and hypertension
7 Fruits and vegetables and cancer of the digestive system
8 Folate and neural tube defect
9 Sugar alcohols do not increase dental caries
10 Soy protein and risk of CHD
11 Plant sterols and stanols and risk of CHD

* Modified from Tee (2009) and Zawistowski (2008).

> healthy meals with appropriate exercise may support healthy bones of young women and reduce the risk of osteoporosis when aged.' Eligible FOSHU products must provide 300–700 mg of calcium daily dose.
>
> • Folic acid and neural tube defect – 'Intake of proper amount of folic acid contained in healthy meals may support women to bear healthy baby by reducing the risk of neural tube defect, such as spondyloschisis, during fetal development.' Eligible FOSHU products should provide 400–1000 μg of folate daily dose.

Some of health functional foods in Korea listed in Table 5.6 are qualified by the Korean Food and Drug administration to bear disease risk reduction claims. Among these are phytosterols, red yeast rice, and soy protein, all associated with the risk reduction of CHD (Kim *et al.*, 2005).

5.5.5   Maintenance claims

Maintenance claims are unique to Taiwan. These types of claims depict foods with 'specific health care abilities' in regards to improve health and/or reduce the risk of disease (HFCA, 2006). Clearly, some of these claims can be also classified as disease reduction claims. The Health Food Control Act permits seven maintenance claims on health foods:

• Regulating blood lipids.
• Regulating the gastrointestinal tract.
• Regulating the immune system.
• Preventing osteoporosis.
• Maintaining dental health.

- Regulating blood sugar.
- Protecting the liver from chemical damage.

The health claim can be made for foods if it is supported by scientific assessments and approved by the Department of Health. The authorized health claims describe a type of health maintenance that foods may provide in a relationship to disease or health-related conditions. In contrast to the USA, Codex and EU regulations, the HFCA does not permit a link between a food bioactive ingredient and a disease. For instance, a recently approved sterol-containing milk drink bears a label claim 'An animal study shows that consumption of this product may help lower blood total cholesterol'. The claim refers to drink and does not state that 'plant sterols have been shown to lower/reduce blood cholesterol' as in the approved claim in the EU (Zawistowski, 2008).

5.5.6   Forbidden claims

Similar to other countries, Asian jurisdictions prohibit claims on functional foods to prevent, mitigate or cure specific diseases. Most of them, with the exception of Taiwan, also forbid claims related to the prevention of diseases. The latter is particularly challenging in conjunction with disease reduction claims, since consumers have difficulties to differentiate between the terms 'disease risk reduction' and 'prevention of diseases'. Some of countries such as Malaysia, Thailand and China deal with this issue by not allowing disease risk reduction claims on foods. However, most jurisdictions have promulgated law and regulations to protect consumers against drug-like claims, misleading claims and claims that can not be substantiated by scientific evidence.

In Japan, any reference to treatment, diagnosis, cure or prevention of human disease, any 'hint' for drug efficacy on a label of functional foods or in advertising is considered to be in violation of the Pharmaceutical Affairs Law (Ohama et al., 2008). Any function/health claims on foods 'must be relevant and substantiated by scientific evidence'. Under Japanese law any claims that are exaggerated and misleading are strictly prohibited (MHLW, 2010). Similarly, Singapore law prohibits 'the use of claims for therapeutic or prophylactic action; claims which could be interpreted as advice of a medical nature from any person; claims that a food will prevent, alleviate or cure any disease or condition affecting the human body; and claims that health or an improved physical condition may be achieved by consuming any food' (AVA, 2010).

The Indonesian Consumer Protection Act contains a provision against misleading claims on foods such as drug claims. It also prohibits claiming enhancement of vitality and improvement of intelligence. The claims 'food with natural fibre content helps improve health and vitality'; 'food for kids and babies with DHA content helps improve brain cells and intelligence'; 'Soy sauce helps to improve IQ' are examples of unacceptable claims (GAIN, 2009).

Malaysian Regulations of the Food Act prohibits the description of any foods, which includes the word 'compounded', 'medicated', 'tonic', 'health' or other descriptions which refer primarily to drugs. The Act also has provisions that prohibit label claims, 'as to the suitability of a food for use in the prevention, alleviation treatment or cure of a disease, disorder, or particular physical condition unless they are permitted in this regulation', and 'which could give rise to doubt the safety of a similar food, or which could arouse or exploit fear in the consumer' (Tee, 2000).

5.6   Labelling of functional foods

Functional foods that are approved for marketing must be labelled according to the standards promulgated under the labelling regulations for conventional foods. In general, labelling information requires the inclusion of the product name, list of ingredients, net content, production date (or best before date), and name and address of the manufacturer or the importer. If a country allows function/health claims, the labeling regulations reflect a claim statement and nutritional information. For imported foods, country of origin should be indicated on the label. The claim wording that is used on a label or in advertising must be approved by the appropriate regulatory authorities. Although there are no mandatory requirements for nutrition labelling of conventional foods in most of the Asian countries, the majority of them enforce nutritional information on foods with nutrition and health claims.

In Thailand, nutrition labelling is mandatory for foods with claims, regardless of whether a food product bears a nutrient function claim or a health claim (MPH, 1988). This policy is also enforced in Indonesia and specific requirements for the labelling of foods with claims are promulgated by the Indonesia Department of Health (PP 69, 2004).

In Japan, nutrition labelling is voluntary for all foods except foods with claims. Nutrition labelling includes declaration of energy value and nutrients in accordance with Nutrition Labelling Standards. Nutrients covered in the standards are protein, fat, carbohydrate, sodium, minerals, and vitamins (MHLW, 2010).

Although in China nutrition labelling is voluntary, it is used *de facto* on packaged foods sold in the domestic market. Currently, Chinese authorities have published a draft which standardizes nutrition labelling to ensure quality of food and to protect consumer health. The core nutrition panel must include four nutrients: energy, protein, fat and carbohydrates expressed per 100 g of 100 ml and/or serving size. Food manufacturers have options to use an extensive food nutrition label which additionally includes cholesterol, sugar, dietary fibre, vitamins and minerals (GAIN, 2008).

In Singapore, mandatory nutrition labelling is required for foods with nutrition claims, vitamin claims, mineral claims and approved health claims. The food regulations (AVA, 2010) require the placement of a nutrition information panel on the label. The panel must include the serving size as well as a list of a core of four nutrients per serving size and per 100 g or 100 ml (AVA, 2010; MHS, 1998).

Functional foods, that are approved as health foods in Taiwan, must be labelled according to the standards promulgated under regulations for food labelling in the Food Administration Act (FAA, 2007) and the Health Food Control Act (HFCA, 2006). The FAA regulations apply to conventional foods sold on the Taiwanese market, while HFCA describes specific instructions for health foods.

Malaysia enacted regulations on nutrition labelling in 2005 and made them mandatory for foods with nutrient content, comparative and nutrient function claims (Tee, 2007). Specific requirements for nutrition labelling in Indonesia are outlined in the food regulations prepared by Department of Health (PP 69, 2004), while the labelling standards for health/functional foods in South Korea are promulgated in the Health Functional Food Act (Kim, 2004).

Most jurisdictions also require specific information regarding functional foods, in addition to general labelling standards. This may include:

- A name of functional foods that is approved by the regulatory authorities.
- A statement about the efficacy claim, using wording that is approved by the regulatory body.
- Serving size and amount of bioactive ingredient intake per serving size.
- Directions of use.
- Warnings and disclaimers that the product does not prevent, cure or mitigate disease.
- Nutrition information, even if nutrition labelling is not required for its conventional food counterpart.
- Reference number of the permit, as required by some countries (e.g. Taiwan).
- Additional information as required by the labelling standards for functional foods in each country.

Moreover, countries such as Japan, China, Taiwan and South Korea required a seal of approval (logo) placed on a label on functional food products once product dossiers are reviewed and products are approved for marketing (Fig. 5.2).

5.7   Health claims and consumer confidence

Health claims on functional foods provide a message from the industry to consumers concerning product effects. If the health claim is recognized and approved by the regulatory body, it makes this message reliable and trustworthy. In a recent survey ($n = 1000$) conducted by Strei and Kapsak (2007) on consumer attitudes toward functional foods, it was observed that a food label is a significant source of information to the consumer. Furthermore, a source of a claim is also of importance, and most consumers gain confidence in a product if health claims are approved by the highest regulatory authorities (Cranfield, 2010). Many modern consumers recognize true value in food products with health claims proven by scientific studies.

A well-defined regulatory framework that protects public health is of paramount importance. As has been mentioned before, Japan is one of the Asian countries that has a strict policy regarding the substantiation of functional foods (FOSHU).

Regulators require that FOSHU efficacy must be supported by the double-blind, placebo-controlled randomized clinical studies conducted on Japanese subjects in addition to elucidation of the mechanism of action. This has been criticized by some experts, who believed that there are no needs for drug-type studies in the support of food products (Bailey, 2005). Nevertheless, the rigid regulations and their enforcement provide confidence in FOSHU to Japanese consumers. Unfortunately, this is not always true in respect to other Asian countries. A survey conducted by the China Consumer Association and China Health Science and Technology Institute on health food advertisements, indicated that 73.5% of advertisements and promotional materials are not in line with law and regulations. About 42% of advertisements depicted false information, while 31% declared health functions without prior approval from the Ministry of Health. The same survey shows that consumer's trust for health product advertisements has significantly decreased over the years and the efficacy of functional foods is being questioned (CN Foods, 2002). In some Asian countries, functional foods promoting health are often based on testimonials rather than scientific evidence. In addition, dishonest marketers advertise products using misleading information.

Over the last decade, many countries in Asia have introduced, and are still in the process of refining, a regulatory framework to protect consumers from misleading claims and false labelling. Other countries such Thailand, Indonesia, Myanmar, Singapore, and Vietnam, recognize the importance of functional foods, but have no specific regulations for such foods (Tee, 2003).

Asian governmental institutions and non-governmental organizations (NGO), through meetings, workshops and conferences, are trying to address the needs for scientific support of functional foods in Asia. This is challenging, but important that health claims are supported by science-based evidence from well designed human clinical studies. Scientifically sound functional foods will most likely gain the confidence of consumers. These issues were a major subject of the Asia-Pacific Economic Cooperation (APEC) meeting in Auckland (APEC, 1999); the Association of Southeast Asian Nations (ASEAN) meeting in Bangkok (Valyasevi, 2004); the 2nd International Conference on East-West Perspectives on Functional Foods: Science, Innovations and Claims in Kuala Lumpur (Florentino, 2008); and the recent conference on food innovation in Bangkok (FIF, 2009). Moreover, the International Life Sciences Institute (ILSI), and its Asian branch have significantly contributed to improving the regulatory situation in the region. ILSI, a Non-Governmental Organization (NGO) that is affiliated with the World Health Organization (WHO) and Food and Agriculture Organization (FAO), is well respected in Asia. Through a series of initiatives such as international meetings, consultations and workshops, ILSI SEA (South-East Asia) has published Guidelines for Scientific Substantiation of Nutrition and Health Claims, and the Proposed Regulatory Framework for Nutrition Labelling and Claims (Binns, 2009). The guidelines focus on key characteristics of functional foods, as well as the major issues for future activities in the region such as criteria for the assessment of health claims, development of biomarkers, research design and methodology that is essential for the study of such foods. In addition, ILSI provides guidelines for the evaluation of safety of functional foods as well as regulatory framework for harmonization of claims (Binns, 2009). The established guidelines can be a significant reference to regulatory agencies in the region for developing and refining national frameworks.

5.8   Future trends: harmonization of law and regulations of functional foods

Asia is endowed with natural products that have been historically used for health benefits. China, India and other countries are the World's biggest provider of potential ingredients for functional foods. Therefore, Asian countries recognize economic opportunities for the functional food market within the region, but they are also aware about significant challenges associated with the regulations of such foods.

The landscape of global regulations in Asia has changed since the introduction of the functional food concept in Japan. Following the Japanese example, China, South Korea, and Taiwan introduced law and regulations to fit specific needs for their countries. Other Asian jurisdictions: Thailand, Indonesia, Malaysia, Philippines, Singapore, and Hong Kong adopted and follow the guidelines of Codex Alimentarius, EU and USA regulations or the food and drug regulations of their own countries. However, there are more differences than similarities in the regulatory approaches among countries of the Asian region. Functional foods have a different meaning in various countries; as foods (e.g. Singapore, Indonesia), dietary supplements in medicinal format (e.g. China), or food–drug interface products (e.g. Malaysia). Differences exist within the approval process and allowed health claims. Disease risk reduction claims are allowed in some countries (Japan, Philippines, and Indonesia), prohibited in others (Malaysia) or are still under review in some other countries.

There is no doubt that harmonization of the regulatory system for manufacturing, approval and sale of functional foods in Asia is a key element of the trading relationships between countries. Fortunately, governmental policy makers and NGO organizations pay attention to global harmonization and collaboration within the region. Recently, the ASEAN proposed a plan of action in regards to science and technology for 2007–2011 that envisions R&D collaboration on functional ingredients between South East Asian countries, Japan and China. Collaborative research involves product development, safety assessment and clinical trials (Valyasevi, 2004). The harmonization of regulations within the region continues to be a major focus of a number of consultation meetings and workshops organized by ILSI Asia during the last decade. As a result of these meetings, a National Expert Committee on Nutrition and Health Claims has been established. The primary focus of the committee is to found a harmonized regulatory framework for functional foods, function claims, health claims, labelling and the approval process. Although ILSI has acknowledged that a lack of harmonization within the region is due to differences 'in philosophy about the role of functional foods and the tensions that exist worldwide between scientific progress and consumer protection', the organization remains optimistic about the harmonization of the scientific substantiation of health claims on functional foods (Binns, 2009).

5.9   Sources of further information and governmental websites

China

- State Food and Drug Administration http://eng.sfda.gov.cn/eng/
- Ministry of Health http://www.moh.gov.cn/publicfiles/business/htmlfiles/wsb/index.htm
- General Administration of Quality Supervision, Inspection and Quarantine of P.R.C. http://english.aqsiq.gov.cn/LawsandRegulations/allenglish/200709/t20070905_38073.htm

Hong Kong

- Hong Kong Special Administrative Region Government http://webstat.cis.gov.hk/webstat/
- Food and Health Bureau http://www.fhb.gov.hk/en/index.html
- Centre for Food Safety http://www.cfs.gov.hk/eindex.html

India

- Health Foods and Dietary Supplements Association http://www.hadsa.com/
- Ministry of Consumers Affairs, Food and Public Distribution – Department of Food and Public Distribution http://www.fcamin.nic.in/dfpd_html/index.asp
- Ministry of Health and Family Welfare http://www.mohfw.nic.in/
- Food Safety India http://foodsafetyindia.nic.in/relevantlinks.htm
- International Law Book Company http://supremecourtcaselaw.com/FS-E.htm

Indonesia

- The National Agency of Drug and Food Control (Badanpom Badan Pengawas Obat dan Makanan) http://www.pom.go.id/e_default.asp

Japan

- Ministry of Health, Labour and Welfare – Food Safety http://www.mhlw.go.jp/english/topics/foodsafety/index.html
- FOSHU http://www.mhlw.go.jp/english/topics/foodsafety/fhc/02.html
- Japan Health, Food and Nutrition Food Association http://www.jhnfa.org/
- Ministry of Agriculture, Forestry and Fisheries http://www.maff.go.jp/e/index.html

Korea

- Korea Food and Drug Administration http://eng.kfda.go.kr
- Ministry of Food, Agriculture, Forestry and Fisheries http://english.mifaff.go.kr/main.tdf

Malaysia

- National Pharmaceutical Control Bureau (Biro Pengawalan Farmaseutikal Kebangsaan) http://portal.bpfk.gov.my/
- Legislation Malaysia http://www.lexadin.nl/wlg/legis/nofr/oeur/lxwemal.htm
- Ministry of Health http://www.moh.gov.my/

Singapore

- Agri-Food & Veterinary Authority of Singapore http://www.ava.gov.sg/FoodSector/FoodLabelingAdvertisement/
- Ministry of Health http://www.sgdi.gov.sg/

Taiwan

- Executive Yuan Republic of China (Taiwan) http://www.ey.gov.tw/mp?mp=11
- Department of Health http://www.doh.gov.tw/EN2006/index_EN.aspx

5.10   Acknowledgements

This chapter is dedicated to my children: Dorota, Robert and Isabela. I would like to thank my son Robert for inciting discussion and proofreading of the manuscript.

5.11   References

Act 368 (1989), 'Sale of drugs act 1952', enacted by Ord No. 28 of 1952, revised 1 July 1989, with latest amendment (Act A1084/2000), 1 November 1952, L.N. 536/1952; Sabah and Sarawak – 1 September 1999, P.U. (A) 380/1992; Federal Territory of Labuan – 1 September 1989, P.U. (A) 381/1992, Malaysia. Available from: http://www.pharmacy.gov.my/aeimages//File/Sales_of_Drug_Act_1952_Act_368.pdf, accessed 4 May 2010.

Act No. 34 of 2006 (2009), 'Genetically modified foods, organic foods, functional foods, proprietary foods', in *Food Safety and Standards Act, 2006 with Comments, Shortnotes and Important Gazette Notifications*, sec 22, subsec 1, 3rd edition, Delhi, India, International Law Book Company, 37–38.

APEC (1999), 'The Auckland challenge. APEC principles to enhance competition and regulatory reform', Asia-Pacific Economic Cooperation (APEC) Meeting, Auckland, New Zealand, 13 September 1999.

Arai S (1996), 'Studies of functional foods in Japan – state of the art', *Biosci Biotechnol Biochem*, **60**, 9–15.

Arai S (2002), 'Global view on functional foods: Asian perspectives', *Br J Nutr*, **88**, S139–S143.

Arai S, Yasuoka A and Abe K (2008), 'Functional food science and food for specified health use policy in Japan: state of the art', *Curr Opin Lipidol*, **19**, 69–73.

Arvantitoyannis I S and Van Houwelingen-Koukaliaroglou M (2005) 'Functional foods: a survey of health claims, pros and cons, and current legislation', *Crit Rev Food Sci Nutr*, **45**, 385–404.

Asp NG (2005), 'Rationale and scientific support for health claims on foods', *Suppl Am J Clin Nutr*, **18**, 98–101.

AVA (2010), 'A guide to food labelling and advertisements', Agri-Food & Veterinary Authority, Singapore, February 2010, pp. 1–38. Available from: http://www.ava.gov.sg/FoodSector/FoodLabelingAdvertisement/, accessed 22 May 2010.

Bailey R (2004), 'Dietary supplements, nutraceuticals, functional foods: the Japanese market', *Nutraceuticals World*, **6**, 52–55.

Bailey R (2005), 'Functional foods in Japan: FOSHU (Foods for specified health uses) and foods with nutrient function claims', in Hasler CM, *Regulation of Functional Foods and Nutraceuticals: A global perspective*, Ames, IA: Blackwell Publishing, 247–261.

Binns N (2009), 'Perspectives on ILSI's international activities on functional foods', *International Life Sciences Institute, Report of ILSI Europe Functional Foods Task Force*, May 2009, 1–57.

Bogor Agricultural University (2003), 'Country Investment Plan for Food Fortification in Indonesia' *Report*, National Fortification Commission, Jakarta, Indonesia.

Canadian Food Inspection Agency (2007), 'Guide to food labelling and advertising', *Health claims*, Chapter 8. Available from: http://www.inspection.gc.ca/english/fssa/ labeti/guide/ch8e.shtml, accessed 5 May 2010.

CFR (2002), 'Health Claims', *Code of Federal Regulations, Food and Drugs*, **21**(2), Chap I, Part 101, Food Labeling, §101.71–101.83, 124–149.

Charoenpong C and Nitithamyong A (2004). 'Review of country status on functional foods: Thailand, Report of the regional expert consultation of the Asia-Pacific network for food and nutrition on functional foods and their implications in the daily diet', FAO Corporate Document Repository, RAP Publication 2004/33.

Chay Y (2005), 'Nutritional supplements', International Natural and Health Products Expo-2005, Seoul, Korea.

CN Foods (2002), 'Market research report on Chinese health products', China Health Food Network Hotline, Nanchang, China, available from: http://www.cnfoods.org/, accessed 15 January 2008.

Codex (2004), 'Guidelines for the Use of Nutrition and Health Claims', *CAC/GL 23–1997 (Rev 1–2004)*, 1–5.

Codex (2008), 'Procedural manual', *Codex Alimentarius Commission*, Joint FAO/WHO Food Standards Programme, 16th Edition, 1–173.

Cranfield J (2010), 'Public perception of values of plant sterols in foods', 101st American Oil Chemical Society Meeting and Expo, Phoenix, AZ, USA, 16–19 May 2010.

Datamonitor (2008), 'Japanese product innovation series market report: FOSHU market', *Research and Markets*, Dublin, Ireland, 1–17.

Doyon M and Labrecque J A (2005), 'Functional foods: a conceptual definition', *Cahier de Recherché HEC Montreal*, 05–09, 1–17.

EC 333 (2004), 'Commission Regulations, EC No 333/2004', *Official J EU* L 105/40, 14 April 2004.

EC 983 (2009), 'Commission Regulations, EC No. 983/2009', *Official J EU* L 277/3, 22 October 2009.

EC 384 (2010), 'Commission Regulations, EC No. 384/2010', *Official J EU* L 113/6, 5 May, 2010.

FDA (2003), 'Claims that can be made for conventional foods and dietary supplements', available from: http://www.fda.gov/Food/LabelingNutrition/LabelClaims/ucm111447. htm, accessed 27 May 2010.

FAA (2007), 'Food Administration Act', Council of Agriculture, Executive Yuan, R.O.C. Taiwan.

FIF (2009), 'Food in the future', InnovAsia 2009 Conference and Exhibition, National Innovation Agency, 17–19 December 2009, Bangkok, Thailand.

Florentino RF (2008), 'The 2nd International Conference on East–West perspectives on functional foods: science, innovations and claims. Special report', *Asia Pac J Clin Nutr* **17**(3), 540–543.

Ford K, Konishi Y, Rajalahti R and Pehu E (2007), 'Health enhancing foods: country case studies of China and India', *Agriculture and Rural Development Discussion Paper 32*. Washington, DC: The World Bank.

FSSAI (2009), 'Food safety and standards regulations, 2009', Food Safety and Standards Authority of India. Available from: http://www.indiaenvironmentportal.org.in/files/ FSSAI%20regulations.pdf, accessed 9 May 2010.

Furukawa T (1993), 'The nutraceutical rules: health and medical claims. Food for specified health use in Japan', *Regulatory Affairs*, **5**, 189–192.

GAIN (2005), 'Food and Agricultural Imports Regulations and Standards Report (FAIRS) Republic of Korea', Global Agriculture Information Network (GAIN) Report Number KS5037', USDA Foreign Agriculture Service, 1–46.

GAIN (2006), 'Indonesia Food and Agricultural Import Regulations and Standards, Country Report', Global Agriculture Information Network (GAIN) Report Number ID6020, USDA Foreign Agriculture Service, 1–22.

GAIN (2008), 'People Republic of China, FAIRS subject report, China notifies draft nutrition labelling regulation 2007', Global Agriculture Information Network (GAIN) Report Number CH8004, USDA Foreign Agriculture Service, 1–20.

GAIN (2009), 'Indonesia Food and Agricultural Import Regulations and Standards – Narrative, FAIRS Country Report', Global Agriculture Information Network (GAIN) Report Number ID9020, USDA Foreign Agriculture Service, 1–29.

Government Regulation of the Republic of Indonesia on Food Safety, Quality and Nutrition (2004), Number 28 Tahun, p. 80. Available from: http://www.pom.go.id/public/hukum_perundangan/pdf/PP28-_in%20English_a.pdf, accessed 5 May 2010.

HFCA (2006), 'Health Food Control Act', Promulgated on 3 February 1999; amended and promulgated on 8 November 2000; amended and promulgated on 30 January 2002, with amended articles of 2, 3, 14, 15, 24 and 28 pursuant to the President's Order Hua Zong Yi Zi No. 09500069821 promulgated on 17 May 2006, Department of Health, Executive Yuan. Taipei, Taiwan.

HK 00.05.52.0685 (2005), 'Basic provisions on functional food supervision', Food and Drug Supervisory Board Republic of Indonesia, Jakarta, Indonesia.

JECFA (2008), 'Phytosterols, phytostanols and their esters', Monograph 5, FAO Joint Expert Committee on Food Additives. Available from: http://www.fao.org/ag/agn/jecfa-additives/specs/monograph5/additive-509-m5.pdf, accessed 15 January 2009.

Kim J (2004), 'The Health Functional Food Act – A new regulatory framework in Korea', Assistant Director, Health Functional Food Division, Korea Food and Drug Administration, Seoul, Korea.

Kim JY, Dai BK and Hyong JL (2005), 'Regulations on health/functional foods in Korea', Nutrition and Functional Food Headquarters, Korea Food and Drug Administration, Seoul 122–704, South Korea, 30 December 2005.

Kongchuntuk H (2000), 'Thailand experience in nutrition labelling regulations and education', in Proceedings of the National Seminar on Nutrition Labelling: Regulations and Education, 7–8 August 2000; Kuala Lumpur 36–45.

Kurowska EM, Spence JD and Jordan J (2000), 'HDL-cholesterol-raising effect of orange juice in subjects with hypercholesterolemia', Am J Clin Nutr, 72, 1095–1100.

Law M (2004), 'Plant sterol and stanol margarines and health', Brit Med J, 320, 861–864.

Law of the People (59) (2005), The People's Republic of China Food Hygiene Law, Available from: http://www.moh.gov.cn/publicfiles/business/htmlfiles/mohzcfgs/s3576/200804/16488.htm, accessed 22 May 2010.

Liu J (2004), Chinese Foods, Beijing, China International Press.

MHLW (2006), 'Food for Specified Health Uses (FOSHU)' Japanese Ministry of Health, Labour and Welfare. Available from: http://www.mhlw.go.jp/english/topics/foodsafety/fhc/02.html, accessed 5 May 2010.

MHLW (2010), 'Food with health claims, food for special dietary uses, and nutrition labeling', Japanese Ministry of Health, Labour and Welfare. Avalilable from: http://www.mhlw.go.jp/english/topics/foodsafety/fhc/index.html, accessed 27 May 2010.

MHS (1998), 'Nutrition labelling: a handbook on the nutrition information panel', Department of Health, Ministry of Health Singapore.

Ministerial Ordinance (1991), The Nutrition Improvement Law Enforcement Regulations, Ministerial Ordinance No. 41, July 1991, Amendment to Ministerial Ordinance No. 33, 25 May 1996.

Ministry of Health China (2003), 'Notification for the adjustment of range of acceptance, examination and approval for the function of health food application', Ministry of Health China P.R., 2003 edition, 1 May 2003, Beijing, China.

Ministry of Health Malaysia (2007), 'Guide to Classification of Food-Drug Interface Products', Standards section food safety and quality division. Available from: http://fsq. moh.gov.my/info_en/Standard_Section2.pdf, accessed 5 May 2010.

MPH (1988). 'Nutrition Labeling', Notification Vol. 182, Ministry of Public Health Thailand, Bangkok, Thailand.

Nakagawa K (2004), 'The history of emergence of "Food for Specified Health Use" and its future prospects', Japan Functional Food Research Association. Healthy Interview. Available from: http://www.jafra.gr.jp/eng/nakagawa.html, accessed 15 December 2009.

Ohama H, Ikeda H and Mariyama H (2008), 'Health foods and foods with health claims in Japan', in Bagchi E, *Nutraceutical and Functional Food Regulations in the United States and Around the World*, Amsterdam, Academic Press, 249–280.

OJ (2009), 'Regulation (EC) No 983/2009 of the European Parliament and of the Council, Official Journal of the European Union L 277/3, 22.10.2009, 1–10.

Patel D, Dufour Y and Domigan N (2008), 'Functional food and nutraceutical registration process in Japan and China: similarities and differences', *J Pharm Pharmaceut Sc*, **11**, 1–11.

PFA (2004) 'The prevention of food adulturation act and rules', as on 01.10.2004. Rule 32A, p. 96. India. Available from: http://mohfw.nic.in/pfa%20acts%20and%20rules.pdf, accessed 12 March 2010.

PP 28 (2004), 'Government regulation of the Republic of Indonesia on food safety, quality and nutrition, Number 28/2004', State Secretariat of the Republic of Indonesia, Jakarta, Indonesia, 1–80.

PP 69 (2004), 'Government regulation of the Republic of Indonesia on food labelling and advertisement, Number 69/1999', Directorate General of Drug and Food Control, Jakarta, Indonesia. 1–31.

Reynolds S (1999), 'China, Peoples Republic of Food and Agricultural Import Regulations and Standards', *GAIN Report #CH9010*, Global Agriculture Information Network, USDA, 1–177.

Singapore Food Regulations (1988), 'Sale of Food Act – Food Regulations', Chapter 283, Section 56 (1), 1–111.

Strei J and Kapsak WR (2007), *Consumer Attitudes Toward Functional Foods/Foods for Health*, International Food Information Council, Washington, DC, USA

Tee ES (2000), 'Proposed new law on nutrition labelling and claims: what should you know? Health claims and advertisement', Nutrition Society of Malaysia, 1–9.

Tee ES (2003). 'Report of ILSI Southeast Asia Region Coordinated Survey of Functional Foods in Asia', ILSI Southeast Asia Region, Singapore.

Tee ES (2007), 'Claims and scientific substantiation: efforts in harmonizing in Asia', Conference on Functional Foods, Malta, May 2007.

Tee ES (2009), 'Nutrition labelling and health claims: Codex guidelines', 8th International Food Data Conference, 1–3 October 2009, Bangkok, Thailand.

Tee ES, Tamin S, Ilyas R, Ramos A, Tan WL, Lai DKS, and Kongchuntuk H (2002), 'Current status of nutritional labelling and claims in the South-East Asian region: are we in harmony?', *Asia Pacific J Clin Nutr*, **11**, S80–S86.

The Government of Hong Kong Special Administrative Region, Food and Environmental Hygiene Department (2006), 'Health and Functional Food'.

UU 7 (1996), 'Act of the Republic of Indonesia on food, Number 7 of 1996', House of People's Representatives of the Republic of Indonesia, Jakarta, Indonesia, 1–38.

Wang L (2002), *Chinese Tea Culture*, Beijing, Foreign Languages Press.

Williams M, Pehu E and Ragasa C (2006) 'Functional foods: opportunities and challenges for developing countries', Agriculture and Rural Development Note of the World Bank, 19, 1–4.

Wong E (2001), 'Regulation of health foods in overseas places: overall comparison', Research and Library Services Division Legislative Council Secretariat, 15 May 2001, Hong Kong.

Wu J (2001), *Regulation of Health Food in Hong Kong*. Hong Kong, Research and Library Services Division Legislative Council Secretariat.

Valyasevi R (2004), 'ASCFST activities on functional foods', Conference of the Association of Southeast Asian Nations Committee on Science and Technology (ASCFST), Bangkok, Thailand.

Xiu Z (2002), *Diseases Treated with Melons, Fruits and Vegetables*. Beijing, Foreign Languages Press.

Yamada K, Sato-Mito N, Nagata J and Umegaki K (2008), 'Health claim evidence requirements in Japan' *J Nutr*, **138**, 1192S–1198S.

Yamaguchi P (2003), 'FOSHU approval – is it worth the price?', NPI Center. Available from: http://www.npicenter.com/anm/templates/newsATemp.aspx, accessed 23 April 2010.

Yang Y (2008), 'Scientific substantiation of functional food health claims in China', *J Nutr*, **138**, 1199S–1205S.

Zawistowski J (2008), 'Regulation of functional foods in selected Asian countries in the Pacific Rim', in Bagchi E, *Nutraceutical and Functional Food Regulations in the United States and Around the World*, Amsterdam, Academic Press, 365–401.

Zawistowski J and Kitts D.D (2004), 'Functional foods – a new step in the evolution of food development', *Clin Nutr Rounds*, **4**, 1–6.

Zeng Q and Liu D (2008), *China's Traditional Way of Health Preservation*, Beijing, Foreign Languages Press.

Zhu L (2005), 'China update', *Squire Sanders*, Beijing, Legal Counsel Worldwide.

6

Consumers and health claims for functional foods

L. Lähteenmäki, Aarhus University, Denmark

Abstract: Consumer responses will determine how effective the health claims will be in promoting the food products in the future. This chapter reviews our current knowledge on factors that affect consumer acceptance and ability to understand health claims. Claim-, product- and consumer-related issues are discussed together with the implications they have for communicating the benefits to consumers.

Key words: health claim, consumer behaviour, food choice, perception of healthiness.

6.1   Introduction

6.1.1   What are health claims?

Health has been named as the most significant trend and innovation driver in the global food and drinks market (Meziane, 2007). Health claims typically promise specific improvements in physiological functions or reduced risks of diseases. In addition to health claims, various other product cues can signal healthiness to consumers, such as low-fat, light, nutritious, organic, natural, enriched and so on. All health-related quality cues are credence attributes that cannot be directly observed from the product and therefore need be conveyed to consumers with information (Grunert *et al.*, 2000). Health claims have thus to compete with other messages, including those with health connotations, in getting the attention of consumers.

Functional food is a commonly used term to describe a product that promises a claimed health-related benefit, and in this chapter the terms 'functional food' and 'food product with a health claim' are used as synonyms, although there is no official definition for the term functional food. One of the most mature functional food markets is Japan where legislation for 'food for specified health use' called FOSHU was established in 1993. In Japan, functional foods are regarded as food products that are eaten as part of an ordinary diet, although not all products that are marketed with health-related claims have been processed through the system and thus gained the official status of FOSHU-foods (Arai, 2002). In the USA the Nutrition Labeling and Education Act (NLEA, 1990) governs presentation of health and nutrition claims. In the European Community health claims were defined by legislation (Regulation (EC) 1924/2006) in 2006 and these rules are also followed by most non-member countries in Europe as well. The legislation states that health claims will be accepted in food products and supplements if they are based on substantiated scientific evidence. The strength of this evidence is assessed by the European Safety Authority (EFSA), and based on EFSA's advice the European Commission will make the decisions on approving claims. In this chapter the reference point in relation to consumer issues is mostly the European legislation.

6.1.2   The implications of regulations to the consumers

Having legislation that governs the use of health claims should be beneficial for the whole food value chain. If we think about the situation in the EU, the positive list of claims that are allowed means that all EU countries have the same rules for using health claims in food products and supplements. From the consumer point of view the EU legislation and approved list of claims should promote consumers' trust in health claims by several aspects. In Nordic countries the health and nutrition experts and authorities were clearly regarded as more trusted sources of information than commercial actors and media in relation to health claims (Fig. 6.1). Verification of the promised benefit from trusted impartial actors should promote consumers' confidence that all the claims used in the market are scientifically valid. The positive list provides authorities a possibility to take action if non-listed health claims are used in marketing. Since health claims are only allowed in products that comply with required nutritional profiles, the products carrying claims should also be nutritionally sound. Furthermore, the new legislation requires that claims should be understandable to an average consumer so that consumers will be able to utilise the benefits of the products as aimed by the manufacturer. However, the assessment of consumer understanding has remained undecided.

   In relation to health claims the term average consumer has created a lot of discussions among stakeholders. The legislation defines an average consumer as 'reasonably well-informed and reasonably observant and circumspect, taking into account social, cultural, and linguistic factors' (Regulation (EC) 1924/2006). This definition implies that the average consumer should be ready to process claim information actively, but the legislation also clearly states that possible vulnerable consumer groups should be taken into account when national authorities make their interpretations. Basically, the assumption is that consumers will make informed choices based on an elaborated decision-making process, but those consumers who may not, for one reason or other, be able to make these informed choices should be protected.

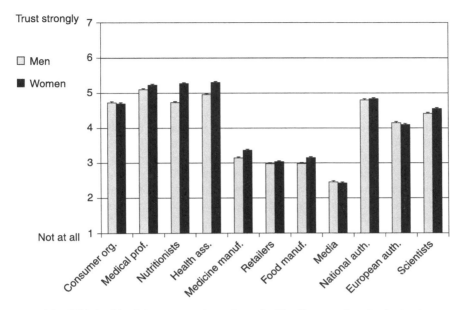

Fig. 6.1 With health claims, respondents from the Nordic countries clearly trust more information that comes from health professionals and consumer organisations than information coming from commercial sources. The authorities are almost as well trusted as health professionals, but there is a clear gap between national and European authorities (figure based on the same data as results reported by Grunert *et al.* (2009) and Lähteenmäki *et al.* (2010)).

6.1.3   Role of health claims in promoting health

Health claims offer a positive health message to the consumers, showing which products to favour in order to gain positive physiological effects on bodily functions or to achieve a reduced level of risk of diseases. The message that promises specific well-defined benefits from single products differs greatly from the advice on nutritionally healthy eating which emphasises the role of whole diet, not single products. The promised reward of following the nutritionally good diet is a higher probability of maintaining a good health status and lowering the risks of life style related diseases, but the reward is unsure and far away, and no direct benefits can be observed or sensed in most cases while pursuing the goal. Functional foods, on the other hand promise outcomes that can be achieved in a reasonably short time. Some effects, such as lowering blood cholesterol levels can be relatively easily measured, whereas others, e.g. improving the immune defence, are mostly based on trust on the promised effect. For many possible functions the problem is that there are no biomarkers that could be verified by consumers and used as indicators of the effects.

Health claims have caused some concerns among health professionals, consumer organisations and authorities. One issue has been whether consumers interpret health claims as a solution for healthy eating with no concern on other components of the diet. When Quaker Oats were testing how consumers understand health-related claims, those receiving an oatmeal or a fibre claim did not more often believe that one does not need to pay attention to the rest of the diet than those who received no claim in the package (Paul *et al.*, 1999). However, a Finnish study that measured indirectly consumers' impressions of buyers of functional foods with a shopping list method found that users of functional foods were perceived as more innovative and more disciplined than buyers of similar conventional products (Saher *et al.*, 2004). The latter was true only when the other food choices in the shopping list contained neutral items. Those shoppers who had a basic list of products with a high health image were rated as more disciplined regardless of their functional choices. Choosing functional foods thus required some discipline but less than buying conventionally healthy foods which suggests that functional foods are regarded as somewhat easier option than choosing healthy options in general.

In the following section (6.2) the consumer perception of health claims will be discussed in more detail. Health claims are linked to different products and the attitudes and acceptability of functional foods depend both on the claim, promised benefit and the carrier product. The factors influencing the acceptability of functional foods will be discussed in section 6.3. Section 6.4 draws together consumer issues in relation to dairy products and reflects on the factors that are especially important for the future success of functional dairy products among consumers, and section 6.5 considers the future perspectives of health claims in foods.

6.2   Consumer perceptions of health claims

6.2.1   Wording of the claim

The research on consumer perception of health claims has used different designs and research questions. The few systematic studies have revealed wide culture-dependent differences among countries depending on the type of benefit promised (van Trijp & van der Lans, 2007) or type of health-related message (Arvola *et al.*, 2007). In a Nordic study (Grunert *et al.*, 2009; Lähteenmäki *et al.*, 2010) the claims were dissected to different components in order to study the impact of claim wording systematically. In addition to splitting health claims in physiological function and risk reduction claims they can also be divided into different categories according to their structure, benefit, ingredient or compound providing the benefit and phrasing of the claim.

Claims can be basically constructed from three components: the active ingredient, effective function and health outcome (Fig. 6.2). When looking at the claim structure or architecture, a claim that consists of all three components contains an explanation of what the health claim is based on. When only ingredient, function or outcome are included in the claim there is less information to assess the credibility of the claim or what the health-related outcome may be. The studies on the consumer perception of claim information have resulted in somewhat

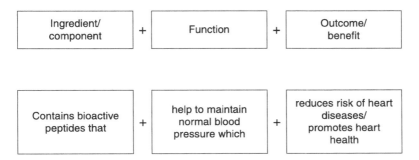

Fig. 6.2   Health claims can be constructed from three different components either separately or by combining them in different ways. The outcome can be framed as promising a gain (a positive outcome) or as avoiding a negative consequence.

contradictory results. In some studies consumers have not made much difference between different types of claims when assessing the possible benefits of products with health claims (Urala *et al.*, 2003; van Trijp & van der Lans, 2007). In a Nordic study, however there were clearly two types of consumers: those who found the claims with the whole chain of ingredient, function and outcome as most credible ('know-all' group) and those who found short claims just stating the outcome benefit as most credible ('benefit-only' group) (Grunert *et al.*, 2009). These consumer groups were approximately equally sized in the study with a large group of respondents (n = 4612) from the five Nordic countries, Denmark, Finland, Iceland, Norway and Sweden. Previous exposure to the claims within the country, positive attitude towards products with health claims and trust in authorities and scientists all contributed to the membership in the 'know-all' group, although these background variables could only explain a small part of the variance.

The promised benefit was important when consumers assessed the appeal and perceived healthiness of the claims (van Trijp & van der Lans, 2007), but the perceptions varied widely between countries. In a cross-cultural study carried out in Denmark, Finland and the USA (Bech-Larsen & Grunert, 2003), the most attractive influences of functional foods were related to heart health or cardiovascular diseases mentioned by 54–59%, followed by prevention of stomach cancer mentioned by 34–48% depending on the country. Similarly products with heart-related benefits were regarded as more healthy than products with memory or weight-related benefits in the Nordic study (Lähteenmäki *et al.*, 2010). Physiological claims were evaluated more positively than psychological claims in Switzerland (Siegrist *et al.*, 2008). These findings support the earlier findings of van Kleef *et al.* (2005) where disease prevention and general health enhancing products were perceived more positively than those improving psychological effects or appearance. These results are likely to reflect the fact that the best known products with health claims in the market have targeted on heart health (e.g. cholesterol lowering products) or other physiological functions, whereas the other benefits are newcomers for most consumers.

Familiarity and earlier knowledge of the component seem to have a great impact on how the claims are perceived. Components familiar from basic nutrition (e.g. calcium) or a topical term (e.g. probiotics) produce positive responses on their own even when their consequences are not mentioned (Urala *et al.*, 2003). Similarly, in many products, using omega-3 as an ingredient was perceived as more convincing in health claims than bioactive peptides that have been available only in some products (Grunert *et al.*, 2009). When the claim contained the function and the health outcome, both increased the perceived healthiness of claims that had the relatively unknown ingredient, but no such improvement could be perceived in product descriptions that had omega-3 as an ingredient (Lähteenmäki *et al.*, 2010). The ingredient *per se* appears to activate the existing health-related beliefs in consumers' minds and the information about the function and/or outcome in the claim is relevant only when it provides new information to the consumers. However, the increase in perceived healthiness was rather low for the bioactive peptides and consumers are not likely to be easily persuaded by the claim on its own.

In order to indicate the level of certainty in scientific knowledge behind the claims the FDA in the United States allows the use of qualifiers. The question on how well consumers make a distinction between these qualifiers is somewhat unsure. In their study, Hooker and Teratanavat (2008) found that consumers do not make a difference between different levels of claim unless there is a visual aid helping to make the judgement. Used qualifiers were based on the categorisation used by the FDA varying from significant scientific agreement (level A) to a very low level of scientific agreement (level D). In the five Nordic countries consumers were not influenced by the qualifier and the importance of having the word 'may' was very low in assessing the convincingness or how easy it is to understand the claim (Grunert *et al.*, 2009). This suggests that qualifiers in the claim on their own do not indicate the scientific strength and agreement behind the claims to the consumers unless they are accompanied by visual aids.

6.2.2   Risk reduction versus functional claims

The claims can be framed either as gaining something positive or as avoiding some negative outcomes. The Prospect Theory states that people are more sensitive towards possible losses than possible gain and therefore the negatively framed health claims should be perceived as more persuasive (Kahnemann & Tversky, 1979). Basically both functional and risk reduction claims can be framed either in positive or negative term, but typically risk reduction claims tend to be avoidance claims: the product should be eaten in order to avoid the higher risk. This may partly explain why risk reduction claims often receive stronger responses from consumers. However, the results from framing have been inconclusive and somewhat contradictory. In the Nordic study (Grunert *et al.*, 2009) the framing had very little importance in how the claim was perceived, although earlier studies indicate that the effect may be dependent on the type of outcome (van Kleef *et al.*, 2005).

Consumer responses to functional and risk reduction claims appear to be rather context specific. Van Kleef *et al.* (2005) observed that consumers (n = 50) find claims that promise to reduce risks of diseases more attractive than those claims that enhance physiological functions. However, there was an interaction between the benefit and its framing. With cardiovascular disease the reduced risk claim increased willingness to buy the products in comparison to enhanced heart function claim, whereas for energy level claims the results were the opposite. In addition to just framing the messages, also the content of the message should be considered: heart-related functions can easily be connected with disease whereas impact on energy/activity level is a function that improves overall well-being. Ability to imagine consequences may influence the effects of framing the messages. Broemer (2004) found that negatively framed messages are more effective when symptoms are easy to imagine, whereas positively framed messages are more effective when picturing outcomes is difficult.

There can also be cultural differences in the ways people like issues to be expressed: in a four-country study, respondents in the UK clearly preferred the claim that stated a positively framed outcome compared to a risk reduction claim; whereas in Finland and Germany the risk reduction claim increased more likelihood to buy (Saba *et al.*, 2010). In a large study carried out in Italy, Germany, the UK and USA (n = 6367) consumer perception of credibility, attractiveness and willingness to buy were driven by the benefit regardless of the type of claim linked to the product (van Trijp & van der Lans, 2007). The results are somewhat contradictory and require further research to improve our understanding of the personal motivation and information processing styles that may have an impact on our perceptions of claims.

6.2.3   Role of carrier product

Functional foods are marketed with health related arguments and although consumer perception of claims is crucial for their acceptability, the reasons for choosing functional products depend on the product categories they belong to (Urala and Lähteenmäki, 2003) and different factors explaining the behavioural responses to individual products (De Jong *et al.*, 2003; Urala and Lähteenmäki, 2004). The health claim, image and role of the carrier product and consumer characteristics all influence on how the functional food is perceived.

The health image of the carrier product has an impact on how beneficial the claim is perceived to be. Products that already have a healthy image for consumers are easier to accept as carriers of functional health claims (Bech-Larsen & Grunert, 2003; Dean *et al.*, 2007; Siegrist *et al.*, 2008; van Kleef *et al.*, 2005), but on the other hand claims in these products can be regarded as unnecessary, since the need to boost the healthiness of something that already is regarded as healthy by nature can be questioned by consumers (Lampila *et al.*, 2009). In a study with four countries from different parts of Europe (Finland, Germany, Italy and the UK; n = 2094) the benefit was perceived as highest when claims were linked with bread and lowest when connected to biscuits with pasta in the middle (Dean *et al.*, 2007) regardless of the type of claim. These products were selected to the study based on their roles as either staple foods (bread and pasta) or foods used as hedonic treats (biscuits).

Consumer perception of health-related claims depends on its suitability to the product in question. In Denmark consumers were more positive about functional effects that were created through adding components that are naturally occurring ingredients or components in that food product (Bech & Grunert, 2003). Adding calcium into milk products may be more acceptable in consumers' minds than adding other minerals that do not originally belong to milk in any significant quantities. Among some Americans, living bacteria are considered as repelling and the idea of beneficial probiotic yoghurt with living bacteria was deemed as an unacceptable product (Bruhn *et al.*, 2002). The bacteria, in the mind of these consumers, were linked with harmful pathogens.

Furthermore, functional foods are a category of foods which may require novel production or processing technologies and consequently, the concerns consumers have for these technologies need to be taken account (Frewer *et al.*, 2003). If achieving the claimed benefits requires such new methods as genetic engineering the products are regarded as low in acceptability (Cox *et al.*, 2004), although with clear health or environmental benefits the products may gain acceptability (Lähteenmäki *et al.*, 2002; Cox *et al.*, 2008).

The food and meal systems are culturally determined and the role of a carrier product in this system is usually well defined. Therefore the products and their health-related claims need to fit into this food system in order to be accepted. In some cases the functional food products have by-passed the food system by offering an additional product that is eaten or drunk separately in small quantity, in the same way as medicines are taken apart from dietary rules. An example of these kind products are the small bottles of probiotic yoghurt drinks originally introduced by Yakult and nowadays containing a wide range of products with new ingredients and claims for other benefits. The acceptability of these products can be built in a different way as they do not require a role in the food system.

6.2.4   Impact of health claims in perception of other quality cues, e.g. taste, convenience and naturalness

Related to consumer understanding of claims, one specific concern has been whether consumers infer from claims unjustified qualities in other product attributes: consumers may think that foods with health-related claims are generally superior. A 'halo effect' occurs if the consumer generalises positive perceptions to other product attributes (Roe *et al.*, 1999). Since health claims promise only health-related benefits they should mainly have an impact on perception of health-related product attributes. In the previous studies health-related claims have resulted in higher ratings of perceived healthiness, but the increase has been small or moderate at the best (Ares *et al.*, 2009; Lyly *et al.*, 2007; Urala *et al.*, 2003; van Trijp & van der Lans, 2007). The results from the Nordic study suggest that consumers can rate the products with health claims even less healthy than those without the claim (Lähteenmäki *et al.*, 2010). In cases where ingredient was new in the market with no previous exposure to health claims the impact on perceived healthiness was negative. Similarly, in Italy the health claims were perceived as lowering the ratings for likelihood to buy the cereal-based product descriptions (Saba *et al.*, 2010).

Taste
Consumers regard health benefits as positive factors, but only as long as they do not have to make any compromises with taste characteristics (Tepper & Trail, 1998). Consumers are not ready to compromise taste for functionality (Tuorila & Cardello, 2002; Verbeke, 2005). In Belgium (n = 245) half of the respondents were ready to accept the concept of functional foods if they taste good, whereas only 9% accepted the concept if the products would taste worse than their conventional counterparts (Verbeke, 2005). In a three country study, health claims added in the willingness to use beverages and ready-to-eat frozen soups slightly, but the acceptability was mostly determined by tasted pleasantness (Lyly *et al.*, 2007).

Naturalness
Naturalness is a valued attribute in food products and closely linked with perceived healthiness (Margetts *et al.*, 1997). Products with specific health benefits are likely to be perceived more positively if the benefit is based on components that are naturally present in the product (Bech-Larsen & Grunert, 2003; Verbeke *et al.*, 2009). Whether functional foods are perceived as natural or not natural varies widely between countries and individuals (Bäckström *et al.*, 2004; De Jong *et al.*, 2003). Yoghurt with lactic acid bacteria was rated as natural by almost half of consumers in a Dutch study (n = 1183) and less than one-third regarded it as not natural (De Jong *et al.*, 2003). Willingness to try modified dairy products including functional yoghurt, functional ice cream and calcium fortified milk was positively associated with both adherence to technology and naturalness and negatively to suspicion towards new foods in a study applying social representations in measuring responses to novel foods in Finland (n = 743) (Bäckström *et al.*, 2004). This suggests that although these foods were regarded with suspicion there was no obvious contradiction between naturalness and technology in the acceptability of functional foods. In the Nordic study health claims had a strong negative impact in perceived naturalness, but the effect depended on the type of product. Adding functional components (omega-3 or bioactive peptides) into yoghurt or bread caused a moderate decrease of around 0.7 on a 7-point scale, but the decrease in adding the same functional components into pork chops was almost −1.4 (Lähteenmäki *et al.*, 2010). A functional component is likely to have a negative impact on perceived naturalness (Lampila *et al.*, 2009), but the extent depends on the relationship between the functional components and target foods.

6.3   Consumer acceptability of health claims

6.3.1   Gender and age
The results on the role of gender, age and education have been contradictory from one study to another. According to some studies the most positive group towards

functional foods have been women (Ares *et al.*, 2009; Dean *et al.*, 2007; Urala *et al.*, 2003). Although women are more positive towards products with health claims, the claim in itself, whether functional or risk reduction, has a bigger positive impact on men's assessment of the product (Ares *et al.*, 2009). In some studies there have been no differences (Verbeke, 2005) or the differences between genders have been product-specific (De Jong *et al.*, 2003; Urala *et al.*, 2003). Although women are in general more health conscious (Rozin *et al.*, 1999), socio-demographic variables do not appear as strong factors in explaining consumer responses to functional foods as a concept, but if the relevance of the health benefit is gender related the role of gender may be crucial and needs to be verified on a product-by-product basis.

Health concerns tend to increase with age. Use of products with health claims is higher among the older age groups than among the younger ones in a study carried out in Canada (Herath *et al.*, 2008). In a study with a population of those who had been diagnosed for high or elevated cholesterol levels in blood (n = 2950), the use of cholesterol-lowering spread became more frequent with age: only 7% of those under 45 used cholesterol-lowering spread, but over 11% of those who were 45 or older used it (De Jong *et al.*, 2004). In Uruguay, the older age group had a higher intention to buy functional milk desserts than the younger age group, although both perceived a similar increase in healthiness (Ares *et al.*, 2009), and in Switzerland age promoted the willingness to buy functional products, including yoghurt (Siegrist *et al.*, 2008).

6.3.2   Country-wise differences

The country-wise differences in the perception of health claims are large (van Trijp & van der Lans, 2007). Foods with health claims are new products in some countries, whereas others have already have these products available in the market for several years. The finding from the Nordic study on health claims (Grunert *et al.*, 2009; Lähteenmäki *et al.*, 2010), that respondents from Denmark were most negative towards health claims and found claims with relatively simple messages more convincing, is likely to reflect lack of consumers' earlier exposure to the claims, whereas the Finnish and Swedish consumers tended to be more positive and find the detailed information in the claims convincing. In Denmark, health claims have not been allowed at all; in Norway only some claims have been allowed; whereas in Finland and Sweden there has been a number of functional products in the market for several years (Mejborn, 2007). Responses to health claims varied also widely among four countries (Finland, Germany, Italy and the UK) in a study that used different kinds of health-related messages in the product description. In all countries claims increased perceived healthiness with a risk reduction claim having a higher impact than a claim promising a general positive outcome with cereal-containing products as carriers. However, the likelihood to buy a product was much less influenced by the claim and both in Italy and the UK the impact of the risk reduction claim was negative, whereas in Finland and Germany it increased the utility of the product. In comparison, the wholegrain label in the products increased likelihood to buy in all other countries, except in Italy where its ability to raise the perceived healthiness was also lower compared to the other three countries (Saba *et al.*, 2010).

6.3.3 Perceived relevance of the benefit

To be able to choose functional foods consumers have to be aware of the health benefits offered by them, but knowledge *per se* is not a sufficient condition for willingness to use these products. One strong promoter for products with health claims has been if there is a perceived personal need for the promised benefit. When the motivational basis is taken into account the socio-demographic differences may exist, but they tend to be rather small. A person's own belief in the effectiveness of the product together with self-efficacy was the strongest predictor for intentions to choose functional products that combat memory loss (Cox *et al.*, 2004). The belief in health benefit increased the acceptance of the concept of functional foods (Verbeke, 2005). The relevance has been reflected in the gender differences. Women have been more responsive than men to products that are associated with breast cancer (Urala *et al.*, 2003) or foods containing extra calcium (De Jong *et al.*, 2003). Relevance can also be related to other people close by, e.g. an ill family member increased the acceptance of the functional food concept (Verbeke, 2005). If a consumer feels a need to lower blood cholesterol level or reduce level of stress then the products promising these effects are appealing. Producers of functional foods have to balance between messages and claims that are highly relevant to a small group of consumers and messages that aim to produce general well-being to most consumers. With the targeted approach one can reach a small number of highly motivated consumers, but with the latter approach the interested group is larger, although the motivation may be lower.

6.3.4 Attitudes towards products with health claims

Foods with health claims are relatively new in many countries so that consumer attitudes towards these so-called functional foods are not yet fully established and tend to change with time (Urala & Lähteenmäki, 2004; 2007). In the Nordic countries with different previous exposure to functional foods, the attitudes towards products with health claims were neutral in all countries, but there was a difference in the mean ratings so that Denmark had the lowest attitude score and Finland the highest, which reflects the earlier exposure to the claims (Fig. 6.3). In many studies, attitudes towards functional foods have been strong predictors for acceptability of these products (Verbeke *et al.*, 2009). In Finland, the strongest attitudinal predictor in willingness to use functional foods was perceived personal reward of taking care of oneself by choosing the functional options (Urala & Lähteenmäki, 2004). This personally felt reward was the best predictor for almost all functional foods used in the study. Whether functional foods were perceived as necessary in general predicted the willingness to use some products and confidence

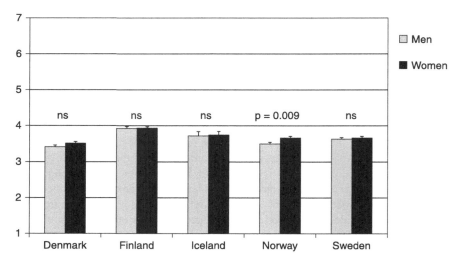

Fig. 6.3 Attitudes towards functional foods are neutral in the Nordic countries, but the minor differences between countries reflect the earlier exposure to health claims in the market (figure based on same data as results reported by Grunert *et al.* (2009) and Lähteenmäki *et al.* (2010)).

in their promised benefits seemed to be important in those products whose effects are hard to verify by measuring any specific outcomes, such as probiotic products or calcium added beverages.

6.3.5   Price and willingness to pay a premium for health claims in products

Functional foods with health-related claims tend to be more expensive than their conventional alternatives. Within such a new product category, consumers' willingness to pay is hard to estimate, since consumers may lack a reference point for making reliable judgements. Price has been regarded as a barrier in adopting functional foods as part of the diet (Wilkinson *et al.*, 2004), but in some studies the price has had very little impact on intention to buy (Bech-Larsen & Grunert, 2003; Verbeke *et al.*, 2009). In a study where two types of products were tasted and tried in three countries consumers in Finland, France and Sweden (n = 1157) were not ready to pay extra for the products that contained a health claim (Lyly *et al.*, 2007).

6.4   Implications for dairy product development

6.4.1   Dairy products as carriers of health claims

Successful functional foods have to be able to compete in product quality with their conventional alternatives. Functional foods are perceived as members of a product category and they need to compete with other alternatives within these product categories (Urala & Lähteenmäki, 2003). The health claim displaying a benefit is just one product characteristic among others and its importance varies among consumers. The studies carried out with functional products demonstrate that consumers are not ready to make sacrifices in hedonic pleasure (Lyly *et al.*, 2007; Tuorila and Cardello, 2002), although the loss of attractiveness cannot always be totally contributed to the expected taste loss (Lähteenmäki *et al.*, 2010). One reason for consumers' lower attractiveness ratings can be contributed to the loss in perceived naturalness. In dairy products naturally occurring ingredients, such as calcium and lactic acid bacteria, can be more easily accepted than ingredients that are not inherently part of the dairy products.

The dairy industry has been the most innovative sector within the food industry, and especially yoghurts have been used as carriers of functional components and health claims. Dairy products include a variety of products that differ in their nutrient content and also in their health image among consumers. The standard functional carrier product, yoghurt has been regarded as healthy product and used in many studies as a model food for health claims (e.g. Lähteenmäki *et al.*, 2010; Saba *et al.*, 2010; Siegrist *et al.*, 2008; van Trijp & van der Lans, 2007) and can be regarded as an attractive carrier for health claims (Williams *et al.*, 2008). The success of small bottles of drinkable yoghurts containing several kind of beneficial components, such as probiotics, and plant sterols and stanols has further made consumers familiar with functional dairy products. Yet, some dairy products are used as delicacies, e.g. dessert cheeses or butter in cooking and baking, and health is not likely to be the main criterion in their choices. This wide range of dairy products means that the role of health claims, and health in general, needs to be assessed separately case-by-case for different dairy products.

Dairy products have several advantages on their side as carriers of health claims. Milk-based products are traditionally considered as part of a healthy diet and recognised as good sources of protein, calcium and other minerals, especially for children. Dairy products are also mostly products that are used on daily basis thus providing suitable carriers for health-beneficial ingredients. Acceptability of health claims in products that are regarded as delicacies seems to be lower than adding health claims to products that are nutritionally wholesome (Dean *et al.*, 2007; Saba *et al.*, 2010). In the EU, the legislation demands that health claims should only be allowed in products that comply with nutritional profiles. Fulfilling the nutrition profiles should be possible for dairy products, since the low-fat products are largely available and accepted in most product categories, although added sugar in some products may cause problems.

6.4.2   Scientific evidence and consumer trust

Substantiating the health effects and ensuring their presence in the final product requires scientifically sound research. From the consumer point of view an impartial assessment of the validity of the health claims is essential to promote consumer trust in the claims. In EU (Regulation (EC) No 1924/2006), all used health claims have to pass the assessment of the European Food Safety Authority. The large number of proposed claims, however, has surprised the authorities in Europe. If the number of claims that will be allowed is large, then consumers will face a new challenge: how to find those benefits that are relevant to oneself. Furthermore, if a large number of claims are allowed, this may inflate the value of claims for consumers, especially if they become standard features and expected norms in many products.

Claims can also be divided into generic claims and product-specific claims. Generic claims are based on the presence of a certain nutrient or compound in the product, whereas product-specific claims refer to benefits derived from that specific product. Generic claims may be less appealing to the manufacturers since they do not provide differentiation between the products and it may be relatively easy for other producers to follow any successful product launches. From the manufacturer's point of view product-specific claims can be more appealing as they link not only the compound or ingredient, but also the specific product with the promised benefit in the claim. The product-specific claim offers better protection against competitors and gives a chance to use the claim effectively in marketing. A product-specific claim has to be proven in clinical studies using that specific product, which makes these claims expensive to companies. The studies should give sufficient support for the evidence that products provide the promised benefits with portions that are eaten as a part of normal diet.

Lately the discussion in Europe has evolved around dairy products containing probiotic bacteria. Although being relatively well-known among consumers and promising versatile consumer benefits, the quality of presented causal scientific evidence behind these claims has been deemed as insufficient by the European Food Safety Authority. The lack of official recognition in the beneficial effects of probiotic bacteria may become a hurdle for consumer acceptability of these products, and thereby slow down the further developments in this product category. The unsupportive opinions from the official body can create a suspicion over the whole product category in consumers' minds and make it impossible to promote the probiotic products with health claims in product label. Using any other channels to convey the message about the possible health benefits to the consumer will become illegal as well. The results from future applications will show how the probiotic field will develop in the EU. The Food Ethics Council in the UK (2009), in the report from a Business Forum meeting in March 2009, has brought forward the viewpoint that consumers may have a right to know about the possible health effects, although the evidence behind them is not yet conclusive.

6.4.3   Informing consumers about the health effects

The further challenge in marketing functional foods is how to make the claims understandable and appealing to consumers. Research on consumer perception of health claims provide support to the idea that consumers are likely to understand the messages in the claims as they are intended by the producers (Lähteenmäki *et al.*, 2010) and are not very sensitive to the wording of the claim (van Trijp & van der Lans, 2007; Grunert *et al.*, 2009). However, these studies are based on study designs which force responding consumers to process the information actively, which may not be the case in the everyday decision-making on food choices that are largely based in routine, habit and heuristic rules we use to solve many everyday problems (Leathwood *et al.*, 2007). The effect of the claim has also been relatively weak emphasising the role of other communication channels and familiarising consumers with the ingredient, function and its outcome. For dairy products with a strong track record as health beneficial food categories this may be easier than in many other product categories. Although having a claim accepted is the prerequisite that gives the impartially approved support to the claim, in order to get the message through the manufacturers need to consider the whole marketing strategy and not to rely too much on the claims *per se*.

The so-called functional food section has had the highest market growth during the past few years and therefore health claims are regarded as a desirable marketing tool for food producers. Health claims represent on alternative for healthier choices and they may appeal to some of the consumer segments that are not responsive to traditional nutritional advice. The socio-demographic differences in willingness to use seem to vary between products and their benefits with perceived relevance appearing as a strong predictor for acceptability. For future success of products with health claims the challenge is to find the right target groups for the products, since the relevance-based segmentation of consumers is likely to be more difficult than that based on socio-demographics.

6.5   Future trends

The best known functional foods at the moment are cholesterol-lowering products, antioxidants, and products containing fibre or beneficial bacteria. Although these products carry a new message, basically they respond to needs that have been recognised in medical and nutritional sciences for a long time. Consumers are becoming more familiar with these products and at the same time, while losing their novelty, they seem to gain acceptance from those who wish to follow nutritional recommendations and are interested in health in food choices in general (Urala & Lähteenmäki, 2007). The question for the future is that what is the role of foods with specific health claims: are they offering an additional benefit to consumers who try to avoid medication, are they just one more issue to consider for those who wish to eat in a healthy way in general, or do they become a standard that most people want to choose in order to enhance their well-being and lower the risks of diseases just as a precautionary measure?

The biggest threat to future acceptability of foods with health claims is a possible clash consumers perceive between these products and naturalness. There seems to be a growing trend of considering how different foods are produced and whether the production and processing methods can be categorised as sustainable. In functional foods the sources of functional components and ingredients are issues that will be likely to raise discussions in the future, e.g. what are the sources of omega-3 fatty acids and how the increased use of extracts from rare plants and fruits will impact on local economies in different parts of the world. If food products, such as milk, are used as raw material for specific functional compounds, this may blur the line between medicines and food. In order to gain further general acceptance and thereby provide true benefits to consumers, the functional healthiness will need to guarantee that the other aspects of healthiness and sustainability are taken into consideration.

6.6   Sources of further information and advice

The websites for authorities give latest information on developments related to health claims and consumers

Europe
List of allowed claims: http://ec.europa.eu/food/food/labellingnutrition/claims/
   community_register/health_claims_en.htm
Scientific opinions on claims by EFSA: http://www.efsa.europa.eu/en/ndaclaims/
   ndaclaims13.htm

USA
Information related to nutrition and health labelling: http://www.fda.gov/Food/
LabelingNutrition/ConsumerInformation/default.htm

6.7   References

Arai S (2002), 'Global view on functional foods: Asian perspectives', *Br J Nutr*, **88** (Suppl. 2), S139–S143.
Ares G, Gimenez A, Gámbaro A (2009), 'Consumers perceived healthiness and willingness to try functional milk desserts. Influence of ingredient, ingredient name and health claim', *Food Qual Preference*, **20**, 50–56.
Arvola A, Lähteenmäki L, Dean M, Vassallo M, Winkelmann M, Claupein, E, Saba A, Shepherd R (2007), 'Consumers' beliefs about whole and refined grain products in UK, Italy and Finland', *J Cereal Sci*, **46**, 197–206.
Bäckström A, Pirttilä-Backman AM, Tuorila H (2004), 'Willingness to try new foods as predicted by social representations and attitude and trait scales', *Appetite*, **43**, 75–83.
Bech-Larsen T, Grunert KG (2003), 'The perceived healthiness of functional foods. A conjoint study of Danish, Finnish and American consumers' perception of functional foods', *Appetite*, **40**, 9–14.
Broemer P (2004), 'Ease of imagination moderates reactions to differently framed messages', *Eur J Soc Psychol*, **34**, 103–119.
Bruhn CM, Bruhn CJ, Cotter A, Garrett M, Klenk M, Powell C, Stanford G, Steinbring Y, West E (2002), 'Consumer attitudes toward use of probiotic cultures', *J Food Sci*, **67**, 1969–1972.
Cox DN, Koster A, Russell CG (2004), 'Predicting intentions to consume functional foods and supplements to offset memory loss using an adaptation of protection memory theory', *Appetite*, **43**, 55–64.
Cox DN, Evans G, Lease HJ (2008), 'Australian consumers' preferences for conventional and novel sources of long chain omega-3 fatty acids: A conjoint study', *Food Qual Preference* **19**, 306–314.

De Jong N, Ocké MC, Branderhorst HAC, Friele R (2003), 'Demographic and lifestyle characteristics of functional food consumers and dietary supplement users', *Br J Nutr*, **89**, 273–281.

De Jong N, Simojoki M, Laatikainen T, Tapanainen H, Valsta L, Lahti-Koski M, Uutela A, Vartiainen E (2004), 'The combined use of cholesterol-lowering drugs and cholesterol-lowering bread spreads; health behavior data from Finland', *Prev Med*, **39**, 849–855.

Dean M, Raats MM, Shepherd R, Arvola A, Lahteenmaki L, Saba A, Vassallo M, Claupein E, Winkelmann M (2007), 'Consumer perceptions and expectations for healthy cereal products', *J Cereal Sci*, **46**, 188–196.

Food Ethics Council (2009), 'Health claims and functional foods. How will EU regulation shape our choices?', A report of the Business Forum meeting on 17 March 2009. http://www.foodethicscouncil.org/system/files/businessforum170309.pdf

Frewer L, Scholderer J, Lambert N (2003), 'Consumer acceptance of functional foods: issues for the future', *Br Food J*, **105**, 714–773.

Grunert K G, Bech-Larsen T, Bredahl L (2000), 'Three issues in consumer quality perception and acceptance of dairy products', *Int Dairy J*, **10**, 575–584.

Grunert KG, Lähteenmäki L, Boztug Y, Martinsdottír E, Ueland Ø, Åström A, Lampila P (2009), 'Perception of health claims among Nordic consumers', *Consumer Policy*, **32**, 269–287.

Herath D, Cranfield J, Henson S (2008), 'Who consumes functional foods and neutraceuticals in Canada? Results of cluster analysis of the 2006 survey of Canadians' demand for food products supporting health and wellness', *Appetite*, **51**, 256–265.

Hooker NH, Teratanavat R (2008), 'Dissecting qualified health claims: evidence from experimental studies', *Critical Rev Food Sci*, **48**, 160–176.

Kahneman D, Tversky A (1979), 'Prospect theory: An analysis of decision under risk', *Econometrica*, **47**, 263–291.

Lähteenmäki L, Grunert K, Ueland O, Åström A, Arvola A, Bech-Larsen T (2002), 'Acceptability of genetically modified cheese presented as real product alternative', *Food Qual Preference*, **13**, 523–533.

Lähteenmäki L, Lampila P, Grunert KG, Boztug Y, Ueland Ø, Åström A, Martinsdóttir E (2010), 'The impact of health-related claims on the perception of other product attributes', *Food Policy*, **35**, 230–239.

Lampila P, van Lieshout M, Gremmen B, Lähteenmäki L (2009), 'Consumer attitudes towards enhanced flavonoid content in fruit', *Food Res Intl*, **42**, 122–129.

Leathwood PD, Richardson DP, Sträter P, Todd PM, van Trijp HCM (2007), 'Consumer understanding of nutrition and health claims: Sources of evidence', *Br J Nutr*, **98**(3), 474–484.

Lyly M, Roininen K, Honkapää K, Lähteenmäki L (2007), 'Factors influencing consumers' willingness to use beverages and ready-to-eat frozen soups containing oat β-glucan in Finland, France and Sweden', *Food Qual Pref*, **18**, 242–255.

Margetts BM. Martinez JA, Saba A, Holm L, Kearney M (1997), 'Definitions of "healthy" eating: a pan-EU survey of consumer attitudes to food, nutrition and health', *Eur J Clin Nutr*, **51** (Suppl. 2), S23–S29.

Mejborn H (2007), *Health Claims on Food and Food Supplements*, National Food Institute, DTU, Copenhagen, Denmark.

Meziane Z (2007), *Future Innovations in Food and Drinks to 2012. NPD, Trend Convergence and Emerging Growth Opportunities*, Business Insights Ltd. http://www.business-insights.com/about

NLEA (1990), 'Nutrition labelling and education act of 1990,' Public law, 101–535 21 USC 301 (8 November 1990).

Paul G L, Ink S L and Geiger C J (1999), 'The Quaker Oats health claim: A case study', *J Nutraceuticals, Funct & Med Foods*, **1**(4), 5–32.

Regulation (EC) No 1924/2006 of the European Parliament and of the Council of 20 December 2006 on nutrition and health claims made on foods. *Official Journal of the European Union* L 404, 9–25.

Roe BE, Levy AS, Derby BM (1999), 'The impact of health claims on consumer search and product evaluation outcomes: Results from FDA experimental data', *J Publ Policy & Marketing*, **18**(1), 89–115.

Rozin P, Fischler C, Imada S, Sarubin A, Wrzesniewski A (1999), 'Attitudes to food and the role of food in life in the USA, Japan, Flemish Belgium and France: possible implications to diet-health debate', *Appetite*, **33**, 163–180.

Saba A, Vassallo M, Shepherd R, Lampila P, Arvola A, Dean M, Winkelmann M, Claupein E, Lähteenmäki L (2010), 'Country-wise differences in perception of health-related messages in cereal-based food products', *Food Qual Preference*, **21**, 385–393.

Saher M, Arvola A, Lindeman M, Lähteenmäki L (2004), 'Impressions of functional food consumers', *Appetite*, **42**, 79–89.

Siegrist M, Stampfli N, Kastenholz (2008), 'Consumers' willingness to buy functional foods. The influence of carrier, benefit and trust', *Appetite*, **51**, 526–529.

Tepper BJ, Trail AC (1998), 'Taste or health: a study on consumer acceptance of corn chips', *Food Qual Preference*, **9**, 267–272.

Tuorila H, Cardello AV (2002), 'Consumer responses to off-flavour in juice in the presence of specific health claims', *Food Qual Preference*, **13**, 561–569.

Urala N, Arvola A, Lähteenmäki L (2003), 'Strength of health-related claims', *Int J Food Sci Tech*, **38**, 1–12.

Urala N, Lähteenmäki L (2003), 'Reasons behind consumers' functional food choices', *Nutr Food Sci*, **33**, 148–158.

Urala N, Lähteenmäki L (2004), 'Attitudes behind consumers' willingness to use functional foods', *Food Qual Preference*, **15**, 793–803.

Urala N, Lähteenmäki L (2007), 'Consumers changing attitudes towards functional foods', *Food Qual Preference*, **18**, 1–12.

Van Kleef E, van Trijp HCM, Luning P (2005), 'Functional foods: health claim – food product compatibility and the impact of health claim framing on consumer evaluation', *Appetite*, **44**, 299–308.

Van Trijp HCM, van der Lans IA (2007), 'Consumer perceptions of nutrition and health claims', *Appetite*, **48**, 305–324.

Verbeke W (2005), 'Consumer acceptance of functional foods: socio-demographic, cognitive and attitudinal determinants', *Food Qual Preference*, **16**, 45–57.

Verbeke W, Scholderer J, Lähteenmäki L (2009), 'Consumer appeal of nutrition and health claims in three existing product concepts', *Appetite*, **52**, 684–692.

Wilkinson SBT, Pidgeon N, Lee J, Pattison C, Lambert N (2004), 'Exploring consumer attitudes towards functional foods: a qualitative study', *J Nutraceut*, **4**(3/4), 5–28.

Williams P, Ridges L, Batterham M, Ripper B, Chi Hung M (2008), 'Australian consumer attitudes to health claim – food product compatibility for functional foods', *Food Policy*, **33**, 640–643.

Part II

Functional foods and health

7

Functional foods and acute gastrointestinal infections

H. Szajewska, The Medical University of Warsaw, Poland

Abstract: Acute gastrointestinal infections are very common, particularly in infants and children, and have an impact on an individual, but also on society and the health service. Currently, functional foods such as probiotics and/or prebiotics are increasingly being used to treat or prevent gastrointestinal infections, driven in large part by the food and pharmaceutical industry. However, uncertainty exists regarding their efficacy. In this chapter, current literature pertaining to the clinical effects of the use of probiotics and/or prebiotics for the treatment and prevention of acute gastrointestinal infections is reviewed.

Key words: probiotics, prebiotics, synbiotics, randomized controlled trial, systematic review, meta-analysis.

7.1 Introduction

Acute gastrointestinal infections are very common, particularly in infants and children. Agents that commonly cause acute gastrointestinal illness include viruses, bacteria, and protozoa. Worldwide, both in developed and developing countries, rotavirus is the major cause of severe acute gastroenteritis (Gray *et al.*, 2008). Approximately 500 000 deaths occur annually due to diarrhoea associated with rotavirus gastroenteritis, primarily in developing countries. In developed countries, while death due to rotavirus infection is rare, it is estimated that each year rotavirus is responsible for a substantial number of medical consultations and hospitalizations. In Europe, by the age of five years, almost every child will experience an episode of rotavirus gastroenteritis; one in seven will require an outpatient visit, and one in 54 will need hospitalization (Soriano-Gabarro *et al.*, 2006). Gastrointestinal infections have an impact on an individual, but they also have a major impact on society and the health service. Therefore, there is interest in developing measures to reduce this disease burden, including the use of functional foods such as probiotics and/or prebiotics.

Probiotics are usually defined as 'live microorganisms which when administered in adequate amounts confer a health benefit on the host' (FAO/WHO, 2002). The term 'prebiotic' refers to 'a nondigestible food ingredient that beneficially affects the host by selectively stimulating the growth and/or activity of one or a limited number of bacteria in the colon and thereby improving host health' (Gibson and Roberfroid, 1995). The term 'synbiotic' refers to a product that contains both probiotics and prebiotics (Schrezenmeir and de Vrese, 2001).

7.2   How the intervention might work

The rationale for the use of probiotics to treat and prevent gastrointestinal infections is based on the assumption that they modify the composition of the gut microbiota and act against enteric pathogens. While the exact mechanism by which probiotics might exert their activity against enteropathogens in humans remains unknown, several possible mechanisms have been proposed based on results of *in vitro* and animal studies. These mechanisms include the synthesis of antimicrobial substances (e.g. *Lactobacillus rhamnosus* GG [LGG] and *Lactobacillus acidophilus* strain LB have been shown to produce inhibitory substances against some gram-positive and gram-negative pathogens) (Coconnier *et al.*, 1997; Goldin *et al.*, 1992; Silva *et al.*, 1987), competition for nutrients required for growth of pathogens (Walker, 2000; Wilson and Perini, 1988), competitive inhibition of adhesion of pathogens (Bernet *et al.*, 1994; Davidson and Hirsch, 1976; Michail and Abernathy, 2002; Rigothier *et al.*, 1994), and modification of toxins or toxin receptors (Czerucka *et al.*, 1994; Pothoulaskis *et al.*, 1993). Additionally, studies have shown that probiotics stimulate or modify nonspecific and specific immune responses to pathogens. In fact, certain probiotics increase the number of circulating lymphocytes (De Simone *et al.*, 1992) and lymphocyte proliferation (Aattour *et al.*, 2002), stimulate phagocytosis, increase specific antibody responses to the rotavirus vaccine strain (Isolauri *et al.*, 1995), and increase cytokine secretion, including interferon γ (Aattour *et al.*, 2002; Kaila *et al.*, 1992; Majamaa *et al.*, 1995; Miettinen *et al.*, 1996). Experimental data have documented that *Lactobacillus* species (LGG as well as *L. plantarum* strain 299v) inhibit, in a dose-dependent manner, the binding of *Escherichia coli* strains to intestinal-derived epithelial cells grown in a tissue culture by stimulation of synthesis and secretion of mucins (glycoproteins known to have a protective effect in intestinal infections) (Mack *et al.*, 1999). Furthermore, probiotics have been shown to enhance mucosal immune defences (Isolauri *et al.*, 1993) and protect against structural and functional damage promoted by enterovirulent pathogens in the brush border of enterocytes, probably by interfering with the cross-talk between the pathogen and host cells (i.e. inhibition of pathogen-induced cell signalling) (Lievin-Le Moal *et al.*, 2002). It is likely that several of the above-described mechanisms operate simultaneously, and they may well differ depending on the properties of the enteric pathogen (e.g. bacterial or viral) and probiotic strain.

Prebiotics present in human milk, found in food, or supplemented to the diet (e.g. inulin-type fructans, galactooligosaccharides) are not hydrolyzed by small intestinal enzymes; thus, they enter the colon and are fermented, resulting in a more acidic luminal pH and an increased concentration of short-chain fatty acids such as lactic, butyric, propionic, and acetic acid. This, in turn, results in the increased proliferation of certain commensal bacteria, mainly but not exclusively bifidobacteria and lactobacilli, which function as probiotics to stimulate intestinal host defences (Forchielli and Walker, 2005). Thus, prebiotics may be indirectly responsible for some of the effects of probiotics. In addition, the produced short-chain fatty acids provide an energy source for colonocytes as well as a stimulus for some of the bacterial–epithelial 'cross-talk' cellular events, e.g. up-regulation of TLR expression (Zapolska-Downar *et al.*, 2004). Several studies have demonstrated the specific effect of prebiotic oligosaccharides in achieving a lower luminal pH and increased concentration of short-chain fatty acids in the colon, as well as increased concentrations of bifidobacteria and lactobacilli; however, long-term studies demonstrating the sustained effects of prebiotics are lacking. In addition, one may assume that since prebiotics stimulate an increase in bifidobacteria and lactobacilli, the effect of this stimulation on health is similar to that observed with use of probiotics. This assumption, however, has to be proven in clinical trials. Prebiotics can interact with receptors on immune cells and, thus, provide direct effects that do not require the proliferation of commensal (probiotic) bacteria (Watzl *et al.*, 2005; Roller *et al.*, 2004). Furthermore, pathologic bacteria must first adhere to the mucosa, as without adherence pathogens cannot act on the gut epithelium to cause disease. Specific terminal sugars on oligosaccharides (e.g. oligofructose) can interfere with the receptors on bacteria by binding to the bacteria and preventing its attachment to the same sugar on microvillus glycoconjugates (Forchielli and Walker, 2005).

7.3   How to assess the effectiveness of probiotics and/or prebiotics

Data from animal models and *in vitro* findings can be used to explain the mechanisms by which probiotics and/or prebiotics work or serve as screening instruments to choose new probiotic strains or prebiotic substrates for preventive or therapeutic use. However, when addressing questions regarding the effects of therapeutic and prophylactic interventions, the gold standard for this is the evaluation of randomized controlled trials (RCTs) and systematic reviews (or meta-analyses) of RCTs.

7.4   What is the aim of this chapter?

Currently, probiotics and/or prebiotics are increasingly being used to treat or prevent gastrointestinal infections, driven in large part by the food and pharmaceutical industry. However, uncertainty exists regarding their efficacy. In this chapter, current literature pertaining to the clinical effects of the use of probiotics and/or prebiotics for the treatment and prevention of acute gastrointestinal infections is reviewed. Data were identified by searches of the Cochrane Database of Systematic Reviews, the Cochrane Controlled Trials Register, and MEDLINE databases (all up until December 2009) as well as references from relevant articles. The search was limited to RCTs or their systematic reviews/meta-analyses, which were identified using relevant keywords. For conditions that had previously been reviewed in a systematic review/meta-analysis, only the findings of those reviews are summarized. In the event that relevant primary RCTs were published after the systematic review/meta-analysis was published, these were also included and reviewed. The MEDLINE database was also searched for published, evidence-based clinical practice guidelines developed by respected scientific societies or expert groups.

7.5   Probiotics

7.5.1   Treatment of acute gastroenteritis

Acute gastroenteritis generally is a self-limited illness lasting five to seven days, and thus, the main aim of treatment is to prevent dehydration, metabolic acidosis, and electrolyte disturbances. In the vast majority of cases of acute gastroenteritis with mild or moderate dehydration, this can be achieved with oral rehydration solutions. Despite the proven efficacy of oral rehydration, it remains underused (Guarino *et al.*, 2001). The main reason for this is that an oral rehydration solution neither reduces the frequency of bowel movements and fluid loss nor shortens the duration of illness, which decreases its acceptance and prompts interest in adjunctive treatments.

Systematic reviews/meta-analyses
Several systematic reviews/meta-analyses of RCTs examining the effectiveness of the use of probiotics compared to a control product in the treatment of acute gastroenteritis have been published (see Table 7.1) (Allen *et al.*, 2003; Huang *et al.*, 2002; Szajewska and Mrukowicz, 2001; Szajewska *et al.*, 2007a; Van Niel *et al.*, 2002). Thus far, the beneficial effects of probiotics in the management of acute infectious diarrhoea seem to be as follows:

- moderate (approximately one day reduction in the duration of diarrhoea);
- strain-dependent;
- dose-dependent (greater for doses $\geq 10^{10}$–10^{12} colony-forming units [CFU]/day);
- significant for watery diarrhoea and viral gastroenteritis but nonexistent for invasive, bacterial diarrhoea;
- more evident when treatment with probiotics is initiated early in the course of the disease;
- more evident in the developed countries.

Table 7.1   Probiotics in the treatment of acute infectious diarrhoea. Outcome: duration of diarrhoea. Results of meta-analyses

Reference	RCTs (n)	Probiotic(s)	Population	WMD (95% CI)
Szajewska *et al.*, 2001	8 (731)	Various	Children	−18 h (−27 to −10)
Van Niel *et al.*, 2002	9 (675)	Lactobacilli	Children	−17 h (−29 to −7)
Huang *et al.*, 2002	18 (1917)	Various	Children	−19 h (−26 to −14)
Allen *et al.*, 2003	12 (970)	Various	Children and adults	−30 h (−42 to −19)
Szajewska *et al.*, 2007	7 (876)	Lactobacillus GG	Children	−26 h (−46 to −7)
Szajewska *et al.*, 2009	7 (944)	*S. boulardii*	Children	−26 h (−39 to −13)

WMD – weighted mean difference (negative values indicate that the duration of diarrhoea was shorter in the probiotic group than in the control group).
CI – confidence interval, RCTs – randomized controlled trials.

Meta-analyses limited to one probiotic microorganism
Some recent meta-analyses have focused exclusively on assessing the efficacy of administering only a single probiotic microorganism. This decision is based on evidence that the beneficial effects of probiotics seem to be strain-specific, thus, pooling data on different strains may result in misleading conclusions. For LGG (Szajewska *et al.*, 2007), eight RCTs, involving 988 participants, met the inclusion criteria for one meta-analysis. Compared with controls, administration of LGG had no effect on the total stool volume (two RCTs, n = 303). However, use of LGG was associated with a significant reduction in diarrhoea duration (seven RCTs, 876 infants, weighted mean difference [WMD] −1.1 days, 95% confidence interval [CI] −1.9 to −0.3), particularly of rotavirus aetiology (WMD −2.1 days, 95% CI −3.6 to −0.6). For *Saccharomyces boulardii* (Szajewska and Skorka, 2009), nine RCTs, involving 1117 participants, were included in another meta-analysis. A meta-analysis of seven RCTs (n = 944) showed a reduction in the duration of diarrhoea (WMD −1.1 day, 95% CI −1.6 to 0.5) in those treated with *S. boulardii* compared with placebo. Both meta-analyses included trials of varying methodological quality, so caution in the interpretation of the results is needed.

Published guidelines
The evidence related to probiotics was recently thoroughly evaluated in evidence-based guidelines on the management of acute gastroenteritis in children developed by the European Society for Paediatric Gastroenterology, Hepatology and Nutrition (ESPGHAN) and the European Society of Paediatric Infectious Diseases (ESPID) (Guarino, 2008a; 2008b). The recommendation was made for the use of probiotics for the management of acute gastroenteritis, particularly those probiotics with documented efficacy such as LGG and *S. boulardii*. Other

probiotics may also be used provided their efficacy is documented in high quality RCTs (or in meta-analyses).

Another recent set of recommendations comes from the National Institute for Health and Clinical Excellence (NICE) (NICE, 2009). Similar to the ESPGHAN/ESPID guidelines, this set of guidelines is based on systematic reviews of the best available evidence. The NICE guidelines concluded that there is evidence from a high quality systematic review suggesting the efficacy of probiotics in regard to shortening of the duration of the diarrhoea and reducing stool frequency. However, in contrast to the ESPGHAN/ESPID recommendations, the position of NICE is that despite some evidence of a possible clinical benefit, currently it is not appropriate to recommend the use of probiotics. It is noteworthy that the NICE guidelines are addressed to health care professionals in the United Kingdom where licensed probiotic preparations are not available in the National Health Service.

In summary, selected probiotic microorganisms may reduce the duration and intensity of symptoms of acute gastroenteritis. The use of probiotics with proven efficacy and in appropriate doses as an adjunct to rehydration therapy is recommended by some scientific societies.

7.5.2   Prevention of nosocomial diarrhoea

Nosocomial diarrhoea is any diarrhoea that a patient contracts in a health-care institution. In children, it is commonly caused by enteric pathogens, especially rotavirus (Matson and Estes, 1990). Depending on the population, type of hospital and standard of care, the reported incidence ranges from 4.5 (Ford-Jones *et al.*, 1990) to 22.6 (Ponce *et al.*, 1995) episodes per 100 admissions. Nosocomial diarrhoea may prolong the hospital stay and increase medical costs.

Lactobacillus rhamnosus GG

Three placebo-controlled RCTs conducted in hospitalized children have evaluated the effectiveness of LGG in the prevention of nosocomial gastrointestinal illnesses (Hojsak *et al.*, 2010a; Mastretta *et al.*, 2002; Szajewska and Mrukowicz, 2001). One double-blind RCT carried out in Poland that involved 81 children aged 1 to 36 months revealed that 6×10^9 CFU of LGG administered orally twice daily significantly reduced the risk of nosocomial diarrhoea compared with the placebo (6.7% *vs.* 33.3%, relative risk [RR] 0.2, 95% confidence interval [CI] 0.06 to 0.6, $P = 0.002$) (Szajewska *et al.*, 2001). Similarly, a study carried out in Croatia in 742 hospitalized children revealed that LGG administration significantly reduced the risk of gastrointestinal infections (RR 0.4, 95% CI 0.25 to 0.7) (Hojsak *et al.*, 2010a). The only RCT that did not document a beneficial effect of LGG administration involved 220 Italian children aged 1 to 18 months. Whereas breast-feeding was effective, oral administration of 10^{10} CFU of LGG once daily did not prevent the development of nosocomial rotavirus infections compared with the placebo (25.4% *vs.* 30.2%, RR 0.8, 95% CI 0.55 to 1.3, P=0.4) (Mastretta *et al.*, 2002).

Bifidobacterium bifidum and Streptococcus thermophilus
Two double-blind RCTs evaluated the effectiveness of *Bifidobacterium bifidum* (recently renamed *B. lactis*) and *Streptococcus thermophilus* in the prevention of nosocomial diarrhoea. The first included infants aged 5 to 24 months (n = 55) who were admitted to a chronic care hospital (relatively long stay). Administration of standard infant formula supplemented with *B. bifidum* and *Streptococcus thermophilus* reduced the prevalence of nosocomial diarrhoea compared with the placebo (7% *vs.* 31%, RR 0.2, 95% CI 0.06 to 0.8) (Saavedra *et al.*, 1994). The second RCT was conducted in 90 healthy infants younger than 8 months, who were living in residential nurseries or foster care centres. In this study, milk formula supplemented with viable *B. lactis strain* Bb 12 did not reduce the prevalence of diarrhoea compared with administration of a placebo (28.3% *vs.* 38.7%, RR 0.7, 95% CI 0.4 to 1.3) (Chouraqui *et al.*, 2004).

In summary, there is currently evidence to recommend the use of LGG, but not enough evidence to recommend the use of *Bifidobacterium lactis* and *Str. thermophilus*, to prevent nosocomial diarrhoea. No published cost-effectiveness analyses were identified. However, this is a field of potential great benefit.

7.5.3   Prevention of community-acquired diarrhoea

Over the past several years, enormous efforts have been made in the development of safe and effective vaccines against enteric infections, mainly rotavirus. The availability of two efficacious and safe rotavirus vaccines with high efficacy against severe rotavirus gastroenteritis, combined with consistent recommendations to include these vaccines in national immunization programmes (Vesikari *et al.*, 2008; Committee of Infectious Diseases, AAP 2009), offers promise in reducing the burden of disease caused by this virus. The effects of these vaccines are very encouraging. However, in some circumstances, effective alternative interventions such as use of probiotics may be considered due to their immediate onset of action, activity against microorganisms other than rotavirus, and lower costs.

Lactobacillus rhamnosus GG
One RCT that involved 204 undernourished infants living in a community with a high burden of diarrhoeal diseases (Peru) revealed fewer episodes of diarrhoea in children who received LGG compared with a placebo (5.21 *vs.* 6.02 episodes/child/year; P = 0.03). This benefit was particularly evident in non-breastfed children aged 18–29 months (4.69 *vs.* 5.86 episodes/child/year; P = 0.005) (Oberhelman *et al.*, 1999).

In contrast, two, double-blind, placebo-controlled RCTs carried out in Europe in children attending day care centres did not demonstrate an effect of LGG administration on the prevention of gastrointestinal infections. The Finnish study conducted in 571 children aged 1–6 years revealed no difference between the LGG and placebo groups in the number of days with gastrointestinal symptoms or in the proportion of children without diarrhoea (Hatakka *et al.*, 2001). However, the incidence of gastroenteritis in this setting was low. Similarly, an RCT conducted in 281 Croatian children revealed no significant reduction in the risk of gastrointestinal infections, vomiting episodes, and diarrhoeal episodes, as well as no reduction in the number of days with gastrointestinal symptoms, in children who received LGG compared with placebo (Hojsak *et al.*, 2010b).

Bifidobacterium breve C50 and Streptococcus thermophilus 065
Compared with placebo, use of a formula containing *B. breve* C50 and *Str. thermophilus* 065 in healthy infants did not reduce the incidence or duration of diarrhoeal episodes, but the episodes were less severe (Thibault *et al.*, 2004).

Lactobacillus reuteri or Bifidobacterium lactis
One double-blind, placebo-controlled RCT that compared *L. reuteri* ATCC 55730 or *B. lactis* (BB-12) treatment with a placebo for the prevention of infections in 201 infants attending child care centres demonstrated a reduction in the number and duration of diarrhoeal episodes in infants treated with the probiotics (Weizman *et al.*, 2005).

In summary, several studies have examined the role of probiotics in the prevention of gastrointestinal infections in healthy individuals, particularly those in children's day care centres. Although RCTs have shown a modest effect for some probiotics, the results are not uniform. Confirmatory RCTs are needed.

7.5.4   Prevention of traveller's diarrhoea
Traveller's diarrhoea is a common problem, occurring in 5% to 50% of travellers. It is usually due to bacterial enteropathogens, with enterotoxigenic *E. coli* (ETEC) representing a major cause. There have been two meta-analyses of the role of probiotics in the prevention of traveller's diarrhoea with conflicting conclusions. The first (McFarland, 2007) (search date: 2005) identified 12 studies with a total of 4709 subjects. The pooled relative risk indicates that probiotics significantly prevent traveller's diarrhoea (RR 0.85, 95% CI 0.79 to 0.91). The authors concluded that several probiotics, such as *S. boulardii* and a mixture of *L. acidophilus* and *B. bifidum*, had significant efficacy and that probiotics may offer a safe and effective method of preventing traveller's diarrhoea. However, opposite conclusions were reached by the authors of the second meta-analysis (Takahashi *et al.*, 2007) (search date: 2005). The pooled results of five RCTs of varying methodological quality involving 3326 subjects showed no significant difference between the probiotic and the control groups in the risk of traveller's diarrhoea (RR 0.93, 95% CI 0.85 to 1.01). The authors concluded that use of probiotics is not effective for the prevention of traveller's diarrhoea.

In summary, the evidence suggests that some probiotics may be effective in preventing traveller's diarrhoea, while others are not. However, data are still limited. If travellers choose to take probiotics, they should take the strain(s) with documented efficacy.

7.5.5   Prevention of antibiotic-associated diarrhoea

A common side effect of antibiotic treatment is antibiotic-associated diarrhoea (AAD), defined as otherwise unexplained diarrhoea that occurs in association with the administration of antibiotics (Bartlett, 2002). AAD occurs in approximately 5% to 40% of patients between the initiation of therapy and up to two months after cessation of treatment (Barbut *et al.*, 1997; Elstner *et al.*, 1983; Turck *et al.*, 2003). This wide range reflects the definition of diarrhoea used, patient ages, host factors, and the inciting antimicrobial agents. Almost all antibiotics, particularly those active against anaerobes, can cause diarrhoea; however, the risk of AAD seems to be higher with aminopenicillins, the combination of aminopenicillins and clavulanate, cephalosporins, and clindamycin (Barbut *et al.*, 1997; McFarland *et al.*, 1990). Although no infectious agent is found in most cases, the bacterial agent commonly associated with AAD, particularly in the most severe episodes (pseudomembranous colitis), is *Clostridium difficile* (Bartlett *et al.*, 1978).

Meta-analyses/systematic reviews in paediatric population
Three systematic reviews/meta-analyses of RCTs involving only children were found (see Table 7.2). The first systematic review with a meta-analysis (Szajewska *et al.*, 2006) (search date: December 2005) identified six RCTs involving 766 children. This review found that treatment with probiotics compared with placebo reduced the risk of AAD from 28.5% to 11.9% (RR 0.4, 95% CI 0.25 to 0.8). Preplanned subgroup analysis showed that reduction in the risk of AAD was associated with the use of LGG (two RCTs, n = 307, RR 0.3, 95% CI 0.15 to 0.6), *S. boulardii* (one RCT, 246 participants, RR 0.2, 95% CI 0.07 to 0.6), or *B. lactis and Str. thermophilus* (one RCT, 157 participants, RR 0.5, 95% CI 0.3 to 0.95).

A more recent systematic review (Johnston *et al.*, 2006) (search date: August 2006) identified ten RCTs (six of them were included in the above-mentioned meta-analysis) involving 1986 participants that compared the effects of treatment with either *Lactobacilli* spp., *Bifidobacterium* spp., *Streptococcus* spp., or *S. boulardii*, alone or in combination, in children up to 18 years of age being treated with antibiotics. The objective of this review was to assess the efficacy of these probiotics for the prevention of AAD in children. Six studies used a single-strain probiotic agent, and four combined two probiotic strains. In seven trials, the intervention was compared to placebo; in two trials, probiotics were compared to a product other than placebo (i.e. diosmectite, infant formula); and in one trial, probiotics were compared to no treatment. The per protocol analysis for nine trials reporting on the incidence of diarrhoea showed statistically significant results favouring probiotics over active/non-active controls (RR 0.49, 95% CI 0.32 to 0.74). In contrast, intention-to-treat analysis showed nonsignificant results overall (RR 0.90, 95% CI 0.50 to 1.63). However, as indicted by the authors of this review, the validity of the intention-to-treat analysis in this review can be questioned due to the high losses to follow-up.

Another meta-analysis (Johnston *et al.*, 2007) (search date: January 2005) covers data included in the Cochrane Review by the same authors and, therefore, is not discussed here.

Table 7.2   Probiotics in the prevention of antibiotic-associated diarrhoea: results of meta-analyses of randomized controlled trials (RCTs)

Study	Probiotics	Number of RCTs (n)	Measure of effect size	Effect (95% CI)	Number needed to treat (95% CI)
Children only					
Szajewska et al., 2006	Various	6 (766)	RR	0.4 (0.25 to 0.8)	7 (5 to 10)
Johnston et al., 2006	Various	6 (707)	RR	0.4 (0.25 to 0.75) (per protocol analysis)	
				1.01 (0.6 to 1.6) (intention-to-treat analysis)	
Johnston et al., 2007	Various	9 (1946)	RR	0.5(0.32 to 0.74)	
Adults and children					
D'Souza et al., 2002	S. boulardii	4 (830)	OR	0.4 (0.25 to 0.6)	11 (8 to 20)
	Lactobacillus spp.	5 (384)	OR	0.3 (0.2 to 0.6)	11 (8 to 18)
	Total	9 (1214)	OR	0.4 (0.3 to 0.5)	
Cremonini et al., 2002	Lactobacillus spp.	4 (446)	RR	0.5 (0.4 to 0.7)	9 (7 to 17)
	S. boulardii	3 (435)	RR	0.6 (0.4 to 0.9)	14 (8 to 108)
	Total	7 (881)	RR	0.4 (0.3 to 0.6)	9 (7 to 14)
Szajewska and Mrukowicz, 2005	S. boulardii	5 (1076)	RR	0.4 (0.2 to 0.8)	10 (7 to 16)
Hawrelak et al., 2005	Lactobacillus GG	6 (692)	No statistical pooling		
Sazawal et al., 2006	Various	19 (no data)	RR	0.5 (0.35 to 0.65)	
McFarland, 2006	Various	25 (2810)	RR	0.4 (0.3 to 0.6)	
Wenus et al., 2008	Lactobacillus GG, La-5, Bb-12	63	RR	0.2 (0.05 to 0.9)	
Hickson et al., 2007	Lactobacillus casei DN-114 001, S. thermophilus, L. bulgaricus	113	RR	0.36 (0.2 to 0.8)	5 (3 to 16)

Ruszczynski et al., 2008	Lactobacillus rhamnosus (strains E/N, Oxy and Pen)	240	RR	0.45 (0.2 to 0.95)	11 (6 to 106)
Szymański et al., 2008	Bifidobacterium longum PL03, Lactobacillus rhamnosus KL53A and Lactobacillus plantarum PL02	78	RR	0.47 (0.04 to 5)	Not significant
Merenstein et al., 2009	Kefir	125	RR	0.8 (0.5 to 1.4)	Not significant

CI – confidence interval, RR – relative risk, OR – odds ratio.

As with almost all meta-analyses/systematic reviews, these meta-analyses/ systematic reviews are limited by the quantity and quality of the existing data. The methodology of the included studies differed and often was suboptimal. Potential limitations included unclear or inadequate allocation concealment and no intention-to-treat analysis. Study limitations also included a small sample size in some trials and no widely agreed upon definition of diarrhoea.

Systematic reviews/meta-analyses in general population
Several other systematic reviews/meta-analyses of RCTs that included both adults and children were found (see Table 7.2). The first (D'Souza et al., 2002), located through searching MEDLINE and the Cochrane Library (search date: 2000), identified nine trials with 1214 patients, including only two trials involving children (Tankanov et al., 1990; Vanderhoof et al., 1999). The objective of this meta-analysis was to evaluate the efficacy of probiotics in the prevention and treatment of diarrhoea associated with the use of antibiotics. The pooled odds ratio (OR) showed that probiotic treatment was more effective than placebo in the prevention of diarrhoea (OR 0.4, 95% CI 0.3 to 0.5). The combined odds ratios for four trials that used *S. boulardii* also favoured probiotic treatment (OR 0.4, 95% CI 0.25 to 0.62), as did studies that used lactobacilli or enterococci (OR 0.3, 95% CI 0.19 to 0.61) (D'Souza et al., 2002).

The second meta-analysis (Cremonini et al., 2002) (search date: 2001) identified seven studies with 881 patients (five of those were also identified in the above-mentioned meta-analysis). Two studies involved children, and the rest were performed in adults. These studies showed a significant overall reduction in the risk of AAD during probiotic administration. The pooled relative risk was 0.4 (95% CI 0.3 to 0.6).

The objective of the third meta-analysis (Sazawal et al., 2006) was to evaluate evidence for the use of probiotics in the prevention of acute diarrhoea. Of 19 trials with data on AAD, 18 had positive point estimates; six of these attained statistical significance, with an overall reduction in AAD of 52% (95% CI 35 to 65%). In some of these trials, probiotics were administered together with eradication therapy for *Helicobacter pylori*. These factors need to be considered when interpreting and extrapolating overall results.

Meta-analyses limited to one probiotic microorganism
Critics of using a meta-analytical approach to assess the efficacy of probiotics argue that the beneficial effects of probiotics seem to be strain-specific, thus, pooling data on different strains may result in misleading conclusions. Given these concerns, the author of this chapter co-reviewed data on the effectiveness and safety of only one probiotic microorganism – *S. boulardii* – in the prevention of AAD (Szajewska and Mrukowicz, 2005). Of 16 potentially relevant clinical trials identified, five RCTs (1076 participants) met the inclusion criteria for this systematic review. Treatment with *S. boulardii* compared with placebo reduced the risk of AAD from 17.2% to 6.7% (RR 0.4, 95% CI 0.2 to 0.8). No side effects were reported. The mechanism by which *S. boulardii*, a nonpathogenic yeast, exerts its action in preventing AAD is unclear. Possible mechanisms, which have been demonstrated in animals, include the production of a protease that inactivates a receptor for toxin A of *C. difficile*, secretion of increased levels of secretory IgA and IgA antitoxin A, and competition for attachment sites (Pothoulakis *et al.*, 1993; Qamar *et al.*, 2001; Wilson and Perini, 1988). *S. boulardii* has also been shown to block *C. difficile* adherence to cells in vitro (Tasteyre *et al.*, 2002).

Another systematic review (Hawrelak *et al.*, 2005) focused on the efficacy of LGG versus placebo in the prevention of AAD. MEDLINE, CINAHL, AMED, the Cochrane Controlled Trials Register and the Cochrane Database of Systematic Reviews were searched up to July 2003 using the reported search terms. The reference lists of identified primary studies were searched for further studies. Six RCTs involving 692 participants (including 307 children) met the inclusion criteria. Two of the included studies were for treatment of *H. pylori* infection. Significant statistical heterogeneity of the trials precluded meta-analysis. Four of the six trials revealed a significant reduction in the risk of AAD with coadministration of LGG. One of the trials revealed a reduced number of days with AAD with LGG administration, while one trial failed to demonstrate a benefit of LGG supplementation.

RCTs published subsequently to the publication of the meta-analyses
The evidence from the above-described analyses is indeed very encouraging. Also, a few of some of the more recent trials, which were not included in the meta-analyses, showed encouraging results.

The first RCT involved 87 adult patients who received a fermented milk drink containing LGG, *Lactobacillus acidophilus* La-5, and *Bifidobacterium* Bb-12 (n = 46) or a placebo with heat-killed bacteria (n = 41) for a period of 14 days. Sixty-three patients completed the study according to the protocol. Eight (27.6%) patients in the placebo group and two (5.9%) patients in the experimental group developed AAD (P = 0.035). The risk of AAD was reduced by 79% (RR 0.21, 95% CI 0.05 to 0.93) with ingestion of the fermented milk drink containing the probiotics (Wenus *et al.*, 2008).

The second, randomized, double-blind, placebo-controlled trial involved 135 hospitalized patients (mean age: 74 years) who were taking antibiotics; 113 of these patients were included in the final analysis. This study demonstrated a reduced risk of diarrhoea associated with antibiotic use in the group who consumed a readily available probiotic drink containing *Lactobacillus casei* DN-114 001, *S. thermophilus*, and *L. bulgaricus* twice daily during the course of antibiotics and for one week after the course was finished compared with the placebo group (7/57 (12%) *vs.* 19/56 (34%), odds ratio 0.25, 95% CI 0.07 to 0.85). The absolute risk reduction was 21.6% (6.6% to 36.6%), and the number needed to treat was 5 (3 to 15). No one in the probiotic group and 9/53 (17%) patients in the placebo group had diarrhoea caused by *C. difficile* (P = 0.001). The absolute risk reduction was 17% (7% to 27%), and the number needed to treat was 6 (4 to 14). It was calculated that the cost to prevent one case of diarrhoea was £50 (€74; $100), and it cost £60 (€87.5; $120) to prevent one case of *C. difficile* (Hickson *et al.*, 2007). The limitations of this trial include highly selective inclusion and exclusion criteria (e.g. exclusion of subjects receiving 'high-risk antibiotics') and a quite liberal definition of diarrhoea.

In children, one, recent, double-blind, randomized, placebo-controlled trial evaluated the effectiveness of kefir, a fermented milk similar to yogurt but containing different fermentation microbes, in preventing AAD. This study conducted in 125 children aged 1 to 5 years found no significant difference in the rates of diarrhoea during the 14-day follow-up period in children receiving antibiotics in the kefir group compared to the placebo group (18% *vs.* 21.9%, RR 0.82, 95% CI 0.5 to 1.4) (Merenstein *et al.*, 2009).

7.5.6   *Clostridium difficile*-associated diarrhoea

In contrast, there is only weak or inconclusive evidence from two systematic reviews regarding the effectiveness of probiotic administration for the prevention and treatment of *C. difficile*-associated diarrhoea (see Table 7.3). The authors of the first review concluded that available evidence (all in adults) does not support the administration of probiotics with antibiotics to prevent or treat *C. difficile* diarrhoea (Dendukuri *et al.*, 2005). The conclusions from the second systematic review (with meta-analysis) support probiotic use (McFarland, 2006). However, the latter meta-analysis has been criticized for combining the results from one study on prevention of *C. difficile* diarrhoea with results from five studies on treatment of *C. difficile* diarrhoea. It also has been criticized for pooling data on different probiotics, different conditions and different patient characteristics, as well as some methodological issues, calling for caution in interpreting the conclusions (Dendukuri and Brophy, 2007; Lewis, 2006). In children, in spite of some anecdotal evidence supporting the efficacy of probiotics (Biller *et al.*, 1995; Buts *et al.*, 1993), no RCT investigating such a possibility has been conducted.

Table 7.3 Probiotics in the prevention and treatment of *Clostridium difficile* diarrhoea: results of meta-analyses of randomized controlled trials (RCTs)

Study	Probiotics	Number of RCTs (n)	Measure of effect size	Effect (95% CI)	Number needed to treat (95% CI)
Treatment					
Dendukuri *et al.*, 2005	Various	3 (No data)	No statistical pooling		
McFarland *et al.*, 2006	Various	6 (354)	RR	0.59 (0.4 to 0.85)	8 (6 to 22)
Prevention					
Dendukuri *et al.*, 2005	Various	5	No statistical pooling		
McFarland *et al.*, 2006	*L. acidophilus* plus *B. bifidum*	1 (No data)	RR	0.33 (0.07 to 1.59)	Not significant

In summary, the currently available evidence suggests a beneficial effect of selected probiotics in the prevention of AAD. The use of probiotics with a documented efficacy, in appropriate doses confirmed in controlled trials, is probably acceptable whenever preventing this usually self-limited complication is important. The available data provide evidence that selected probiotics significantly reduce the risk of diarrhoea in patients being treated with antibiotics in general. However, not all antibiotics are likely to be equally selective in causing AAD. The role of probiotics in the prevention and treatment of *C. difficile*-associated diarrhoea remains unclear, particularly in the paediatric population.

7.6   Prebiotics

7.6.1   Prevention of acute gastrointestinal infections

In a large well-designed study performed in infants aged 6 to 12 months (n = 282), Duggan *et al.* (2003) compared the effect of consuming an infant cereal supplemented with oligofructose (0.55 g/15 g cereal) with a nonsupplemented cereal on the prevalence of diarrhoea. There was no difference in the number of diarrhoeal episodes, episodes of severe diarrhoea, or episodes of dysentery between groups who received the supplemented versus the nonsupplemented cereal. No significant difference was found in the mean duration of diarrhoea between groups. During a second part of the same trial that involved 349 subjects, zinc (1 mg/15 g cereal) was added to both the oligofructose-supplemented and control cereals. Likewise, no significant difference was found in the mean duration of diarrhoea between groups.

More recently, Bruzzese *et al.* (2009) evaluated the effect of ingestion of an infant formula containing prebiotic oligosaccharides (short-chain galactooligosaccharides [GOS] plus long-chain fructooligosaccharides [FOS]) compared with a standard infant formula on the incidence of intestinal and respiratory infections in healthy infants. This open, randomized, placebo-controlled trial involved 342 healthy infants with 12 months of follow-up. Compared with the control formula, the use of the prebiotic-supplemented formula was associated with a significant reduction in the incidence of gastroenteritis (0.12 ± 0.04 vs. 0.29 ± 0.05 episodes/child/12 months; $P = 0.015$). In addition, the number of children with one or more episodes of acute diarrhoea was significantly lower in the GOS/FOS group compared with the control group (10/96 *vs.* 26/109, RR 0.44, 95% CI 0.22 to 0.86). These findings regarding the prevention of gastrointestinal infections are promising. However, there are some methodological limitations to the study, including no allocation concealment, no blinding, and no intention-to-treat analysis; this may result in selection, performance, and/or attrition biases and, eventually, may invalidate the results.

One RCT with follow-up at six months (Arslanoglu *et al.*, 2007) and two years (Arslanoglu *et al.*, 2008) found a similar number of episodes of diarrhoea (secondary outcome measure) in the groups of infants who received extensively hydrolyzed whey formula supplemented either with 0.8 g GOS/FOS or maltodextrin as placebo.

7.6.2   Treatment of acute gastrointestinal infections

A double-blind RCT conducted in Bangladeshi children with acute non-cholera diarrhoea revealed no significant improvement in stool output (except on day 7) in the group of children who received partially hydrolyzed guar gum in their oral rehydration solution (ORS) compared to the controls who received ORS alone. However, the total duration of diarrhoea after treatment was significantly reduced in the experimental group compared with the control group (Alam *et al.*, 2000).

Another RCT conducted in 195 Bangladeshi men examined the effect of supplementing ORS with a partially hydrolyzed guar gum on reducing the stool output and duration of diarrhoea in adults with severe cholera. No significant difference was found in mean stool weights during the first and second 24 hours between the experimental and control groups, although some improvement was observed in a subgroup of moderately purging subjects (Alam *et al.*, 2008).

A randomized, double-blind, placebo-controlled, multicentre study (Hoekstra *et al.*, 2004) conducted in 144 boys aged 1 to 36 months evaluated the efficacy of using a mixture of non-digestible carbohydrates as an adjunct to oral rehydration therapy in the treatment of acute infectious diarrhoea associated with mild or moderate dehydration. Intention-to-treat analysis revealed no significant difference for any of the outcomes studied between those receiving the mixture of non-digestible carbohydrates, including soy polysaccharide 25%, α-cellulose 9%, gum arabic 19%, fructooligosaccharides 18.5%, inulin 21.5%, and resistant starch 7%, as an adjunct to oral rehydration therapy and those receiving unsupplemented oral rehydration solution only. In particular, there was no significant difference between groups in the mean 48-hour stool volume, duration of the diarrhoea after randomization, duration of hospital stay, and unscheduled intravenous rehydration episodes. No significant adverse effects were noted.

7.6.3   Prevention of antibiotic-associated diarrhoea

In contrast to probiotics, there is a paucity of data on the use of prebiotics in the prevention of AAD. The only relevant paediatric double-blind RCT (Brunser *et al.*, 2006) involved 140 children (1 to 2 years of age) who were treated with amoxicillin for acute bronchitis. This study revealed no significant difference in the incidence of diarrhoea in children receiving oligofructose and inulin administered in a milk formula (4.5 g/L) for 21 days after completion of antibiotic treatment compared with control formula (10% *vs.* 6%, RR 0.6, 95% CI 0.2 to 1.8). However, compared with controls, children who received the prebiotics administered in the milk formula had increased faecal bifidobacteria early after amoxicillin treatment.

Another RCT conducted in elderly (>65 years of age) patients evaluated whether the incidence of AAD in elderly patients could be reduced by the oral administration of the prebiotic oligofructose. Patients received either oligofructose (12 g/day) while taking broad-spectrum antibiotics for seven days, followed by another seven days of the prebiotic, or placebo. No difference was observed regarding the incidence of diarrhoea, *C. difficile* infection, and duration of hospital stay between groups. However, oligofructose significantly increased faecal bifidobacteria concentrations (Lewis *et al.*, 2005b).

In contrast, in an RCT in which 145 patients in the experimental group continued consumption of oligofructose (12 g /day) for an additional 30 days after the cessation of *C. difficile*-associated diarrhoea, this treatment reduced the relapse rate (8.3% oligofructose *vs.* 34.3% placebo, P < 0.001) and increased faecal bifidobacteria levels (Lewis *et al.*, 2005a).

7.6.4   Traveller's diarrhoea

One RCT examined the effectiveness of the administration of FOS compared with placebo in the prevention of traveller's diarrhoea. The authors reported that the consumption of 10 g of FOS per day for a two-week pre-travel period that was continued during a two-week travel period to high- and medium-risk destinations had no effect on the prevention of traveller's diarrhoea, although it significantly improved the sense of 'well-being' (Cummings, 2001).

A more recent, double-blind, randomized, placebo-controlled trial was conducted in 159 healthy volunteers who travelled for minimum of two weeks to a country of low or high risk for traveller's diarrhoea. Volunteers were randomized to receive a prebiotic GOS mixture or placebo. The results showed significant differences between the prebiotic GOS mixture group and the placebo group in the incidence (P < 0.05) and duration (P < 0.05) of traveller's diarrhoea, as well as in the overall quality of life assessment (P < 0.05) (Drakoularakou *et al.*, 2009).

In summary, clearly a rationale is present for the use of prebiotics. However, the number of controlled trials that have examined the efficacy of administering prebiotics for the prevention or treatment of gastrointestinal infections is limited. Only some specific prebiotics have been evaluated in RCTs. Some studies have demonstrated positive outcomes with prebiotics, while other studies have demonstrated no effect. Thus, no firm conclusions can be made at this stage. Subjects who choose to take prebiotics should be advised to take only the products with documented efficacy.

7.7   Synbiotics

7.7.1   Prevention of diarrhoea

A recent RCT involving 284 infants evaluated the safety, tolerability, and effect on the incidence of diarrhoea of infant formulas containing probiotics only or synbiotics. In this trial, healthy full-term infants were exclusively fed either a control formula or one of three experimental formulas containing the following:

1. *B. longum* BL999 (BL999) plus *Lactobacillus rhamnosus* LPR (LPR),
2. BL999 + LPR + 4 g/L of 90% galactooligosaccharide/10% short-chain fructooligosaccharide (GOS/SCFOS), or
3. BL999 plus *Lactobacillus paracasei* ST11 plus 4 g/L of GOS/SCFOS.

The study products were administered from ≤2 to 16 weeks of age. Infants fed formulas containing either probiotics or synbiotics showed a weight gain similar to those fed a control formula. There was no significant difference between the study groups regarding the incidence of diarrhoea (Chouraqui *et al.*, 2008).

Another RCT evaluated the safety and long-term effects of administering synbiotics to newborn infants. Of 1018 eligible infants, 925 completed the two-year follow-up assessment. The infants received placebo or synbiotic supplementation (LGG and LC705, *Bifidobacterium breve* Bb99, and *Propionibacterium freudenreichii* ssp. *shermanii* JS plus galactooligosaccharides) daily for 6 months after birth. Compared to placebo, synbiotic supplementation failed to prevent diarrhoea; however, episodes of diarrhoea were uncommon (14%) (Kukkonen *et al.*, 2008).

7.7.2   Prevention of antibiotic-associated diarrhoea

Only one RCT (La Rosa *et al.*, 2003) has investigated the effect of synbiotic administration on the prevention of AAD. This double-blind RCT was conducted in 120 children aged 4 months to 15 years. Children received antibiotic treatment (erythromycin, other macrolides, amoxicillin + clavulanic acid) plus either 250 mg of FOS with *Bacillus sporogenes* [named by the authors *L. sporogenes*] or placebo for ten days. Analyses were based on intention to treat. Patients in the intervention group had a lower prevalence of diarrhoea (two liquid or watery stools per 24 h) than those who received the placebo (43% *vs.* 68%, RR 0.6, CI 0.4 to 0.9). The duration of diarrhoea also was reduced in the intervention group compared with the placebo-treated group (0.7 *vs.* 1.6 days, P = 0.002). Study limitations include a relatively small sample size and the use of a not widely accepted definition of diarrhoea, which is usually defined as three (not two as in this study) liquid or watery stools per 24 hours. Also, there was no extended follow-up period. With a lack of robust evidence, no recommendation can be made currently regarding the efficacy of using synbiotics to prevent AAD in the paediatric population.

7.8   Conclusions and future trends

- Functional foods such as probiotics and/or prebiotics have the potential to prevent and treat gastrointestinal infections.
- Not all probiotics and/or prebiotics are equal. The clinical effects and safety of any single probiotic or prebiotic product or combination of probiotics and/or prebiotics should not be extrapolated to other probiotics and/or prebiotics (single or used in combination). The efficacy and safety should be established for each probiotic and/or prebiotic product.
- Regarding probiotics, best documented is the efficacy of probiotics for the treatment of acute gastroenteritis in children. The use of probiotics with proven efficacy and in appropriate doses as an adjunct to rehydration therapy is recommended by some scientific societies.
- Prebiotics and synbiotics have the potential to prevent and treat gastrointestinal infections. Currently, however, the benefits are largely unproven.
- Health professionals and/or patients (or their carers) who choose to use probiotics and/or prebiotics should be advised to take the product that is sufficiently characterized, with clinical efficacy and safety documented in well-designed and conducted trials, at the dose studied and recommended by the manufacturer.
- The use of products with no documented health benefits should be discouraged until data supporting their use are available.
- Probiotics and/or prebiotics are an important field of further research. Further well-conducted clinical studies using validated outcome measures are recommended. Among others, issues to be addressed are to further identify populations that would benefit most from probiotic(s)/prebiotic(s) administration, to determine the most effective dosing schedules, and to address the cost-effectiveness of using probiotics and/or prebiotics for preventing and treating gastrointestinal infections.

7.9   Sources of further information and advice

- International Scientific Association for Probiotics and Prebiotics. http://www.isapp.net/
- European Food Safety Authority. http://www.efsa.europa.eu/

- WGO Practice Guideline – Probiotics and Prebiotics. http://www. worldgastroenterology.org/probiotics-prebiotics.html

7.10   References

Aattour N, Bouras M, Tome D, Marcos A, Lemonnier D (2002), Oral ingestion of lactic-acid bacteria by rats increases lymphocyte proliferation and interferon-gamma production, *Br J Nutr*, **87**, 367–73.

Alam NH, Ashraf H, Sarker SA, Olesen M, Troup J, Salam MA, Gyr N, Meier R (2008), Efficacy of partially hydrolyzed guar gum-added oral rehydration solution in the treatment of severe cholera in adults, *Digestion*, **78**, 24–9.

Alam NH, Meier R, Schneider H, Sarker SA, Bardhan PK, Mahalanabis D, Fuchs GJ, Gyr N (2000), Partially hydrolyzed guar gum-supplemented oral rehydration solution in the treatment of acute diarrhea in children, *J Pediatr Gastroenterol Nutr*, **31**, 503–7.

Allen SJ, Okoko B, Martinez E, *et al.* (2003), Probiotics for treating infectious diarrhoea, *The Cochrane Database of Systematic Reviews* 2003, Issue 4.

Arslanoglu S, Moro GE, Boehm G (2007), Early supplementation of prebiotic oligosaccharides protects formula-fed infants against infections during the first 6 months of life, *J Nutr*, **137**, 2420–4.

Arslanoglu S, Moro GE, Schmitt J, *et al.* (2008), Early dietary intervention with a mixture of prebiotic oligosaccharides reduces the incidence of allergic manifestations and infections during the first two years of life, *J Nutr*, **138**, 1091–5.

Barbut F, Meynard JL, Guiguet M, *et al.* (1997), *Clostridium difficile*-associated diarrhea in HIV infected patients, epidemiology and risk factors, *J Acq Immun Def Synd*, **16**, 176–81.

Bartlett JG, Chang TW, Gurwith M, *et al.* (1978), Antibiotic-associated pseudomembranous colitis due to toxin producing *Clostridia*, *N Engl J Med*, **298**, 531–4.

Bartlett JG, (2002), Antibiotic-associated diarrhea, *N Engl J Med*, **346**, 334–9.

Bernet MF, Brassart D, Nesser JR, Servin AI (1994), *Lactobacillus acidophilus* LA1 binds to human intestinal cell lines and inhibits cell attachment and cell invasion by enterovirulent bacteria, *Gut*, **35**, 483–9.

Biller JA, Katz AJ, Flores AF, Buie TM, Gorbach SL (1995), Treatment of recurrent *Clostridium difficile* colitis with *Lactobacillus* GG, *J Pediatr Gastroenterol Nutr*, **21**, 224–6.

Brunser O, Gotteland M, Cruchet S, *et al.* (2006), Effect of a milk formula with prebiotics on the intestinal microbiota of infants after an antibiotic treatment, *Pediatr Res*, **59**, 451–6.

Bruzzese E, Volpicelli M, Squeglia V, Bruzzese D, Salvini F, Bisceglia M, Lionetti P, Cinquetti M, Iacono G, Amarri S, Guarino A (2009), A formula containing galacto- and fructo-oligosaccharides prevents intestinal and extra-intestinal infections, an observational study, *Clin Nutr*, **28**, 156–61.

Buts JP, Corthier G, Delmee M (1993), *Saccharomyces boulardii* for *Clostridium difficile*-associated enteropathies in infants, *J Pediatr Gastroenterol Nutr*, **16**, 419–25.

Chouraqui JP, Grathwohl D, Labaune JM, *et al.* (2008), Assessment of the safety, tolerance, and protective effect against diarrhea of infant formulas containing mixtures of probiotics or probiotics and prebiotics in a randomized controlled trial, *Am J Clin Nutr*, **87**, 1365–73.

Chouraqui JP, Van Egroo LD, Fichot MC (2004), Acidified milk formula supplemented with *Bifidobacterium lactis*, impact on infant diarrhea in residential care settings, *J Pediatr Gastroenterol Nutr*, **38**, 288–92.

Coconnier MH, Lievin V, Bernet-Camard MF, Hudault S, Servin AL (1997), Antibacterial effect of the adhering human *Lactobacillus acidophilus* strain LB, *Antimicrob Agents Chemother*, **41**, 1046–52.

Committee on Infectious Diseases, American Academy of Pediatrics (2009), Prevention of rotavirus disease, updated guidelines for use of rotavirus vaccine, *Pediatrics*, **123**, 1412–20.

Cremonini F, di Caro S, Nista EC, *et al.* (2002), Meta-analysis, the effect of probiotic administration on antibiotic-associated diarrhea, *Aliment Pharmacol Ther*, **16**, 1461–7.

Cummings JH, Christie S, Cole TJ (2001), A study of fructo oligosaccharides in the prevention of travellers' diarrhoea, *Aliment Pharmacol Ther*, **15**, 1139–45.

Czerucka D, Roux I, Rampal P (1994), *Saccharomyces boulardii* inhibits secretagogue-mediated adenosine 3′, 5′-cyclic monophosphate induction in intestinal cells, *Gastroenterology*, **106**, 65–72.

Davidson JN, Hirsch DC (1976), Bacterial competition as a mean of preventing diarrhea in pigs, *Infect Immun*, **13**, 1773–4.

De Simone C, Ciardi A, Grassi A, Lambert Gardini S, Tzantzoglou S, Trinchieri V, *et al.* (1992), Effect of *Bifidobacterium bifidum* and *Lactobacillus acidophilus* on gut mucosa and peripheral blood B lymphocytes, *Immunopharmacol Immunotoxicol*, **14**, 331–40.

Dendukuri N, Brophy J (2007), Inappropriate use of meta-analysis to estimate efficacy of probiotics, *Am J Gastroenterol*, **102**, 201, author reply 202–204.

Dendukuri N, Costa V, McGregor M, Brophy J (2005), Probiotic therapy for the prevention and treatment of *Clostridium difficile*-associated diarrhea, a systematic review, *CMAJ*, **173**, 167–70.

Drakoularakou A, Tzortzis G, Rastall RA, Gibson GR (2009), A double-blind, placebo-controlled, randomized human study assessing the capacity of a novel galacto-oligosaccharide mixture in reducing travellers' diarrhoea, *Eur J Clin Nutr*, Sep 16.

D'Souza AL, Rajkumar C, Cooke J, Bulpitt CJ (2002), Probiotics in prevention of antibiotic associated diarrhea, meta-analysis *Br Med J*, **324**, 1361–1364.

Duggan C, Penny ME, Hibberd P, *et al.* (2003), Oligofructose-supplemented infant cereal, 2 randomized, blinded, community-based trials in Peruvian infants, *Am J Clin Nutr*, **77**, 937–42.

Elstner CL, Lindsay AN, Book LS, *et al.* (1983), Lack of relationship of *Clostridium difficile* to antibiotic-associated diarrhea in children, *Pediatr Inf Dis*, **2**, 364–6.

FAO/WHO (2002). Joint FAO/WHO Working Group Report on Drafting Guidelines for the Evaluation of Probiotics in Food, London, Ontario, Canada, April 30 and May 1, 2002.

Forchielli ML, Walker WA (2005), The role of gut-associated lymphoid tissue and mucosal defence, *Br J Nutr*, **93**, S41–S48.

Ford-Jones EL, Mindorff CM, Gold R, *et al.* (1990), The incidence of viral-associated diarrhea after admission to a pediatric hospital, *Am J Epidemiol*, **131**, 711–18.

Gibson GR, Roberfroid MB (1995), Dietary modulation of the human colonic microbiota, Introducing the concept of prebiotics, *J Nutr*, **125**, 1401–12.

Goldin BR, Gorbach SL, Saxelin M, Barakat S, Gaultieri L, Salminen S (1992), Survival of *Lactobacillus* species (strain GG) in human gastrointestinal tract, *Dig Dis Sci*, **37**, 121–8.

Gray J, Vesikari T, Van Damme P, *et al.* (2008), Rotavirus, *J Pediatr Gastroenterol Nutr*, **46**(Suppl 2), S24–31.

Guarino A, Albano F, Ashkenazi S, *et al.* (2008a), The ESPGHAN/ESPID Guidelines for the Management of Acute Gastroenteritis in Children in Europe, *J Pediatr Gastroenterol Nutr*, **46**, S81–S184.

Guarino A, Albano F, Ashkenazi S, *et al.* (2008b), European Society for Paediatric Gastroenterology, Hepatology and Nutrition/European Society for Paediatric Infectious Diseases Evidence-based Guidelines for the Management of Acute Gastroenteritis in children in Europe, Executive summary, *J Pediatr Gastroenterol Nutr*, **46**, 619–21.

Guarino A, Albano F, Guandalini S, for the ESPGHAN Working Group on Acute Diarrhea (2001), Oral rehydration solution, toward a real solution, *J Pediatr Gastroenterol Nutr*, **33**, S2–S12.

Hatakka K, Savilahti E, Ponka A, *et al.* (2001), Effect of long term consumption of probiotic milk on infections in children attending day care centres, double blind, randomised trial, *Br Med J*, **322**, 1327–31.

Hawrelak JA, Whitten DL, Myers SP (2005), Is *Lactobacillus rhamnosus* GG effective in preventing the onset of antibiotic-associated diarrhoea, a systematic review, *Digestion*, **72**, 51–6.

Hickson M, D'Souza AL, Muthu N, Rogers TR, Want S, Rajkumar C, Bulpitt CJ (2007), Use of probiotic *Lactobacillus* preparation to prevent diarrhoea associated with antibiotics, randomised double blind placebo controlled trial, *Br Med J*, **335**, 80–4.
Hoekstra JH, Szajewska H, Zikri MA, *et al.* (2004), Oral rehydration solution containing a mixture of non-digestible carbohydrates in the treatment of acute diarrhea, a multicenter randomized placebo controlled study on behalf of the ESPGHAN working group on intestinal infections, *J Pediatr Gastroenterol Nutr*, **39**, 239–45.
Hojsak I, Abdovic S, Szajewska H, Kolacek S, Milosević M, Krznarić Z, Kolacek S (2010a), *Lactobacillus* GG in the prevention of nosocomial gastrointestinal and respiratory tract infections, *Pediatrics*, **125**, 1171–7.
Hojsak I, Snovak N, Abdović S, Szajewska H, Mišak Z, Koláček S (2010b), *Lactobacillus* GG in the prevention of gastrointestinal and respiratory tract infections in children who attend day care centers: a randomized, double-blind, placebo-controlled trial, *Clin Nutr*, **29**, 312–16.
Huang J S, Bousvaros A, Lee JW, *et al.* (2002), Efficacy of probiotic use in acute diarrhea in children, a meta-analysis, *Dig Dis Sci*, **47**, 2625–34.
Isolauri E, Joensuu J, Suomalainen H, Luomala M, Vesikari T (1995), Improved immunogenicity of oral D × RRV reassortant rotavirus vaccine by *Lactobacillus casei* GG, *Vaccine*, **13**, 310–12.
Isolauri E, Majamaa H, Arvola T, Rantala I, Virtanen E, Arvilommi H (1993), *Lactobacillus casei* strain GG reverses increased intestinal permeability induced by cow milk in suckling rats, *Gastroenterology*, **105**, 1643–50.
Johnston BC, Supina AL, Ospina M, Vohra S (2007) Probiotics for the prevention of pediatric antibiotic-associated diarrhea, *Cochrane Database Syst Rev*, 2007 Apr 18, (2), CD004827.
Johnston BC, Supina AL, Vohra S (2006), Probiotics for pediatric antibiotic-associated diarrhea, a meta-analysis of randomized placebo-controlled trials, *CMAJ*, **175**, 377–383, Erratum in *CMAJ* 2006, **175**, 777.
Kaila M, Isolauri E, Soppi E, Virtanen E, Laine S, Arvilommi H (1992), Enhancement of the circulating antibody secreting cell response in human diarrhea by a human *Lactobacillus* strain, *Pediatr Res*, **32**, 141–4.
Kukkonen K, Savilahti E, Haahtela T, *et al.* (2008), Long-term safety and impact on infection rates of postnatal probiotic and prebiotic (synbiotic) treatment, randomized, double-blind, placebo-controlled trial, *Pediatrics*, **122**, 8–12.
La Rosa M, Bottaro G, Gulino N, *et al.* (2003), Prevention of antibiotic-associated diarrhea with *Lactobacillus* sporogens and fructo-oligosaccharides in children, A multicentric double-blind vs placebo study, *Minerva Pediatr*, **55**, 447–52, Italian.
Lewis S, Burmeister S, Brazier J (2005a), Effect of the prebiotic oligofructose on relapse of *Clostridium difficile*-associated diarrhea, a randomized, controlled study, *Clin Gastroenterol Hepatol*, **3**, 442–8.
Lewis S, Burmeister S, Cohen S, Brazier J, Awasthi A (2005b), Failure of dietary oligofructose to prevent antibiotic-associated diarrhoea, *Aliment Pharmacol Ther*, **21**, 469–77.
Lewis S, Response to the article, McFarland LV (2006), Meta-analysis of probiotics for the prevention of antibiotic-associated diarrhea and the treatment of *Clostridium difficile* disease, *Am J Gastroenterol*, **101**, 812–22; *Am J Gastroenterol* (2007), **102**, 201–2.
Lievin-Le Moal V, Amsellem R, Servin AL, Coconnier M-H (2002), *Lactobacillus acidophilus* (strain LB) from the resident adult human gastrointestinal microflora exerts activity against brush border damage promoted by a diarrheagenic *Escherichia coli* in human enterocyte-like cells, *Gut*, **50**, 803–11.
Mack DR, Michail S, Wei S, McDougall L, Hollingsworth MA (1999), Probiotics inhibit enteropathogenic *E. coli* adherence in vitro by inducing intestinal mucin gene expression, *Am J Physiol*, **276**, G941–G950.

Majamaa H, Isolauri E, Saxelin M, Vesikari T (1995), Lactic acid bacteria in the treatment of acute rotavirus gastroenteritis, *J Pediatr Gastroenterol Nutr*, **20**, 333–8.

Mastretta E, Longo P, Laccisaglia A, Balbo L, Russo R (2002), *Lactobacillus* GG and breast feeding in the prevention of rotavirus nosocomial infection, *J Pediatr Gastr Nutr*, **35**, 527–31.

Matson DO, Estes MK (1990), Impact of rotavirus infection at a large pediatric hospital, *J Infect Dis*, **162**, 598–604.

McFarland LV, Surawicz CM, Stamm WE (1990), Risk factors for *Clostridium difficile* carriage and *C, difficile*-associated diarrhea in a cohort of hospitalized patients, *J Infect Dis*, **162**, 678–84.

McFarland LV (2007), Meta-analysis of probiotics for the prevention of traveler's diarrhea, *Travel Med Infect Dis*, **5**, 97–105.

McFarland LV (2006), Meta-analysis of probiotics for the prevention of antibiotic associated diarrhea and the treatment of *Clostridium difficile* disease, *Am J Gastroenterol*, **101**, 812–22.

Merenstein DJ, Foster J, D'Amico F (2009), A randomized clinical trial measuring the influence of kefir on antibiotic-associated diarrhea, the measuring the influence of Kefir (MILK) Study, *Arch Pediatr Adolesc Med*, **163**, 750–4.

Michail S, Abernathy F (2002), *Lactobacillus plantarum* reduces the in vitro secretory respone of intestinal epithelial cells to enteropathogenic *Escherichia coli* infection, *J Pediatr Gastroenterol Nutr*, **35**, 350–5.

Miettinen M, Vuopio-Varkila J, Varkila K (1996), Production of human tumor necrosis factor alpha, interleukin-6 and interleukin-10 is induced by lactic acid bacteria, *Infect Immun*, **64**, 5403–5.

NICE (2009), National Collaborating Centre for Women's and Children's Health, Diarrhoea and vomiting caused by gastroenteritis, Diagnosis, assessment and management in children younger than 5 years, RCOG Press, http://www.nice.org.uk/nicemedia/pdf/CG84FullGuideline.pdf

Oberhelman RA, Gilman RH, Sheen P, Taylor DN, Black RE, Cabrera L, *et al.* (1999), A placebo-controlled trial of *Lactobacillus* GG to prevent diarrhea in undernourished Peruvian children, *J Pediatr*, **134**, 15–20.

Ponce MF, Rial MJ, Alarcon N, *et al.* (1995), Use of a prospectively measured incidence rate of nosocomial diarrhea in an infant/toddler ward as a meaningful quality assessment tool, *Clin Perform Qual Health Care*, **3**, 128–31.

Pothoulakis C, Kelly CP, Joshi MA, *et al.* (1993), *Saccharomyces boulardii* inhibits *Clostridium difficile* toxin A binding and enterotoxicity in rat ileum, *Gastroenterology*, **104**, 1108–15.

Qamar A, Aboudola A, Warny M, *et al.* (2001), *Saccharomyces boulardii* stimulates intestinal immunoglobulin A immune response to *Clostridium difficile* toxin A in mice, *Infect Immun*, **69**, 2762–5.

Rigothier MC, Maccanio J, Gayral P (1994), Inhibitory activity of *Saccharomyces* yeasts on the adhesion of *Entamoeba histolytica* trophozoites to human erythrocytes in vitro, *Parasitol Res*, **80**, 10–5.

Roller M, Rechkemmer G, Watzl B (2004), Prebiotic inulin enriched with oligofructose in combination with the probiotics *Lactobacillus* rhamnosus and *Bifidobacterium* lactis modulates intestinal immune functions in rats, *J Nutr*, **134**, 153–6.

Ruszczyński M, Radzikowski A, Szajewska H (2008), Clinical trial, effectiveness of *Lactobacillus* rhamnosus (strains E/N, Oxy and Pen) in the prevention of antibiotic-associated diarrhoea in children, *Aliment Pharmacol Ther*, **28**, 154–61.

Saavedra JM, Bauman NA, Oung I, Perman JA, Yolken RH (1994), Feeding of *Bifidobacterium bifidum* and *Streptococcus thermophilus* to infants in hospital for prevention of diarrhea and shedding of rotavirus, *Lancet*, **344**, 1046–9.

Sazawal S, Hiremath G, Dhingra U, Malik P, Deb S, Black RE (2006), Efficacy of probiotics in prevention of acute diarrhoea, a meta-analysis of masked, randomised, placebo-controlled trials, *Lancet Infect Dis*, **6**, 374–82.

Schrezenmeir J, de Vrese M (2001), Probiotics, prebiotics, and synbiotics – approaching a definition, *Am J Clin Nutr*, **73**(2 Suppl), 361S–364S.

Silva M, Jacobus NV, Deneke C, Gorbach SL (1987), Antimicrobial substance from a human *Lactobacillus* strain, *Antimicrob Agents Chemother*, **31**, 1231–3.

Soriano-Gabarró M, Mrukowicz J, Vesikari T, Verstraeten T (2006), Burden of rotavirus disease in European Union countries, *Pediatr Infect Dis J*, **25**(1 Suppl), S7–S11.

Szajewska H, Kotowska M, Mrukowicz J, Armanska M, Mikolajczyk W (2001), *Lactobacillus* GG in prevention of diarrhea in hospitalized children, *J Pediatr*, **138**, 361–5.

Szajewska H, Mrukowicz J (2005), Meta-analysis, non-pathogenic yeast *Saccharomyces boulardii* in the prevention of antibiotic-associated diarrhoea, *Aliment Pharmacol Ther*, **22**, 365–72.

Szajewska H, Mrukowicz J (2001), Probiotics in the treatment and prevention of acute infectious diarrhea in infants and children, a systematic review of published randomized, double-blind, placebo controlled trials, *J Pediatr Gastroenterol Nutr*, **33**, S17–S25.

Szajewska H, Ruszczynski M, Radzikowski A (2006), Probiotics in the prevention of antibiotic-associated diarrhea in children, a meta-analysis of randomized controlled trials, *J Pediatr*, **149**, 367–72.

Szajewska H, Skórka, A, Dylag M (2007a), Meta-analysis, *Saccharomyces boulardii* for treating acute diarrhoea in children, *Aliment Pharmacol Ther*, **25**, 257–64.

Szajewska H, Skórka A, Ruszczyński M, Gieruszczak-Białek D (2007b), Meta-analysis, *Lactobacillus* GG for treating acute diarrhoea in children, *Aliment Pharmacol Ther*, **25**, 871–81.

Szajewska H, Skórka A (2009), *Saccharomyces boulardii* for treating acute gastroenteritis in children, updated meta-analysis of randomized controlled trials, *Aliment Pharmacol Ther*, **30**, 955–63.

Szymański H, Armańska M, Kowalska-Duplaga K, Szajewska H (2008), Bifidobacterium longum PL03, *Lactobacillus* rhamnosus KL53A, and *Lactobacillus* plantarum PL02 in the prevention of antibiotic-associated diarrhea in children, a randomized controlled pilot trial, *Digestion*, **78**, 13–17.

Takahashi O, Noguchi Y, Omata F, Tokuda Y, Fukui T (2007), Probiotics in the prevention of traveler's diarrhea, meta-analysis, *J Clin Gastroenterol*, **41**, 336–7.

Tankanov RM, Ross MB, Ertel IJ, Dickinson DG, McCormick LS, Garfinkel JF (1990), Double blind, placebo-controlled study of the efficacy of Lactinex in the prophylaxis of amoxicillin-induced diarrhea, *DICP, Ann Pharm*, **24**, 382–4.

Tasteyre A, Barc MC, Karjalainen T, *et al.* (2002), Inhibition of in vitro cell adherence of *Clostridium difficile* by *Saccharomyces boulardii*, *Microbiol Pathogens*, **32**, 219–25.

Thibault H, Aubert-Jacquin C, Goulet O (2004), Effects of long-term consumption of a fermented infant formula (with *Bifidobacterium breve* c50 and *Streptococcus thermophilus* 065) on acute diarrhea in healthy infants, *J Pediatr Gastroenterol Nutr*, **39**, 147–52.

Turck D, Bernet JP, Marx J, *et al.* (2003), Incidence and risk factors of oral antibiotic-associated diarrhea in an outpatient pediatric population, *J Pediatr Gastroenterol Nutr*, **37**, 22–6.

Van Niel C, Feudtner C, Garrison MM, Christakis DA (2002), *Lactobacillus* therapy for acute infectious diarrhea in children, a meta-analysis, *Pediatrics*, **109**, 678–84.

Vanderhoof JA, Whitney DB, Antonson DL, Hanner TL, Lupo JV, Young RJ (1999), *Lactobacillus* GG in the prevention of antibiotic-associated diarrhea in children, *J Pediatrics*, **135**, 564–8.

Vesikari T, Van Damme P, Giaquinto C, *et al.* (2008), European Society for Paediatric Infectious Diseases/European Society for Paediatric Gastroenterology, Hepatology, and Nutrition evidence-based recommendations for rotavirus vaccination in Europe, *J Pediatr Gastroenterol Nutr*, **46**(Suppl 2), S38–48.

Walker WA (2000), Role of nutrients and bacterial colonisation in the development of intestinal host defense, *J Pediatr Gastroenterol Nutr*, **30**(suppl), S2–7.

Watzl B, Girrbach S, Roller M (2005), Inulin, oligofructose and immunomodulation, *Br J Nutr*, **93**, S49–S55.

Weizman Z, Asli G, Alsheikh A (2005), Effect of a probiotic infant formula on infections in child care centers, comparison of two probiotic agents, *Pediatrics*, **115**, 5–9.

Wenus C, Goll R, Loken EB, Biong AS, Halvorsen DS, Florholmen J (2008), Prevention of antibiotic-associated diarrhoea by a fermented probiotic milk drink, *Eur J Clin Nutr*, **62**, 299–301.

Wilson KH, Perini I (1988), Role of competition for nutrients in suppression of *Clostridium difficile* by the colonic microflora, *Infect Immunol*, **56**, 2610–14.

Zapolska-Downar D, Siennicka A, Kaczmarczyk M, *et al.* (2004), Butyrate inhibits cytokine-induced VCAM-1 and ICAM-1 expression in cultured endothelial cells, the role of NF-kappaB and PPARalpha, *J Nutr Biochem*, **15**, 220–8.

8

Functional foods and coronary heart disease (CHD)

Julie A. Lovegrove and Kim G. Jackson, University of Reading, UK

Abstract: Public health strategies for reducing the risk of coronary heart disease (CHD) have focused on lowering plasma lipids, particularly cholesterol levels. One approach is to supplement the diet with probiotics, prebiotics and/or synbiotics. These functional foods have been proposed to improve lipid profiles and glycaemic control by promoting the growth of selective health-promoting gut bacteria and the consequence of their metabolic by-products. This chapter reviews the effects, and possible mechanisms, of probiotics in the form of fermented milk products and lactic acid bacteria, non-digestible fermentable prebiotics and synbiotics on circulating lipaemia and glycaemia in humans.

Key words: probiotics, prebiotics, synbiotics, coronary heart disease, glucose, lipids, lactic acid bacteria, short chain fatty acids, inulin.

8.1   Introduction

Cardiovascular disease (CVD), which comprises coronary heart disease (CHD) and stroke, is one of the major causes of death in adults in the Western world. Although there has been a trend over the past 25 years towards a reduction in the rates of CHD in the major industrialised nations (including the USA, Australia and the UK) due to better health screening, drug treatment, smoking and dietary advice, there has been an alarming increase in CHD in the Ukraine, Russian Federation and Kazakhstan.[1]

CHD is a condition in which the main coronary arteries supplying the heart are no longer able to supply sufficient blood and oxygen to the heart muscle (myocardium). The main cause of the reduced flow is an accumulation of plaques, mainly in the intima of arteries, a disease known as atherosclerosis. This is a slow, but progressive disease which usually begins in childhood, but does not usually manifest itself until later life. Depending on the rate of narrowing of the arteries and its ultimate severity, four syndromes may occur during the progression of

CHD. These include angina pectoris, unstable angina pectoris, myocardial infarction and sudden death. Angina pectoris literally means a 'strangling sensation in the chest' and is often provoked by physical activity or stress. This pain, which often radiates from the chest to the left arm and neck, is caused by reduced blood flow in the coronary artery but this pain fades quite quickly when the patient is rested. Unstable angina pectoris occurs as the condition worsens and pain is experienced not only during physical activity but also during rest. This type of angina is thought to involve rupture or fissuring of a fixed lesion, which when untreated leads to an acute myocardial infarction. The condition is responsible for a large proportion of deaths from CHD and occurs as a result of prolonged occlusion of the coronary artery leading to death of some of the heart muscle. Disturbances to the contraction of the heart can lead to disruption in the electrical contraction of heart muscle and the heart may go into an uncoordinated rhythm (ventricular fibrillation) or may stop completely. Sudden death from a severe myocardial infarction occurs within one hour of the attack and is generally associated with advanced atherosclerosis.

A number of risk factors known to predispose an individual to CHD have been categorised into those which are not modifiable, such as age, gender, race and family history and those which are modifiable such as hyperlipidaemia (high levels of lipids (fat) in the blood), hypertension (high blood pressure), obesity, diet, cigarette smoking and lack of exercise. Epidemiological studies examining CHD risks in different populations have observed a positive correlation between an individual's fasting cholesterol level, especially elevated levels of low-density lipoprotein cholesterol (LDL-C), and development of CHD.[2] Low levels of high-density lipoprotein cholesterol (HDL-C) have been shown to be another risk factor for CHD since an inverse relationship exists with CHD development. This lipoprotein is involved in reverse cholesterol transport, carrying cholesterol from cells in the periphery to the liver for removal from the body, and a low level of HDL-C is thought to reflect an impairment in this process.

Elevated levels of triacylglycerol (TAG; a major fat in the blood) in both the fasted and fed (postprandial) state have been demonstrated to be associated with CHD in a number of observational studies.[3] More recently, raised postprandial TAG has been reported to be an independent risk factor for CHD and more discriminatory than fasting TAG.[4,5] The atherogenic lipoprotein phenotype (ALP) and the metabolic syndrome describe a collection of both classical and non-classical risk factors which predispose an apparently healthy individual to an increased CHD risk.[6,7] The lipid abnormalities of these conditions are discussed in more detail in section 8.3.3. The development of techniques by which to characterise the LDL subclass of individuals with CHD and those without CHD has enabled the prevalence of those with ALP to be identified in the population. Heritability studies have revealed that 50% of the variability in expression is due to genetic factors, with the remainder being associated with environmental influences such as diet, smoking and a sedentary lifestyle.

Individuals with CHD and those with a high risk of developing the condition are treated in a number of ways to help lower their total cholesterol, LDL-C and

TAG concentrations whilst elevating their HDL-C. Many lines of evidence suggest that adverse dietary habits are a contributory factor in CHD and so the first line of treatment for individuals with moderately raised cholesterol (5.0–6.5 mmol/l) and/or TAG (1.5–2.2 mmol/l) levels is to modify their diet. This is implemented by reducing the percentage dietary energy derived from fat to approximately 30%, with a reduction of saturated fatty acids (SFAs) to 10% of the dietary energy derived from fat. Candidate fats for the replacement of a large proportion of SFAs include polyunsaturated fatty acids (PUFAs) of the *n*-6 (linoleic) series and monounsaturated fatty acids (MUFAs). Although both PUFAs (*n*-6 series) and MUFAs have both been shown to decrease total cholesterol and LDL-C levels, MUFAs have also been shown to maintain or increase HDL-C concentrations when they are used to substitute SFAs compared with *n*-6 PUFAs. When added to the diet, PUFAs of the *n*-3 series (eicosapentaenoic acid (EPA) and docosahexaenoic acid (DHA)) have been shown to reduce plasma TAG levels in both the fed and fasted states and reduce thrombosis, but they do not usually reduce total and LDL-C levels.

Individuals with total cholesterol levels above 6.5 mmol/l and/or TAG levels greater than 2.2 mmol/l require not only dietary modification but also lipid lowering drugs to help reduce their disorder. Drugs which are available are effective in a number of ways, including:

- enhanced LDL clearance (e.g. cholestyramine) and hydroxy-methyl-glutaryl CoA (HMG-CoA) reductase inhibition (e.g. simvasatin and atorvastatin);
- reduced synthesis of very low density lipoprotein (VLDL) and LDL (e.g. nicotinic acid);
- enhanced VLDL clearance (e.g. benzafibrate).

Fenofibrate, has been shown not only to reduce cholesterol and TAG levels, but also increases HDL-C concentrations and is able to shift the LDL class profile away from the more atherogenic small dense LDL (LDL-III). These drugs are more aggressive and although they cause greater reductions in lipid levels compared with dietary modification, they are often associated with unpleasant side-effects. Therefore, this supports the need for effective dietary strategies which can reduce circulating lipid levels in both the fed and fasted state and which offer long-term efficacy comparable with most effective drug treatments. One dietary strategy which has been proposed to benefit the lipid profile, involves the supplementation of the diet with probiotics, prebiotics and synbiotics which are mechanisms to improve the health of the host by supplementation and/or fortification of certain health-promoting gut bacteria.

A 'probiotic' is a live microbial feed supplement which beneficially affects the host animal by improving its intestinal microbial balance and are generally fermented milk products containing lactic acid bacteria such as bifidobacteria and/or lactobacilli. The putative health benefits of probiotics include improved resistance to gastrointestinal infections, reduction in total cholesterol and TAG levels and stimulation of the immune system.[8] A number of mechanisms have been proposed to explain their putative lipid-lowering capacity and these include a 'milk factor' which has been thought to inhibit HMG-CoA reductase and the assimilation of cholesterol by certain bacteria.

A 'prebiotic' is a non-viable component of the diet that reaches the colon in an intact form and which is selectively fermented by colon bacteria such as bifidobacteria and lactobacilli. The term prebiotic refers to non-digestible oligosaccharides derived from plants and also synthetically produced oligosaccharides. Animal studies have shown that dietary supplementation with prebiotics markedly reduced circulating TAG and to a lesser extent cholesterol concentrations. The generation of short chain fatty acids (SCFAs) during fermentation of the prebiotic by the gut microbiota has been proposed to be one of the mechanisms responsible for their lipid lowering effects via inhibition of enzymes involved in *de novo* lipogenesis. Of the human studies conducted to date, there have been inconsistent findings with respect to changes in lipid levels, although on the whole there have been favourable outcomes.

A combination of a prebiotic and a probiotic, termed a 'synbiotic', is receiving attention at present since this association is thought to improve the survival of the probiotic bacteria in the colon. However, further well-controlled nutrition trials are required to investigate the mechanisms of action and effects of probiotics, prebiotics and synbiotics.

Over the past ten years, manufacturers in the USA and Europe have been exploring the commercial opportunities for foods which contain health-promoting food ingredients (probiotics, prebiotic and synbiotics). Issues considered important to the continuing development of the growing market include safety, consumer education, price and appropriate health claims. Most popular of the food products marketed have been probiotics incorporated into dairy products. However, with the increasing interest in prebiotics, a more diverse food market has been opened up since prebiotics can be incorporated into many long-life foods ranging from bread to ice-cream. Although there is increasing interest in the use of probiotics, prebiotics and synbiotics as supplements to the diet, there is a need to ensure claims for these products are based on carefully conducted human trials, which exploit up-to-date methodologies.

8.2   Coronary heart disease and risk factors

Diseases of the circulatory system account for an appreciable proportion of total morbidity and mortality in adults throughout the world. In 2006, CVD accounted for 35% of all deaths in the United Kingdom, half of these deaths were from CHD (48%) and more than a quarter from stroke (28%).[1] The rates of mortality due to CVD throughout the world vary. For example, a recent review of heart disease and stroke statistics by the American Heart Association has indicated in men aged 35–74 years, the international CVD death rates (per 100 000 population) varied from 149.8 in France (2006) to 1555.2 in the Russian Federation (2002).[9]

Figure 8.1 shows trends in CHD standardised mortality rates for men aged 25–74 years in selected countries in the European Union.[10] Rates in the majority

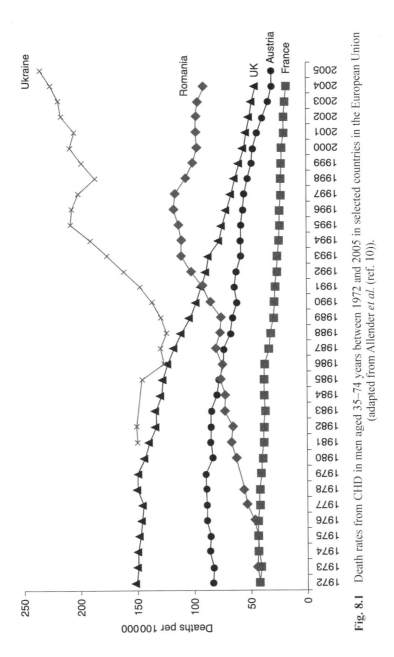

Fig. 8.1 Death rates from CHD in men aged 35–74 years between 1972 and 2005 in selected countries in the European Union (adapted from Allender *et al.* (ref. 10)).

of countries are reducing, but the decline in CHD mortality in the UK began later than in Austria and Denmark. However in the Ukraine, rates of CHD are increasing dramatically, which is in contrast to many other parts of Europe. Improved surgical procedures, more extensive use of cholesterol-lowering drugs and other medication, a reduction in smoking and increased health screening are in part responsible for this downturn. In addition changes in diet, and especially in the type of fat consumed, may also have had a beneficial impact on disease incidence.

8.2.1   Pathology of coronary heart disease development

The underlying basis for clinical CVD is a combination of atherosclerosis and thrombosis. Atherosclerosis is a condition in which the arterial lining is thickened in places by raised plaques as a result of excessive accumulation of modified lipids, and of the proliferation and migration of smooth muscle cells from deeper layers of the arterial wall. The atherosclerotic plaque usually develops at a point of minor injury in the arterial wall. Tissue macrophages (a type of white blood cell) are attracted to this point of damage and engulf and accumulate LDL particles from the blood. Studies have shown that LDL particles that have become oxidised are more likely to be taken up and cause cholesterol accumulation in macrophages. The cholesterol-loaded macrophages are transformed into lipid-laden foam cells, which remain in the arterial wall. At a later stage, the plaque becomes sclerosed and calcified, hence the term 'hardening of the arteries'.

Formation of an atherosclerotic plaque can occlude one or more of the arteries, mainly the coronary and cerebral arteries, resulting in CHD or a stroke, respectively. In addition a superimposed thrombus or clot may further occlude the artery. An example of an artery which has atherosclerotic lesions and has been completely occluded by a thrombus is shown in Fig. 8.2. Blood clot formation is in part determined by a release of eicosanoids from platelets and the vessel walls. PUFA released from platelet membranes are metabolised into thromboxane (an eicosanoid) which stimulate platelet aggregation and vasoconstriction. Simultaneously, the vessel walls also release PUFA which are converted to prostacyclins (antagonistic eicosanoids), leading to an inhibition of platelet aggregation and vasodilation. The balance between production of thromboxane and prostacyclin, and the relative potencies of these two eicosanoids, will determine the extent of the blood clot formed.

Two major clinical conditions are associated with these processes: angina pectoris and coronary thrombosis or myocardial infarction. Angina pectoris is characterised by pain and discomfort in the chest, which is brought on by exertion and stress. It results from a reduction or temporary block in the blood flow through the coronary artery to the heart and seldom lasts for more than 15 minutes. A coronary thrombosis results from prolonged total occlusion of the artery, which causes infarct or death of some of the heart muscle and is associated with prolonged and usually excruciating central chest pain.

A variety of cells and lipids are involved in arterial thrombus, including lipoproteins, cholesterol, TAG, platelets, monocytes, endothelial cells, fibroblasts

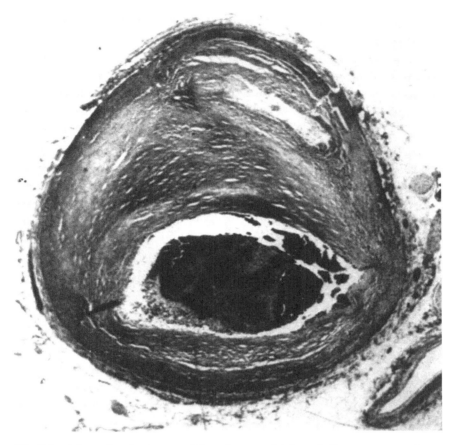

Fig. 8.2   Atherosclerotic plaque and thrombus completely occluding a coronary artery.

and smooth muscle cells. Nutrition may influence the development of CHD by modifying one or more of these factors and this will be discussed in more detail in section 8.4. For the purposes of this chapter the disease of the circulatory system that will be addressed is CHD, with little discussion of other CVD such as strokes.

8.2.2   Risk factors for the development of coronary heart disease

CHD is a multifaceted condition which has no single cause. The term 'risk factor' is used extensively, and often very loosely, to describe features of lifestyle and behaviour, as well as physical activity and biochemical attributes, which predict the likelihood of developing disease. Potential risk factors are continually being refined as research into the aetiology of CHD progresses. The known risk factors for development of CHD can be categorised into those that cannot be modified, those that can be changed, those associated with disease states and those related to geographic distribution, as shown in Table 8.1.

Some risk factors have a greater influence on CHD development than others. It has been demonstrated that there is a strong and consistent relationship between total plasma cholesterol and CHD risk.[11,12] The positive association is largely confined to the LDL fraction, which transports about 70% of cholesterol in the blood. In a large prospective study published in 1986, a five-fold difference in CHD mortality, over a range of plasma cholesterol levels, was observed in the US population.[11] In a large meta-analysis of individual data from 61 prospective studies with 55 000 vascular deaths it was concluded that total cholesterol was positively associated with ischaemic heart disease in both middle and old age and at all blood pressure levels.[12] In a cholesterol-lowering drug trial in a healthy population, a reduction of 20% and 26% in total and LDL-C respectively was associated with a 31% reduction in the five-year incidence of myocardial infarction and CHD death.[13] It is this relationship between the plasma cholesterol levels and its link with CHD, which forms the basis of most dietary guidelines, which recommend reductions in total fat and SFA intakes. There is at present an obesity epidemic within the Western and developing world, with many proposed

Table 8.1   Risk factors for the development of coronary heart disease

Unmodifiable	Being male
	Increasing age
	Genetic traits (including lipid metabolism abnormalities)
	Body build
	Ethnic origin
Modifiable	Cigarette smoking
	Some hyperlipidaemias (increased plasma cholesterol and triacylglycerol)
	Low levels of high-density lipoprotein (HDL)
	Obesity
	Hypertension
	Low physical activity
	Increased thrombosis (ability to clot)
	Stress
	Alcohol consumption
	Diet
Diseases	Diabetes (glucose intolerance)
Geographic	Climate and season: cold weather
	Soft drinking water

initiatives to reduce this serious global challenge. Many studies have reported an association between obesity with chronic disease. A meta-analysis of 57 prospective studies including 900 000 adults confirmed that body mass index (BMI) above 25 kg/m^2 is a strong predictor of vascular disease and is probably largely causal.[14]

If an individual presented with any one, or a combination of, risk factors it is not inevitable that that person will suffer from CHD. The ability to predict the occurrence of a myocardial infarction in individuals is fraught with complications. An obese, middle-aged man, who suffers from diabetes, consumes a high-fat diet, smokes 40 cigarettes a day and has a stressful job, may never suffer from CHD; whereas a slim, physically active, non-smoker who consumes a low-fat diet may die from a myocardial infarct prematurely. Despite this anomaly, individuals and populations are deemed at increasing risk of CHD according to the severity and number of identified risk factors (Table 8.2).[15,16]

The purpose of relative risk scores is in prediction, as it clearly contains factors that cannot be modified. However, for the purpose of intervention, one must go beyond the factors used to predict risk and consider issues such as diet, body weight, physical activity and stress (factors not used in the scoring system), as well as blood pressure and cigarette smoking, which are taken into account. General population dietary recommendations have been provided by a number of bodies which are aimed at reducing the incidence and severity of CHD within the population. Those specifically related to dietary factors are discussed in detail in section 8.4.

Table 8.2 Hazard ratios (with 95% confidence intervals) for 30-year risk of CVD (includes coronary death, myocardial infarction and fatal and non-fatal stroke) in adults

Variables	30-Year risk model
Male sex	1.72 (1.44, 2.05)
Age	2.08 (1.88, 2.31)
Systolic blood pressure	1.26 (1.16, 1.37)
Antihypertensive treatment	1.48 (1.10, 2.00)
Smoking	2.04 (1.74, 2.38)
Diabetes mellitus	2.42 (1.77, 3.31)
Total cholesterol	1.32 (1.22, 1.43)
HDL cholesterol	0.80 (0.73, 0.87)
Body mass index	1.10* (1.00, 1.20)

Notes: Hazard ratios for continuous risk factors are given per one-standard-deviation increase in the natural logarithm. All $P \leq 0.01$ except as notes. $*P = 0.04$.

Source: adapted from Pencina et al.[16]

8.3   Relevant lipid particles

8.3.1   Plasma lipoprotein metabolism

Plasma lipoproteins are macromolecules representing complexes of lipids such as TAG, cholesterol and phospholipids, as well as one or more specific proteins referred to as apoproteins. They are involved in the transport of water-insoluble nutrients throughout the blood stream from their site of absorption or synthesis, to peripheral tissue. For the correct targeting of lipoproteins to sites of metabolism, the lipoproteins rely heavily on apoproteins associated with their surface coat.

The liver and intestine are the primary sites of lipoprotein synthesis and the two major transported lipid components, TAG and cholesterol, follow two separate fates. TAGs are shuttled primarily to adipose tissue for storage, and to muscle, where the fatty acids are oxidised for energy. Cholesterol, in contrast, is continuously shuttled among the liver, intestine and extrahepatic tissues by HDL.[17] Human lipoproteins are divided into five major classes according to their flotation density (Table 8.3). The density of the particles is inversely related to their sizes, reflecting the relative amounts of low-density, non-polar lipid and high-density surface protein present. The two largest lipoproteins contain mainly TAG within their core structures. These are chylomicrons (CMs), secreted by the enterocytes (cells of the small intestine), and VLDL, secreted by the hepatocytes (liver cells). Intermediate-density lipoprotein (IDL) contains appreciable amounts of both TAG and cholesterol esters in their core. The two smallest classes, LDL and HDL, contain cholesterol

Table 8.3   Structure and function of lipoproteins

Lipoprotein	Structural apoproteins	Apoproteins attached	Function
CM	B-48	A-I, A-IV, C-I, C-II and C-III	Carries exogenous TAG from gut to adipose tissue, muscle and liver
CM remnant	B-48	C-I, C-II, C-III and E	Carries exogenous cholesterol to the liver and periphery
VLDL (VLDL$_1$ and VLDL$_2$)	B-100	C-I, C-II, C-III and E	Carries endogenous TAG to the periphery
IDL	B-100	E	Carries endogenous cholesterol to the periphery
LDL	B-100	–	Carries cholesterol to the liver and periphery
HDL$_2$ and HDL$_3$	A-I and A-II	C-I, C-II, C-III, E, LCAT and CETP	Reverse cholesterol transport

Note: CM, chylomicron; VLDL, very low density lipoprotein; IDL, intermediate-density lipoprotein; LDL, low-density lipoprotein; HDL, high-density lipoprotein; LCAT, lecithin cholesterol acyltransferase; CETP, cholesterol ester transfer protein.

Source: adapted from Erkelens.[171]

esters in their core structures and the mature forms of these particles are not secreted directly from the liver but are produced by metabolic processes within the circulation. LDL are produced as end products of the metabolism of VLDL, whereas components of HDL are secreted with CMs and VLDL. The lipid metabolic pathways can be divided into exogenous and endogenous cycle, which are responsible for the transport of dietary and hepatically derived lipids respectively.[18]

Exogenous pathway
Following the digestion of dietary fat in the small intestine, long chain fatty acids are absorbed by the enterocyte. The nascent CM particle consists of a core of TAG (84–89% of the mass) and cholesterol ester (3–5%) and on the surface, free cholesterol (1–2%), phospholipids (7–9%) and apoproteins (1.5–2.5%).[19] Following secretion, the TAG component of the CM particle is hydrolysed by lipoprotein lipase (LPL) bound to the luminal surface of the endothelial cells in adipose tissue and muscle. Approximately 70–90% of the TAG is removed to produce a cholesterol ester-rich lipoprotein particle termed a CM remnant.[20] As the core of the CM remnant particle becomes smaller, surface materials, phospholipids, cholesterol and apoproteins are transferred to HDL to maintain particle stability. Uptake of these particles probably requires interaction with hepatic lipase (HL) which is situated on the surface of the liver. HL further hydrolyses the TAG and phospholipid components of the CM remnant before uptake by a receptor mediated process in the liver.[21] The remnants are endocytosed and catabolised in lysosomes from which cholesterol can enter metabolic pathways in hepatocytes, including excretion into the bile (Fig. 8.3).

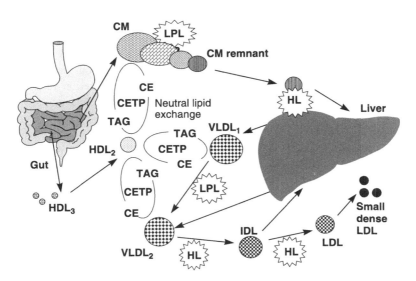

Fig. 8.3   Simplified overview of lipoprotein metabolism showing the inter-relationships between the exogenous and endogenous pathways.

Endogenous pathway
VLDL provides a pathway for the transport of TAG from the liver to the peripheral circulation. Two subclasses of VLDL are released from the liver, $VLDL_1$ (large TAG-rich lipoprotein) and $VLDL_2$ (smaller, denser particles). LPL in the capillary bed extracts TAG from the secreted $VLDL_1$ but less efficiently when compared with CMs.[22] LDL receptors on the surface of the liver, recognise the $VLDL_2$ particles and mediate the endocytosis of a fraction of these particles. Prolonged residency of some VLDL particles in the plasma results in further metabolism by LPL, and to some extent HL, to form the higher-density IDL. HL, on the surface of hepatocytes, further hydrolyses IDL with eventual formation of LDL.[23] LDL is a heterogeneous population consisting of larger LDL species (LDL-I and LDL-II subclass) and smaller denser LDL particles (LDL-III). LDL can be taken up by LDL receptors present on the surface of hepatocytes and on extrahepatic cells.

Reverse cholesterol transport
A function of HDL is to trigger the flux of cholesterol from peripheral cells and from membranes undergoing turnover to the liver for excretion. The process of reverse cholesterol transport is mediated by an enzyme, lecithin cholesterol acyltransferase (LCAT), bound to species of HDL particles. It acts by trapping cholesterol into the core of the nascent HDL following interaction of this particle with a cell surface protein. The cholesterol is transferred to HDL_3, which in turn is converted to HDL_2. This particle can follow one of two pathways (direct or indirect) to deliver the cholesterol to the liver.[24] In the direct pathway, the HDL_2 is removed via receptor mediated endocytosis by the LDL receptor or via selective uptake of cholesterol ester from the HDL particle by the liver. The cholesterol ester transfer protein (CETP), is involved in the indirect pathway and transfers cholesterol ester to lower density lipoproteins (CMs and VLDL), in return for TAG, and is followed by their uptake by the liver (neutral lipid exchange) (Fig. 8.3).

The balance between the forward (exogenous and endogenous pathways) and the reverse pathway, which is tightly regulated by the secretion rates of the lipoproteins, determines the concentration of cholesterol in the plasma.

8.3.2   Classical lipid risk factors in coronary heart disease
Many epidemiological studies have shown a positive correlation between fasting total cholesterol levels, especially LDL-C levels and CHD mortality.[2] Accumulation of LDL in the plasma leads to a deposition of cholesterol in the arterial wall, a process which involves oxidative modification of the LDL particles. The oxidised LDL is taken up by macrophages which eventually become foam cells and forms the basis of the early atherosclerotic plaque. The role of cholesterol-lowering as a public health strategy in the primary prevention of CVD is unequivocally supported by a prospective meta-analysis of data from 90,056 participants in 14 randomised control trials of statins.[25] After one year of treatment, LDL-C concentrations were reduced by approximately 1 mmol/l which equated

to a 19% reduction in coronary mortality. The maintenance of a 1 mmol/l reduction in LDL-C for a period of five years is suggested to contribute to a 23% reduction in major coronary events.

HDL-C levels may influence the relationship between total cholesterol levels and CVD risk. A strong inverse relationship between fasting plasma HDL-C and the risk of development of CHD has been reported.[26] On average, HDL-C levels are higher in women than in men. Factors which may lead to reduced HDL-C levels include smoking, low physical activity and diabetes mellitus; whereas those which increase levels include moderate alcohol consumption. The Münster Heart Study, carried out between 1979 and 1991, investigated CVD risk factors, stroke and mortality in people at work. Examination of fasting lipid parameters at the beginning of the study and with a follow-up six to seven years later, demonstrated that HDL-C concentrations were significantly lower in the group with major coronary events compared to the group which was free of such coronary events. Low HDL-C levels are thought to reflect a compromised pathway for the excretion of cholesterol (reverse cholesterol transport) and have been associated with a five-fold increase in risk of CHD compared with normal HDL-C values.[27]

Currently, the total to HDL-C ratio is considered to be the most sensitive biomarker of CVD risk.[12,28] Findings from the follow up of 302 430 participants (without initial vascular disease) from 68 long-term prospective studies mainly conducted in Europe and North America, have also suggested that the lipid assessment to determine CVD risk could be simplified to the measurement of either total or HDL-C.[29]

8.3.3 Non-classical risk factors
Elevated fasting and postprandial TAG levels
Almost all of the epidemiological evidence for CHD risk has been determined from fasting lipoprotein concentrations, obtained following a 12-hour overnight fast. However, individuals spend a large proportion of the day in the postprandial state when the lipid transport system is challenged by fat-containing meals. The magnitude and duration of postprandial TAG concentrations following a fat load has been correlated with the risk of development of CHD. This relationship has been shown in patients with CHD who show a more pronounced and prolonged TAG response following a meal compared with matched people without CHD, even though both groups showed similar fasting TAG concentrations.[3] The strength of the association between TAG levels and CHD has been demonstrated in a number of observational studies.[30] In 2007, two prospective cohort studies conducted in 26 509 women in the US[4] and 13 981 adults in Denmark[5] have shown elevated non-fasting TAG concentrations to be an independent predictor of CVD risk and more discriminatory than fasting TAG.[4] In the Copenhagen Heart Study, non-fasting TAG levels of ≥ 5, 4–4.99, 3–3.99, 2–2.99, 1–1.99 mmol/l versus < 1 mmol/l predicting a 16.8-, 5.1-, 3.9-, 4.4-, and 2.2-fold, increase in risk of myocardial infarction in females, with equivalent values in males of 4.6-, 3.3-, 3.6-, 2.3-, and 1.6-fold respectively.[5]

Elevated levels chylomicrons and chylomicron remnants

The development of specific methods to differentiate between the exogenous and endogenous TAG-rich lipoproteins, CMs and VLDL, in postprandial samples has enabled the atherogenicity of these lipoproteins to be investigated. Karpe and colleagues[31] provided evidence that a delayed uptake of small CM remnants is associated with the progression of atherosclerosis. Elevated levels of postprandial TAG-rich lipoproteins (CM and CM remnants) circulating after a fat-containing meal are thought to be implicated directly and/or indirectly with the presence of CHD. Evidence from animal studies have shown that CM remnants can directly infiltrate the arterial wall.[32] The mechanisms whereby CM remnants provide the building blocks of arterial lesions are thought to occur by one of two processes. First, the CM remnants may bind and penetrate the arterial surfaces (just in the same way as plasma LDL), therefore the rate of atherogenesis should be proportional to the plasma remnant concentrations. Secondly, CMs may be absorbed and then degraded to remnants on the arterial surface.[33] In each instance, the reaction leading to the endocytosis of remnants by smooth muscle cells may take place at sites where local injury has removed the endothelium.

The magnitude of postprandial lipaemia is dependent on a number of factors including rates of clearance by peripheral tissue and receptor-mediated uptake of the remnants by the liver. Defects in any of these processes will cause an accumulation of CMs and their remnants which in turn can influence endogenous lipoproteins known to be atherogenic. In particular the transfer of TAG from CMs to LDL and HDL and a reciprocal transfer of cholesterol esters to the CMs by CETP may increase the atherogenic lipid profile. This is known as neutral lipid exchange. The transfer of cholesterol ester to CMs and VLDL makes them resistant to lipase action which impedes the normal metabolism of these TAG-rich lipoproteins. The cholesterol ester-enriched CM remnants are then able to be taken up by the macrophages in the arterial lesion. LDL and HDL on the other hand, become suitable substrates for LPL and HL causing a reduction in the size of these particles. This results in the development of an atherogenic lipoprotein profile in which the TAG-rich lipoproteins become cholesterol ester enriched, LDL size is reduced and HDL-C levels are reduced. The small dense nature of the LDL makes it unrecognisable by the LDL receptors in the liver and so makes it a favourable candidate for uptake by scavenger receptors present on macrophages in the arterial lesion.[34]

Elevated levels of small dense LDL (LDL-III)

It has long been established that elevated circulating LDL-C levels represents a major risk factor for the development of CHD. With the use of density gradient ultracentrifugation techniques, LDL has been separated into three major subclasses. These are subdivided as light large LDL (LDL-I), intermediate size LDL (LDL-II) and small dense LDL (LDL-III).[35] In healthy normolipidaemic males, a preponderance of LDL-II is seen, with only a small percentage of LDL-III being present.

A number of case control, cross-sectional and prospective studies has examined the relationship between LDL subclass and risk of CHD with inconsistent findings.[36,37] In studies in men with CHD, or those who had survived a myocardial infarction, it was demonstrated that small dense LDL-III was more common in the men with CHD than without. In 1988, Austin et al.[35] proposed that a preponderance of LDL-III in young men was associated with a three-fold increase in CHD. The increased atherogenicity of small dense LDL-III is thought to be due to the increased residency of these particles in the circulation due to their slow uptake by the LDL receptor in the liver and peripheral tissues. This allows time for the small dense LDL to infiltrate into the intima of the arterial wall where it is thought that these particles are retained by extracellular matrix components before oxidation of the LDL particles occur. The modified small dense LDL-III is then taken up by the scavenger receptor on macrophages leading to the subsequent formation of foam cells.[38] However, Sachs and Campos[37] have suggested that the relationship between small dense LDL and CVD risk may not be independent of other lipid risk markers such as TAG and HDL-C. In the Framingham Heart Offspring Study, small dense LDL was shown to be elevated in the metabolic syndrome and the authors concluded that small dense LDL was not directly correlated with a greater CVD risk but a feature of the atherogenic dyslipidaemia characteristic of the ALP and the metabolic syndrome.[39]

Atherogenic lipoprotein phenotype
The ALP is a collection of lipid abnormalities which confers an increased risk of CHD upon normal, healthy individuals. It has been proposed that between 30–35% of middle-aged men in the Western world may be affected.[6] In the fasting state, this phenotype is characterised by a moderately raised TAG concentration (1.5 to 2.3 mmol/l), low HDL-C (less than 1.0 mmol/l) and a predominance of small dense LDL-III (greater than 35% of LDL mass) and HDL particles. It is important to note that total cholesterol levels are usually in the normal range or are only moderately raised. The atherogenic nature of the ALP may arise from the impairment of the removal of TAG-rich lipoproteins (CMs and VLDL) leading to the conversion of small, atherogenic cholesterol enriched remnants, LDL and HDL by neutral lipid exchange. It is generally considered that this collection of lipid abnormalities is closely associated with the metabolic syndrome, formally referred to as the insulin resistance syndrome.[40]

Metabolic syndrome
The metabolic syndrome is the term given to the collection of metabolic abnormalities which include central obesity, insulin resistance, high blood pressure, low HDL-C and high TAG concentrations. Estimates indicate that 20–25% of the world's adult population have the metabolic syndrome, with an approximate two-three fold increase in CVD risk and a five-fold increase in developing type II diabetes.[7,41] Criteria for identifying individuals with the metabolic syndrome have been published by a number of different expert panels,[42–46] with the general consensus that at least three or more of the five common features are required to determine the presence of this syndrome. However, recent studies have questioned whether a specific feature or combinations

of features associated with the metabolic syndrome can interact leading to a greater relative risk of CVD than the classification of the metabolic syndrome alone.[47–49] Interestingly, in the Guize et al.[48] study, the three- and four-component combinations highly associated with all cause mortality included both increased abdominal obesity and hyperglycaemia, with the addition of either elevated TAG or blood pressure.

8.4   Diet and coronary heart disease risk: the evidence

There is a substantial, diverse, and generally consistent body of evidence linking diet with CVD. The evidence is most extensive for the relationship between CHD and dietary fat. Diet is believed to influence the risk of CHD through its effects on certain risk factors described in Table 8.1, for example blood lipids, and blood pressure, and probably also through thrombogenic mechanisms. More recently, evidence suggests a protective role for dietary antioxidants such as vitamins E and C and carotenes, possibly through a mechanism which prevents the oxidation of LDL particles.

8.4.1   Dietary fat intake

Epidemiological and clinical evidence clearly shows that the likelihood of death from CHD is directly related to the circulating level of total cholesterol, and more specifically LDL-C.[12] Increasing evidence suggests that an exaggerated postprandial TAG response to fat-containing meals is also a significant risk factor for CHD.[3] Numerous studies have shown that the kinds and amounts of fat in the diet significantly influence plasma cholesterol levels. In the Seven Countries Study, mean concentrations of total cholesterol in each population group were highly correlated with percentage energy derived from SFA, and even more strikingly related to a formula which also took into account the intake of PUFA (Fig. 8.4).[50]

Since this research, numerous other studies have supported the relationship between the dietary intake of saturates and the raised plasma lipid concentrations with the hypercholesterolaemic response to a particular SFA varying, depending in part on the TAG structure[51] and in part on LDL receptor activity.[52] The mechanism that is responsible for the increase in plasma cholesterol due to SFAs is at present unclear, but a reduction in the LDL receptor activity is one possibility. It has been recommended that the average contribution of SFA to dietary energy be reduced to no more than 10%.[53] The current UK dietary intake is shown in Table 8.4. A considerable reduction from current levels of intake of dietary SFA (average 13%) would be required to meet this recommendation.[54]

Despite the recommendations to reduce dietary SFA, advice on which fatty acid should replace it, are not given. The effect of the substitution of SFA ingestion with different fatty acids on plasma cholesterol levels is summarised in Table 8.5. Substitution of SFA by MUFA or n-6 PUFA significantly reduces LDL-C levels

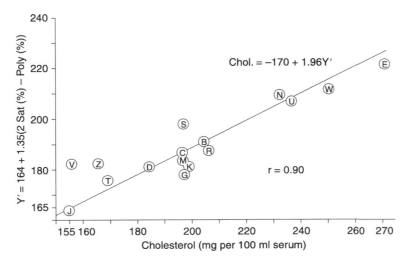

Fig. 8.4 Relationship between the mean cholesterol concentrations of the cohorts of the Seven Countries Study and habitual dietary fat composition (A = Zregnjamin, B = Belgrade, C = Crevalcore, D = Dalmatia, E = East Finland, G = Corfu, J = Ushibuka, K = Crete, M = Montegiorgio, N = Zutphen, R = Rome, S = Slavonia, T = Tanushimara, U = USA, V = Velika Kisna, W = West Finland) (adapted from Keys[2]).

Table 8.4 Dietary intakes of selected nutrients for men and women aged 19–64 years

Nutrient	Men		Women	
	Intake	% Total energy	Intake	% Total energy
Total energy (MJ)	9.72 (2.5)		6.87 (1.8)	
Fat (g)	86.5 (28.2)	35.8 (5.6)	61.4 (21.7)	34.9 (6.5)
SFA (g)	32.5 (12.1)	13.4 (2.9)	23.3 (9.6)	13.2 (3.3)
cis MUFA (g)	29.1 (9.8)	12.1 (2.3)	20.2 (7.4)	11.5 (2.6)
cis n-3 PUFA (g)	2.3 (1.0)	1.0 (0.4)	1.7 (0.8)	1.0 (0.5)
cis n-6 PUFA (g)	12.9 (5.3)	5.4 (1.6)	9.4 (3.3)	5.3 (1.6)
trans FA (g)	2.9 (1.5)	1.2 (0.4)	2.0 (1.0)	1.2 (0.4)
Cholesterol (mg)	304 (128)		213 (95)	
Carbohydrate (g)	275 (79)	47.7 (6.0)	203 (59)	48.5 (6.7)
Protein (g)	88.2 (32.7)	16.5 (3.6)	63.7 (16.6)	16.6 (3.5)
Alcohol (g)	21.9 (24.7)	6.5 (7.2)	9.3 (12.1)	3.9 (5.1)
NSP (g)	15.2 (6.0)		12.6 (5.0)	

Notes: values represent mean (SD).

SFA – saturated fatty acids; MUFA – monounsaturated fatty acids; PUFA – polyunsaturated fatty acids; NSP – non starch polysaccharide.

Source: adapted from Henderson *et al.*[54]

Table 8.5   Effects of fatty acids on fasting plasma lipid concentrations

Fatty acid	Total cholesterol	LDL cholesterol	HDL cholesterol	Triacylglycerol
Saturated FA	Increase ++	Increase ++	Increase +	Increase +
n-6 PUFA	Decrease ++	Decrease +	Decrease +	Neutral
n-3 PUFA (vegetable)	Unchanged	Unchanged	Increased	Decrease +
n-3 PUFA (marine)	Increase +	Increase +	Neutral	Decrease ++
Trans FA	Increase ++	Increase ++	Decrease +	Neutral/increase
MUFA	Decrease +	Decrease +	Neutral/increase	Neutral
Cholesterol (>450 mg/d)	Increase +	Increase +	Increase +	Neutral

Notes: FA – fatty acid; PUFA – polyunsaturated fatty acid; MUFA – monounsaturated fatty acids; NA – not available.

although *n*-6 PUFA are more effective in this respect. There has been doubt as to whether MUFA are effective in cholesterol-lowering or whether the observed decrease in plasma cholesterol was simply due to a replacement of SFA. However it has long been recognised that, in Mediterranean populations, there is a significantly lower risk of CHD.[50] Their diet traditionally contains high amounts of MUFA-containing olive oil in addition to high quantities of fruits and vegetables and long chain *n*-3 PUFA compared to the UK diet. Evidence from intervention studies such as the Lyon Heart Study[55] is supportive of this association. However it is unclear which components of this diet are of paramount importance to CHD risk reduction and to date no specific recommendations are given for dietary MUFA intake.

As regards CHD, *trans* fatty acids appear to act similarly to SFA in their effects on blood cholesterol except that *trans* fatty acids decreased HDL-C, whereas SFA increased HDL-C. In a trial conducted to compare the effects of different fatty acids, elaidic (*trans* 18:1), the principal *trans* fatty acid found in the diet, was reported to significantly decrease HDL-C and increase LDL-C levels.[56] Some epidemiological evidence also supports these findings. Hydrogenated fats are a major dietary source of *trans* fatty acids and are abundant in vegetable margarines and processed foods. However due to the reported link between CHD risk and *trans* fatty acids the level of these fatty acids have been substantially reduced in many margarines and manufactured foods in recent years. Although there is an undisputed link between high ingestion of *trans* fatty acids and CVD there is consistent evidence that the levels of *trans* fatty acids ingested in the UK diet at present do not impact detrimentally on CVD risk, although an increase should be avoided.[57]

The weight of evidence supports the view that raising the cholesterol content of the diet increases plasma cholesterol, primarily LDL-C, although there is considerable inter-individual response. Studies in humans over the past 35 years have indicated a threshold for an effect at an intake of about 95 mg/4300 kJ with a ceiling at about 450 mg/4300 kJ. Excess cholesterol is either not absorbed or suppresses endogenous production. As daily intake (Table 8.4) is at the lower end of this range, it is recommended that current dietary cholesterol intakes, measured per unit of dietary energy, should not rise.[53]

In contrast to dietary SFA, MUFA, n-6 PUFA and *trans* fatty acids whose effects on cardiac health primarily reside in their ability to modify plasma LDL-C and HDL-C levels, the benefits of an increased intake of long chain n-3 PUFA lie in their ability to reduce thrombosis and decrease plasma TAG levels. The low incidence of CHD in Greenland Eskimos and Japanese fisherman, despite a high fat intake (fat providing 80% of dietary energy) has been attributed to their intake of marine foods high in EPA (20:5, n-3) and DHA (22:6, n-3).[58] The DART and GISSI long-term intervention trials lent further evidence that moderate intakes of 1-2 portions of oily fish/week affords a significant reduction in mortality from CHD.[59,60]

Fatty acids from the n-3 PUFA series also have a beneficial effect on thrombogenesis (blood clot formation). The utilisation of n-3 PUFA instead of n-6 PUFA in the production of eicosanoids (substances involved with the formation of blood clotting) can significantly reduce the rate of blood clot formation and thus reduce the risk of myocardial infarction. In addition, n-3 PUFA ingestion may result in the reduction in cardiac arrhythmias.[61] Sudden cardiac death is a serious problem in Western countries and no drug treatment, to date, has had any significant effect on incidence. Epidemiological studies have shown a reduced incidence of sudden death with n-3 PUFA intake, and animal and limited human evidence also suggests an anti-arrythmic effect.[62] The Scientific Advisory Committee on Nutrition (SACN) recommend a daily intake of 0.45 g of long chain n-3 PUFA to reduce the risk of CVD.[63] Table 8.6 shows the dietary guidelines of the European Community[64] and those of the UK Committee of Medical Aspects of Food Policy.[65]

Table 8.6 Recommended daily intakes of dietary fat and fatty acids in the EU and UK

Recommendations	Total fat (% energy)	SFA (% energy)	PUFA (g/day)	MUFA (g/day)	Trans FA (g/day)
European (EEC, 1992)	20–30*	10*	0.5† (LC n-3) 2.0† (n-6)	NR	NR
UK (DH, 1994)	<35	<10	0.45‡ (LC n-3) 5.0 (n-6)	NR	<2

Notes:
* Ultimate goal.
† Population reference intake.
‡ SACN 2004.
NR – no recommendations.

8.4.2   Carbohydrate intake

Recommendations for reductions in total fat in the diet have important implications for dietary carbohydrate intake. There is little variation in the proportion of energy derived from dietary protein; therefore there is a reciprocal relationship between the contributions of dietary fat and carbohydrate to energy. The metabolic effects of exchanging carbohydrate for fat depend mainly on the degree of substitution. Diets in which 60% of food energy is derived from carbohydrate are associated with lower HDL-C levels and higher TAG levels, and despite lower LDL-C levels have been suggested to be associated with a higher risk of CHD.[65,66] However increases in carbohydrate, particularly complex carbohydrates, to accommodate reductions in dietary fat of 35% of energy have not been associated with detrimental changes in TAG and HDL-C, and may benefit CHD health. In addition to the absolute quantity of dietary carbohydrate, there is increasing interest in the quality, with a preference for a diet that contains low glycaemic index (GI) foods (the blood glucose raising ability of carbohydrate-containing foods). Evidence exists for the association between low GI diets and reduced risk of CHD[67] and such diets are favoured for CHD risk reduction.

8.4.3   Dietary fibre intake

A number of prospective studies have shown an inverse relationship between dietary fibre intake and CHD. The studies have varied in the source of fibre which was found to be effective. Morris et al.[68] reported that cereal fibre was inversely related to cases of CHD, whereas others found that vegetable sources of fibre were associated with decreased risk.[69] On the contrary, a two-year intervention study in men who had suffered a previous heart attack found no effect of increasing cereal fibre intake on subsequent risk of mortality from CVD.[59] Although results are inconsistent, a meta-analysis of cohort studies reported that overall higher dietary fibre intakes were significantly associated with reductions in CHD.[70] Much of the benefit of higher fibre intakes has been credited to soluble, rather than insoluble fibre.[71] The effect of a number of soluble fibres which are selectively digested by the colonic gut microbiota (classed as prebiotics) on the blood levels of cholesterol and especially LDL-C will be discussed in detail in section 8.6. Due to the evidence to date the UK recommends the ingestion of 18–24 g/day of dietary fibre. In addition to the beneficial effects of dietary fibre there is increasing evidence from prospective population studies and epidemiological population studies that consumption of wholegrain foods (which contain not only dietary fibres but also antioxidants, vitamins and minerals) is associated with a reduced risk of CVD.[72] This has led to the introduction of a recommendation in the UK to consume at least three servings of wholegrain daily. However despite this strong epidemiological evidence, supportive data from intervention and detailed mechanistic studies is lacking, and the true link between wholegrain ingestion and CVD requires confirmation.

8.4.4   Sodium and potassium intake

Sodium intake appears to be an important determinant of blood pressure in the population as a whole, at least in part by influencing the rise in blood pressure with age.[73–75] A diet lower in common salt and higher in potassium would be expected to result in lower blood pressure and a smaller rise in blood pressure with age. Salt is the predominant source of sodium in the diet, with manufactured foods contributing to 65–85% of the total salt ingested. Blood pressure is an important risk factor for the development of CHD and strokes. It has been recommended that the UK population reduces its salt intake to 6 g/day with specific recommendations introduced in 2003 for infants and children.[76]

8.4.5   Alcohol intake

The debate surrounding the benefits of alcohol consumption and more specifically red wine ingestion and the risk of CHD is one that has been running for many years. Moderate alcohol consumption appears to be associated with relatively low risk of CHD across a variety of study populations. Intakes of 0–20 g/day have been associated with reduced risk and greater than 89 g/day associated with increased risk of CHD,[77] although the risk of stroke in relation to alcohol consumption is less clear.[78] The benefit, which is associated with alcohol consumption, is believed to be almost entirely due to the increased levels of HDL-C.[79] However other factors such as lower platelet activity reducing the risk of thrombosis and antioxidant properties of some drinks such as red wine have also been suggested. A consumption of two units (one unit is equivalent to 8 g of alcohol) of alcohol a day is believed to be beneficial in the risk of CHD, but the debate continues.[80]

8.4.6   Summary

The diet is one of the modifiable risk factors associated with CHD risk. Recommendations for reducing total fat (especially saturated fat), increasing dietary fibre intake and increased consumption of fruits and vegetables is advice that is likely to be associated with overall benefits on health. However, there is great inertia for dietary change, and many new products that claim to reduce the risk of CHD and other chronic diseases, without altering lifestyle factors such as diet, clearly attract a great deal of attention.

8.5   The effects of probiotics including fermented milk products and lactic acid bacteria on coronary heart disease

Due to the low consumer compliance to dietary recommendations, attempts have been made to identify other dietary components that can reduce blood cholesterol levels. These have included investigations into the possible hypocholesterolaemic and hypotriacylglycerolaemic properties of milk products, usually in a fermented form. The role of fermented milk products as hypocholesterolaemic agents in humans is still equivocal, as the studies performed have been of varying quality, design and statistical analysis, with incomplete documentation being the major limitation of most studies. However, since 1974 when Mann and Spoerry[81] showed an 18% fall in plasma cholesterol after feeding four to five litres of fermented milk per day for three weeks in 24 Maasi warriors, there has been considerable interest in the effect of probiotics on human lipid metabolism.

8.5.1   Evidence for the 'milk factor'

As a follow-up to the Maasi trial, Mann[82] fed a small group of US volunteers (n = 4) four litres per day of yoghurt (microbiological activity unspecified) over a 12-day period and reported a significant fall of 37% in serum cholesterol values (however, the tabulated data indicated only a 16.8% fall). When the intake of the yoghurt was reduced to two litres the hypocholesterolaemic effect was maintained, although an intake of one litre per day resulted in a return to baseline cholesterol levels. The rate of cholesterol biosynthesis was monitored by measuring the specific activity of plasma digitonin-precipitated sterols, two hours after a pulse of [^{14}C] acetate. A 28% fall in acetate incorporation into serum cholesterol was reported 16 days after completion of a 12-day trial in which a high dose of yoghurt (four litres per day) was ingested. Mann proposed the presence of a 'milk factor' to explain the fall in serum cholesterol, such as a HMG-CoA reductase inhibitor. Investigating possible candidates for the 'milk factor', Howard and Marks[83] fed lactose ± Ca/Mg, cheese whey or yoghurt, to volunteers over a two-week period. The yoghurt, but not the lactose ± Ca/Mg or cheese whey, significantly reduced plasma cholesterol by 5.5%. However, this trial was subject to a lack of dietary control with substantial changes made to the volunteers' habitual diet resulting in a number of confounding factors.

Most of the early studies introduced confounding factors due to the lack of control of the subjects' diet. Hepner et al.[84] performed a study which attempted to control for these. This was a crossover study in which 720 ml of yoghurt and 750 ml milk were given to the subjects for a four-week period. Significant reductions in plasma cholesterol were observed after the first week of both supplementation periods.[84] The observation that cholesterol levels can significantly fall after acceptance onto a study has been well documented. This is probably due to a conscious or even unconscious modification of the diet by the volunteer due to an acute awareness of dietary assessment. In an attempt to reduce this, baseline run-in periods are essential.[85] Of the early negative studies that have been published, those of Thompson et al.,[86] Massay[87] and McNamara et al.[88] incorporated a run-in period. The study performed by McNamara et al.[88] was one of the more carefully designed interventions. They investigated the effects of the ingestion of 480 ml unspecified yoghurt in a study which included a three-week run-in period and four-week intervention period compared to a non-fermented milk concentrate (as a control). Dietary intake and body weight remained constant and there was no change in serum total, LDL-C, HDL-C or TAG levels.[88] In another well-controlled, double-blind, crossover study using 500 ml of fermented milk product called Kefir (traditionally consumed in Soviet countries for its potential health benefits), no lipid lowering properties were reported when compared to unfermented milk.[89] From the studies mentioned above it can be concluded that there is little evidence that fermented milk products affect serum lipid parameters *per se*.

8.5.2 The effect of viable lactic acid bacteria on lipid parameters

Hepner *et al.*[84] were the first to attempt to discern whether the presence of live bacteria was important for the reported affects of yoghurt on lipid parameters. The aim of the study was to compare the effects of 750 ml of pasteurised and unpasteurised yoghurt, using milk as a placebo. After a 12-week intervention period all treatments significantly reduced plasma cholesterol levels, with milk resulting in a lesser reduction. Unfortunately, the nutritional and microbiological content of the products used was not reported, which severely hampers comparison with other study data. Thompson *et al.*[86] assessed a wide range of milk based products including milk supplemented with *Lactobacillus acidophilus* (undefined, strain code not given – 1.3×10^7 colony forming units (CFU)/ml), buttermilk (a milk product fermented with *Streptococcus cremoris* and *Streptococcus lactis* –6.4×10^8 CFU/ml) and a yoghurt (fermented with *Lactobacillus bulgaricus* and *Streptococcus thermophilus* –1.2×10^9 CFU/ml). One litre of supplement was fed for a three-week period, but no significant change was reported in serum total cholesterol, LDL-C or HDL-C. The possible importance of variation in yoghurt cultures stimulated Jaspers *et al.*[90] to assess the effect of 681 g/day of three strains of a yoghurt fermented with a 1:1 ratio of *Lactobacillus bulgaricus* and *Streptococcus thermophilus*. Two culture strains, CH-I and CH-II (species not given) were taken separately over a 14-day period and two batches of a third strain SH-IIIA and SH-IIIB (species not given) were taken separately over 14 days and seven days running consecutively, with a 21-day 'washout period' between each of the intervention periods. Body weight remained constant in the subjects and there were only differences in the dietary intakes of minerals and vitamins. Significant falls in serum total and LDL-C levels occurred after week one with the CH-II strain and two weeks with the SH-IIIA strain. These transient changes could be explained by the effect of commencing a study as discussed previously, or this could be a true difference between the efficacious properties of different strains. It is evident that the type of lactic acid bacterium or probiotic present in the product is of importance to the physiological effect. Controlled studies using the probiotics *Bifidobacterium longum* BL1 (300 ml/day, 10^8 CFU/ml) for four weeks and *Bifidobacterium lactis* (undefined, strain code not given, 300 g/day) for six weeks in normocholesterolaemic and hypercholesterolaemic subjects respectively, resulted in significant hypocholesterolaemic effects[91,92] which probably reflected the efficacy of the particular probiotic bacteria present.

The subject group studied is an important factor in the physiological effect of lactic acid bacteria. De Roos and colleagues[93] performed a large study (n = 78) investigating the impact of 500 ml/day of yoghurt supplemented with *Lactobacillus acidophilus* L-1 for a six-week period in a parallel study design in normocholesterolaemic subjects. It was reported that there was no significant effect on any lipid parameters determined. This is in contrast to the studies by Anderson and colleagues[94] which investigated a smaller volume (200 ml) of fermented milk (yoghurt-type) containing human *Lactobacillus acidophilus* L-1 or swine *Lactobacillus acidophilus* (ATCC 43121) in 40 hypercholesterolaemic subjects for a four-week period and reported a significant reduction of 4.3% in total cholesterol. These data illustrate the importance of the cholesterol status of study participants on entry.

A number of studies have tested the lipid-lowering effects of a particular probiotic yoghurt Gaio® (MD Foods Aarhus, Denmark) fermented by Causido® consisting of *Enterococcus faecium* (human species, undefined, strain code not given) and two strains of *Streptococcus thermophilus* with varying results. Agerbaek *et al.*,[95] tested the effect of 200 ml (*Enterococcus faecium*, ~2 × 10^8 CFU/ml) per day of Gaio® in a parallel study design, where the active yoghurt was tested against an identical yoghurt that had been chemically acidified with an organic acid (delta-gluco-lactone). The intervention was for a six-week period in 58 middle-aged men with moderately raised cholesterol levels (5.0–6.5 mmol/l). They observed a 9.8% reduction in LDL-C levels for the live yoghurt group, which was sustained over the intervention period (Table 8.7). This was a well-controlled study, which excluded many variables such as age, sex and body weight. However, an unforeseen skew in the randomisation of the subjects resulted in significantly different baseline total and LDL-C levels in the two groups. The fall in these parameters observed in the active yoghurt group could be ascribed to a regression towards the mean. Another study performed using the same yoghurt and a similar design for a longer period (six months) was carried out in 87 men and women aged between 50–70 years.[96] It was reported that at 12 weeks there was a significant drop in LDL-C levels in the group taking the active yoghurt. These reductions were not sustained and this was partly explained by a reduction in the numbers of viable bacteria (*Enterococcus faecium*) in yoghurt at 12 weeks. At the end of the study, no significant reductions in total or LDL-C levels were observed between the two groups. Another publication investigating the same product used a 200 g/day ingestion of the yoghurt, for an eight-week period in a randomised double-blind placebo controlled trial, with 32 patients who had mild to moderate hypercholesterolaemia. The patients were asked to follow a lipid-lowering diet for eight weeks and were then given the test or control product for two eight-week periods. The results showed a significant reduction of 10.3% for total cholesterol and a 6.2% reduction in LDL-C levels after the active product. However, the authors did question whether or not the average reduction of approximately 5% for total and LDL-C was clinically important.[97]

A similar trial of the same Gaio® product containing *Enterococcus faecium* was conducted in 160 middle-aged men and women with moderately raised

Table 8.7 Human studies to evaluate the lipid-lowering properties of fermented milk products

Author	Subjects M/F	Study design	Product (vol/type)	Duration	TC	LDL-C	HDL-C	TAG
Mann and Spoerry[81]	24/0 Normchol	SB/parallel (2 gp)	8.3 l lacto/yog	3 wk	−9.6%***	NA	NA	NA
Mann[82]	3/1 Normchol	Sequential	4 l WMY	12 d	−16.8%*	NA	NA	NA
	3/2 Normchol	Sequential	2 l SMY	12 d	−23.2%*	NA	NA	NA
Howard and Marks[83]	10 NA	Parallel	2 l SMY	3 wk	−5.5%*	NA	NA	NA
Hepner et al.[84]	11/7 Normchol	Crossover	720 ml (A)	4 wk	−5.4%**	NA	NA	NS
	13/23 Normchol	Parallel (4 gp)	720 ml (B)	4 wk	8.9%**	NA	NA	NS
Rossouw et al.[98]	32/0 Normchol	Parallel (3 gp)	2 l yoghurt	3 wk	+16%**	+12%***	NS	NA
Thompson et al.[86]	26/42 Normchol	Parallel (6 gp)	1 l UPY	3 wk	NS	NS	NS	15.7%***
Bazzare et al.[106]	5/16 Normochol	Crossover	550 g yoghurt	1 wk	−8.7%*** Women only	NA	+8.9%*** Women only	NA
Massey[87]	0/30 Normchol	SB/crossover	480 ml yoghurt	4 wk	NS	NS	NS	NS

Continued

Table 8.7 Continued

Author	Subjects M/F	Study design	Product (vol/type)	Duration	TC	LDL-C	HDL-C	TAG
Jaspers et al.[90]	10/0 NA	Sequential	681 g yoghurt	2 wk	−11.6%*†	NS	NS	NS
McNamara et al.[88]	18/0 Normochol	Crossover	16 oz LFY	4 wk	NS	NS	NS	NA
Agerbaek et al.[95]	32/20 Normochol	DB/crossover	200 ml UPY	6 wk	−6.1%***	−9.8%***	NA	NA
Richelsen et al.[96]	47/43 Normochol	DB/crossover	200 ml UPY	24 wk	NA	−9%*†	NS	NS
Sessions et al.[85]	78/76 Hyperchol	DB/crossover	200 ml UPY	12 wk	NS	NS	NS	NS
Bertolami et al.[97]	11/21 Hyperchol	DB/crossover	200 ml UPY	8 wk	−5.3%**	6.2%***	NS	NS
de Roos et al.[93]	78 Normochol	Parallel (2 gp)	500 ml UPY	6 wk	NS	NS	NS	NS
Anderson et al.[94]	9/20 Hyperchol	SB/parallel (2 gp)	200 ml FM	3 wk	−2.4%*	NS	−5.9%***	NA
	18/22 Hyperchol	DB/crossover	200 ml FM	4 wk	−4.3%**	NA	NA	NA
Agerholm-Larsen et al.[99]	20/50 Normochol	DB/parallel	450 ml UPY	8 wk	NS	−8.4%*	NA	NA
St-Onge et al.[89]	13/0 Hyperchol	SB/crossover	500 ml FM	4 wk	NS	NS	NS	NS
Xiao et al.[91]	32/0 Normochol	SB/parallel	3 × 100 ml UPY	4 wk	−5.4%*	NS	NS	NS

Rossi et al.[100]	44 Normochol	DB/parallel (2 gp)	200 ml FM (soy)	6 wk	NS	NS	10%*	NA
Larkin et al.[101]	21/15 Hyperchol	Crossover	100 ml UPY (soy)	5 wk	−4.7%*	NS	NS	NS
Ataie-Jafari et al.[92]	14 Hyperchol	SB/crossover	300 g UPY	6 wk	−5.5*	NS	NS	NS
Karlsson et al.[102]	18/0 Atherosclerotic plaques	DB/parallel (2 gp)	100 ml FM (oat)	4 wk	NS	NS	NS	NS

Notes: F, female; M, male; Normochol, normocholesterolaemic; Hyperchol, hypercholesterolaemic; WMY, whole milk yoghurt; UPY, unpasteurised yoghurt; SMY, skimmed milk yoghurt; PY, pasteurised yoghurt; LFY, low fat yoghurt; NA, data not available; † Transient; SB, single blind; DB, double blind; * P<0.05; ** P<0.01; *** P<0.001.

cholesterol.[85] The study was a randomised, double-blind, multi-centre, placebo controlled parallel study and was the largest performed to date. Volunteers consumed 200 ml per day of either the active or chemically acidified yoghurt for a 12-week period. Stratified randomisation was used to ensure that the groups were comparable for age, sex, BMI and baseline fasting cholesterol levels. The importance of not changing their dietary habits and lifestyle during the study was emphasised and adherence to the protocol confirmed by dietary assessment. Due to the importance of high enough levels of viable bacteria in the yoghurt, viability of *Enterococcus faecium* was monitored throughout the study. The levels were found to be no lower than 1×10^6 CFU/ml at any time tested. During the two-week run-in period, both groups showed significant reductions in blood cholesterol levels, but thereafter there were no further changes in either of the groups or between the groups at any of the time points. These data do not support previous studies discussed but are consistent with the conclusions drawn by Rossouw *et al.*[98] which indicated that apparent effects of some probiotics on blood cholesterol levels may be attributed to reductions in blood lipids observed in subjects who commence an intervention trial. Whilst these reductions are well recognised but are difficult to prevent; they highlight the importance of the inclusion of a run-in period within such studies. In summary, six published studies have investigated whether the addition of Gaio® to the habitual diet can reduce plasma cholesterol. Four studies showed a small beneficial short-term effect of a 6–10% reduction of LDL-C.[95–97,99] Yet the long-term effects were inconclusive[96] and the largest study failed to show any significant effects.[85] However, despite these inconsistent reports after a meta-analysis of these studies was performed, it was concluded that both the total and LDL-C was reduced by 6% and 9% respectively compared to the control yoghurt and provides evidence for a short-term effect of Gaio®.[99]

The majority of the studies investigating the effect of lactic acid bacteria and probiotics have used fermented cow's milk or cow's milk yoghurt. In contrast, two studies have determined the effect of fermented soy milk[100] and soy milk consumed with a probiotic yoghurt[101] on lipid concentrations with conflicting results and one study with fermented oat milk.[102] Although there are discrepancies in relation to the particular components of soy that are active, there is increasing evidence that soy consumption is related to a reduction in plasma lipids.[103] Isoflavones alone generally do not reduce lipids[104] yet in combination with soy proteins appear to be beneficial.[103,105] Consequently the impact of the addition of a probiotic to soy products on the lipid-lowering effects of these products was investigated. Rossi and colleagues[100] determined the impact of the addition of 200 ml of fermented soy milk produced with *Enterococcus faecium* (undefined, strain not given) and *Lactobacillus jugurti* (undefined, strain not given) for a six-week period in normocholesterolaemic middle-aged men. Despite containing isoflavones, soy protein and the same species as Gaio (*Enterococcus faecium*), this fermented soy milk did not significantly affect the total or LDL-C levels, but did result in a 10% increase in HDL-C.[100] These data are in contrast to the observations of a study which investigated the effect of soy milk and either 100 ml probiotic yoghurt (containing 10^8 CFU/serving of each of *Lactobacillus acidophilus* (undefined, strain not given), *Bifidobacterium bifidus* (undefined, strain not given), and *Lactobacillus rhamnosus* GG) or yoghurt containing the typical yoghurt starter cultures. It was reported that the dietary combination of soy with probiotic yoghurt resulted in a significant reduction in total cholesterol (−4.7%) and potential synergistic hypocholesterolaemic actions between soy and probiotic bacteria were suggested.[101] In another study, 100 ml of fermented oat milk containing *Lactobacillus plantarum* (DSM 9843, 10^{11} CFU/ml) was consumed in a double-blind parallel study in 18 men with atherosclerotic plaques. Although it was reported that there was a significant increase in plasma SCFAs and colonic bacterial diversity, there was no significant impact on lipid concentrations compared to a control product.[102]

From the findings available to date, it can be concluded that there is some evidence to support a hypocholesterolaemic effect of a daily consumption of some lactic acid bacteria containing products which is more apparent in those with hypercholesterolaemia and may be gender specific.[106] The most consistent finding is a reduction in total cholesterol, which is associated with a significant LDL-C reduction in some[95,97–99] but not all studies. However none of the studies that have measured plasma TAG (14 out of 26 see Table 8.7) have reported a significant reduction in this lipid level, with one study reporting a significant increase of 16%.[86] Therefore it is apparent that the impact of lactic acid bacteria on CHD lipid risk reduction is in their potential hypocholesterolaemic effects. However results are generally inconsistent and further suitably powered and well controlled studies are required before firm conclusions can be drawn on the efficacy of lactic acid bacterial use and CHD risk reduction.

8.5.3   Possible mechanisms of action of lactic acid bacteria

Before the possible mechanisms are considered, it is important to highlight that since viable and biologically active micro-organisms are usually required at the target site in the host, it is essential that the probiotics not only have the characteristics that are necessary to produce the desired biological effects; but also have the required viability and are able to withstand the host's natural barriers against ingested bacteria. The classic yoghurt starter bacteria, *Streptococcus thermophilus* and *Lactobacillus bulgaricus* are technologically effective, but they do not reach the lower intestinal tract in a viable form. Therefore, intrinsic microbiological properties, such as tolerance to gastric acid, bile and pancreatic juice are important factors when probiotic organisms are considered.[107]

The mechanism of action of lactic acid bacteria and probiotics on cholesterol reduction is unclear, but there are a number of proposed possibilities which may act independently or synergistically. These include physiological actions of the end products of fermentation SCFAs; cholesterol assimilation, deconjugation of bile acids and cholesterol binding to bacterial cell walls. The SCFAs that are produced by the bacterial anaerobic breakdown of carbohydrate are acetic, propionic and butyric acid. The physiological effects of these are discussed in detail in section 8.6.3.

It has been well documented that microbial bile acid metabolism is a peculiar effect involved in the therapeutic role of some bacteria. The deconjugation reaction is catalysed by conjugated bile acid hydrolase enzyme, which is produced exclusively by bacteria. This deconjugation ability is widely found in many intestinal bacteria including genera *Enterococcus, Peptostreptococcus, Bifidobacterium, Fusobacterium, Clostridium, Bacteroides* and *Lactobacillus*.[108] This reaction liberates the amino acid moiety and the deconjugated bile acid thereby reducing cholesterol re-absorption, by increasing faecal excretion of the deconjugated bile acids. Many *in vitro* studies have investigated the ability of various bacteria to deconjugate a variety of different bile acids. Grill *et al.*[109] reported *Bifidobacterium longum* strains (BB536 and OC) as the most efficient bacterium among four *Bifidobacterium* strains (*Bifidobacterium animalis, Bifidobacterium infantis, Bifidobacteriu brev and Bifidobacterium thermophilum*) when tested against six different bile salts. Another study reported that *Lactobacillus* species had varying ability to deconjugate glycocholate and taurocholate[110] with *Lactobacillus fermentum* KC5b reported to have the ability to deconjugate a number of bile salts *in vitro*.[111] Studies performed on *in vitro* responses are useful, but *in vivo* studies in animals and humans are required to determine the full contribution of bile acid deconjugation to cholesterol reduction. Intervention studies in animals and ileostomy patients have shown that oral administration of certain bacterial strains led to an increased excretion of free and secondary bile salts.[91,112,113]

There is also some *in vitro* evidence to support the hypothesis that certain bacteria can assimilate (take up) cholesterol. It was reported that *Lactobacillus acidophilus* (RP32),[114] *Bifidobacterium bifidum* (strains BYU and BPO),[115] and *Lactobacillus fermentum* (KC5b)[116] had the ability to assimilate cholesterol in *in vitro* studies, but only in the presence of bile and under anaerobic conditions. However, despite these reports there is uncertainty whether the bacteria are assimilating cholesterol or whether the cholesterol is co-precipitating with the bile salts. Studies have been performed to address this question. Klaver and Meer[117] concluded that the removal of cholesterol from the growth medium in which *Lactobacillus acidophilus* (RP32) and a *Bifidobacterium* (MUH80) were growing was not due to assimilation, but due to bacterial bile salt deconjugase activity. The same question was addressed by Tahri *et al.*,[118] with conflicting results, and they concluded that part of the removed cholesterol was found in the cell extracts and that cholesterol assimilation and bile acid deconjugase activity could occur simultaneously.

The mechanism of cholesterol binding to bacterial cell walls has also been suggested as a possible explanation for hypocholesterolaemic effects of probiotics. Hosona and Tono-oka[119] reported that *Lactococcus lactis* subsp. *Biovar. Diacylactis* R-43 had the highest binding capacity for cholesterol of bacteria tested in the study. Lin and Chen,[120] after investigating the *in vitro* cholesterol reducing abilities of six *Lactobacillus acidophilus* strains, reported that the *in vivo* hypocholesterolaemic effects of these bacterial cells was due to the direct assimilation by the cells and/or attachment of cholesterol to their surface. It was speculated that the binding differences were due to chemical and structural properties of the cell walls, and that even killed cells may have the ability to bind cholesterol in the intestine. The mechanism of action of probiotics on cholesterol reduction could be one or all of the above mechanisms with the ability of different bacterial species to have varying effects on cholesterol lowering. However, more research is required to fully elucidate the effect and mechanism of probiotics and their possible hypocholesterolaemic action.

8.6   The effects of prebiotics on coronary heart disease

8.6.1   Prebiotics

Over the past ten years, there has been increasing interest in the important nutritional role of prebiotics as functional food ingredients. This interest has been derived from animal studies which showed markedly reduced TAG and total cholesterol levels when diets containing significant amounts of a prebiotic (oligofructose (OFS)) were fed. A prebiotic is defined as 'a non-digestible food ingredient that beneficially affects the host by selectively stimulating the growth and/or the activity of one or a number of bacteria in the colon that has the potential to improve health'.[120] Prebiotics, most often referred to as non-digestible oligosaccharides, are extracted from natural sources (e.g. inulin and OFS) or synthesised from disaccharides (e.g. transgalacto-oligosaccharides). The most commonly studied of the prebiotics include inulin and OFS which are found in many vegetables, including onion, garlic, leek, asparagus, Jerusalem artichoke and chicory root.[122] These consist of between two and 60 fructose molecules joined by β2-1 osidic linkages, which, due to the nature of this type of linkage, escape digestion in the upper gastrointestinal tract and remain intact but are selectively fermented by colonic microbiota. Inulin is currently found as a food ingredient of bread, baked goods, yoghurt and ice-cream because it displays gelling and thickening properties and helps to improve the mouthfeel and appearance of lower energy products.[122] In Europe, the estimated intake of inulin and OFS is between 2 and 12 g per day.[123]

8.6.2   The effect of prebiotics on lipid metabolism in humans

Several studies which have investigated the effects of prebiotics on fasting plasma lipids have generated inconsistent findings (Table 8.8). In studies with individuals with raised blood lipids, one study showed a reduction in fasting total, LDL-C and TAG,[124] three studies showed significant decreases in fasting total and/or LDL-C, with no significant changes in TAG levels[125–127] whereas two studies showed a reduction in TAG only.[128,129] In contrast, two studies in type II diabetics did not observe any change in cholesterol or TAG levels[130,131] (Table 8.8). In normolipidaemic participants, only two studies have demonstrated significant changes in both fasting TAG and total cholesterol levels with inulin[132,133] with a further two studies showing a significant decrease in TAG levels only.[134,135] However, seven studies have reported no effect of OFS or inulin

Table 8.8 Summary of human studies to examine the effects of fructan supplementation on blood lipids

Author	Subjects	Fructan	Dose	Study design	Duration	Vehicle	Significant changes observed in:	
							Blood lipids	Glucose
Yamashita et al.[125]	8 M and 10 F Type II diabetic	OFS	8 g	DB, parallel	2 wk	Coffee drink or jelly	↓TC (8%) ↓LDL-C (10%)	↓Glucose (8%)
Hidaka et al.[126]	37 M and F Hyperlipidaemic	OFS	8 g	DB, parallel	5 wk	Confectionary	↓TC (6%)	NS
Canzi et al.[132]	12 M Normolipidaemic	Inulin	9 g	Sequential	4 wk	Breakfast cereal	↓TAG (27%) ↓TC (5%)	N/A
Luo et al.[136]	12 M Normolipidaemic	OFS	20 g	DB, crossover	4 wk	100 g biscuits	NS	NS
Pedersen et al.[137]	66 F Normolipidaemic	Inulin	14 g	DB, crossover	4 wk	40 g margarine	NS	N/A
Davidson et al.[127]	21 M and F Hyperchol	Inulin	18 g	DB, crossover	6 wk	Chocolate bar, paste or sweetener	↓LDL-C (14%) ↓TC (9%)	N/A
Alles et al.[130]	9 M and 11 F Type II diabetic	OFS	15 g	SB, crossover	3 wk	Not specified	NS	NS
Brighenti et al.[133]	12 M Normolipidaemic	Inulin	9 g	Sequential	4 wk	Breakfast cereal	↓TC (8%) ↓TAG (21%)	NS
Jackson et al.[129]	54 M and F Mod hyperlipid	Inulin	10 g	DB, parallel	8 wk	Sachet	↓TAG (19%)	↓Insulin (15%)
Kruse et al.[138]	8 M and F Normolipidaemic	Inulin	22–34 g	DB, parallel	9 wk	Yoghurt	NS	N/A
van Dokkum et al.[139]	12 M Normolipidaemic	Inulin, OFS or GOS	15 g	DB, crossover	3 wk	Orange juice	NS	NS

Reference	Subjects	Prebiotic	Dose	Study design	Duration	Delivery	Lipid effect	Other
Causey et al.[128]	12 M Hyperchol	Inulin	20 g	DB, crossover	3 wk	Low fat ice-cream	↓TAG (14%)	NS
Luo et al.[131]	6 M and 4 F Type II diabetic	OFS	20 g	DB, crossover	4 wk	Sachet	NS	NS
Balcázar-Munoz et al.[124]	12 M and F Hyperlipidaemic	Inulin	7 g	DB, parallel	4 wk	Not specified	↓TC (22%) ↓LDL-C (17%) ↓TAG (27%)	NS
Letexier et al.[134]	8 M and F Normolipidaemic	Inulin	10 g	DB, crossover	3 wk	Not specified	↓TAG (16%)	NS
Giacco et al.[140]	20 M and 10 F Mod hyperchol	OFS	5.3 g	DB, crossover	8 wk	Sachet	NS	NS
Forcheron et al.[141]	6 M and 11 F Normolipidaemic	Inulin/OFS	10 g	DB, crossover	24 wk	Sachet	NS	NS
Russo et al.[135]	22 M Normolipidaemic	Inulin	11 g	DB, crossover	5 wk	Pasta	↑HDL-C (36%) ↓TAG (23%)	N/A
Vulevic et al.[142]	44 M and F Normolipidaemic	GOS	5.5 g	DB, crossover	10 wk	Sachet	NS	N/A
Genta et al.[147]	35 F mod Hyperlipid	OFS	10 g	DB, parallel	16 wk	Syrup	↓LDL-C (27%)	↓Insulin (49%)

Notes: M, male; F, female; DB, double blind; GOS, galacto-oligosaccharide; Hyperchol, hypercholesterolaemic; N/A, not measured; Mod hyperchol, moderately hypercholesterolaemic; Mod hyperlipid, moderately hyperlipidaemic; NS, not significant; SB, single blind; TC, total cholesterol; LDL-C, low-density lipoprotein cholesterol; OFS, oligofructose; TAG, triacylglycerol.

treatment on plasma lipids levels in young healthy[136–141] or elderly subjects[142]. In the study by Jackson et al.,[129] follow-up blood samples were taken four weeks after completion of the inulin supplementation period by which time the concentrations of TAG had returned to baseline values, supporting the conclusion that inulin feeding may have been responsible. A recent meta-analysis of 15 randomised controlled trials (conducted between 1996 and 2005) has reported that inulin-type fructans can significantly decrease fasting TAG concentrations by 0.17 mmol/l.[143] These findings are in line with observed effects of inulin on lipid levels in animals in which the predominant effect is on TAG rather than cholesterol concentrations.

Raised postprandial TAG concentrations have also been recognised as a risk factor for CHD.[4,5] Data from studies in rats have shown a 40% reduction in postprandial TAG concentrations when diets containing ten per cent OFS (w/v) were fed.[144] However, very little information regarding the effect of prebiotics on postprandial lipaemia in human subjects are available, with two studies reporting a lack of effect of inulin treatment on postprandial TAG levels in middle-aged men and women with moderately raised lipids.[140,145]

The marked reductions in fasting lipid levels observed in animal studies have not been consistently reproduced in human subjects. Only three studies in normolipidaemic subjects has shown significant reductions in fasting TAG levels with inulin[132,133,135] with one study showing a significant effect of inulin treatment over time on fasting TAG levels compared with the placebo group.[129] The amount of fructans used in the human studies in Table 8.8 varies between 5.3–34 g and this amount is small compared to that which is used in animal studies (50–200 g per kg of rat chow of OFS)[146] which is equivalent to a dose in humans of approximately 50–80 g of OFS/inulin per day. The fact that OFS and inulin are fibres restricts its dosage in humans to between 15–20 g per day since doses greater than this can cause gastrointestinal symptoms such as stomach cramps, flatulence and diarrhoea.[137,147] It is not known whether, at the levels used in human studies, significant effects would be observed in animals.[148]

The types of food vehicles used to increase the amount of OFS/inulin in the diet differ. In the case of Luo et al.,[136] 100 g of biscuits were eaten every day and for Pedersen et al.,[137] 40 g of margarine was consumed which may have contributed to the negative findings in blood lipids. In the case of Davidson et al.,[127] significant changes in total and LDL-C levels were observed over six weeks with inulin in comparison with the placebo (sugar) incorporated into a number of study products including a chocolate bar, a chocolate spread and sweeteners for coffee or fruit. The percentage change in each of the lipid parameters was calculated over each of the six-week treatment periods and unexpectedly, there was an increase in total cholesterol, LDL-C and TAG during the placebo phase. Non-significant falls in these variables were observed during inulin treatment and so when the net changes in the variables were calculated (change during inulin minus change during control treatment) there were significant differences in total and LDL-C between the two treatments. The authors attributed the increase in total and LDL-C levels in the placebo phase to be due to the increased intake of SFAs in the chocolate products which were used as two of the vehicles in the study.[127] In later studies, the use of inulin in a powder form has enabled it to be added to many of the foods eaten in the participant's normal diet without any need for dietary advice thus avoiding changes in body weight. Since inulin has water-binding properties, in its powder form inulin could be added to orange juice, tea, coffee, yoghurt and soup.[129,131,140–142]

The significant relationship between the participants initial TAG concentration and percentage change in TAG levels over the eight-week study demonstrated by Jackson et al.[129] lends support to the hypothesis that the initial TAG levels could be important in determining the degree of the TAG response to inulin. The lack of response in some individuals may be as a result of them being less responsive to inulin, variations in their background diet, or non-compliance with the study protocol. Speculation as to possible reasons for variability in response would be aided by a better understanding of the mechanism of action of inulin on plasma TAG levels.

The length of the supplementation period used in the studies in Table 8.8 may be another factor for the inconsistent findings in changes in TAG levels in human subjects with inulin. The studies were conducted over 2 to 24 weeks, with significant effects occurring as early as 3–4 weeks.[124,128,132,134] One study conducted for 26 weeks showed no effect of inulin/OFS on lipid levels in normolipidaemics suggesting that beneficial effects observed in the short-term studies may not persist on a long-term basis. A wash-out period of 4 weeks has been shown to be a sufficient period time for the TAG concentrations to return to baseline values[129]. This may provide an explanation for the significant findings in TAG levels in the studies of Causey et al.[128] and Canzi et al.[132] who used 3- to 4-week sequential and crossover designs with very short wash-out periods.

Whilst some of the studies to date support beneficial effects of inulin on plasma TAG, the findings are by no means consistent and more work is required to provide convincing evidence of the lipid-lowering consequences of prebiotic ingestion.

8.6.3 Mechanism of lipid lowering by prebiotics

Prebiotics have been shown to be an ideal substrate for the health promoting bacteria in the colon, notably bifidobacteria and lactobacilli.[149] During the fermentation process a number of by-products are produced including gases (H_2S, CO_2, H_2, CH_4), lactate and SCFAs (acetate, butyrate and propionate). The SCFAs, acetate and propionate enter the portal blood stream where they are utilised by the liver. Acetate is converted to acetyl CoA in the liver and acts as a lipogenic substrate for de novo lipogenesis, whereas propionate has been reported to inhibit lipid synthesis.[150,151] Butyrate, on the other hand, is taken up by the large intestinal cells (colonocytes) and has been shown to protect against tumour formation in the gut.[152] The type of SCFAs which are produced during the fermentation process is dependent on the microbiota which can be stimulated by the prebiotic. Inulin has been shown to increase both acetate and butyrate levels, whereas synthetically produced prebiotics, for example galacto-oligosaccharides increase the production of acetate and propionate and xylo-oligosaccharides increase acetate only.[152]

Inulin and OFS have been extensively studied to determine the mechanism of action of prebiotics in animals. Early *in vitro* studies using isolated rat hepatocytes suggested that the hypolipidaemic action of OFS was associated with the inhibition of *de novo* cholesterol synthesis by the SCFA propionate following impairment of acetate utilisation by the liver for *de novo* lipogenesis.[151] This is in agreement with human studies in which rectal infusions of acetate and propionate resulted in propionate inhibiting the incorporation of acetate into TAGs released from the liver.[153] Fiordaliso *et al.*[154] demonstrated significant reductions in plasma TAGs, phospholipids and cholesterol in normolipidaemic rats fed a rat chow diet containing ten per cent (w/v) OFS. The TAG-lowering effect was demonstrated after only one week of OFS and was associated with a reduction in VLDL secretion. TAG and phospholipids are synthesised in the liver by esterification of fatty acids and glycerol-3-phosphate before being made available for assembly into VLDL, suggesting that the hypolipidaemic effect of OFS may be occurring in the liver. The reduction observed in cholesterol levels in the rats was only demonstrated after long-term feeding (16 weeks) of OFS. Interestingly, in healthy men and women, ingestion of 10 g of inulin for three weeks led to reduced hepatic lipogenesis and fasting TAG level with no significant effects on plasma cholesterol concentrations.[134] The TAG-lowering effect of OFS is suggested to occur via reduction in VLDL TAG secretion from the liver due to the reduction in activity of all lipogenic enzymes (acetyl-CoA carboxylase, fatty acid synthase, malic enzyme, ATP citrate lyase and glucose-6-phosphate dehydrogenase), and in the case of fatty acid synthase, via modification of lipogenic gene expression[155] (Fig. 8.5).

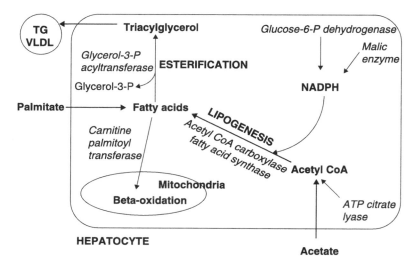

Fig. 8.5 Hepatic fatty acid metabolism.

8.6.4   The effect of prebiotics on glucose and insulin levels

Very little is known about the effects of prebiotics on fasting insulin and glucose levels in humans. Of the supplementation studies conducted in humans, a significant reduction in glucose was observed in type II diabetic subjects[125] and a trend for a reduction in glucose was observed in hyperlipidaemic subjects[126] with OFS. However, two studies have reported no effect of OFS on blood glucose levels in type II diabetics.[130,131] Significant reductions in insulin levels were observed in healthy middle-aged subjects[129] and obese slightly dyslipidaemic women[147] with inulin and OFS, although there was a lack of effect on plasma glucose levels in both studies. The effect of the ingestion of acute test meals containing OFS on blood glucose, insulin and C-peptide levels in healthy adults showed a trend for a lower glycaemic response and peak insulin levels following the OFS-enriched meals.[156]

The mechanism of action of prebiotics on lowering glucose and insulin levels has been proposed to be associated with the SCFAs, especially propionate. A significant reduction in postprandial glucose concentrations was observed following both acute and chronic intakes of propionate-enriched bread.[157] The effect of propionate intake on postprandial insulin levels was not investigated. A recent animal study has shown an attenuation of both postprandial insulin and glucose levels following four weeks of feeding with OFS. These effects were attributed to the actions of OFS on the secretion of the gut hormones, glucose dependent insulinotropic polypeptide (GIP) and glucagon-like peptide 1 (GLP-1).[144] These hormones are secreted from the small intestine (GIP) and the terminal ileum and proximal colon (GLP-1) and contribute to the secretion of insulin following a meal in the presence of raised glucose levels.[158] A recent review has highlighted GLP-1 in particular as an important site of modulation by inulin-type fructans,[159] with a doubling of the serum concentration of this incretin hormone with OFS feeding in mice and rats leading to an improvement in glucose homeostasis. Similar observations have been reported in a human study where plasma GLP-1 levels were increased following ingestion of a mixed meal after feeding 20 g/day of OFS for one week.[160]

In summary, the mechanisms of action of prebiotics, especially inulin and OFS, have been determined largely from animal studies. Present data suggest inhibition of *de novo* lipogenesis as the primary mode of action of prebiotics in mediating their lipid-lowering effects via down regulation of the enzymes involved. If this is the case, more modest or inconsistent effects might be expected in humans, in whom *de novo* lipogenesis is extremely low, or variable depending on their background diet. In animal studies, rats are fed a diet which is low in fat and high in carbohydrate and so *de novo* lipogenesis is an upregulated pathway in these animals for the synthesis of fatty acids. It is interesting to note that when rats are fed OFS along with a high-fat diet typical of the Western-style diet, TAG levels are thought to be decreased by a different mechanism involving the enhanced clearance of TAG-rich lipoproteins. An increased GIP secretion in OFS treated rats was observed by Kok *et al.*[144] and this gut hormone has been shown to enhance the activity of LPL, the principal enzyme involved in the clearance of

TAG-rich lipoproteins following the ingestion of fat.[161] The release of GIP and GLP-1 in the intestine and colon may act as mediators of the systemic effect of prebiotics such as inulin and OFS, on blood lipid, insulin and glucose levels. However, further work is required to determine the metabolic pathways which are influenced by prebiotics. Their effect on gastrointestinal kinetics such as gastric emptying and its modification of the levels of TAG-rich lipoproteins (CMs) and glucose in the circulation has recently been proposed as a potential modulator of systemic effects.[162] Therefore, the design of future studies to investigate the effect of prebiotics in humans should consider the choice of subjects, length of supplementation period and type of vehicle used to increase the intake of prebiotics in the diet, as these variables may influence the outcome of the study.

8.7   The effects of synbiotics including combinations of lactic acid bacteria and prebiotic fibres on coronary heart disease

8.7.1   Synbiotics

A synbiotic is defined as 'a mixture of a prebiotic and a probiotic that beneficially affects the host by improving the survival and the implantation of live microbial dietary supplements in the gastrointestinal tract, by selectively stimulating the growth and/or by activating the metabolism of one or a limited number of health promoting bacteria'.[163] The use of synbiotics (or other combinations of lactic acid bacteria and fibres) as functional food ingredients is a developing area and very few human studies have been performed looking at their effect on risk factors for CHD. A study by Schaafsma et al.[164] reported a significant decrease in total and LDL-C after three weeks of supplementation with a fermented milk product (375 ml) containing 2.5% FOS (~9 g) compared with a control milk fermented by traditional yoghurt starters (375 ml). Levels of HDL-C, TAG and glucose were unchanged, leading to an improvement in the LDL-C to HDL-C ratio. Kießling and colleagues[165] showed the consumption of a fermented milk product with the addition of 1% OFS (~3 g) for six weeks led to no effect on serum total, LDL-C or TAG concentrations. HDL-C and the LDL-C to HDL-C ratio were significantly improved, a finding thought to be attributed to the relatively high intake of milk fat (10.5 g/day) as a result of the consumption of 300 g yoghurt per day. The majority of research conducted so far with synbiotics has looked at their effect on the composition of the gut microbiota. In one study in healthy subjects, a *Bifidobacterium* sp. (undefined, strain not defined) fermented milk product with or without 18 g of inulin was given daily for 12 days.[166] The authors concluded that the administration of the fermented milk product (probiotic) substantially increased the proportion of bifidobacteria in the gut, but that this increase was not enhanced by the addition of 18 g of inulin. The composition of the gut microbiota was then assessed two weeks after completing the supplementation period and it was found that subjects who received the fermented milk product and inulin maintained their bifidobacterial population in the gut compared with the subjects receiving the fermented milk product only. Although a synergistic effect on bifidobacteria in the gut was not observed with the synbiotic, these results suggest that either there was better implantation of the probiotic or a prebiotic effect on indigenous bifidobacteria.[109] A recent study using [1]H Nuclear Magnetic Resonance spectroscopy has reported that feeding healthy individuals with a synbiotic food containing *Bifidobacterium longum* (strain not defined), *L. acidophilus* (strain not defined) and OFS (0.5 g) for 30 days significantly influenced the metabolic activity of the intestinal microbiota. In particular, an increase in specific metabolites such as the SCFA butyrate was positively correlated with the number of bifidobacteria in the faeces after supplementation and negatively correlated with the initial level.[167] Maintenance of high numbers of bifidobacteria in the gut may be beneficial in terms of healthy gut function, however, its effect on the lowering of blood lipid levels remains to be investigated. A lower dose of prebiotic (2.75 g) added to a lactobacillus fermented milk has been shown to significantly increase the number of bifidobacteria when fed over a seven-week period in healthy human subjects.[163] If this effect was a result of the synbiotic product used in this study, the use of lower doses of prebiotics that can be used in synbiotic preparations should help to reduce gastrointestinal complaints observed when a prebiotic is used alone and improve the acceptability of these types of products by the general public.

8.8   Future trends

Over the past 10 years, a number of food manufacturers in the USA and Europe have been interested in the commercial opportunities for foodstuffs containing health promoting probiotics and prebiotics. These food ingredients have received attention for their beneficial effects on the gut microbiota and links to their systemic effects on the lowering of lipids known to be risk factors for CHD, notably cholesterol and TAG. Early attention was given to the incorporation of probiotics into dairy products such as fermented milk products with the recent appearance of these products in breakfast cereals. The market for probiotic products in Europe is currently estimated at €1.4 bn.[168] Prebiotics are also gaining popularity due to the greater versatility of this functional food since they can be baked into bread, breakfast cereals, cakes, biscuits, cereal bars and even added to dairy products, soups and beverages. The slower growth of this market relative to probiotics has been thought to be attributed to the lack of the launch of specific prebiotic products as has been observed with probiotic products such as Yakult and Actimel range of milk drinks. The prebiotic market in Europe is rapidly growing and is valued at approximately €0.9 bn.[169] Synbiotics are also generating interest with some food manufacturers exploiting the combination of a prebiotic with a probiotic in dairy products (e.g. Danone Activia Fibre) and capsule supplements (e.g. Probiotic Plus).

While consumers are interested in the concept of improving their health and well being through diet, this is not quite so straightforward as originally thought. Recent bad press regarding unsubstantiated claims about the health benefits of some strains of probiotics has made the public sceptical about the rapidly growing number of digestive health products. For progress to be made, the consumers need to be educated about the various health benefits and how they will be able to use these products in their own diet without adverse consequences. Although the introduction of functional foods onto the supermarket shelves is gradually being accepted by the UK population, carefully controlled nutrition studies need to be carried out to determine the beneficial effects of prebiotics, probiotics and synbiotics on CHD risk factors before substantial health claims can be made. To further protect the consumer, the European Union adopted a new European Regulation (EC No. 1924/2006) on the use of nutrition and health claims for foods in 2006.[170] The European Food Safety Authority is responsible for ensuring that any health claim made on a food label is clear to the consumer and substantiated by scientific evidence.

Advances in food technology will enable the incorporation of prebiotics and probiotics in a greater range of foods and drink without compromising the quality of the overall product. To make these foods attractive to the consumer, the products also need to be priced in such a way that they are accessible to the general public. The low doses of prebiotics and probiotics needed to help maintain a healthy gut microbiota should be made available to the public at large, whereas products which contain higher amounts of prebiotics in order to help reduce blood lipids (for example, in individuals with a greater risk of developing CHD) will need to be restricted in order for the appropriate population groups to be targeted.

8.9   Sources of further information and advice

General biochemistry and metabolic regulation text books
Frayn, K. N., *Metabolic Regulation: A Human Perspective*, Third edition, J Wiley and Sons Inc., 2010.
Devlin, T. M., *Textbook of Biochemistry with Clinical Correlations*, seventh edition, J Wiley and Sons Inc., 2010.

Published reports on coronary heart disease
Allender, B.A., Peto, V., Scarborough, P., Kaur, A. and Rayner, M., 'Coronary heart disease statistics 2008 edition', British Heart Foundation: London 2008.
Allender, B.A., Scarborough, P., Peto, V., Rayner, M., Leal, J., Luengo-Fernandez, R. and Gray, A. 'European Cardiovascular Disease Statistics 2008 edition', British Heart Foundation: London 2008.

Prebiotic, probiotic and synbiotic information
Roberfroid, M.B., 'Prebiotics and probiotics: are they functional foods?', *Am J Clin Nutr*, 2000, **71** (Suppl), S1682–1.
Inulin and oligofructose: Health benefits and claims – A critical review, *J Nutr*, 2007, **137**, 2489S–2597S (Supplement detailing conference proceedings from the 5th ORAFTI research conference: Inulin and Oligofructose: Proven Health Benefits and Claims).
Jones, P.J.H., Asp, N-G, and Silva, P., 'Evidence for health claims on food: How much is enough? Introduction and general remarks', *J Nutr*, 2008, **138**, S1189S–91.

8.10   References

1. Allender, B.A., Peto, V., Scarborough, P., Kaur, A. and Rayner, M. 'Coronary heart disease statistics 2008 edition', British Heart Foundation: London 2008.
2. Keys, A. 'Coronary artery disease in seven countries', *Circulation*, 1970, **41**, 1–211.
3. Patsch, J.R., Meisenböck, G., Hopferweiser, T., Mulhberger, V., Knapp, E., Dunn, J.K., Gotto, A.M. and Patsch, W. 'Relation of triglyceride metabolism and coronary artery disease. Studies in the postprandial state', *Arterioscler Thromb*, 1992, **12**, 1336–45.
4. Bansal, S., Buring, J.E., Rifai, N., Sacks, F.M. and Ridker, P.M. 'Fasting compared with non-fasting triglycerides and risk of cardiovascular events in women', *JAMA*, 2007, **298**, 309–16.
5. Nordestgaard, B.G., Benn, M., Schnohr, P. and Tybjörg-Hansen, A. 'Nonfasting triglycerides and risk of myocardial infaction, ischamic heart disease, and death in men and women', *JAMA* 2007, **298**, 299–308.
6. Griffin, B.A. and Zampelas, A. 'Influence of dietary fatty acids on the atherogenic lipoprotein phenotype', *Nut Res Rev*, 1995, **8**, 1–26.
7. Lorenzo, C., Hunt, K.J., Williams, K. and Haffner, S.M. 'The National Cholesterol Education Program–Adult Treatment Panel III, International Diabetes Federation, and World Health Organisation definitions of the metabolic syndrome as predictors of incident cardiovascular disease and diabetes', *Diabetes Care*, 2007, **30**, 8–13.
8. Gibson, G.R. and Beaumont, A. *Gut Flora and Health–Past, Present and Future*, London, Royal Society of Medicine Limited, 1996.
9. Lloyd-Jones, D., Adams, R.J., Brown, T.M., *et al.* 'Heart Disease and Stroke Statistics 2010 Update. A report from the American Heart Association', *Circulation*, 2010, **121**, 948–54.
10. Allender, B.A., Scarborough, P., Peto, V., Rayner, M., Leal, J., Luengo-Fernandez, R. and Gray, A. 'European Cardiovascular Disease Statistics 2008 edition', British Heart Foundation: London 2008.
11. Martin, M.J., Browner, W.S., Wentworth, J., Hulley, S.B. and Kuler, L.H. 'Serum cholesterol, blood pressure and mortality: implications from a cohort of 361,662 men', *Lancet*, 1986, **2**, 933–6.
12. The Prospective Studies Collaboration, Lewington, S., Whitlock, G., Clarke, R., Sherliker, P., Emberson, J., Halsey, J., Qizilbash, N., Peto, R. and Collins, R. 'Blood cholesterol and vascular mortality by age, sex, and blood pressure: a meta-analysis of individual data from 61 prospective studies with 55,000 vascular deaths', *Lancet*, 2007, **370**, 1829–39.
13. Shepherd, J. Cobbe, S.M., Ford, I., Isles, C.G., Lorimer, A.R., Macfarlane, P.W., McKillop, J.H. and Packard, C.J. 'Prevention of coronary heart disease with pravastatin in men with hypercholesterolaemia', *New Eng J Med*, 1995, **333**, 1301–7.
14. Prospective Studies Collaboration. 'Body-mass index and cause-specific mortality in 900,000 adults: collaborative analyses of 57 prospective studies'. *Lancet*, 2009, **373**, 1083–96.
15. Shaper, A.G., Pocock, S.J., Philips, A.N. and Walker, M. 'Identifying men at high risk of heart attacks-strategy for use in General Practice.' *BMJ*, 1986, **293**, 474–9.
16. Pencina, M.J., D'Agostino, R.B., Larson, M.G., Massaro, J.M. and Vasan, R.S. 'Predicting the 30-year risk of cardiovascular disease. The Framingham Heart Study', *Circulation*, 2009, **119**, 3078–84.
17. Fielding, P.E. and Fielding, C.J. 'Dynamics of lipoprotein transport in the circulatory system'. In D.E. Vance and J. Vance (eds), *Biochemistry of Lipids, Lipoproteins and Membranes*, pp. 427–59, Amsterdam, Elsevier, 1991.
18. Schneider, W.J. 'Removal of lipoproteins from plasma'. In D.E. Vance and J. Vance (eds), *Biochemistry of Lipids, Lipoproteins and Membranes*, pp. 461–87, Amsterdam, Elsevier, 1991.

19. Devlin, T.M. *Textbook of Biochemistry with clinical correlations*, 3rd edn, New York, John-Wiley, 1992.
20. Redgrave, T.G. *Gastrointestinal Physiology IV*, Baltimore, University Park Press, 1983.
21. Brasaemle, D.L., Cornley-Moss, K. and Bensadoun, A. 'Hepatic lipase treatment of chylomicron remnants increases exposure of apolipoprotein E', *J Lipid Res*, 1993, **34**, 455–63.
22. Karpe, F. and Hultin, M. 'Endogenous triglyceride-rich lipoproteins accumulate in rat plasma when competing with a triglyceride emulsion for a common lipolytic pathway', *J Lipid Res*, 1995, **36**, 1557–66.
23. Griffin, B.A. and Packard, C.J. 'Metabolism of VLDL and LDL subclasses', *Curr Opin Lipidol*, 1994, **5**, 200–6.
24. Tall, A.R. 'Plasma cholesterol ester transfer protein', *J Lipid Res*, 1993, **27**, 361–7.
25. Cholesterol Treatment Trialists' Collaboration. 'Efficacy and safety of cholesterol lowering treatment: prospective meta-analysis of data from 90 056 participants in 14 randomised trials of statins', *Lancet*, 2005, **366**, 1267–78.
26. Third report of the National Cholesterol Education Program (NECP) Expert Panel on Detection, Evaluation and Treatment of High Cholesterol in Adults (Adult Treatment Panel III): Final Report. *Circulation*, **2002**, 3143–3421.
27. Assmann, G., Cullen, P. and Schulte, H. 'The Münster Heart Study (PROCAM). Results of follow-up at 8 years', *Eur Heart J*, 1998, **19** (Suppl. A), A2–A11.
28. Ingelsson, E., Schaefer, E.J., Contois, J.H., McNamara, J.R., Sullivan, L., Keyes, M.J., Pencina, M.J., Schoonmaker, C., Wilson, P.W., D'Agostino, R.B. and Vasan, R.S. 'Clinical utility of different lipid measures for prediction of coronary heart disease in men and women', *JAMA* 2007, **298**, 776–85.
29. The Emerging Factors Collaboration. 'Major lipids, apolipoproteins, and risk of vascular disease', *JAMA*, 2009, **302**, 1993–2000.
30. Austin, M.A. 'Plasma triglyceride and coronary artery disease', *Arterioscl Thromb*, 1991, **11**, 2–14.
31. Karpe, F., Steiner, G., Uffelman, K., Olivecrona, T. and Hamsten, A. 'Postprandial lipoproteins and progression of coronary heart disease', *Atherosclerosis*, 1994, **106**, 83–97.
32. Proctor, S.D., Vine, D.F. and Mamo, J.C.L. 'Arterial permeability and efflux of apolipoprotein B containing lipoproteins assessed by in situ perfusion and three dimensional quantitative confocal microscopy', *Arterioscl Thromb Vasc Biol* 2004, **24**, 2162–7.
33. Zilversmit, D. 'Atherogenesis: A postprandial phenomenon', *Circulation*, 1979, **60**, 473–85.
34. Meisenböck, G. and Patsch, J.R. 'Coronary artery disease: Synergy of triglyceride-rich lipoproteins and HDL', *Cardiovascular Risk Factors*, 1991, **1**, 293–9.
35. Austin, M.A., Breslow, J.L., Hennekens, C.H., Burling, J.E., Willett, W.C. and Krauss, R.M. 'Low density lipoprotein subclass patterns and risk of myocardial infarction', *JAMA*, 1988, **260**, 1917–21.
36. Austin, M.A., Hokanson, J.E. and Brunzell, J.D. 'Characterisation of low-density lipoprotein subclasses: methodological approaches and clinical relevance', *Curr Opin Lipidol*, 1994, **5**, 395–403.
37. Sacks, F.M. and Campos, H. 'Low-density lipoprotein size and cardiovascular disease: A reappraisal', *J Clin Endocrinol Metab*, 2003, **88**, 4525–32.
38. Chapman, M.J., Guérin, M. and Bruckert, E. 'Atherogenic, dense low-density lipoproteins. Pathophysiology and new therapeutic approaches', *Eur Heart J*, 1998, **19** (Suppl. A), A24–A30.
39. Kathiresan, S., Otvos, J.D., Sullivan, L.M., Keyes, M.J., Schaefer, E.J., Wilson, P.W.F., D'Agostino, R.B., Vasan, R.S. and Robins, S.J. 'Increased small low-density lipoprotein particle number. A prominent feature of the metabolic syndrome in the Framingham Heart Study', *Circulation*, 2006, **113**, 20–9.

40. Reaven, G.M., Chen, Y.-D.I., Jeppensen, J., Maheux, P. and Krauss, R.M. 'Insulin resistance and hyperinsulinaemia in individuals with small, dense, low density lipoprotein particles', *J Clin Invest*, 1993, **92**, 141–6.
41. Gami, A.S., Witt, B.J., Howard, D.E., Erwin, P.J., Gami, L.A., Somers, V.K. and Montori, V.M. 'Metabolic Syndrome and Risk of Incident Cardiovascular Events and Death. A systematic review and meta-analysis of longitudinal studies', *J Am Coll Cardiol* 2007, **49**, 403–14.
42. World Health Organisation: Definition, diagnosis and classification of diabetes mellitus and its complications. Report of a WHO consultation. Geneva: World Health Organisation, Department of Noncommunicable Disease Surveilliance; 1999: 1–59.
43. Balkau, B. and Charles, M.A. 'Comment on the provisional report from the WHO consultation. European Group for the study of insulin resistance (EGIR)', *Diabet Med* 1999, **16**, 442–3.
44. Executive Summary of the third report of the National Cholesterol Education Program (NCEP) Expert Panel on detection, evaluation, and treatment of high blood cholesterol in adults (Adult treatment panel III), *JAMA*, 2001, **285**, 2486–97.
45. Einhorn, D., Reaven, G.M. and Cobin, R.H. 'American college of endocrinology position statement on the insulin resistance syndrome.' *Endocr Pract* 2003, **9**, 237–42.
46. Alberti, K.G., Zimmet, P. and Shaw, J. 'Metabolic Syndrome – a new world wide definition. A consensus statement from the International Diabetes Federation', *Diabet Med* 2006, **23**, 469–80.
47. Sunström, J., Vallhagen, E., Risérus, U., Byberg, L., Zethelius, B., Berne, C., Lind, L. and Ingelsson, E. 'Risk associated with the metabolic syndrome versus the sum of its individual components', *Diab Care*, 2006, **29**, 1673–4.
48. Guize, L., Tomas, F., Pannier, B., Bean, K., Jego, B. and Benetos, A. 'All-Cause mortality associated with specific combinations of the metabolic syndrome according to recent definitions', *Diab Care*, 2007, **30**, 2381–7.
49. Sone, H., Tanaka, S., Limuro, S., Oida, K., Yamasaki, Y., Oikawa, S., Ishibashi, S., Katayama, S., Ito, H., Ohashi, Y., Akanuma, Y. and Yamada, N. 'Components of the metabolic syndrome and their components as predictors of cardiovascular disease in Japanese patients with type 2 diabetes. Implications for improved definition. Analysis from Japan Diabetes Complications Study (JDCS)', *J Atheroscler Thromb*, 2009, **16**, 380–7.
50. Keys, A. *Seven Countries: A Multivariate Analysis of Death and Coronary Heart Disease*, Harvard University Press, Cambridge, MA, 1980.
51. Hegsted, D.M., Ansman, L.M., Johnson, J.A. and Dallal, G.E. 'Dietary fat and serum lipids: an evaluation of the experimental data', *Am J Clin Nutr*, 1993, **57**, 875–83.
52. Hayes, K.C. and Khosla, P. 'Dietary fatty acids thesholds and cholesterolaemia', *FASEB J*, 1992, **6**, 2600–7.
53. Department of Health. *Nutritional Aspects of Cardiovascular Disease. Report of the Cardiovascular Review Group Committee on Medical Aspects of Food Policy*. London: HMSO, 1994. Report on Health and Social Subjects 46.
54. Henderson, L., Gregory, J. and Irving, K. '*The Dietary and Nutritional Survey of British Adults: A Survey of the Dietary Behaviour, Nutritional Status and Blood Pressure of Adults aged 19 to 64 living in Great Britain*', Office of Population Census and Surveys, Social Survey Division, London, HMSO, 2003.
55. de Longeril, L.M., Salen, P., Martin, J.L., Monjaud, I., Delaye, J. and Mamelle, N. 'Mediterranean diet, traditional risk factors and the rate of cardiovascular complications after myocardial infarction: Final report of the Lyon Heart Study'. *Circulation*, 1999, **99**, 779–85.
56. Mensink, R.P. and Katan, M.B. 'Effect of dietary *trans* fatty acids in high density and low density lipoprotein cholesterol levels in healthy subjects', *N Eng J Med*, 1990, **323**, 439–45.

57. SACN Position Statement. 'Update on trans fatty acids and health'. TSO (The Stationary Office), 2007.
58. Dyberg, J. and Bang, H.O. 'Haemostatic function and platelet polyunsaturated fatty acids in Eskimos', *Lancet*, 1979, **2**, 433–5.
59. Burr, M.L, Fehily, A.M., Gilbert, J.F. *et al.* 'Effects of changes of fat, fish and fibre intakes on frequency of myocardial infarctions: DART Study', *Lancet*, 1989, **2**, 757–62.
60. GISSI. 'Dietary supplementation with n-3 polyunsaturated fatty acids and vitamin E after myocardial infarction: results of the GISSI-Prevenzione trial. Gruppo Italiano per lo Studio della Sopravvivenza nell'Infarto miocardico', *Lancet*, 1999, **354**, 447–55.
61. Siscovick, D.S., Raghunathan, T.E., King, I. and Weinman, S. 'Dietary intake and cell membrane levels of long chain *n*-3 polyunsaturated fatty acids and the risk of primary cardiac arrest', *J Am Med Assoc*, 1996, **274**, 1363–7.
62. De Deckere, E.A.M., Korver, O., Verschuren, P.M. and Katan, M.B. 'Health aspects of fish and n-3 polyunsaturated fatty acids from plant and marine origin', *Eur J Clin Nutr*, 1998, **52**, 749–53.
63. SACN 'Advice on fish consumption: benefits and risks', TSO (The Stationary Office), 2004.
64. EEC Scientific Committee for Food, *Reference Nutrient Intakes for the European Connumity*, Brussels, EC, 1992.
65. Mensink, R.P. and Katan, M.B. 'Effects of monounsaturated fatty acids versus complex carbohydrates on high density lipoproteins in healthy men and women', *Lancet*, 1987, **1**, 122–5.
66. Grundy, S.M. 'Comparison of monounsaturated fatty acids and carbohydrates for lowering plasma cholesterol', *N Eng J Med*, 1986, **314**, 745–8.
67. Barclay, A.W., Petocz, P. and Millan-Price, J. 'Glycaemic index, glycaemic load and chronic disease risk – a meta analysis of observational studies', *Am J Clin Nutr*, 2008, **87**, 627–37.
68. Morris, J.N., Marr, J.W. and Clayton, D.G. 'Diet and heart: a postscript', *BMJ*, 1977, **2**, 1307–14.
69. Kushi, L.H., Lew, R.A., Stare, F.J. *et al.* 'Diet and 20-year mortality from coronary heart disease: the Ireland-Boston Diet-Heart Study', *N Eng J Med*, 1985, **312**, 811–18.
70. Pereira, M.A., O'Reilly, E., Augustson, K. *et al.* 'Dietary fibre and risk of coronary heart disease: a pooled analysis of cohort studies', *Arch Intern Med*, 2004, **164**, 370–6.
71. Slavin, J.L., Savarino, V., Paredes-Diaz, A. and Fotopoulos, G. 'A review of the role of soluble fiber in health with specific relevance to wheat dextrin', *J Intern Med Res*, 2009, **37**, 1–17.
72. Seal, C.J. 'Wholegrain and CVD', *Proc Nutr Soc*, 2006, **65**, 24–34.
73. Elliot, P., Dyer, A. and Stamler, J. 'Correcting for regression dilution in INTERSALT', *Lancet*, 1993, **342**, 1123.
74. Law, M.R., Frost, C.D. and Wald, N.J. 'By how much does dietary salt reduction lower blood pressure? I–III – Analysis of observational data among populations', *BMJ*, 1991, **302**, 811–24.
75. Sacks, F.M., Svetkey, L.P., Vollmer, W.M., Appel, L.J., Bray, G.A., Harsha, D., Obarzanek, E., Conlin, P.R., Miller, E.R., Simons-Morton, D.G., Karanja, N. and Lin, P.H. 'Effects on blood pressure of reduced dietary sodium and the Dietary Approaches to Stop Hypertention (DASH) diet. DASH-Sodium Collaborative Research Group', *New Eng J Med*, 2001, **344**, 3–10.
76. SACN. 'Salt and health', TSO (The Stationary Office). 2003
77. Corrao, G., Rubbiati, L. and Bagnardi, V. 'Alcohol and coronary heart disease: a meta-analysis', *Addiction*, 2000, **95**, 1505–23.
78. Foster, R.K. and Marriott, H.E. 'Alcohol consumption in the new millennium – weighing up the risks and benefits for our health', *BNF Nutr Bull*, 2006, **31**, 286–331.

79. Gaziano, J.M., Buring, J.E., Breslow, J.L., Goldhaber, S.Z., Rosner, B., Vandenburgh, M., Williet, W.C. and Hennekens, C.H. 'Moderate alcohol intake, increased levels of high density lipoprotein and its subfractions, and decreased risk of myocardial infarction', *New Eng J Med*, 1993, **329**, 1829–34.

80. Law, M. and Wald, N. 'Why heart disease mortality is low in France: the time lag explanation', *BMJ*, 1999, **318**, 1471–80.

81. Mann, G.V. and Spoerry, A. 'Studies of a surfactant and cholesteramia in the Maasai', *Am J Clin Nutr*, 1974, **27**, 464–9.

82. Mann, G.V. 'A factor in yoghurt which lowers cholesteremia in man', *Atherosclerosis*, 1977, **26**, 335–40

83. Howard, A.N. and Marks, J. 'Effect of milk products on serum-cholesterol', *Lancet*, 1979, **II**, 957.

84. Hepner, G., Fried, R., St Jeor, S., Fusetti, L. and Morin, R. 'Hypocholesterolemic effect of yogurt and milk', *Am J Clin Nutr*, 1979, **32**, 19–24.

85. Sessions, V.A., Lovegrove, J.A., Dean, T.S., Williams, C.M., Sanders, T.A.B., Macdonald, I. and Salter, A. 'The effects of a new fermented milk product on plasma cholesterol and apolipoprotein B concentrations in middle aged men and women', *Proc Nutr Soc*, 1997, **56**, 120A.

86. Thompson, L.U., Jenkins, D.J.A., Amer, V., Reichert, R., Jenkins, A. and Kamulsky, J. 'The effect of fermented and unfermented milks on serum cholesterol', *Am J Clin Nutr*, 1982, **36**, 1106–11.

87. Massey, L.K. 'Effect of changing milk and yogurt consumption on human nutrient intake and serum lipoproteins', *J Dairy Sci*, 1984, **67**, 255–62.

88. McNamara, D.J., Lowell, A.E. and Sabb, J.E. 'Effect of yogurt intake on plasma lipid and lipoprotein levels in normolipidemic males', *Atherosclerois*, 1989, **79**, 167–71.

89. St Onge, M.-P., Farnworth, E.R., Savard, T., Chabot, D., Mafu, A. and Jones, P.J.H. 'Kefir consumption does not alter plasma lipid levels or cholesterol fractional synthesis rates relative to milk in hyperlipidemic men: a randomized controlled trial', *BMC Complementary and Alternative Med*, 2002, **2**, 1–6.

90. Jaspers, D.A., Massey, L.K. and Luedecke, L.O. 'Effect of consuming yogurts prepared with thress culture strains on human serum lipoproteins', *J Food Sci* 1984, **49**, 1178–81.

91. Xiao, J.Z., Kondo, S., Takahashi, N., Miyaji, K., Oshida, K., Hiramatsu, A., Iwatsuki, K., Kokubo, S. and Hosono, A. 'Effects of milk products fermented by *Bifidobacterium Longum* on blood lipids in rats and healthy adult male volunteers', *J Dairy Sci*, 2003, **86**, 2452–61.

92. Ataie-Jafari, A., Larijani, B., Alavi Majid, H. and Tahbaz, F. 'Cholesterol-lowering effect of probiotic yogurt in comparison with ordinary yogurt in mildly to moderately hypercholesterolemic subjects', *Ann Nutr Metab*, 2009, **54**, 22–7.

93. de Roos, N.M., Schouten, G. and Katan, M.B. 'Yoghurt enriched with lactobacillus acidophilus does not lower blood lipids in healthy men and women with normal to borderline high serum cholesterol levels', *Eur J Clin Nutr*, 1999, **53**, 277–80.

94. Anderson, J.W. and Gilliland, S.E. 'Effects of fermented milk (yoghurt) containing *Lactobacillus Acidophilus* L1 on serum cholesterol in hypercholesterolaemic humans', *J Am Coll Nutr*, 1999, **18**, 43–50.

95. Agerbaek, M., Gerdes, L.U. and Richelsen, B. 'Hypocholesterolaemic effects of a new product in healthy middle-aged men', *Eur J Clin Nutr*, 1995, **49**, 346–52.

96. Richelsen, B., Kristensen, K. and Pedersen, S.B. 'Long-term (6 months) effect of a new fermented milk product on the level of plasma lipoproteins-a placebo-controlled and double blind study', *Eur J Clin Nutr*, 1996, **50**, 811–15.

97. Bertolami, M.C. 'Evaluation of the effects of a new fermented milk product (Gaio) on primary hypercholesterolemia', *Eur J Clin Nutr*, 1999, **53**, 97–101.

98. Rossouw, J.E., Burger, E.-M., Van Der Vyver, P. and Ferreira, J.J. 'The effect of skim milk yoghurt, and full cream milk on human serum lipids', *Am J Clin Nutr*, 1981, **34**, 351–6.

99. Agerholm-Larsen, L., Raben, A., Haulrik, N., Hansen, A.S.A., Manders, M. and Astrup, A. 'Effect of 8 week intake of probiotic milk products on risk factors for cardiovascular diseases', *Eur J Clin Nutr*, 2000, **54**, 288–97.

100. Rossi, E.A., Vendramini, R.C., Carlos, I.Z., de Oliveira, M.G. and de Valdez, G.F. 'Effect of a new fermented soy milk product on serum lipid levels in normocholesterolemic adult men', *Arch Latinoam Nutr*, 2003, **53**, 47–51.

101. Larkin, T.A., Astheimer, L.B. and Price, W.E. 'Dietary combination of soy with prebiotic or prebiotic food significantly reduces total and LDL cholesterol in mildly hypercholesterolaemic subjects', *Eur J Clin Nutr*, 2009, **63**, 238–45.

102. Karlsson, C., Ahrne, S., Molin, G., Berggren, A., Palmquist, I., Fredrikson, G.N. and Jeppsson, B. 'Probiotic therapy to men with incipient arteriosclerosis initiates increased bacterial diversity in colon: A randomized controlled trial', *Atherosclerosis*, 2010, **208**, 228–33.

103. Steinberg, F., Guthrie, N., Villablanca, A., Kumar, K. and Murray, M. 'Soy protein with isoflavones has favourable effects on endothelial function that are independent of lipid and antioxidant effects in healthy postmenopausal women', *Am J Clin Nutr*, 2003, **78**, 123–30.

104. Hall, W.L., Vafeiadou, K., Hallund, J., *et al*.. 'Soy-isoflavone-enriched foods and markers of lipid and glucose metabolism in postmenopausal women: interactions with genotype and equol production', *Am J Clin Nutr* 2006, **83**, 592–600.

105. Potter, P. 'Soy protein and cardiovascular disease: the impact of bioactive components in soy', *Nutr Rev*, 1998, **56**, 231–5.

106. Bazzare, T.L., Wu, S.-M.L., and Yuhas, J.A. 'Total and HDL-cholesterol concentrations following yogurt and calcium supplementation', *Nutr Reports Int*, 1983, **28**, 1225–32.

107. Huis In't Veld, J.H.J. and Shortt, C. 'Selection criteria for probiotic micro-organisms'. In Leeds AR & Rowland IR (eds) *Gut Flora and Health–Past, Present and Future*. International congress and symposium series No. 219. London, New York: Royal Society of Medicine Press, 1996, 27–36.

108. Hylemond, P.B. 'Metabolism of bile acids in intestinal microflora'. In H. Danielson and J. Sjovall (eds), *Sterols and Bile Acids*, pp. 331–43, New York, Elsevier Science Publishing, 1985.

109. Grill, J.P., Manginot-Durr, C., Schneider, F. and Ballongue, J. 'Bifidobacteria and probiotic effects:action of *Bifidobacterium* species on conjugated bile salts', *Curr Microbiol*, 1995, **31**, 23–7.

110. Gilliland, S.E., Nelson, C.R. and Maxwell, C. 'Assimilation of cholesterol by *Lactobacillus acidophilus*', *Applied Environ Microbiol*, 1985, **49**, 377–81.

111. Pereira, D.I.A., McCartney, A.L. and Gibson, G.R. 'An *in vitro* study of the probiotic potential of a bile-salt-hydrolyzing *Lactobacillus fermentum* strain, and determination of its cholesterol-lowering properties', *Appl & Environ Microbiol*, 2003, **69**, 4743–52.

112. De Smet, I., De Boever, P. and Verstraete, W. 'Cholesterol lowering in pigs through enhanced bacterial bile salt hydrolase activity', *BJN*, 1998, **79**, 185–94.

113. Marteau, P., Gerhardt, M.F., Myara, A., Bouvier, E., Trivin, F. and Rambaud, J.C. 'Metabolism of bile salts by alimentary bacteria during transit in human small intestine', *Microbiol Ecology in Health & Disease*, 1995, **8**, 151–7.

114. Gilliland, S.E., Nelson, C.R. and Maxwell, C. 'Assimilation of cholesterol by *Lactobacillus acidophilus*', *Appl & Environ Microbiol*, 1985, **49**, 377–81.

115. Rasic, J.L., Vujicic, I.F., Skrinjar, M. and Vulic, M. 'Assimilation of cholesterol by some cultures of lactic acid bacteria and bifidobacteria', *Biotech Let*, 1992, **14**, 39–44.

116. Pereira, D.I.A. and Gibson, G.R. 'Cholesterol assimilation by lactic acid bacteria and bifidobacteria isolated from the human gut', *Appl & Environ Microbiol*, 2002, **68**, 4689–93.

117. Klaver, F.A.M. and Van Der Meer, R. 'The assumed assililation of cholesterol by lactobacilli and *Bifidobacterium bifidum* is due to their bile salt-deconjugating activity', *Appl & Environ Microbiol*, 1993, **59**, 1120–4.

118. Tahri, K., Crociani, J., Ballongue, J. and Schneider, F. 'Effects of three strains of bifidobacteria on cholesterol', *Lett Appl Microbiol*, 1995, **21**, 149–51.

119. Hosono, A. and Tono-oka, T. 'Binding of cholesterol with lactic acid bacterial cells', *Milchwissenschaft*, 1995, **50**, 556–60.

120. Lin, M.Y. and Chen, T.W. 'Reduction of cholesterol by *Lactobacillus acidophilus* in culture broth', *J Food Drug Anal*, 2000, **8**, 97–102.

121. Gibson, G.R. and Roberfroid, M.B. 'Dietary modulation of the human colonic microbiota – Introducing the concept of prebiotics', *J Nutr*, 1995, **125**, 1401–12.

122. Dysseler, P. and Hoffem, D. 'Inulin, an alternative dietary fibre. Properties and quantitative analysis', *Eur J Clin Nutr*, 1995, **49**, S145–52.

123. Van Loo, J., Coussement, P., de Leenheer, L., Hoebregs, H. and Smits, G. 'On the presence of inulin and oligofructose as natural ingredients in the Western diet', *Crit Rev Food Sci and Nutr*, 1995, **35**, 525–52.

124. Balcázar-Munoz, B.R., Martinez-Abundis, E. and González-Ortiz, M. 'Effect of oral inulin administration on lipid profile and insulin sensitivity in subjects with obesity and dyslipidemia', *Rev Med Chil*, 2003, **131**, 597–604 (Spanish, abstract only).

125. Yamashita, K., Kawai, K. and Itakura, M. 'Effects of fructo-oligosaccharides on blood glucose and serum lipids in diabetic subjects', *Nutr Res*, 1984, **4**, 961–6.

126. Hidaka, H., Tashiro, Y. and Eida, T. 'Proliferation of bifidobacteria by oligosaccharides and their useful effect on human health', *Bifidobacteria Microflora*, 1991, **10**, 65–79.

127. Davidson, M.H., Synecki, C., Maki, K.C. and Drennen, K.B. 'Effects of dietary inulin in serum lipids in men and women with hypercholesterolaemia', *Nutr Res*, 1998, **3**, 503–17.

128. Causey, J.L., Gallaher, D.D. and Slavin, J.L. 'Effect of inulin consumption on lipid and glucose metabolism in healthy men with moderately elevated cholesterol', *FASEB*, 1998, **12**, 4737.

129. Jackson, K.G., Taylor, G.R.J., Clohessy, A.M. and Williams, C.M. 'The effect of the daily intake of inulin on fasting lipid, insulin and glucose concentrations in middle-aged men and women', *BJN*, 1999, **82**, 23–30.

130. Alles, M.S., de Roos, N.M., Bakx, J.C., van de Lisdonk, E., Zock, P.L. and Hautvast, J.G.A.J. 'Consumption of fructooligosaccharides does not favourably affect blood glucose and serum lipid concentrations in patients with type 2 diabetes', *Am J Clin Nutr*, 1999, **69**, 64–9.

131. Luo, J., Yperselle, M., Rizkalla, S.W., Rossi, F., Bornet, F.R. and Slama, G. 'Chronic consumption of short-chain fructooligosaccharides does not affect basal hepatic glucose production or insulin resistance in type 2 diabetics', *J Nutr*, 2000, **130**, 1572–7.

132. Canzi, E., Brighenti, F., Casiraghi, M.C., Del Puppo, E. and Ferrari, A. 'Prolonged consumption of inulin in ready to eat breakfast cereals: effects on intestinal ecosystem, bowel habits and lipid metabolism', Cost 92. Workshop on dietary fibre and fermentation in the colon, Helsinki, 1995.

133. Brighenti, F., Casiraghi, M.C., Canzi, E. and Ferrari, A. 'Effect of consumption of ready-to-eat breakfast cereal containing inulin on the intestinal milieu and blood lipids in healthy male volunteers', *Eur J Clin Nutr*, 1999, **53**, 726–33.

134. Letexier, D., Diraison, F. and Beylot, M. 'Addition of inulin to a moderately high carbohydrate diet reduces hepatic lipogenesis and plasma triacylglycerol concentrations in humans', *Am J Clin Nutr*, 2003, **77**, 559–64.

135. Russo, F., Chimienti, G., Riezzo, G., Pepe, G., Petrosillo, G., Chiloiro, M. and Marconi, E. 'Inulin-enriched pasta affects lipid profile and Lp(a) concentrations in Italian young healthy male volunteers', *Eur J Nutr* 2008, **47**, 453–9.

136. Luo, J., Rizkalla, S.W., Alamowitch, C., Boussairi, A., Blayo, A., Barry, J.-L., Laffitte, A., Guyon, F., Bornet, F.R.J. and Slama, G. 'Chronic consumption of short-chain

fructooligosaccharides by healthy subjects decreased basal hepatic glucose production but no effect on insulin-stimulated glucose metabolism', *Am J Clin Nutr*, 1996, **63**, 939–45.

137. Pedersen, A., Sandström, B. and van Amelsvoort, J.M.M. 'The effect of ingestion of inulin on blood lipids and gastrointestinal symptoms in healthy females', *BJN*, 1997, **78**, 215–22.

138. Kruse, H.-P., Kleessen, B. and Blaut, M. 'Effect of inulin on faecal bifidobacteria in human subjects', *BJN*, 1999, **82**, 375–82.

139. Van Dokkum, W., Wezendonk, B., Srikumar, T.S. and van den Heuval, E.G.H.M. 'Effect of nondigestible oligosaccharides on large-bowel functions, blood lipid concentrations and glucose absorption in young healthy male subjects', *Eur J Clin Nutr*, 1999, **53**, 1–7.

140. Giacco, R., Clemente, G., Luongo, D., Lasorella, G., Fiume, I., Brouns, F., Bornet, F., Patti, L., Cipriano, P., Rivellese, A.A. and Riccardi, G. 'Effects of short-chain fructo-oligosaccharides on glucose and lipid metabolism in mild hypercholesterolaemic individuals', *Clin Nutr*, 2004, **23**, 331–40.

141. Forcheron, F. and Beylot, M. 'Long-term administration of inulin-type fructans has no significant lipid-lowering effect in normolipidaemic humans', *Metabolism*, 2007, **56**, 1093–8.

142. Vulevic, J., Drakoularakou, A., Yaqoob, P., Tzortzis, G. and Gibson, G.R. 'Modulation of the faecal microflora profile and immune function by a novel trans-galactooligosaccharide mixture (B-GOS) in healthy elderly volunteers', *Am J Clin Nutr*, 2008, **88**, 1438–46.

143. Brighenti, F. 'Dietary fructans and serum triacylglycerols: A meta-analysis of randomised controlled trials', *J Nutr*, 2007, **137**, S2552–6.

144. Kok, N.N., Morgan, L.M., Williams, C.M., Roberfroid, M.B., Thissen, J.-P. and Delzenne, N.M. 'Insulin, glucagon-like peptide 1, glucose dependent insulinotropic polypeptide and insulin-like growth factor 1 as putative mediators of the hypolipidemic effect of oligofructose in rats', *J Nutr*, 1998, **128**, 1099–103.

145. Williams, C.M. 'Effects of inulin on blood lipids in humans', *J Nutr*, 1998, **7**, S1471–3.

146. Roberfroid, M. 'Dietary fiber, inulin and oligofructose: a review comparing their physiological effects', *Crit Rev Food Sci and Nutr*, 1993, **33**, 102–48.

147. Genta, S., Cabrera, W., Habib, N., Pons, J., Carillo, I.M., Grau, A. and Sánchez, S. 'Yacon syrup: beneficial effects on obesity and insulin resistance in humans', *Clin Nutr*, 2009, **28**, 182–7.

148. Delzenne, N.M., Kok, N., Fiordaliso, M.-F., Deboyser, D.M., Goethals, F.M. and Roberfroid, R.M. 'Dietary fructo-oligosaccharides modify lipid metabolism', *Am J Clin Nutr*, 1993, **57**, 820S.

149. Gibson, G.R. and McCartney, A.L. 'Modification of gut flora by dietary means', *Biochem Soc Trans*, 1998, **26**, 222–8.

150. Wolever, T.M.S., Brighenti, F., Royall, D., Jenkins, A.L. and Jenkins, D.J.A. 'Effect of rectal infusion of short chain fatty acids in human subjects', *Am J Gastroenterol*, 1989, **84**, 1027–33.

151. Demigné, C., Morand, C., Levrat, M.-A., Besson, C., Moundras, C. and Rémésey, C. 'Effect of propionate on fatty acid and cholesterol synthesis and on acetate metabolism in isolated rat hepatocytes', *BJN*, 1995, **74**, 209–19.

152. Van Loo, J., Cummings, J., Delzenne, N., Englyst, H., Franck, A., Hopkins, M., Kok, N., Macfarlane, G., Newton, D., Quigley, M., Roberfroid, M., van Vliet, T. and van den Heuval, E. 'Functional food properties of non-digestible oligosaccharides: a consensus report from the ENDO project (DGXII AIRII-CT94-1095)', *BJN*, 1999, **81**, 121–32.

153. Wolever, T.M.S., Spadafora, P.J., Cunnane, S.C. and Pencharz, P.B. 'Propionate inhibits incorporation of colonic [1,2-^{13}C]acetate into plasma lipids in humans', *Am J Clin Nutr*, 1995, **61**, 1241–7.

154. Fiordaliso, M.-F., Kok, N., Desager, J.-P., Goethals, F., Deboyser, D., Roberfroid, R.M. and Delzenne, N. 'Dietary oligofructose lowers triglycerides, phospholipids and cholesterol in serum and very low density lipoproteins in rats', *Lipids*, 1995, **30**, 163–7.

155. Delzenne, N.M. and Kok, N. 'Effect of non-digestible fermentable carbohydrates on hepatic fatty acid metabolism', *Biochem Soc Trans*, 1998, **26**, 228–30.

156. Rumessen, J.J., Bode, S., Hamberg, O. and Gudmand-Hoyer, E. 'Fructans of the Jerusalem artichokes: intestinal transport, absorption, fermentation, and influence on blood glucose, insulin, and C-peptide responses in healthy subjects', *Am J Clin Nutr*, 1990, **52**, 675–81.

157. Todesco, T., Rao, A.V., Bosello, O. and Jenkins, D.J.A. 'Propionate lowers blood glucose and alters lipid metabolism in healthy subjects', *Am J Clin Nutr*, 1991, **54**, 860–5.

158. Morgan, L.M. 'The role of gastrointestinal hormones in carbohydrate and lipid metabolism and homeostasis: effects of gastric inhibitory polypeptide and glucagon-like peptide-1', *Biochem Soc Trans*, 1998, **26**, 216–22.

159. Burcelin, R., Cani, P.D. and Knauf, C. 'Glucagon-like peptide-1 and energy homeostasis', *J Nutr*, 2007, **137**, S2534–8.

160. Delzenne, N., Cani, P.D. and Neyrinck, A.M. 'Modulation of glucagon-like peptide 1 and energy metabolism by insulin and oligofructose: Experimental data', *J Nutr*, 2007, **137**, S2547–51.

161. Knapper, J.M., Puddicombe, S.M., Morgan, L.M. and Fletcher, J.M. 'Investigations into the actions of glucose dependent insulinotrophic polypeptide and glucagon-like peptide-1 (7–36) amide on lipoprotein lipase activity in explants of rat adipose tissue', *J Nutr*, 1995, **125**, 183–8.

162. Delzenne, N. 'The hypolipidaemic effect of inulin: when animal studies help to approach the human problem', *BJN*, 1999, **82**, 3–4.

163. Roberfroid, M.B. 'Prebiotics and synbiotics: concepts and nutritional properties', *BJN*, 1998, **80** (Suppl. 2), S197–202.

164. Schaafsma, G., Meuling, W.J.A., van Dokkum, W. and Bouley, C. 'Effects of a milk product, fermented by Lactobacillus acidophilus and with fructo-oligosaccharides added, on blood lipids in male volunteers', *Eur J Clin Nutr* 1998; **52**, 436–40.

165. Kießling, G., Scheider, J. and Jahreis, G. 'Long-term consumption of fermented dairy products over 6 months increases HDL cholesterol', *Eur J Clin Nutr*, 2002, **56**, 843–9.

166. Bouhnik, Y., Flourie, B., Andrieux, C., Bisetti, N., Briet, F. and Rambaud, J. 'Effect of Bifidobacterium sp fermented milk ingested with or without inulin on colonic bifidobacteria and enzymatic activities in healthy humans', *Eur J Clin Nutr*, 1996, **50**, 269–73.

167. Ndagijimana, M., Laghi, L., Vitali, B., Placucci, G., Brigidi, P. and Guerzoni, M.E. 'Effect of a symbiotic food consumption on human gut metabolic profiles evaluated by 1H nuclear magnetic resonance spectroscopy', *Int J Food Microbiol* 2009, **134**, 147–53.

168. Saxelin, M. 'Probiotic formulations and applications, the current probiotics market, and changes in the marketplace: A European perspective', *Clin Infec Dis*, 2008, **46**, S76–9.

169. Anon. 'The European market for probiotics and prebiotics', http://www.ingredientsdirectory.com/reports/report2.pdf

170. Asp, N.-G. and Bryngelsson, S. 'Health claims in Europe: New legislation and PASSCLAIM for Substantiation', *J Nutr*, 2008, **138**, S1210–15.

171. Erkelens, D.W. 'Apolipoproteins in lipid transport, an impressionist view', *Post Med J*, 1989, **65**, S6–12.

9

Anti-tumour properties of functional foods

I. T. Johnson, Institute of Food Research, UK

Abstract: Diet and other lifestyle factors exert complex effects on the biological processes leading to the development of cancer. The purpose of this chapter is to provide a short overview of the biology of cancer, to illustrate the great variety of mechanisms through which diet can influence its initiation and development, and to consider briefly the potential role of functional foods in its prevention. Among the topics covered are the protective effects of micronutrients and selected phytochemicals, and the potential benefits of dietary fibre, resistant starch and carbohydrate fermentation products.

Key words: cancer prevention, nutrition, phytochemicals, dietary fibre.

9.1   Introduction

Cancer is an ancient disease, as old as human history, but we know almost nothing of the effects of environment and diet on its incidence prior to the twentieth century. In the modern world the incidence of age-related cancers has risen in parallel with average longevity. However, when age is taken into account, it is clear that the life-time risk of most of the most important cancers varies widely between populations, and that these differences are attributable to environmental factors. Industrialisation, increasing prosperity and social progress bring many benefits for public health, but although some cancers become less common as poverty declines, the risk of others rises. For example, during the first half of the twentieth century the incidence of both breast and colorectal cancer in Japan was around 25% of that in the USA and many countries of Northern Europe, whereas stomach cancer was several times more common. Since the 1970s the incidence of both breast and bowel cancer has risen steeply in Japan, whereas the risk of stomach cancer has declined (Key *et al.*, 2002). In their classic epidemiological analysis of the environmental causes of cancer, Doll and Peto estimated that diet was responsible for approximately 35% of cancers in North America and Western Europe (Doll and Peto, 1981). However the uncertainty attached to this estimate was very high, and the mechanisms virtually unknown. More recently, in their two comprehensive reports on nutrition, physical activity and cancer, the World Cancer Research Fund has confirmed the central importance of diet as a major influence on the risk of many forms of cancer across the globe (WCRF, 1997, 2007).

The effects of diet and other lifestyle factors on the biological processes leading to the development of cancer are extremely complex. One obvious mechanism for increased risk is the presence in food of mutagenic compounds directly damaging to DNA. However, contrary to popular perception, this is unlikely to be of great significance in countries with well developed food standards authorities and public health systems. Although there are small quantities of carcinogenic organic compounds in our diets, often derived from natural products or from side reactions in food preparation, the human body is equipped with efficient defenses, and with the exception of alcohol, the level of exposure is thought to be too low to account for more than a few per cent of cancer cases (Lutz and Schlatter, 1992). A second possibility is that the diets of modern Western countries may be deficient in minerals, organic micronutrients or other biologically active food components that exert anti-carcinogenic effects, and that higher levels of consumption would reduce the long-term risk of DNA damage, or suppress the emergence of tumours in other ways (Ames, 2006). A third possibility is that the balance of energy intake and expenditure plays an important role in the aetiology of many cancers, and that rising obesity and declining physical activity levels are major risk factors in modern industrialised societies (Fair and Montgomery, 2009).

Over the past two decades a large body of epidemiological evidence in favour of a protective effect of plant foods against many cancers has accumulated, and the need to promote consumption of fruit and vegetables as a public health strategy has become generally accepted by nutritionists and regulatory bodies (Daviglus *et al.*, 2005). There has also been a remarkable growth of interest in the biological activities of micronutrients and phytochemicals, and in the possibility that they might be usefully incorporated into functional foods. The purpose of this chapter is to provide a short overview of the nature of cancer, to illustrate the great variety of mechanism through which diet can influence its initiation and development, and to consider briefly the potential role of functional food in its prevention.

9.2   Carcinogenesis and the biology of cancer

Both the identity of cancer as a disease, and the distinction between benign and malignant tumours, were recognised by Hippocrates, who is said to have likened the morphology and behaviour of a spreading tumour to the crab (Greek: 'karkinos'). Much more recently, the development of microscopy led to the recognition that tumours contained cells that differed fundamentally in appearance and behaviour from those of the surrounding tissue. The scientific investigation and clinical treatment of tumours began in the early years of the twentieth century, but it is only within the last two decades that the development of the cell and molecular sciences has enabled biologists to begin to acquire a deeper understanding of tumour biology. Much of this knowledge has been gained through the use of isolated tumour cells grown *in vitro*, and from animal models of carcinogenesis, which enable tumours to be studied within the complex environment of living tissue. Further developments have come with the publication of increasingly comprehensive analyses of both the normal human genome, and of human tumours at various stages of development. Cancer is not a single disease. The nature of any particular tumour depends both upon the tissue from which it is derived, and the pattern of genetic abnormalities acquired during its development (Johnson, 2004).

9.2.1   Sequential carcinogenesis

A tumour can be defined as any focal accumulation of cells, beyond the numbers required for the development, repair or function of a tissue. Tumours may be benign or malignant. The former are usually relatively slow growing, but more importantly the cells tend to retain much of the specialisation and spatial localisation of the tissue from which they are derived. In contrast, malignant cells are characterised by a loss of differentiation, faster growth and a tendency to invade surrounding tissues and migrate to other organs to form secondary tumours or metastases (Hanahan and Weinberg, 2000). Thus cancer may be defined as the sequential development, growth and metastatic spread of a malignant neoplasm. Cancer can affect virtually any organ of the body, but tissues such as those of the lungs and gut, which have characteristically high rates of cell division and are chronically exposed to the external environment, are particularly vulnerable. Regardless of their function in the body, all cells carry a complete set of genetic instructions for the development and function of the whole organism. The subset of genes expressed by any particular cell type determines its *phenotype*, a collective term for the specialised structural and functional characteristics that enable it to coexist with other cells in the same tissue. The events that occur during the early stages of cancer development usually involve damage to the DNA coding for such crucial genes (Hanahan and Weinberg, 2000).

9.2.2   Genetics and epigenetics of tumour development

One of the defining characteristics of a tumour cell is the presence of mutations affecting genes controlling the rate at which it is able to divide, differentiate or die, or the efficiency with which DNA damage is repaired (Anderson *et al.*, 1991). In familial cancer syndromes such mutations are inherited though the germ line, whereas in sporadic cancers, which are far more common, they are acquired as somatic mutations during carcinogenesis. Such damage may result from exposure to chemical mutagens or to ionising radiation, or through the effects of free radicals generated by the normal metabolism of the body (Poulsen *et al.*, 2000). Whatever the source of the DNA damage, however, the crucial attribute of a pro-carcinogenic mutation is that it favours the proliferation and survival of an abnormal population of cells that have the potential for further evolution towards the malignant state (Nowell, 1976).

Chemical carcinogens such as those present in tobacco smoke tend to be electrophiles – substances that can react easily with electron-rich regions of cellular proteins and DNA (Wyatt and Pittman, 2006). The products formed by such interactions with DNA are called adducts. These are stable compounds which disrupt the synthesis of new DNA when the cell next divides, so that the sequence of genetic code in that region is damaged and the new cell carries a mutation. Many *procarcinogens* must be activated to an electrophilic form before they can interact with DNA, and this often occurs as part of the sequence of metabolic changes occurring during detoxification of the parent molecule (Androutsopoulos *et al.*, 2009).

Many of the target genes that undergo mutation during carcinogenesis have been identified, and their functions and interactions with other genes are at least partially understood (Todd and Wong, 1999). The *proto-oncogenes* were first identified through their near-homology to the critical DNA sequences present in certain cancer-causing viruses which, when inserted into mammalian cells, would transform them into tumours. These so-called viral oncogenes have evolved through the 'capture' and exploitation of mammalian genes by viruses. In their original form such genes are essential components of normal mammalian cellular physiology and are expressed, usually to facilitate increased cellular proliferation, only at critical stages in the development or function of a tissue. When proto-oncogenes are activated inappropriately within the mammalian genome, without the intervention of a virus, they are termed *oncogenes* (Todd and Wong, 1999). This can occur because of a mutation to the control sequence for the gene, causing over-expression of the normal product, or a mutation in the coding sequence itself, giving rise to a product that functions normally but which cannot be broken down. For example, the K-ras gene, which codes for a protein-regulating cell proliferation, is mutated and hence abnormally expressed early in the development of approximately 40% of human colorectal carcinomas (Bos *et al.*, 1987).

In contrast to the proto-oncogenes, over-expression of which creates conditions that favour tumour growth, it is the loss of expression of a tumour-suppressor gene that facilitates development of malignant characteristics in a cell. The p53 gene is a good example (Donehower and Bradley, 1993). The p53 product is a protein of molecular weight 53 kD, which functions as a regulator of cell proliferation, and as a mediator of programmed cell death in response to unrepaired DNA damage. The absence of p53, or its presence in a mutated and therefore non-functional form, allows cells bearing other forms of DNA damage to continue dividing rather than undergoing apoptosis (Gerwin *et al.*, 1992). There are familial forms of cancer caused by an inherited p53 defect, and acquired mutations of this gene are among the most common genomic abnormalities found in a variety of human cancers.

According to the 'two-hit hypothesis' for the functional role of tumour-suppressor genes, mutations at both alleles are required to fully inactivate the tumour suppressor activity of such genes (Knudson, 1989). However, another important mechanism for the induction of genetic abnormalities has attracted attention in recent years. Cytosine bases in the DNA backbone can acquire a methyl group which, if they lie within the promoter region of a gene, can cause it to be 'silenced' or, in effect, switched off (Kass *et al.*, 1997). This is a normal mechanism for the regulation of gene expression, but abnormal DNA methylation can develop as a result of various metabolic or environmental effects, and once established, can be transmitted across successive cell divisions. Such *epigenetic* effects can lead to the inactivation of genes regulating tumour suppression or DNA repair, and thereby contribute to the complex series of events leading to the development of a tumour (Issa, 2000).

The simplest sequential model of carcinogenesis divides the process into three basic stages of initiation, promotion and progression (Pitot and Dragan, 1994). At the *initiation* stage, a single cell is thought to acquire a mutation and then divide repeatedly so that the mutation is passed on to a clone of daughter cells, forming a focal lesion that can survive and grow at the expense of neighbouring cells. During *promotion* the appearance of further genetic damage leads to a progressive loss of differentiation and orderly growth. At the *progression* stage, the lesion has made the transition to malignancy, and can give rise to secondary tumours at remote sites. Animal models have been used to identify various types of carcinogen which can, for example, act as mutagens at the initiation stage but do not induce malignancy on their own, promoters which cannot initiate tumours but do accelerate tumour development after initiation, and complete carcinogens, which can do both. This approach has also been used to identify food-borne inhibitors of carcinogenesis, and to delineate their mode of action (Wattenberg, 1985).

Because carcinogenesis is a prolonged multi-stage process, which usually occurs over many years, there are many critical steps at which food-related substances or metabolic processes might interact with the development of a tumour, perhaps to accelerate it, or conversely, to delay or even reverse the process. Anti-carcinogenic mechanisms can usefully be classified into *blocking effects*, which operate during the initiation phase of carcinogenesis, and *suppressing effects*, which delay or reverse tumour promotion at a later stage (Johnson *et al.*, 1994; Wattenburg, 1990). A schematic illustration of these concepts and a summary of the mechanisms through which they may act are given in Fig. 9.1.

The principal blocking mechanism through which dietary constituents are thought to act is modulation of the Phase I and Phase II biotransformation enzymes, which are expressed strongly in the gastrointestinal mucosa and in the liver, and act as a first line of defence against toxic substances in the environment (Greenwald *et al.*, 1990). Phase I enzymes include the cytochrome P450 complex (Nelson *et al.*, 1993), a group of enzymes that catalyse oxidation, reduction and hydrolytic reactions, and which render toxins and carcinogens more water soluble and hence more readily excreted. However some of these products are electrophilic intermediates, with a greater potential to damage DNA than the parent compound

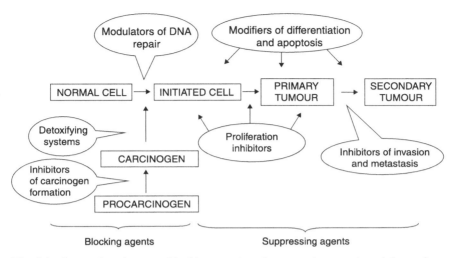

Fig. 9.1 Interactions between blocking agents and suppressing agents and the various stages in the sequence of events associated with the stepwise development of neoplasia. Blocking agents act immediately before or during the initiation of carcinogenesis, and suppressing agents act after initiation, during the prolonged stages of promotion and progression. (From Johnson, 2007.)

from which they are derived. Phase II enzymes, such as glutathione S-transferase, act on the products of Phase I metabolism, forming conjugates with lower reactivity. Thus the actual biological activity of a potential carcinogen will often depend upon the relative activities of the Phase I and II enzymes involved in its metabolism. Pharmacological and dietary treatments can be used to block Phase I enzymes and enhance Phase II activity, so as to minimise the activation of carcinogens and increase their excretion (Prochaska and Talalay, 1988). There is good evidence from experimental animal studies that this strategy can reduce DNA damage and tumour yield. Experimental animal studies have also shown that some substances can inhibit the appearance of tumours, even when given days or weeks after exposure to a chemical carcinogen (Wattenberg, 1981). Hence their mechanism of action cannot involve protection against DNA damage, but must instead be due to some reduction in the rate at which initiated cells develop into tumours (Fig. 9.1). Suppression of carcinogenesis may involve inhibition of mitosis and increased expression of the differentiated phenotype in the target tissure, which serves to reduce the clonal expansion of initiated cells, or it may result from an increased susceptibility to undergo programmed cell death (apoptosis), which tends to favour deletion of pre-cancerous cells from the tissue (West *et al.*, 2009).

9.2.3 Dietary impact on carcinogenesis
Prolonged malnutrition does increase an individual's risk of developing cancer, perhaps by reducing the effectiveness of the immune system, but life expectancy in

societies with large malnourished populations tends to be low, and the principal causes of illness and mortality are usually infectious diseases rather than cancers. In contrast, prosperous Western populations tend to suffer the adverse effects of over-consumption of energy, coupled with inadequate exercise, and these are major risk factors for cancer in later life. The most recent World Cancer Research Fund report on Food, Nutrition, Physical Activity and the Prevention of Cancer recommended that individuals maintain body weight within the normal range and consume energy-dense foods only sparingly (WCRF, 2007). Further recommendations included the consumption of 400 g of non-starchy vegetables and fruits per day, regular consumption of minimally processed cereals and legumes, and only limited intake of red meat. The advice on energy intake is broadly similar to that for the avoidance of heart disease, and is not in itself very relevant to the concept of functional foods. However the recommendation to consume a variety of fruits, vegetables and unprocessed cereals was based partly on the presence in such foods of potentially anticarcinogenic micronutrients, and other biologically active protective factors in plant foods (Johnson *et al.*, 1994). These recommendations do perhaps provide, at least in principle, a rationale for the development of functional food products, but it should be noted that the WCRF report did not recommend any consumption of dietary supplements for cancer prevention (WCRF, 2007).

9.3   Protective effects of nutrients

Nutrients are substances that have been shown to be essential to normal growth, development and function, and for which specific deficiency diseases have been demonstrated. They include a variety of minerals, vitamins and fatty acids that are required in relatively small quantities, as well as protein, and the various macronutrients that provide metabolic energy. A full consideration of the role of nutrients in the development of cancer would require a much more lengthy review than is appropriate here, but several micronutrients that seem particularly relevant in the context of functional foods are discussed below.

9.3.1   Polyunsaturated fatty acids

The polyunsaturated fatty acids (PUFA) are a large and diverse group of plant-derived lipids, several of which are essential for the normal growth and development of humans and other mammals. These *essential fatty acids* fall into two structural groups, the n-3 PUFA, derived from alpha-linolenic acid, and the n-6 PUFA, derived from linoleic acid. The n-3 PUFA are synthesised by marine plankton, and enter the human food chain primarily as seafood, or as supplements or functional food products containing fish oil. The n-6 PUFA are synthesised by terrestrial plants, and are particularly plentiful in the diets of populations consuming large quantities of vegetable oils and products derived from them. One of the most important aspects of PUFA metabolism is their role as substrates for the production of the *eicosanoids*, a group of lipids with a host of important endocrine functions, including the regulation of inflammation. The levels of n-3 and n-6 PUFA in adipose tissue, plasma lipids and cell membranes are to a large extent determined by dietary intake, and there is much interest in the use of diet to manipulate both the production and downstream effects of of the eicosanoids. There is for example good evidence that high intakes of n-3 PUFA can inhibit inflammatory activity in a range of tissues, and thereby suppress a number of pathological mechanisms including cardiovascular disease and cancer (Calder, 2009).

Epidemiological studies have provided evidence for protective effects of n-3 fatty acids against prostate cancer, and breast cancer, though the evidence remains inconclusive. Perhaps the most convincing evidence at present is that for a reduced risk of colorectal cancer in populations consuming relatively large quantities of fish (Norat et al., 2005). One possible explanation for these findings is that a high dietary intake of n-3 polyunsaturated fatty acids from oily fish exerts anticarcinogenic effects on the colorectal mucosa, perhaps by reducing the production of pro-inflammatory eicosanoids via the metabolic activity of the enzyme COX-2. The strongest evidence available at present comes from the European Prospective Investigation into Cancer and Nutrition (EPIC) study on fish consumption and colorectal cancer risk, which has revealed a highly significant reduction in risk in those consuming more than 40 g of fish per day. It should be noted however that in a meta-analysis of the literature then available, MacLean and co-workers collated data from nine studies in which the relationship between CRC risk and n-3 fatty acid intake was assessed, and concluded that there was no statistically significant association between n-3 fatty acid intake and risk of colorectal cancer (MacLean et al., 2006).

There is some evidence that any protective effects of n-3 PUFA may be associated with particular genetic polymorphisms affecting the expression of key proteins involved in peroxisome proliferator-activated receptors (PPAR) signalling and COX-2 expression. Individuals carrying a specific polymorphism of PPARδ have an increased risk of colorectal adenoma but not carcinoma, and the protective effects of fish consumption in relation to tumour are more significant in those carrying a particular COX-2 polymorphism (Siezen et al., 2005). These genes are associated with the control and metabolism of fatty acids and the formation of inflammatory eicosanoids, which supports the hypothesis that the PUFA content of fish is essential to the protective effects of fish. Further support is provided by experimental data showing anti-proliferative and pro-apoptotic effects of eicosapentaenoic acid (EPA) in colorectal epithelial cells in vitro and in vivo (Latham et al., 2001), and by intervention studies with pharmacological quantities of fish oils, showing that EPA and docosahexaenoic acid (DHA) both suppress mitosis and increase apoptosis in the crypts of the human rectal mucosa (Anti et al., 1994). Another possibility is that the ratio of the n-3 fatty acids EPA (C20:5) and DHA (C22:6) relative to arachidonic acid (C20:4) is the more critical factor (Busstra et al., 2003). Western diets contain up to 30 times as much n-6 fatty acid compared to n-3 fatty acids, whereas a ratio nearer 1:2 may be optimal for health. Dietary supplements or functional food products rich in n-3 PUFA can help to improve the ratio of n-3 to n-6 PUFA in the diet. However the most recent WCRF review on diet and cancer made no specific recommendation for increased intakes of n-3 PUFA as a means of reducing the risk of any cancer.

9.3.2   Antioxidant nutrients

Fruits, vegetables and cereals are the main sources of the antioxidant nutrients ascorbic acid and alpha-tocopherol, and of the carotenoids, including beta-carotene. During the 1980s and 1990s a considerable body of epidemiological evidence suggesting a protective effect of fruits and vegetables against cancer was acquired, and one hypothesis proposed to explain these observations was that the protective effects were mainly due to suppression of damage to DNA caused by free radicals such as the hydroxyl radical ($\cdot$ OH) released from H_2O_2 in the presence of iron, nitric oxide (NO$\cdot$) and peroxynitrite (ONOO$^-$). These highly reactive species are generated by a variety of biological mechanisms including inflammation (Hussain et al., 2003), or simply as a side-product of ordinary oxidative metabolism (Poulsen et al., 2000). Cells have evolved an arsenal of antioxidant mechanisms to defend macromolecules from free-radical mediated damage but the steady-state level of oxidative DNA adduct formation in laboratory rats has been estimated to be about 66 000 adducts per cell (Helbock et al., 1998). The cumulative effects of such damage include mutations resulting from faulty DNA repair, and double strand-breaks (Bjelland and Seeberg, 2003). Free-radical reactions can also cause oxidative damage to proteins such as p53 that are involved in the regulation of cellular proliferation and apoptosis, and can thereby contribute directly to tumour promotion (Hofseth et al., 2003).

Epidemiological evidence has shown that both the dietary intake of carotenoids and the concentration of carotenoids in the blood, are inversely related to relative risk of cancers of the oropharyngeal tissues, lung and other sites in a number of case-control studies, but attempts to reproduce the protective effects of fruits and vegetables using carotenoid supplements have largely failed (Musa-Veloso et al., 2009). The Alpha-Tocopherol, Beta-Carotene Cancer Prevention Study (ABCP) was designed to test the hypothesis that prolonged dietary supplementation with the antioxidants alpha-tocopherol (50 mg/d), beta-carotene (20 mg/d) or both, would reduce the incidence of lung cancer in smokers (ABCP, 1994). Over 29 000 male Finnish smokers were randomly assigned to four groups receiving the supplements or a placebo, and followed up for 5–8 years. A total of 876 new cases of lung cancer occurred in the cohort; there was no protective effect of any treatment, and there was a statistically significant increase in the incidence of lung cancer amongst the participants receiving beta-carotene (P = 0.01). Somewhat similar findings were reported later from the Beta-Carotene and Retinol Efficacy (CARET) trial (Omenn et al., 1996). It is now generally accepted that whereas alpha-tocopherol exerts no protective effect against lung cancer in smokers, beta-carotene appears to promote the disease process to a significant degree. More generally, a major review conducted by the International Agency for Research on Cancer in 1998 concluded that the evidence for a protective effect of beta-carotene and other carotenoids against cancer was inadequate (IARC, 1998).

Turning now to colorectal cancer, in a series of analyses of case-control studies conducted in Northern Italy, LaVecchia and co-workers observed a protective effect of fruit and vegetable consumption against colorectal cancer (La Vecchia *et al.*, 1988) and estimated, on the basis of multivariate odds ratios adjusted for total calorie intake, that the combined effect of a low intake of beta-carotene and ascorbic acid accounted for 43% of all colorectal cancer cases in their target population. West *et al.* (1989) also observed a protective effect of beta-carotene of around this magnitude in a case-control study conducted in Utah. Satia-Abouta *et al.* (2003) explored the influence of micronutrient intakes on risk of colorectal cancer in a relatively large group of both white and black Americans. High intakes of vitamin C and beta-carotene were protective in both groups, whereas vitamin E was only shown to be protective in the African Americans.

Most colorectal cancers develop relatively slowly via the adenoma–carcinoma sequence. Patients whose pre-cancerous polyps have been removed are routinely screened for recurrence by endoscopy, and this provides a convenient means of assessing the efficacy of dietary or pharmacological interventions designed to inhibit the development of adenomas. McKeown-Eyssen *et al.* (1988) used this method to assess the effect of supplementation with ascorbic acid (400 mg/d) and alpha-tocopherol (400 mg/d) in 200 patients. After two years of supplementation, 157 subjects had completed the study, and recurrence of polyps was observed in 41.4% of 70 subjects on vitamin supplements and in 50.7% of 67 subjects on placebos. After adjustment for various demographic and dietary factors, the relative risk of polyp occurrence was 0.86, with 95% confidence limits from 0.51 to 1.43. The authors concluded that any effect of the intervention with antioxidants was too small to measure under the conditions of their trial. Similarly Greenberg *et al.* (1994) randomly assigned 864 patients to four treatment groups to receive a placebo; beta-carotene (25 mg daily); vitamin C (1 g daily) and vitamin E (400 mg daily); or a combined dose of both beta-carotene and vitamins C and E. Complete colonoscopic examinations were performed one year and four years after they entered the study. A total of 751 patients completed the study but there was no evidence that beta-carotene or vitamins C and E reduced the incidence of adenomas. Hofstad *et al.* (1998) carried out an intervention study in 116 polyp-bearing patients who received placebo or a mixture of beta-carotene (15 mg), vitamin C (150 mg), vitamin E (75 mg), selenium (101 µg) and calcium carbonate (1.6 g daily) for a period of three years, with annual colonoscopy. All polyps of <10 mm at enrolment or follow-up were left un-resected until the end of the study, so that both recurrence and growth could be quantified. No differences in the growth of adenomas were observed between the intervention and placebo groups, either from year to year, or for the total study period, but there was a reduced recurrence of polyps in the intervention group, compared to the placebo group. However this effect could well have been due to the calcium, which has been shown convincingly to inhibit adenoma recurrence in other trials (Baron *et al.*, 1999).

The failure of intervention with antioxidants during a relatively short period of disease development cannot entirely rule out the possibility that prolonged exposure to antioxidants prior to the appearance of precancerous lesions may be protective. However it should be noted that Connelly *et al.* (2003) reported that adenoma patients with high levels of ascorbic acid in their plasma are much less likely to have high levels of crypt cell apoptosis. This programmed cell death pathway is an important mechanism for the destruction of precancerous cells (Johnson, 2001) and so this finding raises the possibility that antioxidant supplements might actually inhibit the ability of the colonic mucosa to resist the development of pre-neoplastic lesions in patients already at risk of adenomas.

Gastric cancer is strongly associated with inflammatory effects resulting from infection with the bacterium *Helicobacter pylori*, and a chronic inflammatory response to reflux oesophagitis is the major risk factor for oesophageal adenocarcinoma (Ambrus *et al.*, 1984). Case-control studies suggest a protective effect of plant foods intake against tumours of the upper gastrointestinal tract (Kono and Hirohata, 1996), but it is not clear whether the protective effects can be attributed specifically to the presence in such foods of ascorbic acid or other antioxidants. Serafini and colleagues explored the importance of antioxidant effects by using food intake data derived from a food frequency questionnaire to calculate total antioxidant potential of foods consumed (Serafini *et al.*, 2002). There was a strong, statistically significant protective effect of total antioxidant potential against gastric cancers of both the cardia and more distal sites (odds ratio 0.65; 95% confidence interval 0.48–0.89; for the highest quartile of antioxidant activity). However the approach used in this study makes it impossible to distinguish antioxidant effects of nutrients from those of non-nutrient secondary plant metabolites such as flavonoids. As discussed later, these compounds may themselves exert protection against cancer of the stomach and oesophagus via other, non-antioxidant effects (Sun *et al.*, 2002).

Turning from the gastrointestinal tract to the prostate, the SELECT trial (Selenium and Vitamin E Cancer Prevention Trial) has provided important new evidence in relation to antioxidant vitamins and cancer. The trial was designed to test the hypothesis that supplementation with the lipid soluble antioxidant vitamin E, or with selenium (see below) or with a combination of the two, could protect against prostate cancer. A total of 35 533 men aged over 50, from the USA, Canada, and Puerto Rico, were randomly assigned to four double-blinded groups (selenium, vitamin E, selenium + vitamin E and placebo) between 2001 and 2004. Follow-up is still in progress at the time of writing (2010) with prostate cancer as the primary outcome and lung, colorectal, and overall primary cancer as secondary outcomes. As of 2008, the median follow-up time was 5.46 years, and no protective effect of selenium or vitamin E, alone or in combination, against cancer of the prostate or of any other site had been detected (Lippman *et al.*, 2009).

In parallel with these epidemiological and intervention studies, a number of mechanistic experiments have been conducted in recent years to test the hypothesis that fruits and vegetables or antioxidant vitamin supplements can prevent potentially carcinogenic DNA damage in free-living human subjects. The mutation frequency of the hypoxanthine-guanine phosphorybosyltransferase gene (*HPRT*) in T-lymphocytes is used as a biomarker of somatic mutation in humans exposed to genotoxins. Nyberg *et al.* (Nyberg *et al.*, 2003) used this approach to search for evidence of protective effects of fruits and vegetables against somatic mutations in 312 volunteers, of whom 158 were lung cancer patients and 154 were healthy controls. Dietary intakes of various categories of vegetables and fruits, carotenoids, vitamin A and ascorbic acid were calculated using food composition tables and a food-frequency questionnaire. Protective effects against risk of mutation were observed in subjects with relatively high intakes of vegetables, citrus fruits, berries and ascorbic acid. However the effect of beta-carotene was more complex in that there was a U-shaped relationship between exposure and mutation frequency, implying that both high and low intakes may increase the risk of mutation. This is consistent with the adverse effects of beta-carotene supplementation on risk of lung cancer in the ABCP and CARET studies.

Other biomarkers used to detect effects on oxidative DNA damage in humans include the quantification of 8-oxodG in urine to provide a quantitative estimate of the formation of DNA adducts (Loft and Poulsen, 1998), and detection of DNA strand-breaks by use of single-cell gel electrophoresis, the so-called comet assay (Collins, 2002). However the results obtained in human studies using such techniques remain generally inconclusive. In an extensive review of intervention studies designed to quantify the effects of antioxidant supplements on oxidative damage to human white blood cells, Möller and Loft identified a large number of technical limitations and inconclusive results, and concluded that the case for the long-term efficacy of antioxidants as a means of preventing DNA damage remained unproven (Möller and Loft, 2002). The same authors attempted to test the putative role of antioxidant micronutrients directly by means of a placebo-controlled intervention study with 43 human volunteers (Möller et al., 2003). The subjects were randomised into three groups and given an antioxidant-free basal diet plus 600 g of fruits and vegetables, or a supplement containing the corresponding amounts of vitamins and minerals, or a placebo, for 24 days. Blood and urine samples were collected before, during and after the intervention, and the comet assay, excretion of 8-oxodG and markers of DNA-repair activity were used to assess oxidative damage in leukocytes. At the end of the intervention period there was no clear evidence that either the fruits and vegetables, or the vitamins and minerals had significantly reduced the level of oxidative DNA damage detected in mononuclear cell DNA, or via urine biomarkers. Similarly, Jacob et al. (2003) assessed lipid and protein oxidation in 39 healthy male non-smokers and 38 smokers whose typical diet provided only 2.6 servings/d of fruits and vegetables. The volunteers received a daily supplement (272 mg vitamin C, 31 mg α-tocopherol, and 400 μg folic acid), or placebo, for 90 d with their usual diet. Lipid peroxidation products, including F(2)-total and 8-isoprostanes, and protein carbonyls were determined in urine before and after the interventions. Supplementation increased plasma ascorbate and tocopherol, but had no effect on the oxidant biomarkers. It is arguable that the biomarkers currently available for the detection of changes in oxidative damage in human intervention trials are insufficiently sensitive, but at best, the hypothesis that supplementation with antioxidant nutrients provides protection against potentially carcinogenic oxidative damage to DNA in healthy human subjects remains unproven.

9.3.3   Folates

Folate is a collective term for the naturally occuring derivatives of pteroylglutamic acid. The folates are synthesised by plants and yeast, but must be obtained from dietary sources by humans and other mammals, because they are essential for the synthesis, maintenance and repair of DNA. Conversion of deoxyuridylate to thymidylate requires the reduction of 5,10-methylenetetrahydrofolate to 5-methyl-tetrahydrofolate by the enzyme methyltetrahydrofolate reductase (MTHFR). An inadequate supply of 5,10-methylenetetrahydrofolate leads to an imbalance in deoxynucleoside triphosphate (dNTP) pools. The presence of excess dUMP can cause misincorporation of uracil into DNA, faulty DNA repair and excess double-strand breaks (Wickramasinghe and Fida, 1994). Moreover, low levels of 5-methyltetrahyfrofolate within the cell can compromise the availability of the universal methyl-donor S-adenosyl methionine (SAM) and hence interfere with the normal methylation of cytosine residues in DNA. Suboptimal folate levels may be a major cause of genetic damage leading to cancer (Ames, 2001), and convincing epidemiological evidence has emerged to suggest that chronic folate deficiency may indeed contribute to both the initiation and promotion of epithelial neoplasias.

A case-control study conducted in Hawaii showed inverse relationship between lung cancer and intake of green vegetables and beta-carotene, but failed to find any protective effects of folate (Le Marchand et al., 1989). Jatoi et al. (2001) found no evidence of any relationship between risk of lung cancer and plasma or red cell folate, after making adjustments for possible confounding effects of treatment. However, Shen et al. reported that in former smokers, folate intake was significantly higher amongst controls than amongst lung cancer cases, and folate intake above the control median value was associated with a statistically significant, 40% lower risk of lung cancer (Shen et al., 2003). At least one large study has produced evidence that folate intake is inversely related to risk of lung cancer (Voorrips et al., 2000), but a recent cohort study failed to confirm this, and even suggested an adverse effect of folate, which might however have been due to confounding issues (Roswall et al. 2010b).

Folate intake has been shown to be inversely related to the risk of colorectal adenomas in both case-control and prospective studies. The relationship was assessed in both the Health Professionals Follow-Up Study and the Nurses Health Study; the relative risk of adenoma was found to be 0.66 (95% confidence interval = 0.46–0.95 between high and low quintiles of intake) for women and 0.63 (95% confidence interval = 0.41–0.98) for men, independently of dietary fibre or vitamins C and E (Giovannucci et al., 1993). The findings of other smaller studies have generally been consistent with these conclusions (Tseng et al., 1996). In some studies the risk of adenomas has been compared directly with folate status, and an inverse relationship between blood folate levels and adenoma risk has been observed (Bird et al., 1995). Giovannucci and colleagues concluded that the epidemiological evidence from eleven case-control and cohort studies strongly suggested that, within westernised populations, there is a reduction in risk of colon cancer of around 40% in the highest consumers of folate compared to the lowest (Giovannucci, *et al.*, 1993). However genetic factors appear to modify the effects of folate on susceptibility to cancer in subgroups of the population. The enzyme methylenetetrahydrofolate reductase (MTHFR) catalyses the reduction of 5,10-methylenetetrahydrofolate to 5-methyltetrahydrofolate. In about 35% of Caucasians there is a polymorphism at position 677 of the *MTHR* gene, involving a cytosine-to-thymine transition (C677T), which results in reduced enzyme activity. Homozygous individuals (TT) comprise about 11% of the population and have been reported to show abnormal folate metabolism, elevated levels of homocysteine (Frosst *et al.*, 1995), and evidence of hypomethylation of genomic DNA in some tissues (Stern *et al.*, 2000). Three studies have explored the risk of colorectal cancer in subgroups with the CC, CT and TT genotypes. Individuals with the CC and CT derive less protective effect from a high folate diet than those with the TT genotype, but all three genotypes are at similar risk from diets low in folate and methionine, or high in alcohol (Giovannucci, 2002).

Apart from the complexity of genetic variation as a factor influencing the individual metabolic response to dietary folate, controversy has arisen recently as to the possible hazards of over-consumption of folic acid from supplements or fortified foods. The proven role of folate supplementation prior to conception as a preventative measure against the developmental disorder spina bifida has prompted legislation to ensure that wheat-flour is fortified with folic acid in North America. On the basis of epidemiological evidence, some have argued that this has become a risk factor for the progression of cancer, at least in some vulnerable individuals harbouring pre-cancerous polyps (Mason *et al.*, 2007). This problem, coupled with the continuing uncertainty about the protective effects of supplementary folates – as opposed to dietary folate – at the population level (Roswall *et al.*, 2010), seems likely to limit the scope for the development of functional foods in this area for the forseeable future.

9.3.4   Vitamin D

The major source of vitamin D in human metabolism is the photo-conversion of provitamin D3 in skin during exposure to bright sunlight (Webb and Holick, 1988). Vitamin D3 is a hydrophobic lipid, but the metabolite 25-hydroxyvitamin D3 is formed in the liver and is present at significant concentrations in the plasma, bound to vitamin D binding protein. Further hydroxylation of 25-hydroxyvitamin D3 to 1,25-hydroxyvitamin D3, which is the most biologically active metabolite, occurs in the kidney and a few other tissues (DeLuca, 1988). The major biological function of vitamin D is the regulation of calcium homeostasis. Vitamin D deficiency therefore leads to failure of bone formation during growth and development (rickets). In recent years, however, it has been recognised that vitamin D also plays a role in various other aspects of epithelial growth and development (DeLuca, 1988), and that the optimum plasma concentration for the maintenance of cell proliferation and differentiation may be substantially higher than that needed for normal bone development. If so, it is unlikely that even fair-skinned individuals can maintain adequate levels of vitamin D during the winter months at high latitudes. Vitamin D is also present naturally in some foods. Most developed countries set recommended dietary allowances but there is some risk of toxicity, and both target levels of intake and the desirability of dietary supplementation are matters of controversy (Mosekilde, 2008).

From the perspective of cancer prevention, the most active area of research has been concerned with the possibility that relatively high levels of plasma vitamin D protect against colorectal cancer. Several relatively small prospective cohort studies have suggested statistically non-significant inverse relationships between risk of colorectal cancer and plasma levels of 25-hydroxyvitamin D or 1,25-hydroxyvitamin D (Garland *et al.*, 1989; Tangrea *et al.*, 1997). These findings, though inconclusive, are consistent with experimental data showing that supplementation with vitamin D (800 IU/day) promotes differentiation of human colorectal epithelial cells, and may be regarded as a potential suppressor of precancerous changes (Fedirko *et al.*, 2009). Recently a large nested case-control study has been undertaken within the EPIC European cohort, so that the risk of colorectal cancer could be compared with pre-diagnostic levels of vitamin D in plasma, and dietary intakes of vitamin D and calcium (Jenab *et al.*, 2010). There was a strong inverse dose-response relationship between plasma 25-hydroxyvitamin D and risk of colorectal cancer, such that patients in the highest quintile experienced a 40% lower risk than those in the lowest quintile ($p < 0.001$), but there was no evidence of any relationship with vitamin D intake. One particularly important feature of the study was the observation that the relationship between plasma vitamin D levels and colorectal cancer risk was not linear. Most of the excess risk was associated with individuals with levels lower than 75 nmol/l. Individuals with plasma levels in excess of this figure experienced a further reduction in risk but not significantly so. The authors concluded that whereas raising low plasma levels of vitamin D to the mid-range is likely to be beneficial, it is unclear whether the possible risks of raising plasma levels to the 75–100 nmol/l range through dietary supplementation would be worth the relatively small further advantage.

The issue of the relative risks and benefits of maintaining high vitamin D levels by dietary supplementation has been addressed directly by Bischoff-Ferrari and colleagues, who reviewed a number of double-blind randomised controlled trials of vitamin D supplementation, with falls or non-vertebral fractures as endpoints (Bischoff-Ferrari *et al.*, 2009). Their meta-analysis provided evidence for a statistically significant dose-related protective effects, with the strongest protective effect at the highest dose levels used (700–1000 IU vitamin D per day) or the highest range of plasma concentration attained (75–110 nmol/l). There was no evidence that such levels of supplementation had caused significant hypercalcaemia or other adverse health effects in any of the intervention trials reviewed. The authors concluded that dietary supplementation to achieve blood levels of vitamin D consistent with protection against a range of diseases including colorectal cancer could be achieved without side-effects, but they conceded that further work to confirm these conclusions is essential, and the issue remains controversial.

9.3.5   Mineral micronutrients

As in the case of organic micronutrients, there are many who argue that sub-optimal intakes of mineral micronutrients have a long-term adverse effect upon human metabolism, which ultimately leads to an increased risk of cancers (Ames, 1998). This field of research is largely beyond the scope of the present chapter. The discussion will be restricted to selenium, which has gained a special significance in recent years, partly because of the apparent strength of the early evidence, and partly because dietary selenium levels are particularly low in the UK and some other western European countries (Rayman, 2008).

Selenium

The element selenium is an essential nutrient that occurs in the form of selenocysteine as a component in around 12 selenoproteins. In experimental animal models, selenium deficiency is associated with evidence of oxidative damage. In humans, a low intake of dietary selenium (<12 μg/day) is associated with Keshan disease, a specific type of cardiomyopathy (Tan *et al.*, 2002). The selenoprotein glutathione peroxidase is a cytosolic antioxidant enzyme that catalyses the reduction of organic peroxides by reduced glutathione. This is an essential component of the mammalian antioxidant defence system and glutathione peroxidase is expressed in tissues throughout the body. Rosa *et al.* (1998) studied the effects of the synthetic anticarcinogenic organoselenium compound 1,4-phenylenebis(methylene)selenocyanate (p-XSC) (el-Bayoumy *et al.*, 1995) on the formation of DNA adducts in rodent lung tissue after administration of the tobacco-smoke carcinogen 4-(methylnitrosamino)-1-(3-pyridyl)-1-butanone (NNK). This compound forms mutagenic covalent DNA adducts, but also causes oxidative damage to DNA, resulting in the formation of 8-OH-dG which can be measured directly in lung tissue. Dietary supplementation with p-XSC (15 ppm), before and after treatment with NNK prevented the increased levels of 8-OH-dG that occurred in control rats.

Selenium compounds also exert other biological effects that may serve to inhibit the development of cancer. For example the synthetic anticarcinogenic organoselenium compound p-XSC inhibits the formation of DNA adducts in the mammary tissue of rodents treated with the carcinogen 7,12-dimethylbenz(a)anthracene (DMBA) (el-Bayoumy *et al.*, 1992). Inorganic selenium compounds can themselves cause DNA strand breaks at high concentrations, but low molecular weight organic selenium compounds have been shown to induce apoptosis in tumour cells *in vitro* (Lu *et al.*, 1995). Selenium is therefore one of a growing set of food components that have been shown in experimental models to selectively enhance apoptosis of cells carrying genomic damage, and thus delete cells that would otherwise go on to develop into malignant tumours (Johnson, 2001). Selenium also suppresses tumour cell proliferation, may enhance DNA repair, and suppresses aberrant methylation of DNA in experimental models (Fiala *et al.*, 1998). In the context of human nutrition, the functional significance of these various mechanisms of will depend upon a number of factors, including the chemical form in which it enters cellular metabolism.

Studies on the relationship between selenium and cancer began with epidemiology exploring the effect of dietary exposure to selenium on mortality from leukaemia and cancers of colon, rectum, prostate, breast, ovary and lung (Schrauzer *et al.*, 1977). Willett *et al.* (1983) studied the relationship between pre-diagnostic serum selenium levels in patients developing cancer over a five-year period, and in matched healthy controls. The mean selenium levels of cases were about 5% lower than that of the controls, and the risk of cancer was twice as high for subjects in the lowest quintile of serum selenium compared to subjects in the highest. The association between low selenium level and cancer was strongest for gastrointestinal and prostate cancers.

Toenail selenium has been used as a biomarker of long-term selenium status in studies on selenium as a putative protective factor against lung cancer. Van den Brandt *et al* investigated this relationship in a cohort of 120 852 Dutch men and women aged 55–69 years (van den Brandt *et al.*, 1993). The rate ratio of lung cancer for subjects in the highest compared to the lowest quintile of toenail selenium was 0.50 (95% confidence interval, 0.30–0.81), with a significant inverse trend across quintiles. A nested case-control study conducted on a large cohort of subjects in Finland, where dietary levels of selenium are low, provided good evidence of enhanced risk of lung cancer amongst smokers with low levels of selenium in the plasma (Knekt *et al.*, 1998). However, other prospective studies have provided only weak, statistically non-significant evidence of an inverse relationship between selenium status and risk of lung cancer (Epplein *et al.*, 2009).

Human intervention trials with selenium have been carried out in Linxian, China, which has low levels of selenium in the soil, coupled with some of the highest rates of squamous cell carcinoma of the oesophagus in the world (Wei *et al.*, 2004). Evidence for a reduction in mortality from oesophageal and gastric cancers in the supplemented groups was obtained from these trials, although the effects were relatively modest (Li *et al.*, 1993). The strongest current evidence for a protective effect of selenium against colorectal cancer is provided by the data from the Nutritional Prevention of Cancer Trial. This randomised, double-blind, placebo-controlled intervention study was carried out on patients with a history of non-melanoma skin cancer, in regions of the USA with low levels of selenium in the soil (Clark *et al.*, 1996). Patients were randomised to receive either 200 µg/day of selenium in the form of a high-selenium yeast supplement, or a yeast placebo. The primary purpose of the study was to test the hypothesis that selenium supplementation would reduce the re-occurrence of skin cancer, but overall mortality, and incident cases of lung, prostate and colorectal cancers were included as secondary endpoints. After a total follow-up of 8271 person-years, there were no significant differences in the incidence of basal cell or squamous cell skin cancer between groups. However, compared to the controls, patients treated with selenium had a significantly lower risk of mortality from all cancers (relative risk, 0.50; 95% CI, 0.31–0.80), and specifically from cancers of lung, colon and prostate. As a result of these findings, the study was terminated early.

The most recent attempt to test the hypothesis that intervention with selenium could substantially reduce the risk of prostate cancer was the SELECT trial

(Selenium and Vitamin E Cancer Prevention Trial) mentioned earlier, in which the effect of selenium (200 μg/d from L-selenomethionine) alone, or in combination with vitamin E, was investigated in 35 533 men. After approximately 5.5 years of follow-up so far, the study has failed to find evidence for a protective effect of selenium supplements against prostate or any other cancer (Lippman *et al.*, 2009). This study does not entirely refute the hypothesis that lifelong dietary exposure to adequate selenium levels minimises the risk of prostate cancer, but it seriously undermines the case for selenium supplementation, whether from functional foods or pharmaceutical preparations, in middle-aged men.

9.4   Protective effects of phytochemicals

For much of the last two decades there has been growing interest in the role of biologically active secondary plant metabolites from fruits and vegetables in the prevention of cancer. The initial impetus was provided by a wealth of epidemiological evidence suggesting a protective effect of diets rich in fruits and vegetables against cancer, and this led to a substantial body of research on the biological effects of plant constituents in experimental systems based on animal models, and in tissue culture studies. In the early 1990s, Block and colleagues published an influential review of the epidemiological literature, and showed that in many populations, the lowest consumers of fruits and vegetables experienced about twice the risk of many different types of cancer compared to the highest (Block *et al.*, 1992). In a later review of the growing literature, Steinmetz and Potter came to a similar conclusion (Steinmetz and Potter, 1991), and the World Cancer Research Fund report on Food, Nutrition and the prevention of Cancer published in 1997 found 'convincing' evidence for protective effects of fruits and vegetables against cancers of the alimentary tract and lung (WCRF, 1997). Much of this original evidence was based on case-control studies, which are generally considered to be less reliable than prospective studies, and in recent years there has been some weakening of the evidence, mainly as a result of several large prospective studies focusing on the main causes of death from cancer in Western countries (Boffetta *et al.*, 2010). A comprehensive report by the International Agency for Research on Cancer concluded that:

> There is *limited evidence* for a cancer-preventive effect of consumption of fruit and of vegetables for cancers of the mouth and pharynx, oesophagus, stomach colon-rectum, larynx, lung, ovary (vegetables only), bladder (fruit only) and kidney. There is *inadequate* evidence for a cancer-preventive effect of consumption of fruit and vegetables for all other sites.
>
> (IARC, 2003)

Nevertheless, although both the strength and statistical significance of the epidemiological evidence for anticarcinogenic effects of diets rich in fruits and vegetables appear to have diminished recently, interest in the biological effects of their biologically active constituents has grown. Many of these compounds are secondary metabolites that have evolved to repel, or in some cases to attract invertebrate species, but which also exert coincidental biological effects in humans (Johnson, 2007). The anticarcinogenic effects of some of the main groups of these so-called *phytochemicals*, many of which are commonly consumed in fruits and vegetables of various types, will be briefly reviewed below.

9.4.1   Phenolic compounds

The flavonoids comprise a large and complex group of polyphenolic compounds found in a wide variety of plants used as foods and beverages. Collectively they provide much of the flavour and aroma of cocoa products, tea, coffee and wine. Among the most common flavonoids in the human diet are the flavonols, all of which consist of a three-ring structure with two aromatic rings and a central oxygenated heterocycle. They include quercetin, myricetin and kaempferol (Hollman and Katan, 1999).

Detoxification of environmental carcinogens is probably the most thoroughly studied and well-characterised anticarcinogenic mechanism associated with food-borne phytochemicals. Drugs and other substances that act in this way in animal models are often classified as *blocking agents* according to the scheme of Wattenberg (Wattenberg, 1992), because their mode of action is to block the first step in carcinogenesis, either by inhibiting the formation of active carcinogens from procarcinogens, or by enhancing their detoxification and excretion. These effects are achieved primarily through the modulation of Phase I and Phase II metabolic enzymes in the gut, liver, or lung. As mentioned previously, Phase II metabolism leads to the formation of less reactive, water-soluble conjugates, which are readily excreted. Many flavonoids are potent inducers of Phase II enzymes, and amongst these one of the most thoroughly investigated is the flavanol epigallocatechin gallate (EGCG), the principal biologically active component of green tea (Chou et al., 2000).

Another potentially important anticarcinogenic effect of the flavonoids lies in their ability to modulate inflammatory activity in tissues vulnerable to cancer. Inflammation of various types is strongly implicated in the aetiology of many types of cancer, and it is well established that chronic use of anti-inflammatory drugs such as aspirin reduces the risk of cancers of the gastrointestinal tract, and particularly of the colon and oesophagus (Cuzick et al., 2009). This observation has led to a search for naturally occurring anti-inflammatory compounds, and one important focus of interest is the ability of certain phytochemicals to interact with nuclear transcription factor κB (NF-κB). In its inactive form NF-κB is present in the cytoplasm as a complex with IκB. Activation of NF-κB occurs via IκB kinase (IKK)-dependent phosphorylation, ubiquitination and proteolysis of IκB, which frees NF-κB to enter the nucleus and bind to the κB sequence motif in DNA. NF-κB is involved in the regulation of a large number of genes, but is particularly important as an up-regulator of the inflammatory response. Phenolic substances found in plant foods and beverages inhibit NF-κB activation at various stages. Curcumin for example suppresses TNF-induced activation of IKK (Singh and Aggarwal, 1995), whereas caffeic acid phenethyl ester specifically prevents binding of NF-κB to its target DNA sequence (Natarajan et al., 1996).

The cyclooxygenase (prostaglandin H synthase) pathway includes two distinct isoforms; COX-1, which is constitutively expressed, produces prostaglandins essential to platelet aggregation and the maintenance of gastric mucosal integrity, whereas COX-2 is induced by tumour promoters and endogenous cytokines, and produces prostaglandins involved in inflammation. Many flavonoids have been shown to be COX-2 enzyme inhibitors and some, including apigenin, chrysin, and kaempferol, can suppress COX-2 transcription (Liang *et al.*, 2001).

A further possible mechanism whereby phytochemicals or pharmaceutical agents may inhibit the development of cancer after the initial damage to the genome is by enhancing the deletion of pre-cancerous cells from the tissue (Johnson, 2001). The survival of tumour cells depends critically upon their ability to divide continuously, and to evade apoptosis. Compounds that can stimulate cell death at biologically achievable concentrations *in vivo* are of great interest both as chemotherapeutic drugs, and as chemo-protective agents, particularly if they act selectively against transformed cells. Many phytochemicals, including flavonoids, have been shown to inhibit tumour cell proliferation and enhance apoptosis *in vitro* (Johnson, 2001), but it has proven difficult to establish that food-borne flavonoids act in this way in animals or humans.

Ultimately the significance of these various mechanisms for human health depends upon their impact on disease processes at work in human populations. This can only be assessed by randomised clinical trials, which have yet to be carried out. In the mean time, epidemiological studies continue to provide somewhat contradictory messages. For example, in a large-scale case-control study, Theodoratou *et al.* (2007) observed significant dose-dependent reductions in the risk of colorectal cancer associated with high consumption of the flavonols quercetin, catechin and epicatechin.

9.4.2   Glucosinolates

The glucosinolates are a group of water-soluble glycosides found exclusively in cruciferous plants. All glucosinolates contain the same sulphur group, but they differ in their physical properties and breakdown products because of the presence of a variable side-chain (Mithen *et al.*, 2000). About 100 glucosinolates have been identified, and they are present in significant quantities in human diets rich in brassica vegetables, and cruciferous salad herbs including mustard (*Brassica juncea*), rocket (*Eruca sativa*), and radishes (*Raphanus sativus*). Glucosinolates are thought to have evolved as natural pesticides. They are biologically inactive in the intact plant tissue, but physical disruption brings the glucosinolates into contact with the plant enzyme myrosinase. The resulting hydrolysis yields free glucose and an unstable sulphur compound that undergoes spontaneous rearrangements to give a variety of active products, which vary, both with the structure of the parent glucosinolate and the ambient conditions. The major products include isothiocyanates (ITC), indole-3-carbinols (derived from indolyl glucosinolates), nitriles, cyano-epithioalkanes and thiocyanates. Glucosinolate breakdown products can be formed in food processing, during digestion of uncooked vegetables in the upper gastrointestinal tract, or by exposure to bacterial myrosinase in the colon (Verkerk *et al.*, 2009).

The significance of the isothiocyanates lies both in their ability to induce apoptosis in cancer cells, both *in vitro* (Musk *et al.*, 1995) and *in vivo* (Smith *et al.*, 2003), and in their activation of Phase I and II enzymes in mammalian tissues (Yoxall *et al.*, 2005) via direct effects on regulatory sequences in the mammalian genome, including the xenobiotic response element (XRE) and the antioxidant response element (ARE). Certain isothiocyanates have the valuable effect of selectively inducing Phase II enzymes, which favour excretion of carcinogens, without simultaneously inducing Phase I enzymes (Wilkinson and Clapper, 1997). A considerable amount of experimental and epidemiological work has been done to explore the significance of these effects, both in animal models, and in humans exposed to carcinogens from cigarette smoke. Both indole-3-carbinol and phenethyl isothiocyanate (PEITC) have been shown to modify the metabolism of tobacco-smoke carcinogens in rat models, and inhibit the development of lung tumours (Hecht *et al.*, 1996; Morse *et al.*, 1990). In humans, increased urinary excretion of two tobacco carcinogen breakdown products was seen in smokers consuming approximately 170 g of watercress (*Rorippa nasturtium-aquaticum*) per day for three days (Hecht *et al.*, 1995, 1999). Hecht and co-workers studied the excretion of tobacco carcinogen metabolites in Singapore Chinese smokers, and observed a correlation between cruciferous vegetable consumption and excretion of carcinogen metabolites that appeared consistent with the known metabolic effects of indole-3-carbinol (Hecht *et al.*, 2004). In general these observations seem to provide a plausible biological mechanism to explain epidemiological studies showing a protective effect of brassica vegetable consumption against cancers of the lung and colon. However it must be noted that both the protective effects of glucosinolates (London *et al.*, 2000) and their metabolic handling by humans (Steck *et al.*, 2007) depends heavily upon the genetic profile of the individual, with respect to patterns of Phase II enzyme expression. Understanding the implications of such genetic factors, in relation both to the development of dietary advice and to the design and marketing of functional food products, will require a great deal of further work. The most recent WCRF report on Food, Nutrition, Physical Activity and the Prevention of Cancer made no particular recommendation favouring increased consumption of cruciferous vegetables (WCRF, 2007).

9.5   Carbohydrates and their fermentation products

Ever since the work of Burkitt and his collaborators who observed in the 1950s that the rural populations Africa and Asia enjoyed a very low incidence of colorectal cancer and other diseases of the bowel, there has been interest in the supposed benefits of bulky, poorly digested components of unprocessed plant foods. During the 1970s this early work became one of the main drivers for the development of the dietary fibre hypothesis, which states that the non-digestible cell wall polysaccharides found in complex carbohydrate foods exert a range of physiological effects and health benefits. Decades of both epidemiological and laboratory research have lent support to this hypothesis, and public health bodies everywhere now provide recommended minimum levels of intake for dietary fibre. Nevertheless the importance of fibre in the prevention of cancer remains surprisingly controversial.

9.5.1 Dietary fibre

During the earliest stages of development of the dietary fibre hypothesis, neither the physical properties of undigested cell wall polysaccharides, nor their susceptibility to fermentation in the large bowel were understood in any detail. The earliest definition of dietary fibre included only cell wall polysaccharides and lignin (Trowell *et al.*, 1976), which together provide the structural skeleton of plant cell walls. However modern definitions are moving toward the inclusion of all dietary carbohydrates that reach the colon intact, regardless of their molecular weight (Cummings *et al.*, 2009). It is now well established that lignified polysaccharides resist bacterial degradation, whereas soluble cell wall polymers such as pectins and beta-glucans are more readily fermented. However all unabsorbed carbohydrates provide increased faecal bulk, either in the form of a physically intact water-retentive polymers, or as increased bacterial mass following anaerobic fermentation. It is also clear that a significant fraction of ordinary dietary starch escapes hydrolysis by pancreatic enzymes during human digestion, and in future it seems likely that estimates of this fraction will be included within the definition of fibre (Muir *et al.*, 2004).

Early theories of cancer prevention by dietary fibre emphasised the importance of faecal bulk, which was thought to be important both for its ability to dilute faecal carcinogens, and for the increased rate of transit through the colon (Burkitt, 1973). However studies on the fermentation of dietary fibre by the colonic microbiota later prompted interest in the metabolic effects of short chain fatty acids derived from this process. Amongst these, butyrate is the principal source of metabolic energy for colonic epithelial cells, whereas acetate and propionate are absorbed, and then metabolised in the liver and peripheral tissues of the human body. There is now abundant evidence from *in vitro* studies to suggest that butyrate plays a major role in the regulation of the growth, proliferation and programmed death of the intestinal epithelial cells, which form the lining of the intestine, and from which most colon cancers develop (Wong *et al.*, 2006). Research with colorectal and other cancer cell lines *in vitro* has established that butyrate exerts potentially anticarcinogenic effects, including slowing of cell division, promotion of differentiation, and induction of apoptosis. There is still considerable uncertainty about the precise effects of butyrate on the epithelial cells of the healthy mucosa *in vivo*, but some animal studies do provide evidence for an inhibitory effect of butyrate against experimental models of cancer. Thus there are now at least two plausible mechanisms for anticarcinogenic effects in humans, and the protective effects of high-fibre diets against obesity and hyperinsulinaemia may provide a third (Slavin, 2003).

The dietary fibre hypothesis was amongst the earliest theories suggesting that diet could be used to reduce the risk of cancer in humans, and an enormous amount of research has been done in the last three decades to test it. It is disappointing therefore that the issue has not yet been entirely resolved. The conclusions drawn from the promising early epidemiology of Burkitt and others have not always been supported by later large and more carefully controlled trials. For example, Fuchs and colleagues observed no protective effects of fibre in a large prospective study of 88 757 middle-aged North American women (Fuchs *et al.*, 1999), whereas the results of the European Prospective Investigation of Cancer and Nutrition (EPIC) project, which was designed to overcome the limitations of smaller trials conducted within relatively homogeneous populations, have been much more supportive. In 2003 Bingham *et al.* (2003) reported that the relative risk of colorectal cancer in EPIC participants within the highest quintile of fibre intake (mean 35 g/d) versus those in the lowest the lowest (mean 15 g/d) was 0.58. This is a very substantial protective effect, which has been confirmed by subsequent analysis of further data (Bingham *et al.*, 2005). The most recent systematic review of dietary fibre and colorectal cancer is that of the World Cancer Research Fund, which included a formal meta-analysis of eight studies, including EPIC. The results indicated a dose-dependent protective effect, with a reduction in risk of about 10% for each increment in fibre intake of 10 g per day (WCRF, 2007). The overall judgement of the report was that foods containing dietary fibre 'probably protect against colon cancer', though confounding effects due to other risk factors could not be entirely excluded.

For obvious reasons, colorectal cancer has been the main focus of research on dietary fibre and cancer prevention, but there is some sporadic evidence for protective effects against other cancers, particularly in the upper gastrointestinal tract. During the last few decades, adenocarcinoma of the oesophagus has become increasingly common in industrialised countries. This tumour develops at the base of the oesophagus, close to the junction with the stomach, as a complication of chronic gastroesophageal reflux disease. The risk of both conditions is strongly linked to obesity. The 2007 WCRF report concluded that there was 'limited evidence from sparse and inconsistent case-control studies only, suggesting that foods containing dietary fibre protect against oesophageal cancer', but the report's authors were not able to distinguish between oesophageal adenocarcinoma and other cancers of the oesophagus (WCRF, 2007). It is to be hoped that one or more large cohort studies will examine this issue in the future.

9.5.2   Pre- and probiotics

The biological effects of the bacterial species normally resident in the human gastrointestinal tract have long been of interest to those the scientific community interested in maximizing health over the human lifespan (Metchnikoff, 1907), and recently also to both consumers and manufacturers of food products (Saulnier *et al.*, 2009a). *Probiotics* are live bacterial cultures which, when consumed as foods, survive their passage through the upper alimentary tract, and then go on to modify the composition of the complex microbiota of the colon. *Prebiotics* are readily fermentable carbohydrates that resist digestion in the small intestine, but are preferentially fermented by supposedly beneficial bacteria in the colon, and *synbiotics* are preparations of the two (Saulnier *et al.*, 2009b). The biological effects and benefits of probiotics and prebiotics are thoroughly reviewed in other chapters, and no detailed discussion is needed here. However it is worth noting that a number of potentially anticarcinogenic effects are proposed for both pro- and prebiotics, based on the displacement of potentially carcinogenic bacterial species from the colon, the suppression of potential carcinogenic enzyme activity in the faecal stream, the induction of detoxification systems such as the Phase II enzymes, and various modifications to the gastrointestinal and systemic immune systems (Kumar *et al.*, 2010). Almost all of the evidence for these effects is based on *in vitro* studies, or on animal models carrying very restricted bacterial populations, and although intriguing, the hypotheses developed from this work await properly controlled intervention trials in humans. Such studies are difficult and expensive, particularly if the endpoint is recurrence of cancer, and so much of the work that has been done in humans relies on the identification and measurement of cancer biomarkers.

In one recent randomised, double-blind, placebo-controlled trial *Bifidobacterium animalis lactis* and resistant starch were given either alone or as a combined synbiotic preparation, to 20 human volunteers (Worthley *et al.*, 2009). A comprehensive set of mucosal, faecal and systemic biomarkers were analysed including markers of epithelial cell proliferation and epigenetic change, short-chain fatty acid concentrations, pH, ammonia, and microbiological profiles and measures of cytokine profile and inflammatory status in the serum. The authors observed significant changes in the colonic bacterial profile in response to the synbiotic, but no potentially beneficial changes in the other biomarkers. At present there seems little evidence to suggest that a reduction in the risk of colorectal cancer can be achieved by manipulation of the colorectal microbiota by consuming pre- or probiotics to an extent compatible with normal dietary practice.

9.6   Conclusion: the role of functional foods and future trends

This necessarily brief overview of the various mechanisms by which diet, and more particularly specific food components, may influence human susceptibility to cancer has touched upon what may seem to be a bewildering array of plausible, yet often unproven biological mechanisms. Epidemiology reveals huge differences in the incidence of certain cancers – and particularly those of the alimentary tract – across populations, and there seems little doubt that these differences are linked to diets and nutrition. However neither the more focused epidemiology designed to explore the importance of particular components of food, nor the laboratory research that has developed in parallel with them, have yet provided clear evidence for any single dominant nutrition-related mechanism that can confidently be harnessed for the development of functional foods. Although the possibility of effective chemoprevention remains an area of active interest, it may be that the dominant effects of diet act through metabolic pathways associated with energy balance, adiposity and perhaps inflammatory mechanisms which modify tissue homeostasis over decades, and are most readily manipulated by pharmaceutical strategies. Nevertheless opportunities for further product development do exist. For example, consumers seem particularly receptive to the provision of novel high-fibre products, and it seems likely that a prudent consumption of non-starch polysaccharides and other carbohydrates capable of modifying various aspects of colonic function will continue to find favour amongst advisory and regulatory bodies. Research on phytochemicals has revealed many new and unexpected biological mechanisms, which may yet prove to be important in the prevention of specific types of cancer. There are intriguing efforts being made to develop new plant varieties that can deliver increased levels of such chemicals (Mithen *et al.*, 2003). Similarly the opportunities provided by the ever-expanding fields of human and bacterial genomics seem likely, in the longer term, to drive developments in the fields of both personalised nutrition and 'smart' prebiotics. It remains clear however that the full acceptance of such products will require searching analyses both of their efficacy and their safety.

9.7   Sources of further information and advice

Knasmuller S, DeMarini DM, Johnson I and Gerhauser C. (2009) *Chemoprevention of Cancer and DNA Damage by Dietary Factors*. WILEY-VCH Verlag GmbH & Co. KGaA, Weinheim.

World Cancer Research Fund Report on Food, Nutrition, Physical Activity and the Prevention of Cancer: a Global Perspective. American Institute for Cancer Research, Washington, 2007.

World Health Organization (2003) *IARC Handbook of Cancer Prevention Volume 8, Fruits and Vegetables*. IARC Press, Lyon.

World Health Organization (2004) *IARC Handbook of Cancer Prevention Volume 9, Cruciferous Vegetables, Isothiocyanates and Indoles*. IARC Press, Lyon.

9.8   References

ABCP (1994) The effect of vitamin E and beta carotene on the incidence of lung cancer and other cancers in male smokers. The Alpha-Tocopherol, Beta Carotene Cancer Prevention Study Group. *N Engl J Med* **330**, 1029–1035.

Ambrus JL, Ambrus CM, Lillie DB, Johnson RJ, Gastpar H, *et al.* (1984) Effect of sodium meclofenamate on radiation-induced esophagitis and cystitis. *J Med* **15**, 81–92.

Ames BN (1998) Micronutrients prevent cancer and delay aging. *Toxicol Lett* **102–103**, 5–18.

Ames BN (2001) DNA damage from micronutrient deficiencies is likely to be a major cause of cancer. *Mutat Res* **475**, 7–20.

Ames BN (2006) Low micronutrient intake may accelerate the degenerative diseases of aging through allocation of scarce micronutrients by triage. *Proc Natl Acad Sci U S A* **103**, 17589–17594.

Anderson MW, You M and Reynolds SH (1991) Proto-oncogene activation in rodent and human tumors. *Adv Exp Med Biol* **283**, 235–243.

Androutsopoulos VP, Tsatsakis AM and Spandidos DA (2009) Cytochrome P450 CYP1A1: wider roles in cancer progression and prevention. *BMC Cancer* **9**, 187.

Anti M, Armelao F, Marra G, Percesepe A, Bartoli GM, *et al.* (1994) Effects of different doses of fish oil on rectal cell proliferation in patients with sporadic colonic adenomas. *Gastroenterology* **107**, 1709–1718.

Baron JA, Beach M, Mandel JS, van Stolk RU, Haile RW, *et al.* (1999) Calcium supplements and colorectal adenomas. Polyp Prevention Study Group. *Ann N Y Acad Sci* **889**, 138–145.

Bingham SA, Day NE, Luben R, Ferrari P, Slimani N, *et al.* (2003) Dietary fibre in food and protection against colorectal cancer in the European Prospective Investigation into Cancer and Nutrition (EPIC): an observational study. *Lancet* **361**, 1496–1501.

Bingham SA, Norat T, Moskal A, Ferrari P, Slimani N, *et al.* (2005) Is the association with fiber from foods in colorectal cancer confounded by folate intake? *Cancer Epidemiol Biomarkers Prev* **14**, 1552–1556.

Bird CL, Swendseid ME, Witte JS, Shikany JM, Hunt IF, *et al.* (1995) Red cell and plasma folate, folate consumption, and the risk of colorectal adenomatous polyps. *Cancer Epidemiol Biomarkers Prev* **4**, 709–714.

Bischoff-Ferrari HA, Shao A, Dawson-Hughes B, Hathcock J, Giovannucci E, *et al.* (2009) Benefit-risk assessment of vitamin D supplementation. *Osteoporos Int* **21**, 1121–1132.

Bjelland S and Seeberg E (2003) Mutagenicity, toxicity and repair of DNA base damage induced by oxidation. *Mutat Res* **531**, 37–80.

Block G, Patterson B and Subar A (1992) Fruit, vegetables, and cancer prevention: a review of the epidemiological evidence. *Nutr Cancer* **18**, 1–29.

Boffetta P, Couto E, Wichmann J, Ferrari P, Trichopoulos D, *et al.* (2010) Fruit and vegetable intake and overall cancer risk in the European Prospective Investigation into Cancer and Nutrition (EPIC). *J Natl Cancer Inst* **102**, 529–537.

Bos JL, Fearon ER, Hamilton SR, Verlaan-de Vries M, van Boom JH, *et al.* (1987) Prevalence of ras gene mutations in human colorectal cancers. *Nature* **327**, 293–297.

Burkitt DP (1973) The role of refined carbohydrate in large bowel behaviour and disease. *Plant Foods For Man* **1**, 5–9.

Busstra MC, Siezen CL, Grubben MJ, van Kranen HJ, Nagengast FM, *et al.* (2003) Tissue levels of fish fatty acids and risk of colorectal adenomas: a case-control study (Netherlands). *Cancer Causes Control* **14**, 269–276.

Calder PC (2009) Polyunsaturated fatty acids and inflammatory processes: new twists in an old tale. *Biochimie*.

Chou FP, Chu YC, Hsu JD, Chiang HC and Wang CJ (2000) Specific induction of glutathione S-transferase GSTM2 subunit expression by epigallocatechin gallate in rat liver. *Biochem Pharmacol* **60**, 643–650.

Clark LC, Combs GF, Jr., Turnbull BW, Slate EH, Chalker DK, *et al.* (1996) Effects of selenium supplementation for cancer prevention in patients with carcinoma of the skin. A randomized controlled trial. Nutritional Prevention of Cancer Study Group *Jama* **276**, 1957–1963.

Collins AR (2002) The comet assay. Principles, applications, and limitations. *Methods Mol Biol* **203**, 163–177.

Connelly AE, Satia-Abouta J, Martin CF, Keku TO, Woosley JT, *et al.* (2003) Vitamin C intake and apoptosis in normal rectal epithelium. *Cancer Epidemiol Biomarkers Prev* **12**, 559–565.

Cummings JH, Mann JI, Nishida C and Vorster HH (2009) Dietary fibre: an agreed definition. *Lancet* **373**, 365–366.

Cuzick J, Otto F, Baron JA, Brown PH, Burn J, *et al.* (2009) Aspirin and non-steroidal anti-inflammatory drugs for cancer prevention: an international consensus statement. *Lancet Oncol* **10**, 501–507.

Daviglus ML, Liu K, Pirzada A, Yan LL, Garside DB, *et al.* (2005) Relationship of fruit and vegetable consumption in middle-aged men to medicare expenditures in older age: the Chicago Western Electric Study. *J Am Diet Assoc* **105**, 1735–1744.

DeLuca HF (1988) The vitamin D story: a collaborative effort of basic science and clinical medicine. *Faseb J* **2**, 224–236.

Doll R and Peto R (1981) The causes of cancer: quantitative estimates of avoidable risks of cancer in the United States today. *J Natl Cancer Inst* **66**, 1191–1308.

Donehower LA and Bradley A (1993) The tumor suppressor p53. *Biochim Biophys Acta* **1155**, 181–205.

el-Bayoumy K, Chae YH, Upadhyaya P, Meschter C, Cohen LA, *et al.* (1992) Inhibition of 7,12-dimethylbenz(a)anthracene-induced tumors and DNA adduct formation in the mammary glands of female Sprague-Dawley rats by the synthetic organoselenium compound, 1,4-phenylenebis(methylene)selenocyanate. *Cancer Res* **52**, 2402–2407.

el-Bayoumy K, Upadhyaya P, Chae YH, Sohn OS, Rao CV, *et al.* (1995) Chemoprevention of cancer by organoselenium compounds. *J Cell Biochem Suppl* **22**, 92–100.

Epplein M, Franke AA, Cooney RV, Morris JS, Wilkens LR, *et al.* (2009) Association of plasma micronutrient levels and urinary isoprostane with risk of lung cancer: the multiethnic cohort study. *Cancer Epidemiol Biomarkers Prev* **18**, 1962–1970.

Fair AM and Montgomery K (2009) Energy balance, physical activity, and cancer risk. *Methods Mol Biol* **472**, 57–88.

Fedirko V, Bostick RM, Flanders WD, Long Q, Sidelnikov E, *et al.* (2009) Effects of vitamin D and calcium on proliferation and differentiation in normal colon mucosa: a randomized clinical trial. *Cancer Epidemiol Biomarkers Prev* **18**, 2933–2941.

Fiala ES, Staretz ME, Pandya GA, El-Bayoumy K and Hamilton SR (1998) Inhibition of DNA cytosine methyltransferase by chemopreventive selenium compounds, determined by an improved assay for DNA cytosine methyltransferase and DNA cytosine methylation. *Carcinogenesis* **19**, 597–604.

Frosst P, Blom HJ, Milos R, Goyette P, Sheppard CA, *et al.* (1995) A candidate genetic risk factor for vascular disease: a common mutation in methylenetetrahydrofolate reductase. *Nat Genet* **10**, 111–113.

Fuchs CS, Giovannucci EL, Colditz GA, Hunter DJ, Stampfer MJ, *et al.* (1999) Dietary fiber and the risk of colorectal cancer and adenoma in women. *N Engl J Med* **340**, 169–176.

Garland CF, Comstock GW, Garland FC, Helsing KJ, Shaw EK, *et al.* (1989) Serum 25-hydroxyvitamin D and colon cancer: eight-year prospective study. *Lancet* **2**, 1176–1178.

Gerwin BI, Spillare E, Forrester K, Lehman TA, Kispert J, *et al.* (1992) Mutant p53 can induce tumorigenic conversion of human bronchial epithelial cells and reduce their responsiveness to a negative growth factor, transforming growth factor beta 1. *Proc Natl Acad Sci U S A* **89**, 2759–2763.

Giovannucci E (2002) Epidemiologic studies of folate and colorectal neoplasia: a review. *J Nutr* **132**, 2350S–2355S.

Giovannucci E, Stampfer MJ, Colditz GA, Rimm EB, Trichopoulos D, *et al.* (1993) Folate, methionine, and alcohol intake and risk of colorectal adenoma. *J Natl Cancer Inst* **85**, 875–884.

Greenberg ER, Baron JA, Tosteson TD, Freeman DH, Jr., Beck GJ, *et al.* (1994) A clinical trial of antioxidant vitamins to prevent colorectal adenoma. Polyp Prevention Study Group. *N Engl J Med* **331**, 141–147.

Greenwald P, Nixon DW, Malone WF, Kelloff GJ, Stern HR, *et al.* (1990) Concepts in cancer chemoprevention research. *Cancer* **65**, 1483–1490.

Hanahan D and Weinberg RA (2000) The hallmarks of cancer. *Cell* **100**, 57–70.

Hecht SS, Carmella SG, Kenney PM, Low SH, Arakawa K, *et al.* (2004) Effects of cruciferous vegetable consumption on urinary metabolites of the tobacco-specific lung carcinogen 4-(methylnitrosamino)-1-(3-pyridyl)-1-butanone in singapore chinese. *Cancer Epidemiol Biomarkers Prev* **13**, 997–1004.

Hecht SS, Carmella SG and Murphy SE (1999) Effects of watercress consumption on urinary metabolites of nicotine in smokers. *Cancer Epidemiol Biomarkers Prev* **8**, 907–913.

Hecht SS, Chung FL, Richie JP, Jr., Akerkar SA, Borukhova A, *et al.* (1995) Effects of watercress consumption on metabolism of a tobacco-specific lung carcinogen in smokers. *Cancer Epidemiol Biomarkers Prev* **4**, 877–884.

Hecht SS, Trushin N, Rigotty J, Carmella SG, Borukhova A, *et al.* (1996) Complete inhibition of 4-(methylnitrosamino)-1-(3-pyridyl)-1-butanone- induced rat lung tumorigenesis and favorable modification of biomarkers by phenethyl isothiocyanate. *Cancer Epidemiol Biomarkers Prev* **5**, 645–652.

Helbock HJ, Beckman KB, Shigenaga MK, Walter PB, Woodall AA, *et al.* (1998) DNA oxidation matters: the HPLC-electrochemical detection assay of 8-oxo-deoxyguanosine and 8-oxo-guanine. *Proc Natl Acad Sci U S A* **95**, 288–293.

Hofseth LJ, Saito S, Hussain SP, Espey MG, Miranda KM, *et al.* (2003) Nitric oxide-induced cellular stress and p53 activation in chronic inflammation. *Proc Natl Acad Sci U S A* **100**, 143–148.

Hofstad B, Almendingen K, Vatn M, Andersen SN, Owen RW, *et al.* (1998) Growth and recurrence of colorectal polyps: a double-blind 3-year intervention with calcium and antioxidants. *Digestion* **59**, 148–156.

Hollman PC and Katan MB (1999) Dietary flavonoids: intake, health effects and bioavailability. *Food Chem Toxicol* **37**, 937–942.

Hussain SP, Hofseth LJ and Harris CC (2003) Radical causes of cancer. *Nat Rev Cancer* **3**, 276–285.

IARC (1998) *Carotenoids*. Lyon: IARC Press.

IARC (2003) *Fruit and Vegetables*. Lyon: IARC Press.

Issa JP (2000) CpG-island methylation in aging and cancer. *Curr Top Microbiol Immunol* **249**, 101–118.

Jacob RA, Aiello GM, Stephensen CB, Blumberg JB, Milbury PE, *et al.* (2003) Moderate antioxidant supplementation has no effect on biomarkers of oxidant damage in healthy men with low fruit and vegetable intakes. *J Nutr* **133**, 740–743.

Jatoi A, Daly BD, Kramer G and Mason JB (2001) Folate status among patients with non-small cell lung cancer: a case-control study. *J Surg Oncol* **77**, 247–252.

Jenab M, Bueno-de-Mesquita HB, Ferrari P, van Duijnhoven FJ, Norat T, *et al.* (2010) Association between pre-diagnostic circulating vitamin D concentration and risk of colorectal cancer in European populations: a nested case-control study. *Bmj* **340**, b5500.

Johnson I, Williamson G and Musk S (1994) Anticarcinogenic factors in plant foods: a new class of nutrients? *Nutrition Research Reviews*. **7**, 175–204.

Johnson IT (2001) Mechanisms and possible anticarcinogenic effects of diet related apoptosis in colorectal mucosa. *Nutrition Research Reviews* **14**, 229–256.

Johnson IT (2004) New approaches to the role of diet in the prevention of cancers of the alimentary tract. *Mutat Res* **551**, 9–28.

Johnson IT (2007) Phytochemicals and cancer. *Proc Nutr Soc* **66**, 207–215.

Kass SU, Pruss D and Wolffe AP (1997) How does DNA methylation repress transcription? *Trends Genet* **13**, 444–449.

Key TJ, Allen NE, Spencer EA and Travis RC (2002) The effect of diet on risk of cancer. *Lancet* **360**, 861–868.

Knekt P, Marniemi J, Teppo L, Heliovaara M and Aromaa A (1998) Is low selenium status a risk factor for lung cancer? *Am J Epidemiol* **148**, 975–982.

Knudson AG, Jr. (1989) The ninth Gordon Hamilton-Fairley memorial lecture. Hereditary cancers: clues to mechanisms of carcinogenesis. *Br J Cancer* **59**, 661–666.

Kono S and Hirohata T (1996) Nutrition and stomach cancer. *Cancer Causes Control* **7**, 41–55.

Kumar M, Kumar A, Nagpal R, Mohania D, Behare P, *et al.* (2010) Cancer-preventing attributes of probiotics: an update. *Int J Food Sci Nutr*.

La Vecchia C, Negri E, Decarli A, D'Avanzo B, Gallotti L, *et al.* (1988) A case-control study of diet and colo-rectal cancer in northern Italy. *Int J Cancer* **41**, 492–498.

Latham P, Lund EK, Brown JC and Johnson IT (2001) Effects of cellular redox balance on induction of apoptosis by eicosapentaenoic acid in HT29 colorectal adenocarcinoma cells and rat colon in vivo. *Gut* **49**, 97–105.

Le Marchand L, Yoshizawa CN, Kolonel LN, Hankin JH and Goodman MT (1989) Vegetable consumption and lung cancer risk: a population-based case-control study in Hawaii. *J Natl Cancer Inst* **81**, 1158–1164.

Li JY, Taylor PR, Li B, Dawsey S, Wang GQ, *et al.* (1993) Nutrition intervention trials in Linxian, China: multiple vitamin/mineral supplementation, cancer incidence, and disease-specific mortality among adults with esophageal dysplasia. *J Natl Cancer Inst* **85**, 1492–1498.

Liang YC, Tsai SH, Tsai DC, Lin-Shiau SY and Lin JK (2001) Suppression of inducible cyclooxygenase and nitric oxide synthase through activation of peroxisome proliferator-activated receptor-gamma by flavonoids in mouse macrophages. *FEBS Lett* **496**, 12–18.

Lippman SM, Klein EA, Goodman PJ, Lucia MS, Thompson IM, *et al.* (2009) Effect of selenium and vitamin E on risk of prostate cancer and other cancers: the Selenium and Vitamin E Cancer Prevention Trial (SELECT). *Jama* **301**, 39–51.

Loft S and Poulsen HE (1998) Estimation of oxidative DNA damage in man from urinary excretion of repair products. *Acta Biochim Pol* **45**, 133–144.

London SJ, Yuan JM, Chung FL, Gao YT, Coetzee GA, *et al.* (2000) Isothiocyanates, glutathione S-transferase M1 and T1 polymorphisms, and lung-cancer risk: a prospective study of men in Shanghai, China. *Lancet* **356**, 724–729.

Lu J, Jiang C, Kaeck M, Ganther H, Ip C, *et al.* (1995) Cellular and metabolic effects of triphenylselenonium chloride in a mammary cell culture model. *Carcinogenesis* **16**, 513–517.

Lutz WK and Schlatter J (1992) Chemical carcinogens and overnutrition in diet-related cancer. *Carcinogenesis* **13**, 2211–2216.

MacLean CH, Newberry SJ, Mojica WA, Khanna P, Issa AM, *et al.* (2006) Effects of omega-3 fatty acids on cancer risk: a systematic review. *Jama* **295**, 403–415.

Mason JB, Dickstein A, Jacques PF, Haggarty P, Selhub J, *et al.* (2007) A temporal association between folic acid fortification and an increase in colorectal cancer rates may be illuminating important biological principles: a hypothesis. *Cancer Epidemiol Biomarkers Prev* **16**, 1325–1329.

McKeown-Eyssen G, Holloway C, Jazmaji V, Bright-See E, Dion P, *et al.* (1988) A randomized trial of vitamins C and E in the prevention of recurrence of colorectal polyps. *Cancer Res* **48**, 4701–4705.

Metchnikoff E (1907) *The Prolongation of Life*. London: Heinemann.

Mithen R, Faulkner K, Magrath R, Rose P, Williamson G, *et al.* (2003) Development of isothiocyanate-enriched broccoli, and its enhanced ability to induce phase 2 detoxification enzymes in mammalian cells. *Theor Appl Genet* **106**, 727–734.

Mithen RF, Dekker M, Verkerk R, Rabot S and Johnson IT (2000) The nutritional significance, biosynthesis and bioavailability of glucosinolates in human foods. *Journal of the Science of Food and Agriculture* **80**, 967–984.

Möller P and Loft S (2002) Oxidative DNA damage in human white blood cells in dietary antioxidant intervention studies. *Am J Clin Nutr* **76**, 303–310.

Möller P, Vogel U, Pedersen A, Dragsted LO, Sandstrom B, *et al.* (2003) No effect of 600 grams fruit and vegetables per day on oxidative DNA damage and repair in healthy nonsmokers. *Cancer Epidemiol Biomarkers Prev* **12**, 1016–1022.

Morse MA, LaGreca SD, Amin SG and Chung FL (1990) Effects of indole-3-carbinol on lung tumorigenesis and DNA methylation induced by 4-(methylnitrosamino)-1-(3-pyridyl)-1-butanone (NNK) and on the metabolism and disposition of NNK in A/J mice. *Cancer Res* **50**, 2613–2617.

Mosekilde L (2008) Vitamin D requirement and setting recommendation levels: long-term perspectives. *Nutr Rev* **66**, S170–177.

Muir JG, Yeow EG, Keogh J, Pizzey C, Bird AR, *et al.* (2004) Combining wheat bran with resistant starch has more beneficial effects on fecal indexes than does wheat bran alone. *Am J Clin Nutr* **79**, 1020–1028.

Musa-Veloso K, Card JW, Wong AW and Cooper DA (2009) Influence of observational study design on the interpretation of cancer risk reduction by carotenoids. *Nutr Rev* **67**, 527–545.

Musk SR, Stephenson P, Smith TK, Stening P, Fyfe D, *et al.* (1995) Selective toxicity of compounds naturally present in food toward the transformed phenotype of human colorectal cell line HT29. *Nutr Cancer* **24**, 289–298.

Natarajan K, Singh S, Burke TR, Jr., Grunberger D and Aggarwal BB (1996) Caffeic acid phenethyl ester is a potent and specific inhibitor of activation of nuclear transcription factor NF-kappa B. *Proc Natl Acad Sci U S A* **93**, 9090–9095.

Nelson DR, Kamataki T, Waxman DJ, Guengerich FP, Estabrook RW, *et al.* (1993) The P450 superfamily: update on new sequences, gene mapping, accession numbers, early trivial names of enzymes, and nomenclature. *DNA Cell Biol* **12**, 1–51.

Norat T, Bingham S, Ferrari P, Slimani N, Jenab M, *et al.* (2005) Meat, fish, and colorectal cancer risk: the European Prospective Investigation into cancer and nutrition. *J Natl Cancer Inst* **97**, 906–916.

Nowell PC (1976) The clonal evolution of tumor cell populations. *Science* **194**, 23–28.

Nyberg F, Hou SM, Pershagen G and Lambert B (2003) Dietary fruit and vegetables protect against somatic mutation in vivo, but low or high intake of carotenoids does not. *Carcinogenesis* **24**, 689–696.

Omenn GS, Goodman GE, Thornquist MD, Balmes J, Cullen MR, *et al.* (1996) Effects of a combination of beta carotene and vitamin A on lung cancer and cardiovascular disease. *N Engl J Med* **334**, 1150–1155.

Pitot HC and Dragan YP (1994) The multistage nature of chemically induced hepatocarcinogenesis in the rat. *Drug Metab Rev* **26**, 209–220.

Poulsen HE, Jensen BR, Weimann A, Jensen SA, Sorensen M, *et al.* (2000) Antioxidants, DNA damage and gene expression. *Free Radic Res* **33 Suppl**, S33–39.

Prochaska HJ and Talalay P (1988) Regulatory mechanisms of monofunctional and bifunctional anticarcinogenic enzyme inducers in murine liver. *Cancer Res* **48**, 4776–4782.

Rayman MP (2008) Food-chain selenium and human health: emphasis on intake. *Br J Nutr* **100**, 254–268.

Rosa JG, Prokopczyk B, Desai DH, Amin SG and El-Bayoumy K (1998) Elevated 8-hydroxy-2'-deoxyguanosine levels in lung DNA of A/J mice and F344 rats treated with 4-(methylnitrosamino)-1-(3-pyridyl)-1-butanone and inhibition by dietary 1,4-phenylenebis(methylene)selenocyanate. *Carcinogenesis* **19**, 1783–1788.

Roswall N, Olsen A, Christensen J, Dragsted LO, Overvad K, *et al.* (2010a) Micronutrient intake and risk of colon and rectal cancer in a Danish cohort. *Cancer Epidemiol* **34**, 40–46.

Roswall N, Olsen A, Christensen J, Dragsted LO, Overvad K, *et al.* (2010b) Source-specific effects of micronutrients in lung cancer prevention. *Lung Cancer* **67**, 275–281.

Satia-Abouta J, Galanko JA, Martin CF, Potter JD, Ammerman A, *et al.* (2003) Associations of micronutrients with colon cancer risk in African Americans and whites: results from the North Carolina Colon Cancer Study. *Cancer Epidemiol Biomarkers Prev* **12**, 747–754.

Saulnier DM, Kolida S and Gibson GR (2009a) Microbiology of the human intestinal tract and approaches for its dietary modulation. *Curr Pharm Des* **15**, 1403–1414.

Saulnier DM, Spinler JK, Gibson GR and Versalovic J (2009b) Mechanisms of probiosis and prebiosis: considerations for enhanced functional foods. *Curr Opin Biotechnol* **20**, 135–141.

Schrauzer GN, White DA and Schneider CJ (1977) Cancer mortality correlation studies – III: statistical associations with dietary selenium intakes. *Bioinorg Chem* **7**, 23–31.

Serafini M, Bellocco R, Wolk A and Ekstrom AM (2002) Total antioxidant potential of fruit and vegetables and risk of gastric cancer. *Gastroenterology* **123**, 985–991.

Shen H, Wei Q, Pillow PC, Amos CI, Hong WK, *et al.* (2003) Dietary folate intake and lung cancer risk in former smokers: a case-control analysis. *Cancer Epidemiol Biomarkers Prev* **12**, 980–986.

Siezen CL, van Leeuwen AI, Kram NR, Luken ME, van Kranen HJ, *et al.* (2005) Colorectal adenoma risk is modified by the interplay between polymorphisms in arachidonic acid pathway genes and fish consumption. *Carcinogenesis* **26**, 449–457.

Singh S and Aggarwal BB (1995) Activation of transcription factor NF-kappa B is suppressed by curcumin (diferuloylmethane). *J Biol Chem* **270**, 24995–25000.

Slavin J (2003) Why whole grains are protective: biological mechanisms. *Proc Nutr Soc* **62**, 129–134.

Smith TK, Mithen R and Johnson IT (2003) Effects of Brassica vegetable juice on the induction of apoptosis and aberrant crypt foci in rat colonic mucosal crypts in vivo. *Carcinogenesis* **24**, 491–495.

Steck SE, Gammon MD, Hebert JR, Wall DE and Zeisel SH (2007) GSTM1, GSTT1, GSTP1, and GSTA1 polymorphisms and urinary isothiocyanate metabolites following broccoli consumption in humans. *J Nutr* **137**, 904–909.

Steinmetz KA and Potter JD (1991) Vegetables, fruit, and cancer. I. Epidemiology. *Cancer Causes Control* **2**, 325–357.

Stern LL, Bagley PJ, Rosenberg IH and Selhub J (2000) Conversion of 5-formyltetrahydrofolic acid to 5-methyltetrahydrofolic acid is unimpaired in folate-adequate persons homozygous for the C677T mutation in the methylenetetrahydrofolate reductase gene. *J Nutr* **130**, 2238–2242.

Sun CL, Yuan JM, Lee MJ, Yang CS, Gao YT, *et al.* (2002) Urinary tea polyphenols in relation to gastric and esophageal cancers: a prospective study of men in Shanghai, China. *Carcinogenesis* **23**, 1497–1503.

Tan J, Zhu W, Wang W, Li R, Hou S, *et al.* (2002) Selenium in soil and endemic diseases in China. *Sci Total Environ* **284**, 227–235.

Tangrea J, Helzlsouer K, Pietinen P, Taylor P, Hollis B, *et al.* (1997) Serum levels of vitamin D metabolites and the subsequent risk of colon and rectal cancer in Finnish men. *Cancer Causes Control* **8**, 615–625.

Theodoratou E, Kyle J, Cetnarskyj R, Farrington SM, Tenesa A, *et al.* (2007) Dietary flavonoids and the risk of colorectal cancer. *Cancer Epidemiol Biomarkers Prev* **16**, 684–693.

Todd R and Wong DT (1999) Oncogenes. *Anticancer Res* **19**, 4729–4746.

Trowell HC, Southgate DAT, Wolever TMS, Leeds AR, Gassull MA, *et al.* (1976) Dietary fibre redefined. *Lancet* **i**, 967.

Tseng M, Murray SC, Kupper LL and Sandler RS (1996) Micronutrients and the risk of colorectal adenomas. *Am J Epidemiol* **144**, 1005–1014.

van den Brandt PA, Goldbohm RA, van 't Veer P, Bode P, Dorant E, *et al.* (1993) A prospective cohort study on toenail selenium levels and risk of gastrointestinal cancer. *J Natl Cancer Inst* **85**, 224–229.

Verkerk R, Schreiner M, Krumbein A, Ciska E, Holst B, *et al.* (2009) Glucosinolates in Brassica vegetables: the influence of the food supply chain on intake, bioavailability and human health. *Mol Nutr Food Res* **53 Suppl 2**, S219.

Voorrips LE, Goldbohm RA, Brants HA, van Poppel GA, Sturmans F, *et al.* (2000) A prospective cohort study on antioxidant and folate intake and male lung cancer risk. *Cancer Epidemiol Biomarkers Prev* **9**, 357–365.

Wattenberg LW (1981) Inhibition of carcinogen-induced neoplasia by sodium cyanate, tert-butylisocyanate and benzyl isothiocyanate administered subsequent to carcinogen exposure. *Cancer Research* **41**, 2991–2994.

Wattenberg LW (1985) Chemoprevention of cancer. *Cancer Res* **45**, 1–8.

Wattenberg LW (1992) Inhibition of carcinogenesis by minor dietary constituents. *Cancer Res* **52**, 2085s–2091s.

Wattenburg L (1990) Inhibition of carcinogenesis by minor anutrient constituents of the diet. *Proceedings of the Nutition Society* **49**, 173–183.

WCRF (1997) Food, Nutrition and the Prevention of Cancer: a Global Perspective, pp. 216–251. Washington DC: American Institute for Cancer Research.

WCRF (2007) *Food, Nutrition, Physical Activity and the Prevention of Cancer: A Global perspective*. Washington: American Institute for Cancer Research.

Webb AR and Holick MF (1988) The role of sunlight in the cutaneous production of vitamin D3. *Annu Rev Nutr* **8**, 375–399.

Wei WQ, Abnet CC, Qiao YL, Dawsey SM, Dong ZW, *et al.* (2004) Prospective study of serum selenium concentrations and esophageal and gastric cardia cancer, heart disease, stroke, and total death. *Am J Clin Nutr* **79**, 80–85.

West DW, Slattery ML, Robison LM, Schuman KL, Ford MH, *et al.* (1989) Dietary intake and colon cancer: sex- and anatomic site-specific associations. *Am J Epidemiol* **130**, 883–894.

West NJ, Courtney ED, Poullis AP and Leicester RJ (2009) Apoptosis in the colonic crypt, colorectal adenomata, and manipulation by chemoprevention. *Cancer Epidemiol Biomarkers Prev* **18**, 1680–1687.

Wickramasinghe SN and Fida S (1994) Bone marrow cells from vitamin B12- and folate-deficient patients misincorporate uracil into DNA. *Blood* **83**, 1656–1661.

Wilkinson Jt and Clapper ML (1997) Detoxication enzymes and chemoprevention. *Proc Soc Exp Biol Med* **216**, 192–200.

Willett WC, Polk BF, Morris JS, Stampfer MJ, Pressel S, *et al.* (1983) Prediagnostic serum selenium and risk of cancer. *Lancet* **2**, 130–134.

Wong JM, de Souza R, Kendall CW, Emam A and Jenkins DJ (2006) Colonic health: fermentation and short chain fatty acids. *J Clin Gastroenterol* **40**, 235–243.

Worthley DL, Le Leu RK, Whitehall VL, Conlon M, Christophersen C, *et al.* (2009) A human, double-blind, placebo-controlled, crossover trial of prebiotic, probiotic, and synbiotic supplementation: effects on luminal, inflammatory, epigenetic, and epithelial biomarkers of colorectal cancer. *Am J Clin Nutr* **90**, 578–586.

Wyatt MD and Pittman DL (2006) Methylating agents and DNA repair responses: Methylated bases and sources of strand breaks. *Chem Res Toxicol* **19**, 1580–1594.

Yoxall V, Kentish P, Coldham N, Kuhnert N, Sauer MJ, *et al.* (2005) Modulation of hepatic cytochromes P450 and phase II enzymes by dietary doses of sulforaphane in rats: Implications for its chemopreventive activity. *Int J Cancer* **117**, 356–362

10

Functional foods and obesity

S. B. Myrie and P. J. H. Jones, University of Manitoba, Canada

Abstract: Obesity is a global epidemic; associated with decreased life expectancy, partly due to an increased rate of comorbidities from diseases such as cardiovascular diseases, type 2 diabetes and some cancers. Functional foods can be used strategically as weight management tools in the fight against obesity. Functional foods for obesity should be able to influence energy intake by regulating appetite and satiety, and/or energy output by controlling energy efficiency through regulation of thermogenesis and adipogenesis. The overall objective of this chapter is to review clinical studies that examine the roles of functional food components as weight management tools. Dietary lipids account for over 35% of the daily caloric content of an individual's diet in most industrialized societies, thus it would be advantageous to have dietary lipid components with anti-obesogenic properties. Lipid components, including medium-chain triglycerides, diacylglycerols, conjugated linoleic acid and omega-3 fatty acids, as well as dietary fibre and polyphenols, lead the way in the area of research on weight management. Inclusion of these dietary components in food formulation may categorize such foods as functional foods targeted for weight loss, because of their effects on energy intake and expenditure.

Key words: conjugated linoleic acids (CLA), diacylglycerols (DAG), fibre, green tea, medium-chain triglycerides (MCT), omega-3 fatty acids, resistant starch, polyphenols.

10.1   Introduction

The World Health Organization has labelled obesity as a global epidemic; with more than a billion overweight adults, at least 300 million of them obese (WHO, 2000). Obesity is known to be associated with decreased life expectancy (Fontaine *et al.*, 2003; Peeters *et al.*, 2003; Mann, 2005; Reynolds *et al.*, 2005; Stewart *et al.*, 2009). For example, Peeters and colleagues estimated that overweight or obesity shortened life expectancy by 3.1 to 7.1 years (Peeters *et al.*, 2003). Overall, overweight and obesity are seen as global health problems because they are risk factors for obesity comorbidities including diet-related chronic diseases such as cardiovascular disease, type 2 diabetes mellitus and some cancers (WHO, 2000). Food can contribute to overweight and obesity; thus, strategically it can be used as a weight management tool. The overall objective of this chapter is to review clinical studies that examine the roles of functional components in foods as weight management tools.

10.1.1   Food and diet contribution to overweightness and obesity

With the dramatic increase in the global prevalence of obesity, treatment and prevention of overweight and obesity have become major public health issues. The aetiology of obesity is multi-factorial, ranging from lifestyle choices such as excess food intake and insufficient physical activity, to metabolic factors, which can also be compounded by the use of medications that have weight gain as undesirable side effects. Each factor is further influenced by genetic traits (Aronne *et al.*, 2009; Weinsier *et al.*, 1998). Overall, dietary factors, particularly fat and energy intake are strongly and positively associated with body weight gain (Dubnov-Raz and Berry, 2008; Paradis *et al.*, 2009; Weinsier *et al.*, 1998). Excessive caloric intake and low levels of physical activity over many years promote the development of subcutaneous, perivisceral and intravisceral fat depots with increased risks for various chronic diseases (Ferrari, 2007). Conversely, studies have shown that small weight losses can have large health benefits. For instance, a five to ten percent reduction in initial weight has been shown to be associated with significant improvement in blood pressure, cholesterol levels and glycemic control (Knowler *et al.*, 2002; Pasanisi *et al.*, 2001).

Treatment options for obesity include behavioural therapy, pharmacotherapy and/or bariatric surgery. Behavioural therapy focuses on making lifestyle changes which are aimed at reducing energy intake by increasing physical activity with proper diet and/or low calorie diets. Social and psychological support are emphasised as important components in behavioural therapy. In cases of severe obesity pharmacotherapy and/or surgical procedures may be required to complement behavioural therapy. A recent review by Wieringa and colleagues (Wieringa *et al.*, 2008) suggests a paradigm shift occurring in the approach to prevent and treat overweight and obesity, from a former emphasis on educational and behavioural strategies in public health policies toward a focus on changes in the quality of food products and supply. These authors argue that nutritional factors and food product supply are the most prominent points of intervention for prevention strategies for combating overweight and obesity. More importantly, portion size, which is a product of the food industry, plays a critical role in the fight against obesity (Wansink, 2007). Based on results of their review, Wieringa and colleagues conclude that their findings indicate a certain level of societal pressure directing responsibility towards the food industry and governments in order to change the obesogenic food environment. Examples of such policies involve the development and provision of healthier foods, including functional foods and novel regulations for nutrition labelling (Wieringa *et al.*, 2008).

10.1.2   Functional foods and weight management

Functional food research and development is a rapidly expanding field, with obesity as one of the key target areas. Functional foods are defined broadly as foods and food components that provide more than simple nutrition; supplying additional physiological benefit beyond their inherent nutritional values. For instance, the International Food Information Council (IFIC) defines functional foods as foods and food components that provide a health benefit beyond basic nutrition. The IFIC definition includes conventional foods, fortified, enriched, or enhanced foods, and dietary supplements (IFIC, 2009). The health claim benefits from functional foods may be related to enhanced body function or it may refer to reduced risk of disease as measured by an intermediate biomarker such as serum cholesterol concentration, blood pressure or satiety (Wieringa *et al.*, 2008). In general, functional foods for obesity should be able to influence an individual's energy balance by contributing to a lower intake and/or a higher energy expenditure (Palou *et al.*, 2004).

10.2   Functional foods contribution to weight management

Functional foods that affect energy metabolism and fat partitioning may be helpful adjuncts as part of the dietary approach to body weight control. Foods that have been studied for their effects on body weight, energy expenditure and/or satiety have the potential to be effective functional foods. The purpose of this section is to examine human research that illustrates the potential usefulness of functional food components in the prevention of weight gain or as adjuncts to weight loss efforts. In defining functional foods, it is important to identify the specific components that have potential health benefits. The primary functional food components associated with weight management, particularly weight loss, can be classified according to major nutrient groups as well as nutrient components, including lipids such as medium-chain triglycerides, diacylglycerides, conjugated linoleic acid, docosahexaenoic acid and eicosapentaenoic acid (see Table 10.1), dietary insoluble and soluble fibres and resistant starches (see Table 10.2), and polyphenols including catechins.

10.2.1   Dietary lipid components associated with weight loss and weight control

Modification of dietary fat type represents one strategy for weight management. Dietary lipids account for over 35% of the daily caloric content of an individual's diet in most industrialized societies (Donahoo *et al.*, 2008), thus it would be advantageous to have dietary lipid components with anti-obesogenic properties. Some research suggest that diets high in fats such as medium-chain triglycerides, diacylglycerols, conjugated linoleic acid, docosahexenoic acid and eicosapentoenoic acid may have a greater beneficial impact on energy metabolism and/or satiety compared to diets high in saturated fatty acids.

Medium-chain triglycerides

Medium-chain triglycerides (MCT) are a class of lipids in which three intermediate carbon length saturated fats are bound to a glycerol backbone; the structure is called triacylglycerols or triglycerides (Fig. 10.1). MCT are distinguished from other triacylglycerols in that each fat molecule (R groups in Fig. 10.1) is between six and twelve carbons in length (Table 10.1). The absorption and transport of MCT differ from long chain triglycerides (LCT). Within the gastrointestinal tract, MCT and LCT are digested to their respective fatty acids; however, LC fatty acids are repackaged as LCT into chylomicrons for transport via the lymphatic system via the peripheral circulation. Medium-chain fatty acids (MCFA) because of their shorter chain lengths do not require chylomicron formation for their absorption and transport (Marten *et al.*, 2006). Therefore, MCFA travel directly to the liver via the portal circulation, bypassing peripheral tissues such as adipose tissue. The different mode of transport for MCT compared to LCT allow for quicker absorption and utilization of MCT. MCFA are mostly oxidized by the liver for use as energy source and therefore have been reported to act more like glucose than fats (Anonymous, 2002). Research indicates that MCT can up-regulate energy expenditure (Papamandjaris *et al.*, 1998, 2000); MCT have a greater thermogenic effect compare to LCT thereby leading to an energy imbalance that may assist in weight loss or in the prevention of obesity (Ogawa *et al.*, 2007; Scalfi *et al.*, 1991). Furthermore, MCT consumption may increase satiety more than do LCT consumption, thus promoting weight loss (St-Onge and Jones, 2002).

MCT have been proposed as a tool in the prevention of human obesity due to their overall effect on body weight through mechanisms such as increased energy expenditure and increased satiety resulting in negative energy balance, decreased food intake and decreased adiposity (St-Onge and Jones, 2002; St-Onge *et al.*, 2003a, 2003b). Animal and human studies assessing the effects of MCT vs. LCT have found that body weight is reduced with MCT consumption compared with LCT, and that feed efficiency was reduced (St-Onge and Jones, 2002).

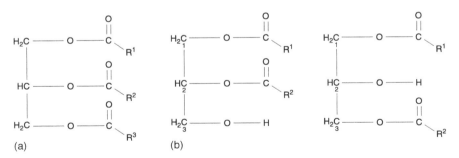

Fig. 10.1 (a) General structure of medium-chain triacylglycerol, which has three saturated fatty acids attached to a glycerol backbone. R groups represent fatty acid molecules, which are six to twelve carbon lengths for MCT. (b) Diacylglycerol (DAG) structure, which has two fatty acid molecules attached to a glycerol backbone. The fatty acids can be attached in the 1,2, or 1,3 position. Oleic (C18:1), linoleic (C18:2) and linolenic (C18:3) acids represent the main fatty acid constituents of DAG.

Table 10.1 Lipid components as functional food components in the potential treatment of overweight and obesity

Common name	Systematic name	Physiological mechanisms that contribute to weight management	Major food source
Saturated fatty acids (medium-chain triacylglycerols: MCT)			
Caproic acid	Hexanoic acid (C6:0)	• Up-regulate energy expenditure	Coconut oil, palm kernel oil, milks from ruminants (cow, sheep, goats)
Caprylic acid	Octanoic acid (C8:0)	• Enhanced fat oxidation	
Capric acid	Decanoic acid (C10:0)	• Increase satiety (leading to decreased food intake)	
Lauric acid	Dodecanoic acid (C12:0)		
Saturated fatty acids (diacylglycerols: DAG)			
Diacylglycerols	1-Palmitoyl-2-oleoyl-glycerol	• Up-regulate energy expenditure • Enhanced fat oxidation	Soybean and canola oil
Polyunsaturated fatty acids (omega-6)			
Conjugated linoleic acid (CLA)	Cis9,trans11-octadecadienoic acid (C18:2) Trans10,cis12-octadecadienoic acid (C18:2)	Prevent lipogenesis (leading to enhanced lean muscle mass and decrease adiposity)	Milk, cheese and meat primarily from ruminants
Polyunsaturated fatty acids (omega-3)			
Eicosapentaenoic acid (EPA)	All cis-5,8,11,14,17-eicosapentaenoic acid (C20:5 n-3)	Suppress appetite (via influence on adipocytokines such as adiponectin and leptin)	Fish and fish oil
Docosahexaenoic acid (DHA)	All cis-4,7,10,13,16,19-docosahexaenoic acid (C22:6 n-3)		Fish, fish oil, specialty eggs

Nagao and Yanagita (2009) conducted a recent systematic review of 26 clinical studies that assess the physiological effects of dietary MCFA/MCT. Some of these clinical studies showed that even a single dose (range from 5 to 48 g) (Binnert *et al.*, 1998; Dulloo *et al.*, 1996; Kasai *et al.*, 2002; Scalfi *et al.*, 1991; Seaton *et al.*, 1986) of MCT can increase fat oxidation and/or postprandial energy expenditure in both normal weight and obese individuals.

Clinical studies have also suggested that MCT may lead to a greater suppression of appetite compared to LCT (Stubbs and Harbron, 1996; Van Wymelbeke *et al.*, 1998, 2001). One study (Stubbs and Harbron, 1996) found that food intake was suppressed ($p < 0.001$) when two-thirds of the fat content of a high fat diet was derived from MCT, although body weight was not affected. Other studies found that the addition of MCT to a meal delay the request for the subsequent meal ($p = 0.05$), and food intake was also smaller ($p < 0.01$) during the meal (Van Wymelbeke *et al.*, 1998, 2001). An increase in satiety due to MCT may be related to direct hepatic access via the portal vein, where most of the MCT is quickly oxidized by the liver, compared to LCT. Expression of satiety hormones such as cholecystokinin (CCK) and gastric inhibitory polypeptide (GIP) may also contribute to the satiety effects from MCT (see review by St-Onge and Jones, 2002).

MCT are a component of many foods including coconut oil, palm kernel oil, butter, milk, yogurt and cheese (Nagao and Yanagita, 2009), with coconut and palm oils representing the richest dietary source of MCT (Anonymous, 2002; Marten *et al.*, 2006). Edible MCT oils are obtained through lipid fractionation from sources such as coconut oil and milk (Nagao and Yanagita, 2009; Marten *et al.*, 2006). These MCT oils contain almost exclusively octanoic and decanoic acid, at a ratio from 50:50 to 80:20 (Marten *et al.*, 2006). General uses for MCT have been limited due to the low smoking point, easy foaming during deep frying and high cost. Recently, medium-chain and long-chain triacylglycerol (MLCT) molecules have been developed by transesterification of MCT with LCT (Aoyama *et al.*, 2007; Takeuchi *et al.*, 2008). The structural conversion of MCT to MLCT is said to broaden their uses and may attract more attention to MCFA/MCT functions (Aoyama *et al.*, 2007; Takeuchi *et al.*, 2008). MLCT possess higher smoking temperatures and are better for cooking than a physical mixture of MCT and LCT. Human studies have shown that MLCT consumption significantly decreases body weight and body fat mass (Kasai *et al.*, 2003; Matsuo *et al.*, 2001; Takeuchi *et al.*, 2002; Xue *et al.*, 2009a, 2009b).

Despite their metabolic benefits, some concerns exist regarding effects of MCT consumption on plasma lipid concentrations. MCT significantly increase serum cholesterol in individuals with prior mild hypercholesterolemia (Cater *et al.*, 1997). In another study, MCT significantly increased serum triglycerides and decreased HDL-cholesterol compared to LCT (Swift *et al.*, 1992). Conversely, other studies have shown that MCT lead to significantly lower plasma triglycerides compared to LCT (Calabrese *et al.*, 1999). Furthermore, it has been suggested that experiments that reported increased plasma triglycerides were due to the very high amount of MCT in the diet, and in some cases the supply of polyunsaturated fatty acids in these diets was critically low (Marten *et al.*, 2006). MCFA consumption, especially when fed in excess of caloric needs, might increase *de novo* lipogenesis. This in turn, would increase triglyceride secretion, and could thus account for the elevated fasting plasma triglyceride levels.

In summary, experimental studies suggest that dietary MCFA/MCT enhances thermogenesis and fat oxidation, as well as suppress appetite in human subjects, thus contributing to weight loss. Such results provide promising news for the use of MCT as a functional food for weight management. However, beneficial effects of MCFA/MCT on obesity/overweight has have not been apparent in some clinical studies, with some studies reporting dyslipidemic profiles attributed to MCT consumption. Thus, more research is required to provide a consensus regarding the health benefits of MCFA/MCT on obesity.

Diacylglycerols
Diacylglycerols (DAG) possess two fatty acids attached to a glycerol backbone represented in conformation as 1,2-diacylglycerol and 1,3-diacylglycerol (Fig. 10.1). Diacylglycerols are catabolized to two free fatty acids and a glycerol moiety, as opposed to two free fatty acids and a 2-monacylglycerol molecule after hydrolysis of triacylglycerol (Morita and Soni, 2009). The 2-monacylglycerol molecule acts as a backbone for the reformation of a triacylglycerol molecule for packaging into chylomicrons. In the absence of 2-monacylglycerol molecules, diacylglycerols cannot be reformed for packaging into chylomicrons, and therefore the free fatty acid and glycerol molecules travel via the portal circulation to the liver where they are rapidly oxidized. The main fatty acid constituents of DAG are oleic, linoleic and linolenic acids (Maki *et al.*, 2002). Diacylglycerols do not increase serum TG levels, so have been used to study weight loss and to decrease body fat accumulation. DAG reportedly increase thermogenic effects, and therefore have the potential to assist in weight loss. DAG thermogenic effects are said to be similar to those of MCT in that they are absorbed and transported directly to the liver rather through the lymphatic system. Diacylglycerols are naturally occurring compounds found in varied amount in many dietary oils and fats. DAG can also be commercially synthesized by enzyme-catalysed esterification of glycerol with fatty acids from oils such as canola, soybean, corn, olive and cottonseed oil (Flickinger and Matsuo, 2003).

Several short-term studies have observed greater fat oxidation with DAG oil consumption compared with TAG oil. For instance, Nagao and colleagues (Nagao *et al.*, 2000) conducted a 16-week study in 38 healthy males with BMI of 24 kg/m². Test diets were given at breakfast as either 10 g of DAG or TAG oil, with total daily lipid intake of 50 g/d. Body weight and BMI decreased (−2.6 kg) in the DAG test group (p < 0.1) while weight increased in the TAG group (1.1 kg). Body fat decreased similarly in the 2 groups, but abdominal fat decreased more significantly in the DAG group (p < 0.05). There were no differences in serum lipid or glucose concentrations between the groups. The researchers concluded that DAG supplementation suppresses body weight and regional fat deposition. A weight-loss study by Maki and colleagues (Maki *et al.*, 2002), found that body weight and fat mass decreased to a greater extent in subjects consuming DAG than in those consuming TAG. The study included overweight and obese men (25) and women (40) in a randomized, parallel-arm trial. Participants were asked to reduce their caloric intakes by 500–800 kcal/d (2090–3344 kJ/d) for a 24-week period. During this period they incorporated foods containing DAG or TAG (oils were consumed as muffins, crackers, soups, cookies and granola bars); foods provided 16–45 g/d of either DAG or TAG, or 15% of the participant's energy requirements. Body composition was assessed by dual-energy X-ray absorptiometry and single-slice computed tomography scanning at the level of the L4–L5 vertebrae. Both groups lost a significant amount of body weight and fat mass, but the changes were greater in participants who were supplementing their diets with DAG containing foods compared to those who supplemented with TAG foods (−3.6 and −2.5%, respectively). The percentage change in intra-abdominal adipose tissue did not differ significantly between groups. A study by Kamphuis and colleagues (Kamphuis *et al.*, 2003c) found that when 12% of the total daily energy intake was provided by DAG in foods, fat oxidation was greater than when the energy intake was provided by TAG in foods. Energy expenditure did not differ between the groups but the participants reported being less hungry after DAG consumption compared to TAG consumption (area under the curve score: 281 and 472 mm.h, respectively).

A recent meta-analysis by Xu and colleagues concluded that DAG was efficacious for reducing body weight compared to TAG, and the effect was influenced by the daily dose of DAG (Xu *et al.*, 2008). The meta-analysis assessed the effects of DAG on body weight from randomized controlled clinical trials. Their statistical analyses included five published trials, showing a significant difference in body weight reduction between groups receiving DAG compared to TAG (−0.75 kg; 95% CI: −1.11 to −0.39; $p < 0.00001$). Moreover, linear regression analysis showed significant correlation between daily dose of DAG and body weight reduction ($p = 0.044$, $R^2 = 0.889$) (Xu *et al.*, 2008). Additionally, a more recent study from our group (Yuan *et al.*, 2010) found that consumption of DAG oil by overweight women (n = 26; BMI: 30.0 ± 0.7 kg/m^2) reduced the accumulation of body fat compared to a control oil blend (composed of sunflower, safflower and rapeseed oils). The study used a single-blind, crossover design; each study phase was of four weeks' duration, with participants consuming 40 g/d of DAG or control oil. Body fat was assessed by DEXA analysis, with the results showing a reduction ($p < 0.05$) in total body fat and fat in trunk, android and gynoid areas, with no change in lean mass when consuming DAG compared to control oil (Yuan *et al.*, 2010). The study found no changes in energy expenditure, fat oxidation or lipogenesis between DAG and control oils, thus, the mechanisms of action of DAG oil in modulating body fat were not identified.

All cooking oils naturally contain small quantities of DAG, ranging from 0.8% in canola oil, 5.5% in olive oil, to 9.5% in cottonseed oil (Flickinger and Matsuo, 2003). Commercial production of DAG oil results from the enzymatic esterification of fatty acids from natural edible plant oils. Commercially produced vegetable-derived DAG oil contains >80% DAG, <20% TAG, <5% monoacylglycerols, and a small amounts of emulsifiers ad antioxidants to maintain quality (Morita and

Soni, 2009). In 1998 the Japanese Ministry of Health, Labour and Welfare (MHLW) approved the use of DAG as a 'food for specified health use' (JMHLW, 1998), and in 2000 the US Food and Drug Administration (FDA) classified DAG as a food ingredient that is generally recognized as safe (GRAS) (FDA, 2000). Reviews assessing the safety of DAG oil found that clinical studies indicated that DAG oil is well tolerated; with no significant toxicity effects noted (Morita and Soni, 2009; Rudkowska *et al.*, 2005). However, in September, 2009, Kao Corporation, the producer of *Econa Cooking Oil*, voluntarily suspended sales of all their DAG oil products in Japan as well as shipment of their products *Envoa Brand Oil* sold in North America (Kao, 2009). On their website, Kao Corporation cited issues raised by European research related to the safety of glycidol fatty acid esters contained in fats and oils (Kao, 2009). The concern arose from research findings from the Chemical and Veterinary Test Agency in Stuttgart, German, who detected glycidol fatty acid esters in refined vegetable fats on a palm oil base (BfR, 2009). The report stated that based on findings from animals experiments, glycidol is classified as probably carcinogenic to humans, thus, the German Federal Institute for Risk Assessment (BfR) is taking the finding seriously (BfR, 2009). Kao Corporation stated that the glycidol fatty acid esters content in their DAG products are introduced as a by-product of deodorization process during production of fats and oils, but they maintained that the main ingredient, DAG, in their products is proven safe, and thus plans to resume sale after reducing the amount of glycidol fatty acid esters introduced in its production method (Kao, 2009).

In summary, accumulated clinical evidence indicate that DAG may be a beneficial functional food component for weight loss. Diacylglycerols have been shown repeatedly to decrease body weight via reduced adiposity and enhanced fat oxidation. DAG is oxidized primarily in the liver, which may also influence satiety. Research results to date indicate the potential for future popularity in the market place for DAG products for weight management. However, there is a need for research to study the safety of long-term consumption of DAG.

Conjugated linoleic acid
Conjugated linoleic acid (CLA) refers to a group of conjugated dienoic isomers of linoleic acid. CLA is formed when reactions shift the location of one or both of the double bonds of linoleic acid; generating various cis- and trans-isomeric combinations (Fig. 10.2). At least 13 CLA isomers have been reported, with the two most predominant occurring CLA isomer found in the diet are cis-9, trans-11 linoleic acid (c9,t11-octadecadienoic acid), followed by c7,t9 CLA, c11,t13 CLA, c8,t10 CLA and t10,c12 CLA (Li *et al.*, 2008). The CLA isomer c9,t11 appears to be responsible for improving muscle growth, while the t10,c12 isomer primarily prevents lipogenesis, that is, the storage of fat in adipose tissue. Early investigations using CLA led to the realization that this set of compounds has multiple biological effects such as reductions in plasma lipoproteins and lipids and atherosclerosis and body fat accumulation (Kennedy *et al.*, 2010). The latter biological effects have led to more research addressing the use of CLA for weight loss in overweight

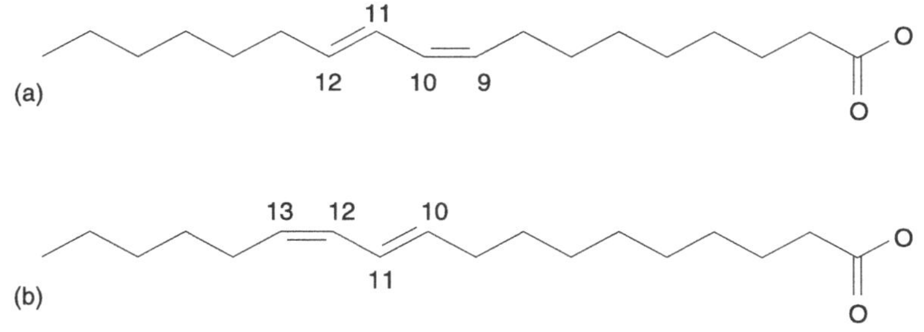

Fig. 10.2 Chemical structure of the two most common synthetic conjugated linoleic acids: (a) 18:2 cis-9,trans-11 linoleic acid and (b) 18:2 trans-10,cis-12 linoleic acid.

and obese humans. There have been extensive studies on the effects of CLA on body composition, specifically on the loss of body fat mass and a possible increase in lean body mass. Unfortunately, these effects have been shown primarily in animals studies with less consistency in results from human studies (see reviews: Kennedy *et al.*, 2010; Li *et al.*, 2008; Whigham *et al.*, 2004). A study by our group (Venkatramanan, 2010) found that consumption of CLA-enriched milk had no effect on lipid profile, body weight or body composition. The study was conducted in moderately overweight, hyperlipidemic individuals (n = 15), using a crossover design. Treatments were control milk low in c9,t11 CLA, milk naturally enriched with c9,t11 CLA, and milk synthetically enriched with t10,c12 CLA and c9,t11 CLA. Each treatment phase was of eight weeks duration. However, some studies (Blankson *et al.*, 2000; Gaullier *et al.*, 2004, 2007; Riserus *et al.*, 2001; Watras *et al.*, 2007) reported that 0.7 to 6.8 g/d of CLA resulted in decreases in body fat.

Gaullier and colleagues (Gaullier *et al.*, 2004) conducted a one-year study of CLA supplementation. The study included 180 men and women with BMIs of 25 to 30 kg/m^2 who were randomly assigned to one of two forms of CLA (50:50 isomer ratio) or placebo (olive oil). There were no restrictions in lifestyle or caloric intake. The primary outcome was a reduction in body fat mass; at 12 months, body fat mass was significantly lower in the CLA-supplemented subjects than in those supplemented with placebo. Secondary outcomes included effects on lean body mass; lean body mass increased slightly with CLA relative to placebo. Adverse events were equally distributed between groups; abdominal discomfort, loose stools, and dyspepsia were most commonly reported. No difference was seen in serum lipid concentrations at 12 months. Conversely, other studies reported no effects of CLA supplementation on body weight (Eyjolfson *et al.*, 2004; Kreider *et al.*, 2002; Lambert *et al.*, 2007; Malpuech-Brugere *et al.*, 2004; Petridou *et al.*, 2003; Riserus *et al.*, 2002, 2004b; Taylor *et al.*, 2006).

Some studies have examined the effect of CLA on weight and fat regain or maintenance after weight loss on an energy-restricted diet. These studies found no effect on those parameters using CLA (Kamphuis *et al.*, 2003a, 2003b; Larsen *et al.*, 2006; Whigham *et al.*, 2004). Conversely, other research has indicated that CLA supplementation increases insulin resistance and serum glucose levels in patients with abdominal obesity without significant decreases in body fat or weight (Riserus et al., 2002, 2004a). Others have also indicated that CLA supplementation can worsen endothelial function, possibly increasing risk for cardiovascular morbidity (Taylor et al., 2006); however, more studies are required to confirm this finding.

Most studies that investigated the effect of CLA in humans were conducted using commercially formulated oral supplements made from a mixture of synthetic CLA isomers (Desroches et al., 2005). These sources usually contain more of the cis-9, trans-11 isomer in a ratio of 30–70:1. For instance, milk fat CLA is synthesized endogenously via Δ-9 desaturase from trans-vassenic acid, an intermediate in the biohydrogenation of linoleic and linolenic acids in the rumen. CLA is also synthesized commercially for human and laboratory use. CLA isomers c9,t11 and t10,c12 are the most common types of synthetic CLA products, constituting 80–90% of the mixture (Li et al., 2008). These two isomers are believed to be the major effectors representing the various biological functions of CLA (Li et al., 2008). Naturally occurring CLA in foods are present only in small quantities, with animal products as the major sources. CLA are present only in milligram quantities in meats and dairy products (Combe and Morin, 2005). The average intake of CLA from naturally occurring CLA in food is estimated to be about 0.3 g/d (EFSA, 2004).

On 30 April 2010 the European Food Safety Authority approved the products *Tonalin TG 80*, a CLA-oil produced by Cognis, and *Clarinol* produced by Lipid Nutrition, as a food ingredients in the context of Regulation (EC) No. 258/97 (EFSA, 2010a, 2010b). Both products are manufactured from safflower oil via saponification and isomeration (conjugation) to yield two CLA isomers c9,t11:t10c,c12 in a 1:1 ratio (EFSA, 2010a, 2010b). *Tonalin TG 80* is comprised of approximately 80% of the two CLA isomers c9,t11:t10,c12 in a 1:1 ratio. *Tonalin TG 80* was registered for intended use as an ingredient in milk-, yogurt- or fruit-type products and other unspecified products, with a suggested daily intake of 4.5 g *Tonalin TG 80*, equivalent to 3.5 g CLA (EFSA, 2010a). Lipid Nutrition has submitted approval for their CLA product, *Clarinol*, which was reviewed for use in beverages, cereal products, dietary supplements, milk products and dry weight beverages, at a daily intake of 3.75 g *Clarinol*, equivalent to 3 g CLA (EFSA, 2010b).

In summary, clinical studies suggest that CLA may be beneficial for weight management; unfortunately, there were inconsistency in these results. The discrepancy is believed to be due to CLA doses and isomers. For instance, a recent review (Plourde et al., 2008) concluded that human studies with CLA that report significant changes in body weight and body fat used doses that was more than ten times above human habitual intake, i.e. 3.2 g/d vs. 0.1–0.3 g/d. Furthermore, as mentioned above, different CLA isomers exert various effects on weight management. Since most CLA supplements are chemically synthesized it would be beneficial to work on improving the purification of CLA isomer mixtures, with more clinical studies required to develop recommendations about the consumption of CLA for weight management.

Omega-3 fatty acids
Omega-3 fatty acids found in fish oil have been shown to decrease TG levels (Harris, 1997), and have been studied in overweight and obese individuals as part of a weight loss strategy (Kratz *et al.*, 2008; Parra *et al.*, 2008). Human and animal studies suggest that omega-3 fatty acids may contribute to improvements in body composition by suppressing appetite, by influencing hormones such as adiponectin and leptin, and by promoting adipocytes apoptisis (Parra *et al.*, 2008; Winnicki *et al.*, 2002). Two specific omega-3 long-chain unsaturated fatty acids that are studied are docosahexaenoic acid (DHA; 22:6 n-3) and eicosapentaenoic acid (EPA; 20:5 n-3) (Fig. 10.3). In humans, both DHA and EPA can be produced endogenously using the essential fatty acid alpha-linolenic acid, derived from sources such as flaxseed and hemp oils, however, this capacity is impaired. Thus, fish represents the most natural abundant source of DHA and EPA; comprising 15–30% of the lipid content of high fat (10–15%), cold-water fish such as salmon, sardines, mackerel, herring, trout and pilchards (Li *et al.*, 2008).

Relatively few studies in humans have examined effects of omega-3 supplementation alone, primarily related to obesity; most studies have focused mainly on cardiovascular health. Couet and colleagues (Couet *et al.*, 1997) conducted a single-blind fish oil supplement trial. Six healthy adults consumed a control diet for three weeks, and after a 10- to 12-week washout, consumed the same diet for three weeks with 6 g/d of visible fat replaced with DHA-rich fish oil. Resting fat oxidation increased (1.06 ± 0.17 vs. 0.87 ± 0.13 mg/kg/min; $p < 0.05$), and body fat was reduced (-0.88 ± 0.16 vs. -0.3 ± 0.34 kg; $p < 0.05$) on the fish oil diet compared with control. However, a major limitation of this study was that all volunteers consumed the control diet followed by the fish oil diet, which may have introduced an order effect and potentially confounded the outcome (Buckley and Howe, 2009). Kabir and colleagues (Kabir *et al.*, 2007) studied the effects of omega-3 intake on body composition in overweight and obese female postmenopausal participants with type 2 diabetes. Participants consumed 3 g/d of EPA-rich fish oil or 3 g/d of paraffin oil for two months. No reduction was observed in body weight nor in subcutaneous or visceral fat between groups. However, a reduction in total body fat mass was observed, primarily as a result of loss of trunk

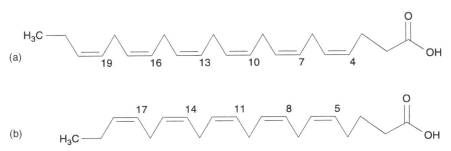

Fig. 10.3   Chemical structure of (a) docosahexaenoic acid (DHA; 22:6 n-3) and (b) eicosapentaenoic acid (EPA; 20:5 n-3).

fat. Furthermore, this reduction was associated with a decrease in adipocyte diameter in subcutaneous periumbilical fat. Mori and colleagues (Mori *et al.*, 1999) randomized 69 overweight (BMI > 25 kg/m^2), hypertensive patients to one to four 16-week treatment arms: control group, daily fish meal, energy-restricted diet, energy-restricted diet plus daily fish. The daily fish meal provided approximately 3.7 g of omega-3 fatty acids. Both energy-restricted diets resulted in an average weight loss of 5.6 kg (p < 0.0001); there were no significant changes in the other two groups. TG concentrations decreased by 29% in the fish group, 26% in the energy-restricted groups, and 38% in the energy-restricted plus fish group (p < 0.001). A study by Hill and colleagues (Hill *et al.*, 2007a) examined the effects of omega-3 fatty acids with exercise on body composition and cardiovascular disease risk factors. The study included 75 adults with BMI > 25 kg/m^2. Study volunteers were randomized to one of four groups: fish oil (6 g), fish oil + regular physical activity, placebo oil, or placebo oil + regular physical activity. Fish oil capsules provided 260 mg DHA and 60 mg EPA per 1 g capsule, and sunflower oil was the placebo oil. The exercise groups were required to run or walk three times per week for 45 minutes. 65 volunteers completed the 12-week study. Fish oil reduced TG and increased HDL concentrations significantly greater than did sunflower oil, 14% versus 5% and 10% versus 3%, respectively (p < 0.05). No differences were seen in blood pressure, heart rate and body weight or body composition in the fish oil groups.

Omega-3 incorporation into tissues such as erythrocyte membranes, has been shown to increase by 150% when provided at a dosage of 4/d of fish oil over a five-week period (Buckley *et al.*, 2009) and can remain elevated for up to 18 weeks (Brown *et al.*, 1991). This extended elevation in plasma omega-3 levels has major implications in terms of the design of fish oil supplementation clinical studies. Any metabolic effects resulting from tissue incorporation of omega-3 in participants who are fed fish oil during a dosage period of 35 days will be likely to persist during a second 35-day period when a control treatment is consumed, potentially confounding the ability to identify a difference between the omega-3 fish oil supplement and control treatment (Buckley and Howe, 2009).

In summary, few clinical studies have assessed the effects of omega-3 fatty acids on weight, and shown evidence that omega-3 may reduce body fat in human. Unfortunately, there are relatively few clinical studies assessing the effects of omega-3 for weight management, thus, more studies are required for more conclusive recommendation about omega-3 as a functional food for weight management.

10.2.2   Dietary fibre and weight loss, weight control

Dietary fibre is defined as the edible parts of plants or analogous carbohydrates that are resistant to digestion and absorption in the human small intestine, with complete or partial fermentation in the human large intestine (DeVries *et al.*, 2001). Dietary fibres are usually classified according to various physical–chemical and physiological criteria including solubility, viscosity, and fermentability (James *et al.*, 2003).

Soluble and insoluble fibres

Traditionally, the two main grouping for dietary fibres are soluble and insoluble fibre. Insoluble fibres are made up of substances which do not dissolve in water; this includes cellulose, hemicelluloses and lignin. Insoluble fibre components resist the action of intestinal microbes, thus this type of fibre can be classified as non-fermentable. Soluble fibres, such as inulin, pectins, mucilages and gums, are composed of water-soluble elements and highly viscous. Soluble fibres are readily fermented to short-chain fatty acids (SCFA) by intestinal microbes and are therefore known as fermentable fibre.

Soluble fibres are predominantly found in pulses, cereals and some fruits. Foods high in insoluble fibre include whole wheat breads, wheat cereals, wheat bran, rye, rice, barley, and vegetables such as cabbage, beets, carrots, brussels sprouts, turnips, cauliflower and apple skins (Shewmake and Huntington, 2009). Good sources of soluble fibre include oat bran, oatmeal, beans, peas, rice bran, barley, citrus fruits, apple pulp, psyllium, carrots, strawberries, peaches with skin, and apples with the skin (Shewmake and Huntington, 2009).

Dietary fibre is known to have numerous health benefits including the ability to aid in weight loss (Anderson *et al.*, 2009; Papathanasopoulos and Camilleri, 2010). Epidemiological, clinical and animal studies indicate that higher fibre intake is associated with less weight gain compared with lower fibre intake. Systematic reviews of cross-sectional and prospective studies by Anderson and colleagues suggest that high fibre consumption reduces the risk for gaining weight or developing obesity by approximately 30% (Anderson *et al.*, 2009). A summary of five randomized controlled trials (RCTs) assessing the effects of high-fibre diets indicated that there was approximately 1 kg greater weight loss with high fibre diets compared to control diets over an eight-week period (Anderson, 2008). The majority of evidence related to clinical markers such as serum lipoprotein changes, weight loss, improved glycemic control in diabetes, improved gastrointestinal function, and enhanced immune function has been documented with fibre supplements rather than with high fibre foods (Anderson *et al.*, 2009). A review of sixteen RCTs studies assessing the effects of fibre supplement on weight loss found

Table 10.2   Dietary fibre components for functional foods

Fibre component	Chemical names	Source
Hemicelluloses	Arabinoxylans, glucuronoarabinoxylans	Fruits and vegetables
Pectins	Methyl esterified rhamnoglacturonan	Apple, citrus peel
Guar gum	Galactomannans	
Fructo-oligosaccharides (FOS)	Galactooligosaccharides, mannan-oligosaccharides	Fruits and vegetables such as banana, onion, garlic, asparagus, barley, wheat, tomatoes, leeks
Resistant starches (RS1–4)	Amylose and amylopectin	Grain legumes, whole cereals, beans and lentils, banana, potato

significant reduction with fibre supplement groups at four and eight weeks compared to placebo/control groups (Anderson, 2008). In these fibre supplement studies the amount of fibre provided ranged from 4.5 to 20 g/d; average 7.5 g/d, representing predominantly insoluble fibre, but guar gum or glucomannan was also used in some studies (Anderson et al., 2009). Other meta-analyses of RCTs on fibre also reported only minor effects on weight loss for commonly used dietary fibre supplements (Papathanasopoulos and Camilleri, 2010). A more recent study by Maki and colleague (Maki et al., 2010) examined the effect of beta-glucan on weight loss. Free-living, overweight and obese adults ($n = 204$) consumed 3 g/d oat beta-glucan or a control for twelve weeks; weight loss was not different between the treatment group and control; however, waist circumference decreased more with oat beta-glucan, which was evident as early as week 4.

Resistant starches

Although widely used, the soluble/insoluble categorization of dietary fibre has been recognized to be misleading because some insoluble fibres are actually fermented in the large intestine and solubility in water does not always predict physiological effects (Buttriss and Stokes, 2008). Particularly, resistant starches and oligosaccharides are carbohydrate-derived components with physiological properties of dietary fibres, but neither fit completely into either soluble or insoluble fibre category (Buttriss and Stokes, 2008). Indeed, resistant starch (RS) is considered the third category of dietary fibre as it has dual benefits of insoluble and soluble fibre. Resistant starches are so named because of the inability of human a-amylase to digest these starches (Sajilata et al., 2006) (see Table 10.3).

Resistant starches have received lots of recent attention for their potential weight management benefits. Some studies have shown that RS have the ability to influence satiety, thus they could potentially be used to manage obesity. 20 healthy individuals who ate a muffin with about 9 g (8.0–9.6 g) of RS reported greater satiety, using a visual analogue scale questionnaire, over 180 min post consumption, compared to the same group who consumed a non-RS muffin (Willis

Table 10.3 Dietary fibre components: categories of resistance starch

Resistant starch type	Description	Examples
RS1	Physically inaccessible in cell or tissues structure because surrounded by plant cell wall material	Unprocessed whole grain (e.g. brown rice), legumes
RS2	Occurs in its natural granular form, i.e. high amylase; long chains, little branching	Raw potato, green banana, high amylase corn starch
RS3	Forms when starch containing foods are cooked and cooled, i.e. retrograded amylase; long chain double helices	Sushi rice, potato salad, bread, cornflakes
RS4	Chemically modified (e.g. heat processing rearrangement of bonding)	Modified maltodextrins

et al., 2009). 15 healthy individuals who consumed an evening meal containing 50 g of available carbohydrate with 30 g as RS from barley-kernel based bread reported increased satiety score after breakfast, as measured by questionnaire, compared with an evening meal of 50 g available carbohydrate with only 1.3 g RS (Nilsson *et al.*, 2008). Additionally, RS can influence body fat. 30 overweight individuals consuming a *Phaseolus vulgaris* (kidney bean) extract that inhibited a-amylase, exhibited greater reduction in BMI, fat mass, adipose thickness, and waist/hip/thigh circumferences while maintaining lean body mass compared with 30 individuals consuming a placebo for 30 d (Celleno *et al.*, 2007).

Various chemically modified resistant starches such as resistant maltodextrins, are currently used as food ingredients. Foods such as legumes have a high percentage of RS (~3.5%) (Englyst *et al.*, 2007), thus representing an effective strategy for increasing dietary RS.

Physiological mechanisms of action of fibres
Dietary fibre may influence body weight regulation through physiologic mechanisms involving intrinsic, hormonal and colonic effects (Pereira and Ludwig, 2001; Papathanasopoulos and Camilleri, 2010). Intrinsic effects refer to high fibre foods' ability to decrease food intake by promoting satiation, i.e. lower meal energy content (Pereira and Ludwig, 2001; Rolls, 2009). Dietary fibre may promote satiety through several hormonal pathways such as the effect on insulin secretion and blood glucose levels and secretion of gut hormones including CCK and glucagon-like-peptide-1. Fibre, especially viscous soluble fibre, may increase intraluminal viscosity, slow gastric emptying, and provide a mechanical barrier to enzymatic digestion of starch in the small intestine. Consequently, postprandial blood glucose concentration tend to be lower on high-fibre meals, resulting in reduced insulin secretion and avoidance of postabsorptive reactive hypoglycemia (Pereira and Ludwig, 2001; Papathanasopoulos and Camilleri, 2010). Cholecystokinin (CCK) is secreted from cells in the proximal small intestine and is involved in regulation of gastric emptying and central inducement of satiety. The biologic actions of fibre in the large intestine may have implications for body weight regulation. The production of SCFAs in the large intestine enters portal circulation and may affect glucose homeostasis. Short-chain fatty acids seem to decrease hepatic output of glucose and circulating concentrations of free fatty acids and stimulate secretion of glucagon-like peptide-1. These actions alter insulin sensitivity, insulin secretion patterns, partitioning of metabolic fuels and regulation of satiety (Pereira and Ludwig, 2001; Rolls, 2009).

In summary, clinical studies have shown that dietary fibre types such as RS and beta-glucan have anti-obesogenic properties. Some of these studies suggest that long-term (as in months to years) interventions are required to effectively contribute to beneficial health impact.

10.2.3   Polyphenols and weight loss, weight control
Polyphenols exist as a group of chemicals found in many fruits, vegetables and other plants such as nuts and tea leaves such as green tea. Green tea is a rich

source of polyphenols, particularly catechins. Only recently is green tea gaining an interest in Western countries, although people in Asia have been aware of the health effects of green tea for hundreds of years, and is one of the most widely consumed beverages in Asian countries (Shixian *et al.*, 2006). Green tea is made by rapid stream processing of fresh leaves of *Camellia sinensis*. Black tea is made from the same plant as green tea but during processing the leaves endure an extra enzymatic oxidation step (Shixian *et al.*, 2006).

Catechins belong to the group of compounds generally classified as flavonoids. A growing body of research shows that green tea catechins may reduce BMI and body weight (Phung *et al.*, 2010; Wolfram *et al.*, 2006). The catechins in green tea include epicatechin (EC), epicatechin gallate (ECG), epigallocatechin (EGC), epigallocatechin gallate (EGCG), gallocatechin (GC), catechin gallate (CG), gallocatechin gallate (GCG), and catechin (C). EGCG is believed to be the most pharmacologically active catechin and constitutes >50% of the total catechin content in most green tea products (Yang and Landau, 2000). Potential mechanisms by which green tea catechins exert anthropometric effects involve inhibition of adipocyte differentiation and proliferation, reduced fat absorption, inhibition of catechol-o-methyl-transferase, increased energy expenditure, and increased utilization of fat.

Hursel and colleagues (Hursel *et al.*, 2009) conducted a meta-analysis to evaluate the effects of green tea (GT) on body weight regulation. Final analyses included 11 randomized, blinded, placebo-controlled clinical trials (Auvichayapat *et al.*, 2008; Diepvens *et al.*, 2005; Hsu *et al.*, 2008; Kovacs *et al.*, 2004; Nagao *et al.*, 2007; Wang *et al.*, 2009; Westerterp-Plantenga *et al.*, 2005) ($n = 616$ GT and $n = 610$ placebo) which assessed weight loss or maintenance after GT supplementation, with or without regular caffeine intake, consumed for 12 or 13 weeks. Green tea treatment dosages range from 440 to 1207 mg/d. These studies, published between 2001 to 2008, included either Asian or Caucasian populations, with BMI ranges of 18.5 to 35 kg/m^2. Results indicated that catechins from green tea significantly decrease body weight and significantly maintained body weight after a period of weight loss (û = −1.31 kg, 95% CI: −2.05 to −0.57; $p < 0.001$). Hursel and colleagues (Hursel *et al.*, 2009) concluded that green tea catechins or an EGCG-caffeine mixture have a small positive effect on weight loss and weight maintenance. Habitual caffeine intake and ethnicity may be moderators, as they may influence the effect of catechins.

Phung and colleagues (Phung *et al.*, 2010) also conducted a meta-analysis to assess the effects of green tea catechins with and without caffeine on anthropometric measures including BMI, body weight, waist circumference and waist-to-hip ratio. Final analysis included 15 randomized placebo-controlled, clinical trials (Auvichayapat *et al.*, 2008; Chan *et al.*, 2006; Diepvens *et al.*, 2006; Frank *et al.*, 2009; Fukino *et al.*, 2005; Hill *et al.*, 2007b; Hsu *et al.*, 2008; Maki *et al.*, 2009; Maron *et al.*, 2003; Matsuyama *et al.*, 2008; Nagao *et al.*, 2005, 2007, 2009) ($n = 1243$) which assessed health effects of GTCs with or without caffeine which were consumed from three to 24 weeks (median: 12 weeks). Treatment groups received GTCs dose range of 141 to 1207 mg/d. These studies, published between

2002 to 2009, included participants with BMI range of 24 to 32.2 kg/m². Results indicated that GTCs significantly reduced BMI, body weight and waist circumference. GTCs with caffeine decreased BMI (-0.55 kg/m², 95% CI: -0.65 to -0.40), body weight (-1.38 kg, 95% CI: -1.70 to -1.06), and waist circumference (-1.93 cm, 95% CI: -2.82 to -1.04) compared with caffeine alone. GTCs with caffeine also significantly decreased body weight (-0.44 kg, 95% CI: -0.72 to -0.15) when compared with a caffeine-free control. Phung and colleagues (Phung *et al.*, 2010) concluded that GTCs with caffeine may positively affect BMI, body weight and waist circumference. However, the magnitude of the effect is small and not likely clinically relevant.

In summary, most of the clinical studies have shown that GTCs have a positive effect on weight loss and weight maintenance.

10.3   Formulating food products for weight control

The studies reviewed in this chapter show that some food components have the potential to manage body weight. Dietary factors, particular fat and energy intake are strongly and positively associated with body weight gain. However, the link between fat intake and overweight is not limited to high energy content. Functional foods that affect energy metabolism and fat portioning may be helpful adjuncts to a dietary approach to body weight control.

Some of the challenges associated with formulating food product with functional lipid components may be relate to the structural stability of the molecules due to the application of temperature and other factors. For instance, general uses for MCT have been limited due to low smoking point. Another issue is the production of the correct isomers for effective metabolic functions, for instance CLA. Challenges also exist with matrixing omega-3 fatty acids into foods, for instance there are issues related to taste and stability if fish oils are used to fortify foods. Some food scientists have opted to use vegetarian sources such as algae as a solution to fish source for omega-3. Omega-3 from algae grown outside the ocean do not have the same sensory, stability and formulation issues that are associated with omega-3 from fish and flax oils.

Not all dietary fibres are created equally. It has been concluded that gel-forming fibres such as guar gum and pectin are more effective in promoting weight loss than non-gel forming fibres such as wheat bran (Krotkiewski and Smith, 1985). The addition of gel-forming fibres to a normal diet leads to increased satiation probably due to slow gastric emptying. A long-term study by Smith (1989) suggested the usefulness of viscous fibres as an adjunct to regular dietary treatment of obesity. Resistant starches have been shown to be anti-obesogenic, thus, one of the future directions in this area would be to design new foods that incorporate significant RS content, while maintaining palatability and minimize any negative side-effects. Overall, more research is needed to expand the use of formulating functional components for widespread use in various food products.

10.4   Future trends

Currently, the weight loss market is undergoing changes as consumer focus shifts from dieting and weight loss programmes to portion control, specific food restrictions and incorporation of functional foods with increased satiating, and other weight management properties (Maletto, 2009). Many weight loss brands focus on the stimulant route to speed up metabolism; however, some are branching out into functional fats such as CLA, MCT and DAG. Overall, satiety seems to lead the area in the formulation of weight loss/ maintenance products. Satiety is new strategy for weight loss. Global sales of satiety foods reached US $7.5 billion in 2005 (Sloan, 2008). Dannon's *Light & Fit Curve Control* yogurt and *LightFull's Satiety Smoothies* are based on protein/fibre blends. Slim-Fast launched *Slim-Fast Hunger Shot* daily dose drink in the UK (Sloan, 2008). PepsiCo's new *Aquafina Alive Satisfy* has 10 calories and 10% daily value of fibre to 'help lightly fill you up' (Sloan, 2008). General Mills has been quite successful with *Fiber One* cereal and bars, and Mott's has introduced fibre-fortified applesauce cups (Anonymous, 2010). Foods that stimulate metabolism are also a growing area. Coca-Coca/Nestle's *Enviga* green tea drink reported a US $24 million sales in 2007 and *Steaz Sparkling Green Tea* now comes in a diet version (Sloan, 2008).

In 2010 despite the recession, in the United States, functional products still outpaced the overall food industry growth rate of 1.6%. Sales of functional foods and beverages reached $37.4 billion in 2009, up 2.7% from the previous year (Anonymous, 2010). Beverages remain the largest functional products segment, at $21.6 billion, up 3% from the previous year. The $6.7 billion functional breads/grain category also grew by 3%; the $2.7 billion snack food and $1.8 billion dairy segments were both up 2% (Sloan, 2010). In the US, 36% of consumers said they consumed a functional food in 2009 for weight loss. Satiety remains the primary strategy for weight loss, with 53% of adult wanting weight control food products focused on satiety. Indeed, fibre remains in the top five ingredients consumers in the US sought in 2009; the list also includes omega-3 fatty acids (Sloan, 2010), but this may be related more to heart health rather than weight management.

Makers of functional beverages are now providing products with multiple benefits in a single product. For example, sports drinks with weight loss (Sloan, 2010). There remains considerable capacity for growth in the weight management functional food market. Nearly two-thirds (64%) of adults want more functional foods that help them to maintain/lose weight (Sloan, 2010). Indeed, there is also lots of room for introduction of functional foods related to lipid components. Research results to date indicate the potential for future popularity in the market place for CLA and omega-3 products for weight management. For instance, EFSA's recent approval of the CLA products, *Tonalin TG 80*, by Cognis, and *Clarinol* by Lipid Nutrition, as a food ingredients (EFSA, 2010a, 2010b) will likely pave the way for approval by other countries such as US FDA and Asian countries. *Tonalin TG 80* was registered for use as an ingredient in milk-, yogurt- or fruit-type products and other unspecified products (EFSA, 2010a), and *Clarinol*, for use in beverages, cereal products, dietary supplements, milk products and dry weight beverages

(EFSA, 2010b); thus, these food products containing CLA will likely be introduced in European markets by the end of year. To conclude, functional food and obesity is a vibrant growing area, with many bioactive components being explored for utilization in the fight against overweight and obesity.

10.5   Sources of further information and advice

Agriculture and Agri-Food Canada – http://www4.agr.gc.ca/AAFC-AAC/

Asian Food Information Centre (AFIC) – http://www.afic.org/. See also Global view of functional foods: Asian perspective (Arai, 2002)

European Food Safety Authority (EFSA) – http://www.efsa.europa.eu/

International Food Information Council Foundation (IFIC) – http://www.foodinsight.org/

US Food and Drug Administration (FDA) Generally Recognized as Safe (GRAS) – http://www.fda.gov/Food/FoodIngredientsPackaging/GenerallyRecognizedasSafeGRAS/default.htm

Consumer acceptance of functional foods (Grunert, 2010; Labrecque *et al.*, 2006; Peng *et al.*, 2006; Verbeke, 2006).

Top 10 functional food trends in the United States; see 2008 and 2010 features (Sloan, 2008, 2010).

10.6   References

Anderson, J. W. (2008) Dietary fiber and associated phytochemicals in prevention and reversal of diabetes. In Pasupuleti, V. K. A. (ed.) *Nutraceuticals, Glycemic Health and Type 2 Diabetes* Iowa, Blackwell Publishing Professional.

Anderson, J. W., Baird, P., Davis, R. H., Jr., Ferreri, S., Knudtson, M., *et al.* (2009) Health benefits of dietary fiber. *Nutr Rev*, **67**, 188–205.

Anonymous (2002) Medium chain triglycerides. Monograph. *Altern Med Rev*, **7**, 418–20.

Anonymous (2010) U.S. functional sales slow, but category outpaces overall food sector in '09. *Nutrition Business Journal*, 1 February, http://nutritionbusinessjournal.com.

Aoyama, T., Nosaka, N. and Kasai, M. (2007) Research on the nutritional characteristics of medium-chain fatty acids. *J Med Invest*, **54**, 385–8.

Arai, S. (2002) Global view on functional foods: Asian perspectives. *British Journal of Nutrition*, **88**, S139–S143.

Aronne, L. J., Nelinson, D. S. and Lillo, J. L. (2009) Obesity as a disease state: a new paradigm for diagnosis and treatment. *Clin Cornerstone*, **9**, 9–25; discussion 26–9.

Auvichayapat, P., Prapochanung, M., Tunkamnerdthai, O., Sripanidkulchai, B. O., Auvichayapat, N., *et al.* (2008) Effectiveness of green tea on weight reduction in obese Thais: A randomized, controlled trial. *Physiol Behav*, **93**, 486–91.

BfR (2009) Intial evaluation of the assessment of levels of glycidol fatty acid esters detected in refined vegetable fats. *BfR Opinion No. 007/2009.* http://www.bfr.bund.de/cm/245/initial_evaluation_of_the_assessment_of_levels_of_glycidol_fatty_acid_esters.pdf

Binnert, C., Pachiaudi, C., Beylot, M., Hans, D., Vandermander, J., *et al.* (1998) Influence of human obesity on the metabolic fate of dietary long- and medium-chain triacylglycerols. *Am J Clin Nutr*, **67**, 595–601.

Blankson, H., Stakkestad, J. A., Fagertun, H., Thom, E., Wadstein, J. and Gudmundsen, O. (2000) Conjugated linoleic acid reduces body fat mass in overweight and obese humans. *J Nutr*, **130**, 2943–8.

Brown, A. J., Pang, E. and Roberts, D. C. (1991) Persistent changes in the fatty acid composition of erythrocyte membranes after moderate intake of n-3 polyunsaturated fatty acids: study design implications. *Am J Clin Nutr*, **54**, 668–73.

Buckley, J. D., Burgess, S., Murphy, K. J. and Howe, P. R. (2009) DHA-rich fish oil lowers heart rate during submaximal exercise in elite Australian Rules footballers. *J Sci Med Sport*, **12**, 503–7.

Buckley, J. D. and Howe, P. R. (2009) Anti-obesity effects of long-chain omega-3 polyunsaturated fatty acids. *Obes Rev*, **10**, 648–59.

Buttriss, J. L. and Stokes, C. S. (2008) Dietary fibre and health: An overview. *Nutrition Bulletin*, **33**, 186–200.

Calabrese, C., Myer, S., Munson, S., Turet, P. and Birdsall, T. C. (1999) A cross-over study of the effect of a single oral feeding of medium chain triglyceride oil vs. canola oil on post-ingestion plasma triglyceride levels in healthy men. *Altern Med Rev*, **4**, 23–8.

Cater, N. B., Heller, H. J. and Denke, M. A. (1997) Comparison of the effects of medium-chain triacylglycerols, palm oil, and high oleic acid sunflower oil on plasma triacylglycerol fatty acids and lipid and lipoprotein concentrations in humans. *Am J Clin Nutr*, **65**, 41–5.

Celleno, L., Tolaini, M. V., D'amore, A., Perricone, N. V. and Preuss, H. G. (2007) A Dietary supplement containing standardized Phaseolus vulgaris extract influences body composition of overweight men and women. *Int J Med Sci*, **4**, 45–52.

Chan, C. C., Koo, M. W., Ng, E. H., Tang, O. S., Yeung, W. S. and Ho, P. C. (2006) Effects of Chinese green tea on weight, and hormonal and biochemical profiles in obese patients with polycystic ovary syndrome—a randomized placebo-controlled trial. *J Soc Gynecol Investig*, **13**, 63–8.

Combe, N. and Morin, O. (2005) Conjugated linoleic acid: Dietary intake and sources. *Sources alimentaires et consommation estime#t2e de CLA*, **12**, 22–25.

Couet, C., Delarue, J., Ritz, P., Antoine, J. M. and Lamisse, F. (1997) Effect of dietary fish oil on body fat mass and basal fat oxidation in healthy adults. *Int J Obes Relat Metab Disord*, **21**, 637–43.

Desroches, S., Chouinard, P. Y., Galibois, I., Corneau, L., Delisle, J., *et al.* (2005) Lack of effect of dietary conjugated linoleic acids naturally incorporated into butter on the lipid profile and body composition of overweight and obese men. *Am J Clin Nutr*, **82**, 309–19.

DeVries, J. W., Camire, M. E., Cho, S., Craig, S., Gordon, D., *et al.* (2001) The definition of dietary fiber. *Cereal Foods World*, **46**, 112–29.

Diepvens, K., Kovacs, E. M., Nijs, I. M., Vogels, N. and Westerterp-Plantenga, M. S. (2005) Effect of green tea on resting energy expenditure and substrate oxidation during weight loss in overweight females. *Br J Nutr*, **94**, 1026–34.

Diepvens, K., Kovacs, E. M., Vogels, N. and Westerterp-Plantenga, M. S. (2006) Metabolic effects of green tea and of phases of weight loss. *Physiol Behav*, **87**, 185–91.

Donahoo, W., Wyatt, H. R., Kriehn, J., Stuht, J., Dong, F., *et al.* (2008) Dietary fat increases energy intake across the range of typical consumption in the United States. *Obesity (Silver Spring)*, **16**, 64–9.

Dubnov-Raz, G. and Berry, E. M. (2008) The dietary treatment of obesity. *Endocrinol Metab Clin North Am*, **37**, 873–86.

Dulloo, A. G., Fathi, M., Mensi, N. and Girardier, L. (1996) Twenty-four-hour energy expenditure and urinary catecholamines of humans consuming low-to-moderate amounts of medium-chain triglycerides: a dose-response study in a human respiratory chamber. *Eur J Clin Nutr*, **50**, 152–8.

EFSA (2004) Opinion of the Scientific Panel on Dieteric Products, Nutrition and Allergies on a request from the Commission related to the presence of trans fatty acids in foods and the effect on human health of the consumption of trans fatty acids (EFSA-Q-2003–022). *European Food Safety Authority*, 8 July.

EFSA (2010a) EFSA Panel on Dietetic Products, Nutrition and Allergies (NDA) Scientific Opinion on the safety of 'conjugated linoleic acid (CLA)-rich oil' (Cognis) as a Novel Food ingredient. *European Food Safety Authority*, **8**(5): 1600, 43 pp.

EFSA (2010b) EFSA Panel on Dietetic Products, Nutrition and Allergies (NDA) Scientific Opinion on the safety of 'conjugated linoleic acid (CLA)-rich oil' (Lipid Nutrition) as a Novel Food ingredient. *European Food Safety Authority*, **8**(5): 1601, 41 pp.

Englyst, K. N., Liu, S. and Englyst, H. N. (2007) Nutritional characterization and measurement of dietary carbohydrates. *Eur J Clin Nutr*, **61** (Suppl 1), S19–39.

Eyjolfson, V., Spriet, L. L. and Dyck, D. J. (2004) Conjugated linoleic acid improves insulin sensitivity in young, sedentary humans. *Med Sci Sports Exerc*, **36**, 814–20.

FDA (2000) US Food and Drug Administration, GRAS Notification #115. http://www.cfsan.fda.gov/≈rdb/opa-gn02.html

Ferrari, C. K. (2007) Functional foods and physical activities in health promotion of aging people. *Maturitas*, **58**, 327–39.

Flickinger, B. D. and Matsuo, N. (2003) Nutritional characteristics of DAG oil. *Lipids*, **38**, 129–32.

Fontaine, K. R., Redden, D. T., Wang, C., Westfall, A. O. and Allison, D. B. (2003) Years of life lost due to obesity. *JAMA*, **289**, 187–93.

Frank, J., George, T. W., Lodge, J. K., Rodriguez-Mateos, A. M., Spencer, J. P., *et al.* (2009) Daily consumption of an aqueous green tea extract supplement does not impair liver function or alter cardiovascular disease risk biomarkers in healthy men. *J Nutr*, **139**, 58–62.

Fukino, Y., Shimbo, M., Aoki, N., Okubo, T. and Iso, H. (2005) Randomized controlled trial for an effect of green tea consumption on insulin resistance and inflammation markers. *J Nutr Sci Vitaminol (Tokyo)*, **51**, 335–42.

Gaullier, J. M., Halse, J., Hoivik, H. O., Hoye, K., Syvertsen, C., *et al.* (2007) Six months supplementation with conjugated linoleic acid induces regional-specific fat mass decreases in overweight and obese. *Br J Nutr*, **97**, 550–60.

Gaullier, J. M., Halse, J., Hoye, K., Kristiansen, K., Fagertun, H., *et al.* (2004) Conjugated linoleic acid supplementation for 1 y reduces body fat mass in healthy overweight humans. *Am J Clin Nutr*, **79**, 1118–25.

Grunert, K. G. (2010) European consumers' acceptance of functional foods. *Annals of the New York Academy of Sciences*, **1190**, 166–173.

Harris, W. S. (1997) n-3 fatty acids and serum lipoproteins: human studies. *Am J Clin Nutr*, **65**, 1645S–1654S.

Hill, A. M., Buckley, J. D., Murphy, K. J. and Howe, P. R. (2007a) Combining fish-oil supplements with regular aerobic exercise improves body composition and cardiovascular disease risk factors. *Am J Clin Nutr*, **85**, 1267–74.

Hill, A. M., Coates, A. M., Buckley, J. D., Ross, R., Thielecke, F. and Howe, P. R. (2007b) Can EGCG reduce abdominal fat in obese subjects? *J Am Coll Nutr*, **26**, S396–402.

Hsu, C. H., Tsai, T. H., Kao, Y. H., Hwang, K. C., Tseng, T. Y. and Chou, P. (2008) Effect of green tea extract on obese women: a randomized, double-blind, placebo-controlled clinical trial. *Clin Nutr*, **27**, 363–70.

Hursel, R., Viechtbauer, W. and Westerterp-Plantenga, M. S. (2009) The effects of green tea on weight loss and weight maintenance: a meta-analysis. *Int J Obes (Lond)*, **33**, 956–61.

IFIC (2009) International Food Information Council Foundation: Background on functional foods, http://www.foodinsight.org/Content/6/FINAL-IFIC-Fndtn-Functional-Foods-Backgrounder-with-Tips-and-changes-03-11-09.pdf.

James, S. L., Muir, J. G., Curtis, S. L. and Gibson, P. R. (2003) Dietary fibre: a roughage guide. *Intern Med J*, **33**, 291–6.

JMHLW (1998) Japanese Ministry of Health, Labour and Welfare, Current FOSHU List. http://www.mhlw.go.jp/topics/0102/tp0221-2.html

Kabir, M., Skurnik, G., Naour, N., Pechtner, V., Meugnier, E., *et al.* (2007) Treatment for 2 mo with n 3 polyunsaturated fatty acids reduces adiposity and some atherogenic factors but does not improve insulin sensitivity in women with type 2 diabetes: a randomized controlled study. *Am J Clin Nutr*, **86**, 1670–9.

Kamphuis, M. M., Lejeune, M. P., Saris, W. H. and Westerterp-Plantenga, M. S. (2003a) Effect of conjugated linoleic acid supplementation after weight loss on appetite and food intake in overweight subjects. *Eur J Clin Nutr*, **57**, 1268–74.

Kamphuis, M. M., Lejeune, M. P., Saris, W. H. and Westerterp-Plantenga, M. S. (2003b) The effect of conjugated linoleic acid supplementation after weight loss on body weight regain, body composition, and resting metabolic rate in overweight subjects. *Int J Obes Relat Metab Disord*, **27**, 840–7.

Kamphuis, M. M., Mela, D. J. and Westerterp-Plantenga, M. S. (2003c) Diacylglycerols affect substrate oxidation and appetite in humans. *Am J Clin Nutr*, **77**, 1133–9.

Kao (2009) Kao to Temporarily Refrain from Selling Econa Products. http://www.kao.com/jp/en/corp_news/2009/20090916_002.html

Kasai, M., Nosaka, N., Maki, H., Negishi, S., Aoyama, T., *et al.* (2003) Effect of dietary medium- and long-chain triacylglycerols (MLCT) on accumulation of body fat in healthy humans. *Asia Pac J Clin Nutr*, **12**, 151–60.

Kasai, M., Nosaka, N., Maki, H., Suzuki, Y., Takeuchi, H., (2002) Comparison of diet-induced thermogenesis of foods containing medium- versus long-chain triacylglycerols. *J Nutr Sci Vitaminol (Tokyo)*, **48**, 536–40.

Kennedy, A., Martinez, K., Schmidt, S., Mandrup, S., Lapoint, K. and Mcintosh, M. (2010) Antiobesity mechanisms of action of conjugated linoleic acid. *Journal of Nutritional Biochemistry*, **21**, 171–9.

Knowler, W. C., Barrett-Connor, E., Fowler, S. E., Hamman, R. F., Lachin, J. M., *et al.* (2002) Reduction in the incidence of type 2 diabetes with lifestyle intervention or metformin. *N Engl J Med*, **346**, 393–403.

Kovacs, E. M., Lejeune, M. P., Nijs, I. and Westerterp-Plantenga, M. S. (2004) Effects of green tea on weight maintenance after body-weight loss. *Br J Nutr*, **91**, 431–7.

Kratz, M., Swarbrick, M. M., Callahan, H. S., Matthys, C. C., Havel, P. J. and Weigle, D. S. (2008) Effect of dietary n-3 polyunsaturated fatty acids on plasma total and high-molecular-weight adiponectin concentrations in overweight to moderately obese men and women. *American Journal of Clinical Nutrition*, **87**, 347–53.

Kreider, R. B., Ferreira, M. P., Greenwood, M., Wilson, M. and Almada, A. L. (2002) Effects of conjugated linoleic acid supplementation during resistance training on body composition, bone density, strength, and selected hematological markers. *J Strength Cond Res*, **16**, 325–34.

Krotkiewski, M. and Smith, U. (1985) Dietary fiber in obesity, in A. R. Leeds (ed.) Dietary Fibre Perspectives. London/Paris, Libbey.

Labrecque, J., Doyon, M., Bellavance, F. and Kolodinsky, J. (2006) Acceptance of functional foods: A comparison of French, American, and French Canadian consumers. *Canadian Journal of Agricultural Economics*, **54**, 647–61.

Lambert, E. V., Goedecke, J. H., Bluett, K., Heggie, K., Claassen, A., *et al.* (2007) Conjugated linoleic acid versus high-oleic acid sunflower oil: effects on energy metabolism, glucose tolerance, blood lipids, appetite and body composition in regularly exercising individuals. *Br J Nutr*, **97**, 1001–11.

Larsen, T. M., Toubro, S., Gudmundsen, O. and Astrup, A. (2006) Conjugated linoleic acid supplementation for 1 y does not prevent weight or body fat regain. *Am J Clin Nutr*, **83**, 606–12.

Li, J. J., Huang, C. J. and Xie, D. (2008) Anti-obesity effects of conjugated linoleic acid, docosahexaenoic acid, and eicosapentaenoic acid. *Mol Nutr Food Res*, **52**, 631–45.

Maki, K. C., Beiseigel, J. M., Jonnalagadda, S. S., Gugger, C. K., Reeves, M. S., *et al.* (2010) Whole-grain ready-to-eat oat cereal, as part of a dietary program for weight loss, reduces low-density lipoprotein cholesterol in adults with overweight and obesity more than a dietary program including low-fiber control foods. *Journal of the American Dietetic Association*, **110**, 205–14.

Maki, K. C., Davidson, M. H., Tsushima, R., Matsuo, N., Tokimitsu, I., *et al.* (2002) Consumption of diacylglycerol oil as part of a reduced-energy diet enhances loss of body weight and fat in comparison with consumption of a triacylglycerol control oil. *Am J Clin Nutr*, **76**, 1230–6.

Maki, K. C., Reeves, M. S., Farmer, M., Yasunaga, K., Matsuo, N., *et al.* (2009) Green tea catechin consumption enhances exercise-induced abdominal fat loss in overweight and obese adults. *J Nutr*, **139**, 264–70.

Maletto, P. (2009) Functional Food Formulation: Growing demand for functional foods is overriding concerns about the dismal economy. *Nutraceuticals World*, 1 May.

Malpuech-Brugere, C., Verboeket-van de Venne, W. P., Mensink, R. P., Arnal, M. A., Morio, B., *et al.* (2004) Effects of two conjugated linoleic acid isomers on body fat mass in overweight humans. *Obes Res*, **12**, 591–8.

Mann, C. C. (2005) Public health. Provocative study says obesity may reduce U.S. life expectancy. *Science*, **307**, 1716–17.

Maron, D. J., Lu, G. P., Cai, N. S., Wu, Z. G., Li, Y. H., *et al.* (2003) Cholesterol-lowering effect of a theaflavin-enriched green tea extract: a randomized controlled trial. *Arch Intern Med*, **163**, 1448–53.

Marten, B., Pfeuffer, M. and Schrezenmeir, J. (2006) Medium-chain triglycerides. *International Dairy Journal*, **16**, 1374–82.

Matsuo, T., Matsuo, M., Kasai, M. and Takeuchi, H. (2001) Effects of a liquid diet supplement containing structured medium- and long-chain triacylglycerols on bodyfat accumulation in healthy young subjects. *Asia Pac J Clin Nutr*, **10**, 46–50.

Matsuyama, T., Tanaka, Y., Kamimaki, I., Nagao, T. and Tokimitsu, I. (2008) Catechin safely improved higher levels of fatness, blood pressure, and cholesterol in children. *Obesity (Silver Spring)*, **16**, 1338–48.

Mori, T. A., Bao, D. Q., Burke, V., Puddey, I. B., Watts, G. F. and Beilin, L. J. (1999) Dietary fish as a major component of a weight-loss diet: effect on serum lipids, glucose, and insulin metabolism in overweight hypertensive subjects. *Am J Clin Nutr*, **70**, 817–25.

Morita, O. and Soni, M. G. (2009) Safety assessment of diacylglycerol oil as an edible oil: A review of the published literature. *Food and Chemical Toxicology*, **47**, 9–21.

Nagao, K. and Yanagita, T. (2009) Medium-chain fatty acids: functional lipids for the prevention and treatment of the metabolic syndrome. *Pharmacol Res*, **61**, 208–12.

Nagao, T., Hase, T. and Tokimitsu, I. (2007) A green tea extract high in catechins reduces body fat and cardiovascular risks in humans. *Obesity (Silver Spring)*, **15**, 1473–83.

Nagao, T., Komine, Y., Soga, S., Meguro, S., Hase, T., *et al.* (2005) Ingestion of a tea rich in catechins leads to a reduction in body fat and malondialdehyde-modified LDL in men. *Am J Clin Nutr*, **81**, 122–9.

Nagao, T., Meguro, S., Hase, T., Otsuka, K., Komikado, M., *et al.* (2009) A catechin-rich beverage improves obesity and blood glucose control in patients with type 2 diabetes. *Obesity (Silver Spring)*, **17**, 310–17.

Nagao, T., Watanabe, H., Goto, N., Onizawa, K., Taguchi, H., *et al.* (2000) Dietary diacylglycerol suppresses accumulation of body fat compared to triacylglycerol in men in a double-blind controlled trial. *J Nutr*, **130**, 792–7.

Nilsson, A. C., Ostman, E. M., Holst, J. J. and Bjorck, I. M. (2008) Including indigestible carbohydrates in the evening meal of healthy subjects improves glucose tolerance, lowers inflammatory markers, and increases satiety after a subsequent standardized breakfast. *J Nutr*, **138**, 732–9.

Ogawa, A., Nosaka, N., Kasai, M., Aoyama, T., Okazaki, M., *et al.* (2007) Dietary medium- and long-chain triacylglycerols accelerate diet-induced thermogenesis in humans. *J Oleo Sci*, **56**, 283–7.

Palou, A., Pico, C. and Bonet, M. L. (2004) Food safety and functional foods in the European Union: obesity as a paradigmatic example for novel food development. *Nutr Rev*, **62**, S169–81.

Papamandjaris, A. A., Macdougall, D. E. and Jones, P. J. (1998) Medium chain fatty acid metabolism and energy expenditure: obesity treatment implications. *Life Sci*, **62**, 1203–15.

Papamandjaris, A. A., White, M. D., Raeini-Sarjaz, M. and Jones, P. J. (2000) Endogenous fat oxidation during medium chain versus long chain triglyceride feeding in healthy women. *Int J Obes Relat Metab Disord*, **24**, 1158–66.

Papathanasopoulos, A. and Camilleri, M. (2010) Dietary fiber supplements: effects in obesity and metabolic syndrome and relationship to gastrointestinal functions. *Gastroenterology*, **138**, 65–72.

Paradis, A. M., Godin, G., Perusse, L. and Vohl, M. C. (2009) Associations between dietary patterns and obesity phenotypes. *Int J Obes (Lond)*, **33**, 1419–26.

Parra, D., Ramel, A., Bandarra, N., Kiely, M., Martãnez, J. A. and Thorsdottir, I. (2008) A diet rich in long chain omega-3 fatty acids modulates satiety in overweight and obese volunteers during weight loss. *Appetite*, **51**, 676–680.

Pasanisi, F., Contaldo, F., De Simone, G. and Mancini, M. (2001) Benefits of sustained moderate weight loss in obesity. *Nutrition, Metabolism and Cardiovascular Diseases*, **11**, 401–6.

Peeters, A., Barendregt, J. J., Willekens, F., Mackenbach, J. P., Al Mamun, A. and Bonneux, L. (2003) Obesity in adulthood and its consequences for life expectancy: a life-table analysis. *Ann Intern Med*, **138**, 24–32.

Peng, Y., West, G. E. and Wang, C. (2006) Consumer attitudes and acceptance of CLA-enriched dairy products. *Canadian Journal of Agricultural Economics*, **54**, 663–84.

Pereira, M. A. and Ludwig, D. S. (2001) Dietary fiber and body-weight regulation: Observations and mechanisms. *Pediatric Clinics of North America*, **48**, 969–80.

Petridou, A., Mougios, V. and Sagredos, A. (2003) Supplementation with CLA: isomer incorporation into serum lipids and effect on body fat of women. *Lipids*, **38**, 805–11.

Phung, O. J., Baker, W. L., Matthews, L. J., Lanosa, M., Thorne, A. and Coleman, C. I. (2010) Effect of green tea catechins with or without caffeine on anthropometric measures: a systematic review and meta-analysis. *Am J Clin Nutr*, **91**, 73–81.

Plourde, M., Jew, S., Cunnane, S. C. and Jones, P. J. (2008) Conjugated linoleic acids: why the discrepancy between animal and human studies? *Nutr Rev*, **66**, 415–21.

Reynolds, S. L., Saito, Y. and Crimmins, E. M. (2005) The impact of obesity on active life expectancy in older American men and women. *Gerontologist*, **45**, 438–44.

Riserus, U., Arner, P., Brismar, K. and Vessby, B. (2002) Treatment with dietary trans10cis12 conjugated linoleic acid causes isomer-specific insulin resistance in obese men with the metabolic syndrome. *Diabetes Care*, **25**, 1516–21.

Riserus, U., Berglund, L. and Vessby, B. (2001) Conjugated linoleic acid (CLA) reduced abdominal adipose tissue in obese middle-aged men with signs of the metabolic syndrome: a randomised controlled trial. *Int J Obes Relat Metab Disord*, **25**, 1129–35.

Riserus, U., Vessby, B., Arner, P. and Zethelius, B. (2004a) Supplementation with trans10cis12-conjugated linoleic acid induces hyperproinsulinaemia in obese men: close association with impaired insulin sensitivity. *Diabetologia*, **47**, 1016–19.

Riserus, U., Vessby, B., Arnlov, J. and Basu, S. (2004b) Effects of cis-9,trans-11 conjugated linoleic acid supplementation on insulin sensitivity, lipid peroxidation, and proinflammatory markers in obese men. *Am J Clin Nutr*, **80**, 279–83.

Rolls, B. J. (2009) The relationship between dietary energy density and energy intake. *Physiol Behav*, **97**, 609–15.

Rudkowska, I., Roynette, C. E., Demonty, I., Vanstone, C. A., Jew, S. and Jones, P. J. (2005) Diacylglycerol: efficacy and mechanism of action of an anti-obesity agent. *Obes Res*, **13**, 1864–76.

Sajilata, M. G., Singhal, R. S. and Kulkarni, P. R. (2006) Resistant starch – A review. *Comprehensive Reviews in Food Science and Food Safety*, **5**, 1–17.

Scalfi, L., Coltorti, A. and Contaldo, F. (1991) Postprandial thermogenesis in lean and obese subjects after meals supplemented with medium-chain and long-chain triglycerides. *Am J Clin Nutr*, **53**, 1130–3.

Seaton, T. B., Welle, S. L., Warenko, M. K. and Campbell, R. G. (1986) Thermic effect of medium-chain and long-chain triglycerides in man. *Am J Clin Nutr*, **44**, 630–4.

Shewmake, R. A. and Huntington, M. K. (2009) Nutritional treatment of obesity. *Primary Care – Clinics in Office Practice*, **36**, 357–77.

Shixian, Q., Vancrey, B., Shi, J., Kakuda, Y. and Jiang, Y. (2006) Green tea extract thermogenesis-induced weight loss by epigallocatechin gallate inhibition of catechol-O-methyltransferase. *J Med Food*, **9**, 451–8.

Sloan, A. E. (2008) The top 10 functional food trends. *Food Technology*, **62**, 24–44.

Sloan, A. E. (2010) The top 10 functional food trends. *Food Technology*, **64**, 22–41.

St-Onge, M. P., Bourque, C., Jones, P. J., Ross, R. and Parsons, W. E. (2003a) Medium- versus long-chain triglycerides for 27 days increases fat oxidation and energy expenditure without resulting in changes in body composition in overweight women. *Int J Obes Relat Metab Disord*, **27**, 95–102.

St-Onge, M. P. and Jones, P. J. (2002) Physiological effects of medium-chain triglycerides: potential agents in the prevention of obesity. *J Nutr*, **132**, 329–32.

St-Onge, M. P., Ross, R., Parsons, W. D. and Jones, P. J. (2003b) Medium-chain triglycerides increase energy expenditure and decrease adiposity in overweight men. *Obes Res*, **11**, 395–402.

Stewart, S. T., Cutler, D. M. and Rosen, A. B. (2009) Forecasting the effects of obesity and smoking on U.S. life expectancy. *N Engl J Med*, **361**, 2252–60.

Stubbs, R. J. and Harbron, C. G. (1996) Covert manipulation of the ratio of medium- to long-chain triglycerides in isoenergetically dense diets: effect on food intake in ad libitum feeding men. *Int J Obes Relat Metab Disord*, **20**, 435–44.

Swift, L. L., Hill, J. O., Peters, J. C. and Greene, H. L. (1992) Plasma lipids and lipoproteins during 6 d of maintenance feeding with long-chain, medium-chain, and mixed-chain triglycerides. *Am J Clin Nutr*, **56**, 881–6.

Takeuchi, H., Kasai, M., Taguchi, N., Tsuji, H. and Suzuki, M. (2002) Effect of triacylglycerols containing medium- and long-chain fatty acids on serum triacylglycerol levels and body fat in college athletes. *J Nutr Sci Vitaminol (Tokyo)*, **48**, 109–14.

Takeuchi, H., Sekine, S., Kojima, K. and Aoyama, T. (2008) The application of medium-chain fatty acids: edible oil with a suppressing effect on body fat accumulation. *Asia Pac J Clin Nutr*, **17** (Suppl 1), 320–3.

Taylor, J. S., Williams, S. R., Rhys, R., James, P. and Frenneaux, M. P. (2006) Conjugated linoleic acid impairs endothelial function. *Arterioscler Thromb Vasc Biol*, **26**, 307–12.

Van Wymelbeke, V., Himaya, A., Louis-Sylvestre, J. and Fantino, M. (1998) Influence of medium-chain and long-chain triacylglycerols on the control of food intake in men. *Am J Clin Nutr*, **68**, 226–34.

Van Wymelbeke, V., Louis-Sylvestre, J. and Fantino, M. (2001) Substrate oxidation and control of food intake in men after a fat-substitute meal compared with meals supplemented with an isoenergetic load of carbohydrate, long-chain triacylglycerols, or medium-chain triacylglycerols. *Am J Clin Nutr*, **74**, 620–30.

Venkatramanan, S., Joseph, S. V., Chouinard, P. Y., Jacques, H., Farnworth, E. R. and Jones, P. J. (2010) Milk enriched with conjugated linoleic acid fails to alter blood lipids or body composition in moderately overweight, borderline hyperlipidemic individuals. *J Am Coll Nutr*, **29**, 152–9.

Verbeke, W. (2006) Functional foods: Consumer willingness to compromise on taste for health? *Food Quality and Preference*, **17**, 126–31.

Wang, H., Wen, Y., Du, Y., Yan, X., Guo, H., *et al.* (2009) Effects of Catechin Enriched Green Tea on Body Composition. *Obesity (Silver Spring)*, **18**, 773–9.

Wansink, B. (2007) Helping consumers eat less. *Food Technology*, **61**, 34–8.

Watras, A. C., Buchholz, A. C., Close, R. N., Zhang, Z. and Schoeller, D. A. (2007) The role of conjugated linoleic acid in reducing body fat and preventing holiday weight gain. *Int J Obes (Lond)*, **31**, 481–7.

Weinsier, R. L., Hunter, G. R., Heini, A. F., Goran, M. I. and Sell, S. M. (1998) The etiology of obesity: relative contribution of metabolic factors, diet, and physical activity. *Am J Med*, **105**, 145–50.

Westerterp-Plantenga, M. S., Lejeune, M. P. and Kovacs, E. M. (2005) Body weight loss and weight maintenance in relation to habitual caffeine intake and green tea supplementation. *Obes Res*, **13**, 1195–204.

Whigham, L. D., O'shea, M., Mohede, I. C., Walaski, H. P. and Atkinson, R. L. (2004) Safety profile of conjugated linoleic acid in a 12-month trial in obese humans. *Food Chem Toxicol*, **42**, 1701–9.

WHO (2000) Obesity: preventing and managing the global epidemic. Report of a WHO consultation. *World Health Organ Tech Rep Ser*, **894**, i–xii, 1–253.

Wieringa, N. F., Van der windt, H. J., Zuiker, R. R., Dijkhuizen, L., Verkerk, M. A., *et al.* (2008) Positioning functional foods in an ecological approach to the prevention of overweight and obesity. *Obes Rev*, **9**, 464–73.

Willis, H. J., Eldridge, A. L., Beiseigel, J., Thomas, W. and Slavin, J. L. (2009) Greater satiety response with resistant starch and corn bran in human subjects. *Nutr Res*, **29**, 100–5.

Winnicki, M., Somers, V. K., Accurso, V., Phillips, B. G., Puato, M., *et al.* (2002) Fish-rich diet, leptin, and body mass. *Circulation*, **106**, 289–91.

Wolfram, S., Wang, Y. and Thielecke, F. (2006) Anti-obesity effects of green tea: from bedside to bench. *Mol Nutr Food Res*, **50**, 176–87.

Xu, T., Li, X., Zhang, Z., Ma, X. and Li, D. (2008) Effect of diacylglycerol on body weight: a meta-analysis. *Asia Pac J Clin Nutr*, **17**, 415–21.

Xue, C., Liu, Y., Wang, J., Zhang, R., Zhang, Y., *et al.* (2009a) Consumption of medium- and long-chain triacylglycerols decreases body fat and blood triglyceride in Chinese hypertriglyceridemic subjects. *Eur J Clin Nutr*, **63**, 879–86.

Xue, C., Liu, Y., Wang, J., Zheng, Z., Zhang, Y., *et al.* (2009b) Chinese hypertriglycerideamic subjects of different ages responded differently to consuming oil with medium- and long-chain fatty acids. *Biosci Biotechnol Biochem*, **73**, 1711–17.

Yang, C. S. and Landau, J. M. (2000) Effects of tea consumption on nutrition and health. *J Nutr*, **130**, 2409–12.

Yuan, Q., Ramprasath, V. R., Harding, S. V., Rideout, T. C., Chan, Y. M. and Jones, P. J. (2010) Diacylglycerol oil reduces body fat but does not alter energy or lipid metabolism in overweight, hypertriglyceridemic women. *J Nutr*, **140**, 1122–6.

11

Functional foods and prevention of diabetes

J. Lindström, National Institute for Health and Welfare, Finland and
S. M. Virtanen, National Institute for Health and Welfare, Finland and
Tampere School of Public Health, Finland

Abstract: The most common types of diabetes mellitus are type 1 (formerly known as 'juvenile diabetes' or 'insulin-dependent diabetes') and type 2 (formerly known as 'adult-onset diabetes' or 'non-insulin-dependent diabetes'). In the aetiology of both type 1 and 2 diabetes hereditary factors are needed for the disease to develop, but environmental factors are decisive in who finally develops the disease. In type 1 diabetes the factors that may affect beta-cell destruction are thought to be crucial in this process of probable autoimmune nature. Early age at introduction of cow's milk, cereals, potatoes and roots, and fruits may increase the risk of type 1 diabetes. Vitamins D and E and n-3 fatty acids may be protective from type 1 diabetes. Nitrates, nitrites and N-nitroso compounds from food and drinking water could cause type 1 diabetes. Type 2 diabetes and other disorders of glycaemia are characterised by insulin resistance and impaired insulin secretion. Obesity and physical inactivity are the most important behavioural risk factors for type 2 diabetes, but other factors also have a role in its aetiology. Epidemiological studies have suggested that several dietary factors may either increase (such as intake of refined grains, red and processed meat, sugar-sweetened beverages, heavy alcohol consumption) or decrease (such as intake of fruits, vegetables, legumes, nuts, coffee, moderate alcohol consumption) the risk. Intervention studies including lifestyle counselling for people with high risk of developing type 2 diabetes have consistently shown that moderate weight reduction, diet following general recommendations and emphasising moderate fat intake and increase in wholegrain and fruit and vegetable consumption efficiently prevent type 2 diabetes.

Key words: type 1 diabetes, type 2 diabetes, aetiology, diet, lifestyle, prevention.

11.1 Introduction

The term 'diabetes mellitus' is used to characterise a group of diseases which share a common symptom, chronic hyperglycaemia. However, the pathogenetic background for the observed hyperglycaemia varies greatly. The two most common types of diabetes, covering majority of the cases of diabetes mellitus, are called type 1 and type 2 diabetes. Type 1 diabetes is considered an autoimmune disease for which the necessary genetic background is required. It is characterised by progressive beta-cell destruction which leads to complete insulin deficiency. Type 2 diabetes develops as a result of interaction between genes and lifestyle and takes years or even decades to manifest. It is characterised by gradual increase in insulin resistance, which when combined with gradual beta-cell failure leads to increased blood glucose values. Type 2 diabetes typically clusters with other metabolic disturbances such as dyslipidaemia and hypertension.

During the last decades a continuous increase has been seen in the incidence of type 1 diabetes especially in several high and middle income countries (Patterson *et al.*, 2009). For example in Finland, the country with the highest incidence of the disease, the increase has been more than five-fold during the last five decades from 12 to 64 per 100 000 persons per year (Somersalo, 1954; Harjutsalo *et al.*, 2008). This increase has been steepest in the youngest age group, in younger than five-year-olds (Harjutsalo *et al.*, 2008; Patterson *et al.*, 2009). Environmental factors such as diet, nutritional status and microbial infections may determine who finally develops the disease. The higher incidence observed in high and middle income, as opposed to low income countries supports the hypothesis that lifestyle factors and/or hygiene could play a role in the disease process (Kondrashova *et al.*, 2005).

The prevalence of type 2 diabetes has also increased steadily during the past decades. The International Diabetes Federation has estimated that 55 million adults in Europe have type 2 diabetes, and by 2030, the number is predicted to rise to 66 million (International Diabetes Federation, 2009). A study completed on Finnish 'young adults' (age 15–39 years) revealed alarming results. Although absolute incidence and thus also prevalence of type 2 diabetes was still low between 1992 and 1996 (11.8 cases per 100 000/year) the incidence increased on average by 7.9% per year (Lammi *et al.*, 2007). Up to the age of 30–34 years the incidence of type 1 diabetes is greater than that of type 2 diabetes. After this age, type 2 becomes more common in Finland (Lammi *et al.*, 2007).

Type 2 diabetes develops as a result of a complex multifactorial process with both lifestyle and genetic origins. When genetically predisposed individuals become insulin resistant due to environmental exposures such as obesity or physical inactivity, they may develop post-prandial hyperglycaemia. Finally, when beta-cell capacity is not sufficient to compensate for insulin resistance, hyperglycaemia worsens and overt diabetes will develop. It is estimated that in Caucasian populations the proportion of people with genetic predisposition to type 2 diabetes is between 20% and 50% (Valle *et al.*, 1997). The most important risk factors for type 2 diabetes are (abdominal) obesity and a sedentary lifestyle (Hu *et al.*, 2003, 2004; World Health Organization, 2003). A dietary pattern predisposing a person to obesity increases the risk of type 2 diabetes. In addition, several dietary components have been associated with type 2 diabetes risk independently of obesity.

11.2   Food and diet as contributing factors to the rise in diabetes

11.2.1   Diet in the aetiology of type 1 diabetes

Cow's milk, cereals, potatoes and roots, and fruits have been suspected to be connected with the aetiology of type 1 diabetes. Vitamins D and E and n-3 fatty acids may protect from type 1 diabetes. Nitrates, nitrites and N-nitroso compounds from food or drinking water could cause type 1 diabetes. There is some animal evidence suggesting that probiotics could prevent immune-mediated diabetes (Calcinaro *et al.*, 2005), while some microbial toxins could be causative (Myers *et al.*, 2001; Virtanen *et al.*, 2008). Evidence whether increased weight or height gain would be associated with increase risk of type 1 diabetes is inconclusive (Virtanen and Knip, 2003; Knip *et al.*, 2010).

There are more and more clues that the process leading to type 1 diabetes may start very early, i.e. during the foetal stage. A high nitrite intake by the mother during pregnancy may increase the risk of type 1 diabetes in the offspring (Virtanen *et al.*, 1994). The findings of studies investigating whether vitamin D during the foetal stage protects the offspring from beta-cell autoimmunity are inconsistent (Fronczak *et al.*, 2003; Brekke and Ludvigsson, 2007; Marjamaki *et al.*, 2010). Maternal antioxidant intake during pregnancy seems not to be associated with the risk of advanced beta-cell autoimmunity of the child (Uusitalo *et al.*, 2008a). Foetal exposure to microbial toxins available in root vegetables was connected to immune-mediated diabetes in non-obese diabetic (NOD) mice (Hettiarachchi *et al.*, 2004). Contrasting this observation, in the US mother–child cohort with increased genetic susceptibility to type 1 diabetes (DAISY study), high intake frequency of potatoes was related to smaller risk of early beta-cell autoimmunity (Lamb *et al.*, 2008). Finnish prospective findings from a birth cohort with increased genetic susceptibility suggest that maternal intake of butter, low-fat margarines, berries and coffee during pregnancy would protect from advanced beta-cell autoimmunity (Virtanen *et al.*, n.d.). High birth weight is associated with slightly increased risk of type 1 diabetes (Harder *et al.*, 2009).

The associations between infant feeding and development of beta-cell autoimmunity and clinical type 1 diabetes, has been the most studied area in the efforts of trying to reveal nutritional risk factors of this disease (Virtanen and Knip, 2003; Knip *et al.*, 2010). Early introduction of cow's milk, gluten-containing and other cereals, fruits and root vegetables have been connected to the risk of beta-cell autoimmunity and clinical type 1 diabetes in prospective studies (Norris *et al.*, 2003; Ziegler *et al.*, 2003; Virtanen *et al.*, 1991, 2006). There is some suggestion that breastfeeding could protect from beta-cell autoimmunity and/or type 1 diabetes (Holmberg *et al.*, 2007; Knip *et al.*, 2010). Findings from the pilot study of a randomised double-blind trial suggest, that the emergence of type 1 diabetes-associated autoantibodies can be prevented or delayed by giving highly hydrolysed infant formula instead of a normal cow's milk based one over the first six to eight months of life in first-degree relatives of subjects with type 1 diabetes (Akerblom *et al.*, 2005). Vitamin D supplementation during infancy has been connected with decreased risk of type 1 diabetes according to both case-control (The EURODIAB Substudy 2 Study Group, 1999; Stene and Joner, 2003) and cohort (Hypponen *et al.*, 2001) findings. Increased weight gain during infancy has been consistently associated with increased risk of type 1 diabetes (Hypponen *et al.*, 1999).

A child's dietary intake of N-nitroso compounds and nitrite are potential risk determinants of type 1 diabetes (Dahlquist *et al.*, 1990; Virtanen *et al.*, 1994). Dietary antioxidants such as vitamin C and α-tocopherol inhibit the formation of N-nitroso compounds from nitrites (Leaf *et al.*, 1989). Low groundwater zinc and acidity were suggested as risk determinants of type 1 diabetes (Haglund *et al.*, 1996; Stene *et al.*, 2002). Findings whether vitamin E and/or vitamin C would protect from type 1 diabetes are inconsistent (Glatthaar *et al.*, 1988; Dahlquist *et al.*, 1990; Knekt *et al.*, 1999; Uusitalo *et al.*, 2005; Uusitalo *et al.*, 2008b). Recent prospective findings suggest that dietary n-3 fatty acids during childhood protect the child from β-cell autoimmunity (Norris *et al.*, 2007). There is evidence that the amount of cow's milk used could be related to the risk of type 1 diabetes (Verge *et al.*, 1994; Virtanen *et al.*, 1998, 2000).

Increased relative weight and obesity may be risk factors for type 1 diabetes (Hypponen *et al.*, 2000). There is no knowledge based on cohort studies of the effects of childhood growth and obesity on the risk of type 1 diabetes or pre-type 1 diabetes.

Overall the majority of the studies on the aetiology of type 1 diabetes have been hypothesis generating: animal studies and ecological comparisons. Among the observational studies, there are still quite few prospective cohort studies which can give better picture on causal relationships. Very few randomised trials findings have been reported so far (e.g. Akerblom *et al.*, 2005).

The identification of type 1 diabetes-associated autoantibodies have made large prospective cohort studies feasible (Knip, 1997) as the number of subjects needed can be smaller and the follow-up time shorter with these intermediate endpoints than with clinical type 1 diabetes.

11.2.2   Diet in the aetiology of type 2 diabetes

Epidemiological cross-sectional studies have suggested high total fat intake to be a risk factor for insulin resistance, glucose intolerance or type 2 diabetes (Marshall *et al.*, 1991). Data from prospective studies are less consistent. In the San Luis Valley Diabetes Study high fat intake predicted conversion from impaired glucose tolerance, which is an intermediate category between normal and diabetic glucose tolerance, to type 2 diabetes (Marshall *et al.*, 1994) and hyperinsulinaemia (Marshall *et al.*, 1997). In the Finnish and Dutch cohorts of the Seven Countries Study baseline intakes of total fat, saturated fat and monounsaturated fat were higher among those who were diagnosed with diabetes in the follow-up study 20 years later (Feskens *et al.*, 1995). In the Health Professionals Follow-up Study total fat intake was associated with diabetes risk during the 12-year follow-up, but the association was attenuated after adjustment for BMI (van Dam *et al.*, 2002b).

The type of fat, rather than total fat intake, has in several studies been associated with increased type 2 diabetes risk, as reviewed by Hu and co-workers (Hu *et al.*,

2001b). While saturated fat has been associated with increased diabetes risk in some studies (Feskens *et al.*, 1995; van Dam *et al.*, 2002b), in the Nurses' Health Study (Salmeron *et al.*, 1997b, 2001) no association between saturated fat and diabetes was found; however, intake of trans fatty acids was associated with increased diabetes risk and intake of polyunsaturated fatty acids with decreased diabetes risk (Salmeron *et al.*, 2001). In the Iowa Women's Health Study, high intake of vegetable fat and polyunsaturated fatty acids decreased diabetes risk (Meyer *et al.*, 2001). On the other hand, the omega-3 polyunsaturated fatty acids increased and trans fatty acids decreased diabetes risk, which is in controversy with the results from other studies (Adler *et al.*, 1994; Salmeron *et al.*, 2001). The mixed findings may originate from the fact that in different food cultures, the sources of nutrients differ. In typical Western diet monounsaturated fat comes mainly from animal sources (meat, milk products) and thus is highly correlated with saturated fat intake, whereas in the Mediterranean diet the dominant source of monounsaturated fat is olive oil. Furthermore, the effect of trans fatty acids on metabolism may depend on whether the trans fat is from natural (milk and ruminant meat) or industrial (partially hydrogenated vegetable oil) origin (Chardigny *et al.*, 2006) or simply on the intake level (van de Vijver *et al.*, 2000).

Fibre intake, especially from cereal origin, has consistently been shown to be inversely associated with type 2 diabetes risk. The early analyses from the Nurses' Health Study I (Salmeron *et al.*, 1997b) showed an association; however, the later analyses with longer follow-up did not (Salmeron *et al.*, 2001). In the younger cohort (Nurses' Health Study II) the association was apparent (Schulze *et al.*, 2004a), as also in the Health Professionals Follow-up Study (Salmeron *et al.*, 1997a), the Iowa Women's Health Study (Meyer *et al.*, 2000), the Atherosclerosis Risk in Communities Study (Stevens *et al.*, 2002) and the Finnish Mobile Clinic Health Examination Survey (Montonen *et al.*, 2003).

However, when associations between dietary intake and type 2 diabetes risk are assessed focusing on single nutrients, there is always the possibility that the observed effect is explained by confounding by some other nutrient, dietary characteristic, or even other related behaviour (e.g. smoking, physical activity). Therefore it is important also to examine the associations between food items and type 2 diabetes risk (Table 11.1). High intake of red and/or processed meat products has been associated with higher diabetes risk (van Dam *et al.*, 2002b; Fung *et al.*, 2004; Song *et al.*, 2004b; Aune *et al.*, 2009). Protective effects of high wholegrain (Liu *et al.*, 2000; Meyer *et al.*, 2000; Fung *et al.*, 2002; Pereira *et al.*, 2002a; Montonen *et al.*, 2003) fruit and vegetable (Sargeant *et al.*, 2001; Liu *et al.*, 2004; Montonen *et al.*, 2005a; Villegas *et al.*, 2008b) and dairy consumption (Pereira *et al.*, 2002b; Choi *et al.*, 2005) have been reported. Intake of alcohol seems to have protective effect associated with moderate consumption but increased risk with high consumption (Stampfer *et al.*, 1988; Holbrook *et al.*, 1990; Ajani *et al.*, 2000; Hodge *et al.*, 2006). A relatively new finding is the association of high coffee consumption (~6 cups/day or more) and reduced diabetes risk (Salazar-Martinez *et al.*, 2004; Tuomilehto *et al.*, 2004; van Dam *et al.*, 2006).

Table 11.1   Association between consumption of some foods and type 2 diabetes risk: epidemiological evidence

Food	Effect on risk*	Reference
Whole grains	↓	Meyer *et al.*, 2000; Pereira *et al.*, 2002a; Montonen *et al.*, 2003; Fung *et al.*, 2002; Liu *et al.*, 2000
Refined grains	↑	Liu *et al.*, 2000
Sugar-sweetened beverages	(↑)	Bray, 2004; Paynter *et al.*, 2006
Red and processed meat	↑	Aune *et al.*, 2009; van Dam *et al.*, 2002b; Fung *et al.*, 2004; Song *et al.*, 2004b
Milk and milk products	(↓)	Choi *et al.*, 2005; Pereira *et al.*, 2002b
Fruit and vegetables	↓	Sargeant *et al.*, 2001; Liu *et al.*, 2004; Montonen *et al.*, 2005a; Villegas *et al.*, 2008b
Nuts	(↓)	Villegas *et al.*, 2008a; Jiang *et al.*, 2002; Parker *et al.*, 2003
Legumes (e.g. soy products)	(↓)	Nanri *et al.*, Villegas *et al.*, 2008a
Alcohol beverages	↓ (Moderate consumption) ↑ (High consumption)	Holbrook *et al.*, 1990; Stampfer *et al.*, 1988; Ajani *et al.*, 2000; Hodge *et al.*, 2006
Coffee	↓	Salazar-Martinez *et al.*, 2004; Tuomilehto *et al.*, 2004; van Dam *et al.*, 2006; Paynter *et al.*, 2006

* ↓ Reduced risk, consistent evidence; (↓) reduced risk, suggestive (controversial) evidence; ↑ increased risk, consistent evidence; (↑) increased risk, suggestive (controversial) evidence

During the past decade there has been a shift in the research from single nutrients or food items towards dietary patterns. In general, studies completed among different populations and food cultures have consistently shown that changing from traditional dietary patterns (typically including unrefined grains and vegetables) to a Western dietary pattern (characterised by high intakes of refined grains, sugar, and red meat) has lead to increase in type 2 diabetes incidence (Hu *et al.*, 2001a; van Dam *et al.*, 2002a; Fung *et al.*, 2004; Montonen *et al.*, 2005b; Nettleton *et al.*, 2008).

11.3   Effects of different food components on insulin secretion, insulin resistance and development of diabetes

It is unclear whether dietary factors that affect insulin secretion and/or insulin resistance could play a role in the development of type 1 diabetes. According to the accelerator hypothesis the overload of the beta cells caused by increased insulin demand may accelerate the process of beta-cell destruction and lead to earlier development of type 1 diabetes (Wilkin, 2001).

Regarding to the role of specific food components in the pathway to type 2 diabetes, there is more evidence. In a three-month clinical study (KANWU) substituting dietary saturated fat for monounsaturated fat impaired insulin sensitivity in healthy individuals, but the beneficial effect of monounsaturated fat was only seen at total fat intake below median intake of 37% of total energy (Vessby *et al.*, 2001). Omega-3 polyunsaturated fatty acids given as fish oil supplement did not have any effect on insulin sensitivity. In another study completed in Finland an eight-week diet enriched in monounsaturated fat (19 E%) improved glucose metabolism after a high-saturated fat (18 E%) diet in individuals with impaired glucose tolerance (Sarkkinen *et al.*, 1996).

Several mechanisms may be behind the observed effects of quality of fat on insulin sensitivity and subsequent type 2 diabetes risk. Dietary fat composition modifies the composition of the cell membrane phospholipids, and saturated fat seems to decrease the membrane fluidity and impair insulin sensitivity (Storlien *et al.*, 1996). Polyunsaturated fat also decreases triacylglycerol accumulation into muscle and pancreatic beta-cells, compared with saturated fatty acids, and may thus modify the lipotoxisity effect (Clarke, 2001). Dietary fatty acids may have an effect on the low-grade systemic inflammation and endothelian dysfunction, which in turn may induce insulin resistance. In a subgroup analysis of the Nurses' Health Study, trans fatty acid intake was directly and omega-3 fatty acid intake was inversely associated with inflammation markers C-reactive protein and interleukin-6 (Lopez-Garcia *et al.*, 2004, 2005). Furthermore, fatty acid composition of diet may modulate insulin secretion, monounsaturated fat appearing to have the most beneficial effect (Rojo-Martinez *et al.*, 2006).

The protective effect of dietary fibre against type 2 diabetes may result from the ability of fibre to lower post-prandial glucose peak, which leads to decreased insulin demand and protects the pancreas from exhaustion. Fibre is known to slow down the digestion and absorption of carbohydrates, but this applies mostly on soluble fibre (Jenkins *et al.*, 1978); however, specifically unsoluble (cereal) fibre has in several studies been associated with decreased diabetes risk (Salmeron *et al.*, 1997a, 1997b; Meyer *et al.*, 2000; Stevens *et al.*, 2002; Montonen *et al.*, 2003; Schulze *et al.*, 2004a). A possible mediator of the effect is the enhanced secretion of gut-hormones (glucoincretins) glucagon-like peptide-1 and gastric inhibitory peptide. They are intestinal peptides secreted in response to glucose, lipid, or non-digestible carbohydrate ingestion, and are responsible for the rapid insulin response to a meal (Burcelin, 2005). In a clinical study the consumption of highly purified insoluble dietary fibres accelerated the acute gastric inhibitory peptide and insulin response, and was further associated with enhanced postprandial carbohydrate handling the following day (Weickert *et al.*, 2005). Short-term (three days) ingestion of purified insoluble fibre has also been shown to increase whole-body insulin sensitivity in overweight women (Weickert *et al.*, 2006).

Total carbohydrate intake has typically not been associated with type 2 diabetes risk, when other dietary factors have been adjusted for. It is probable that the quality of carbohydrates is more important than total amount. It is well established that carbohydrates from different sources produce different glycaemic (Jenkins *et al.*, 1994; Wolever *et al.*, 1994; Wolever and Mehling, 2002) or insulinogenic responses (Juntunen *et al.*, 2003a, 2003b) and may have an effect on insulin resistance (Pereira *et al.*, 2002a). The effect of carbohydrate on blood glucose depends on how fast it is digested. The glycaemic index refers to the ability of carbohydrate contained in a specific food item to raise blood glucose, compared with same amount of carbohydrate (typically 50g) as glucose. Dietary glycaemic load is estimated from glycaemic index by multiplying it with the amount of carbohydrates. In prospective studies dietary glycaemic index has been more consistent than glycaemic load associated with increased diabetes risk (Salmeron *et al.*, 1997a, 1997b; Meyer *et al.*, 2000; Hodge *et al.*, 2004; Schulze *et al.*, 2004a). However, diet high in cereal fibre is usually also high in carbohydrates and usually (but not always) has low glycaemic index, and this may confound the observed associations.

Intake of sucrose has in general not been associated with type 2 diabetes (Daly, 2003; Hodge *et al.*, 2004). In the Nurses' Health Study II, high intake of sugar-sweetened beverages increased diabetes risk (Schulze *et al.*, 2004b), however in the Atherosclerosis Risk in Communities (ARIC) Study such association was not found (Paynter *et al.*, 2006). In the USA beverages are typically sweetened with high-fructose corn syrup (Bray, 2004), and a high consumption of soft drinks can thus lead to unnaturally high intake of fructose, which in turn may disturb glucose and lipid metabolism (Basciano *et al.*, 2005; Nakagawa *et al.*, 2006). Fructose may increase diabetes risk also indirectly through weight gain (Elliott *et al.*, 2002). Fructose ingestion does not stimulate insulin or leptin secretion; as these hormones are major regulators of energy intake, high fructose consumption may lead to energy overconsumption and obesity.

Other dietary factors that have been proposed to have a protective effect in progression to type 2 diabetes include vitamin C (Feskens *et al.*, 1995), vitamin D (Boucher, 1998; Pittas *et al.*, 2006; Knekt *et al.*, 2008), vitamin E (Montonen *et al.*, 2004), several tocopherols (Montonen *et al.*, 2004), calcium (Pittas *et al.*, 2006), and magnesium (Colditz *et al.*, 1992; Salmeron *et al.*, 1997a, 1997b; Lopez-Ridaura *et al.*, 2004; Song *et al.*, 2004a). There is some evidence linking high sodium intake with increased type 2 diabetes risk (Hu *et al.*, 2005).

11.4   Formulating food products for diabetes prevention

11.4.1   Type 1 diabetes

No specific dietary recommendations can yet be given to prevent type 1 diabetes. We must be careful not to cause unnecessary concern among the families before we really know.

11.4.2   Type 2 diabetes

Convincing evidence from intervention studies to prevent type 2 diabetes among high-risk individuals shows that weight reduction and adopting healthy diet and physical activity can significantly reduce type 2 diabetes incidence (Pan *et al.*, 1997; Tuomilehto *et al.*, 2001; The Diabetes Prevention Program Research Group, 2002; Kosaka *et al.*, 2005; Ramachandran *et al.*, 2006; Roumen *et al.*, 2008; Penn *et al.*, 2009). Common features in these lifestyle intervention studies included moderate weight reduction, diet following general recommendations and emphasising moderate fat intake and increase in wholegrain and fruit and vegetable consumption.

Functional foods specifically to prevent type 2 diabetes would be foods or ingredients that have an effect on either insulin secretion or insulin resistance. At the moment we can identify several natural foods that can have such properties, such as whole grains, vegetables, vegetable fat, and coffee. Currently, there is no compelling evidence showing that adding components of these foods (e.g. cereal fibre) into processed foods has long-term effects on diabetes risk. Therefore, the consumption of these 'whole foods' as part of everyday diet should be emphasised.

11.5   Future trends

In the aetiology of type 1 diabetes interactions between genes and environmental factors seem to be important although still today they are largely unknown. The rapid increase in the incidence of this disease during the last five decades may be also explained by epigenetic regulation. Environmental factors may cause epigenetic changes in the regulation of genes which then would affect the disease risk (Litherland, 2008; MacFarlane *et al.*, 2009). The ongoing large prospective cohort studies following individuals with increased disease susceptibility (Norris *et al.*, 2003; Virtanen *et al.*, 2006; The TEDDY Study Group, 2007) and randomised clinical trials (The TRIGR Study Group, 2007) will hopefully give clues on the way to the prevention of type 1 diabetes.

On the contrary to type 1 diabetes, today we know that type 2 diabetes can be prevented among high-risk individuals by lifestyle change. However, the suggested prudent diet does not work for everybody, and more research on the complex association between diet and type 2 diabetes is warranted. Specifically, nutrigenomic and nutrigenetic research may clarify why different people and populations react differently to nutritional environment. We know that specific dietary features have differing effects on metabolism, depending on genetic background. Better knowledge on the interaction between diet and genes might enable the development of more tailored dietary regimes.

11.6   References

Adler, A. I., Boyko, E. J., Schraer, C. D. and Murphy, N. J. (1994) Lower prevalence of impaired glucose tolerance and diabetes associated with daily seal oil or salmon consumption among Alaska Natives. *Diabetes Care*, **17**, 1498–501.
Ajani, U. A., Hennekens, C. H., Spelsberg, A. and Manson, J. E. (2000) Alcohol consumption and risk of type 2 diabetes mellitus among US male physicians. *Arch Intern Med*, **160**, 1025–30.

Akerblom, H. K., Virtanen, S. M., Ilonen, J., Savilahti, E., Vaarala, O., *et al.* (2005) Dietary manipulation of beta cell autoimmunity in infants at increased risk of type 1 diabetes: a pilot study. *Diabetologia*, **48**, 829–37.

Aune, D., Ursin, G. and Veierod, M. B. (2009) Meat consumption and the risk of type 2 diabetes: a systematic review and meta-analysis of cohort studies. *Diabetologia*, **52**, 2277–87.

Basciano, H., Federico, L. and Adeli, K. (2005) Fructose, insulin resistance, and metabolic dyslipidemia. *Nutr Metab (Lond)*, **2**, 5.

Boucher, B. J. (1998) Inadequate vitamin D status: does it contribute to the disorders comprising syndome 'X'? *Br J Nutr*, **79**, 315–27.

Bray, G. A. (2004) The epidemic of obesity and changes in food intake: the Fluoride Hypothesis. *Physiol Behav*, **82**, 115–21.

Brekke, H. K. and Ludvigsson, J. (2007) Vitamin D supplementation and diabetes-related autoimmunity in the ABIS study. *Pediatr Diabetes*, **8**, 11–14.

Burcelin, R. (2005) The incretins: a link between nutrients and well-being. *Br J Nutr*, **93** (Suppl 1), S147–56.

Calcinaro, F., Dionisi, S., Marinaro, M., Candeloro, P., Bonato, V., *et al.* (2005) Oral probiotic administration induces interleukin-10 production and prevents spontaneous autoimmune diabetes in the non-obese diabetic mouse. *Diabetologia*, **48**, 1565–75.

Chardigny, J. M., Malpuech-Brugere, C., Dionisi, F., Bauman, D. E., German, B., *et al.* (2006) Rationale and design of the TRANSFACT project phase I: a study to assess the effect of the two different dietary sources of trans fatty acids on cardiovascular risk factors in humans. *Contemp Clin Trials*, **27**, 364–73.

Choi, H. K., Willett, W. C., Stampfer, M. J., Rimm, E. and Hu, F. B. (2005) Dairy consumption and risk of type 2 diabetes mellitus in men: a prospective study. *Arch Intern Med*, **165**, 997–1003.

Clarke, S. D. (2001) Polyunsaturated fatty acid regulation of gene transcription: a molecular mechanism to improve the metabolic syndrome. *J Nutr*, **131**, 1129–32.

Colditz, G. A., Manson, J. E., Stampfer, M. J., Rosner, B., Willett, W. C. and Speizer, F. E. (1992) Diet and risk of clinical diabetes in women. *Am J Clin Nutr*, **55**, 1018–23.

Dahlquist, G. G., Blom, L. G., Persson, L. A., Sandstrom, A. I. and Wall, S. G. (1990) Dietary factors and the risk of developing insulin dependent diabetes in childhood. *BMJ*, **300**, 1302–6.

Daly, M. (2003) Sugars, insulin sensitivity, and the postprandial state. *Am J Clin Nutr*, **78**, S865–72.

Elliott, S. S., Keim, N. L., Stern, J. S., Teff, K. and Havel, P. J. (2002) Fructose, weight gain, and the insulin resistance syndrome. *Am J Clin Nutr*, **76**, 911–22.

Feskens, E. J., Virtanen, S. M., Räsänen, L., Tuomilehto, J., Stengård, J., *et al.* (1995) Dietary factors determining diabetes and impaired glucose tolerance. A 20-year follow-up of the Finnish and Dutch cohorts of the Seven Countries Study. *Diabetes Care*, **18**, 1104–12.

Fronczak, C. M., Baron, A. E., Chase, H. P., Ross, C., Brady, H. L., *et al.* (2003) In utero dietary exposures and risk of islet autoimmunity in children. *Diabetes Care*, **26**, 3237–42.

Fung, T. T., Hu, F. B., Pereira, M. A., Liu, S., Stampfer, M. J., *et al.* (2002) Whole-grain intake and the risk of type 2 diabetes: a prospective study in men. *Am J Clin Nutr*, **76**, 535–40.

Fung, T. T., Schulze, M., Manson, J. E., Willett, W. C. and Hu, F. B. (2004) Dietary patterns, meat intake, and the risk of type 2 diabetes in women. *Arch Intern Med*, **164**, 2235–40.

Glatthaar, C., Whittall, D. E., Welborn, T. A., Gibson, M. J., Brooks, B. H., *et al.* (1988) Diabetes in Western Australian children: descriptive epidemiology. *Med J Aust*, **148**, 117–23.

Haglund, B., Ryckenberg, K., Selinus, O. and Dahlquist, G. (1996) Evidence of a relationship between childhood-onset type I diabetes and low groundwater concentration of zinc. *Diabetes Care*, **19**, 873–5.

Harder, T., Roepke, K., Diller, N., Stechling, Y., Dudenhausen, J. W. and Plagemann, A. (2009) Birth weight, early weight gain, and subsequent risk of type 1 diabetes: systematic review and meta-analysis. *Am J Epidemiol*, **169**, 1428–36.

Harjutsalo, V., Sjoberg, L. and Tuomilehto, J. (2008) Time trends in the incidence of type 1 diabetes in Finnish children: a cohort study. *Lancet*, **371**, 1777–82.

Hettiarachchi, K. D., Zimmet, P. Z. and Myers, M. A. (2004) Transplacental exposure to bafilomycin disrupts pancreatic islet organogenesis and accelerates diabetes onset in NOD mice. *J Autoimmun*, **22**, 287–96.

Hodge, A. M., English, D. R., O'dea, K. and Giles, G. G. (2004) Glycemic index and dietary fiber and the risk of type 2 diabetes. *Diabetes Care*, **27**, 2701–6.

Hodge, A. M., English, D. R., O'dea, K. and Giles, G. G. (2006) Alcohol intake, consumption pattern and beverage type, and the risk of Type 2 diabetes. *Diabetic Medicine*, **23**, 690–7.

Holbrook, T., Barret-Connor, E. and Wingard, D. (1990) A prospective population-based study of alcohol use and non-insulin-dependent diabetes mellitus. *Am J Epid*, **132**, 902–9.

Holmberg, H., Wahlberg, J., Vaarala, O. and Ludvigsson, J. (2007) Short duration of breast-feeding as a risk-factor for beta-cell autoantibodies in 5-year-old children from the general population. *Br J Nutr*, **97**, 111–16.

Hu, F. B., Manson, J. E., Stampfer, M. J., Colditz, G., Liu, S., *et al.* (2001a) Diet, lifestyle, and the risk of type 2 diabetes mellitus in women. *N Engl J Med*, **345**, 790–7.

Hu, F. B., Van Dam, R. M. and Liu, S. (2001b) Diet and risk of Type II diabetes: the role of types of fat and carbohydrate. *Diabetologia*, **44**, 805–17.

Hu, G., Jousilahti, P., Peltonen, M., Lindström, J. and Tuomilehto, J. (2005) Urinary sodium and potassium excretion and the risk of type 2 diabetes: a prospective study in Finland. *Diabetologia*, **48**, 1477–83.

Hu, G., Lindström, J., Valle, T. T., Eriksson, J. G., Jousilahti, P., *et al.* (2004) Physical activity, body mass index, and risk of type 2 diabetes in patients with normal or impaired glucose regulation. *Arch Intern Med*, **164**, 892–6.

Hu, G., Qiao, Q., Silventoinen, K., Eriksson, J. G., Jousilahti, P., *et al.* (2003) Occupational, commuting, and leisure-time physical activity in relation to risk for Type 2 diabetes in middle-aged Finnish men and women. *Diabetologia*, **46**, 322–9.

Hypponen, E., Kenward, M. G., Virtanen, S. M., Piitulainen, A., Virta-Autio, P., *et al.* (1999) Infant feeding, early weight gain, and risk of type 1 diabetes. Childhood Diabetes in Finland (DiMe) Study Group. *Diabetes Care*, **22**, 1961–5.

Hypponen, E., Laara, E., Reunanen, A., Jarvelin, M. R. and Virtanen, S. M. (2001) Intake of vitamin D and risk of type 1 diabetes: a birth-cohort study. *Lancet*, **358**, 1500–3.

Hypponen, E., Virtanen, S. M., Kenward, M. G., Knip, M. and Akerblom, H. K. (2000) Obesity, increased linear growth, and risk of type 1 diabetes in children. *Diabetes Care*, **23**, 1755–60.

International Diabetes Federation (2009) *Diabetes Atlas*, fourth edition. http://www.eatlas.idf.org/.

Jenkins, D. J., Jenkins, A. L., Wolever, T. M., Vuksan, V., Rao, A. V., *et al.* (1994) Low glycemic index: lente carbohydrates and physiological effects of altered food frequency. *Am J Clin Nutr*, **59**, S706–9.

Jenkins, D. J., Wolever, T. M., Leeds, A. R., Gassull, M. A., Haisman, P., *et al.* (1978) Dietary fibres, fibre analogues, and glucose tolerance: importance of viscosity. *Br Med J*, **1**, 1392–4.

Jiang, R., Manson, J. E., Stampfer, M. J., Liu, S., Willett, W. C. and Hu, F. B. (2002) Nut and peanut butter consumption and risk of type 2 diabetes in women. *Jama*, **288**, 2554–60.

Juntunen, K. S., Laaksonen, D. E., Autio, K., Niskanen, L. K., Holst, J. J., *et al.* (2003a) Structural differences between rye and wheat breads but not total fiber content may explain the lower postprandial insulin response to rye bread. *Am J Clin Nutr*, **78**, 957–64.

Juntunen, K. S., Laaksonen, D. E., Poutanen, K. S., Niskanen, L. K. and Mykkänen, H. M. (2003b) High-fiber rye bread and insulin secretion and sensitivity in healthy postmenopausal women. *Am J Clin Nutr*, **77**, 385–91.

Knekt, P., Laaksonen, M., Mattila, C., Harkanen, T., Marniemi, J., *et al.* (2008) Serum vitamin D and subsequent occurrence of type 2 diabetes. *Epidemiology*, **19**, 666–71.

Knekt, P., Reunanen, A., Marniemi, J., Leino, A. and Aromaa, A. (1999) Low vitamin E status is a potential risk factor for insulin-dependent diabetes mellitus. *J Intern Med*, **245**, 99–102.

Knip, M. (1997) Disease-associated autoimmunity and prevention of insulin-dependent diabetes mellitus. *Ann Med*, **29**, 447–51.

Knip, M., Virtanen, S. M. and Akerblom, H. K. (2010) Infant feeding and risk of type 1 diabetes. *Am J Clin Nutr* (In press).

Kondrashova, A., Reunanen, A., Romanov, A., Karvonen, A., Viskari, H., *et al.* (2005) A six-fold gradient in the incidence of type 1 diabetes at the eastern border of Finland. *Ann Med*, **37**, 67–72.

Kosaka, K., Noda, M. and Kuzuya, T. (2005) Prevention of type 2 diabetes by lifestyle intervention: a Japanese trial in IGT males. *Diabetes Res Clin Pract*, **67**, 152–62.

Lamb, M. M., Myers, M. A., Barriga, K., Zimmet, P. Z., Rewers, M. and Norris, J. M. (2008) Maternal diet during pregnancy and islet autoimmunity in offspring. *Pediatr Diabetes*, **9**, 135–41.

Lammi, N., Taskinen, O., Moltchanova, E., Notkola, I. L., Eriksson, J. G., *et al.* (2007) A high incidence of type 1 diabetes and an alarming increase in the incidence of type 2 diabetes among young adults in Finland between 1992 and 1996. *Diabetologia*, **50**, 1393–400.

Leaf, C. D., Wishnok, J. S. and Tannenbaum, S. R. (1989) Mechanisms of endogenous nitrosation. *Cancer Surv*, **8**, 323–34.

Litherland, S. A. (2008) Immunopathogenic interaction of environmental triggers and genetic susceptibility in diabetes: is epigenetics the missing link? *Diabetes*, **57**, 3184–6.

Liu, S., Manson, J. E., Stampfer, M. J., Hu, F. B., Giovannucci, E., *et al.* (2000) A prospective study of whole-grain intake and risk of type 2 diabetes mellitus in US women. *Am J Public Health*, **90**, 1409–15.

Liu, S., Serdula, M., Janket, S. J., Cook, N. R., Sesso, H. D., *et al.* (2004) A prospective study of fruit and vegetable intake and the risk of type 2 diabetes in women. *Diabetes Care*, **27**, 2993–6.

Lopez-Garcia, E., Schulze, M. B., Manson, J. E., Meigs, J. B., Albert, C. M., *et al.* (2004) Consumption of (n-3) fatty acids is related to plasma biomarkers of inflammation and endothelial activation in women. *J Nutr*, **134**, 1806–11.

Lopez-Garcia, E., Schulze, M. B., Meigs, J. B., Manson, J. E., Rifai, N., *et al.* (2005) Consumption of trans fatty acids is related to plasma biomarkers of inflammation and endothelial dysfunction. *J Nutr*, **135**, 562–6.

Lopez-Ridaura, R., Willett, W. C., Rimm, E. B., Liu, S., Stampfer, M. J., *et al.* (2004) Magnesium intake and risk of type 2 diabetes in men and women. *Diabetes Care*, **27**, 134–40.

Macfarlane, A. J., Strom, A. and Scott, F. W. (2009) Epigenetics: deciphering how environmental factors may modify autoimmune type 1 diabetes. *Mamm Genome*, **20**, 624–32.

Marjamaki, L., Niinisto, S., Kenward, M. G., Uusitalo, L., Uusitalo, U., *et al.* (2010) Maternal intake of vitamin D during pregnancy and risk of advanced beta-cell autoimmunity in the offspring. *Diabetologia* (In press).

Marshall, J. A., Bessesen, D. H. and Hamman, R. F. (1997) High saturated fat and low starch and fibre are associated with hyperinsulinaemia in a non-diabetic population: the San Luis Valley Diabetes Study. *Diabetologia*, **40**, 430–8.

Marshall, J. A., Hamman, R. F. and Baxter, J. (1991) High-fat, low-carbohydrate diet and the etiology of non-insulin-dependent diabetes mellitus: the San Luis Valley Diabetes Study. *Am J Epidemiol*, **134**, 590–603.

Marshall, J. A., Hoag, S., Shetterly, S. and Hamman, R. F. (1994) Dietary fat predicts conversion from impaired glucose tolerance to NIDDM. The San Luis Valley Diabetes Study. *Diabetes Care*, **17**, 50–6.

Meyer, K. A., Kushi, L. H., Jacobs, D. R., Jr and Folsom, A. R. (2001) Dietary fat and incidence of type 2 diabetes in older Iowa women. *Diabetes Care*, **24**, 1528–35.

Meyer, K. A., Kushi, L. H., Jacobs, D. R, Jr, Slavin, J., Sellers, T. A. and Folsom, A. R. (2000) Carbohydrates, dietary fiber, and incident type 2 diabetes in older women. *Am J Clin Nutr*, **71**, 921–30.

Montonen, J., Järvinen, R., Heliövaara, M., Reunanen, A., Aromaa, A. and Knekt, P. (2005a) Food consumption and the incidence of type II diabetes mellitus. *Eur J Clin Nutr*, **59**, 441–8.

Montonen, J., Knekt, P., Härkänen, T., Järvinen, R., Heliövaara, M., *et al.* (2005b) Dietary patterns and the incidence of type 2 diabetes. *Am J Epidemiol*, **161**, 219–27.

Montonen, J., Knekt, P., Järvinen, R., Aromaa, A. and Reunanen, A. (2003) Whole-grain and fiber intake and the incidence of type 2 diabetes. *Am J Clin Nutr*, **77**, 622–9.

Montonen, J., Knekt, P., Järvinen, R. and Reunanen, A. (2004) Dietary antioxidant intake and risk of type 2 diabetes. *Diabetes Care*, **27**, 362–6.

Myers, M. A., Mackay, I. R., Rowley, M. J. and Zimmet, P. Z. (2001) Dietary microbial toxins and type 1 diabetes – a new meaning for seed and soil. *Diabetologia*, **44**, 1199–200.

Nakagawa, T., Hu, H., Zharikov, S., Tuttle, K. R., Short, R. A., *et al.* (2006) A causal role for uric acid in fructose-induced metabolic syndrome. *Am J Physiol Renal Physiol*, **290**, F625–31.

Nanri, A., Mizoue, T., Takahashi, Y., Kirii, K., Inoue, M., *et al.* (2010) Soy Product and Isoflavone Intakes Are Associated with a Lower Risk of Type 2 Diabetes in Overweight Japanese Women. *J Nutr*, **140**(3), 580–6.

Nettleton, J. A., Steffen, L. M., Ni, H., Liu, K. and Jacobs, D. R., Jr (2008) Dietary patterns and risk of incident type 2 diabetes in the Multi-Ethnic Study of Atherosclerosis (MESA). *Diabetes Care*, **31**, 1777–82.

Norris, J. M., Barriga, K., Klingensmith, G., Hoffman, M., Eisenbarth, G. S., *et al.* (2003) Timing of initial cereal exposure in infancy and risk of islet autoimmunity. *Jama*, **290**, 1713–20.

Norris, J. M., Yin, X., Lamb, M. M., Barriga, K., Seifert, J., *et al.* (2007) Omega-3 polyunsaturated fatty acid intake and islet autoimmunity in children at increased risk for type 1 diabetes. *Jama*, **298**, 1420–8.

Pan, X. R., Li, G. W., Hu, Y. H., Wang, J. X., Yang, W. Y., *et al.* (1997) Effects of diet and exercise in preventing NIDDM in people with impaired glucose tolerance. The Da Qing IGT and Diabetes Study. *Diabetes Care*, **20**, 537–44.

Parker, E. D., Harnack, L. J. and Folsom, A. R. (2003) Nut consumption and risk of type 2 diabetes. *Jama*, **290**, 38–9; author reply 39–40.

Patterson, C. C., Dahlquist, G. G., Gyurus, E., Green, A. and Soltesz, G. (2009) Incidence trends for childhood type 1 diabetes in Europe during 1989–2003 and predicted new cases 2005–20: a multicentre prospective registration study. *Lancet*, **373**, 2027–33.

Paynter, N. P., Yeh, H.-C., Voutilainen, S., Schmidt, M. I., Heiss, G., *et al.* (2006) Coffee and Sweetened Beverage Consumption and the Risk of Type 2 Diabetes Mellitus: The Atherosclerosis Risk in Communities Study. *Am. J. Epidemiol.*, **164**, 1075–84.

Penn, L., White, M., Oldroyd, J., Walker, M., Alberti, K. G. and Mathers, J. C. (2009) Prevention of type 2 diabetes in adults with impaired glucose tolerance: the European Diabetes Prevention RCT in Newcastle upon Tyne, UK. *BMC Public Health*, **9**, 342.

Pereira, M. A., Jacobs, D. R., Jr, Pins, J. J., Raatz, S. K., Gross, M. D., *et al.* (2002a) Effect of whole grains on insulin sensitivity in overweight hyperinsulinemic adults. *Am J Clin Nutr*, **75**, 848–55.

Pereira, M. A., Jacobs, D. R., Jr, Van Horn, L., Slattery, M. L., Kartashov, A. I. and Ludwig, D. S. (2002b) Dairy consumption, obesity, and the insulin resistance syndrome in young adults: the CARDIA Study. *JAMA*, **287**, 2081–9.

Pittas, A. G., Dawson-Hughes, B., Li, T., Van Dam, R. M., Willett, W. C., *et al.* (2006) Vitamin D and calcium intake in relation to type 2 diabetes in women. *Diabetes Care*, **29**, 650–6.

Ramachandran, A., Snehalatha, C., Mary, S., Mukesh, B., Bhaskar, A. D. and Vijay, V. (2006) The Indian Diabetes Prevention Programme shows that lifestyle modification and metformin prevent type 2 diabetes in Asian Indian subjects with impaired glucose tolerance (IDPP-1). *Diabetologia*, **49**, 289–97.

Rojo-Martinez, G., Esteva, I., Ruiz de Adana, M. S., Garcia-Almeida, J. M., Tinahones, F., *et al.* (2006) Dietary fatty acids and insulin secretion: a population-based study. *Eur J Clin Nutr*.

Roumen, C., Corpeleijn, E., Feskens, E. J. M., Mensink, M., Saris, W. H. M. and Blaak, E. E. (2008) Impact of 3-year lifestyle intervention on postprandial glucose metabolism: the SLIM study. *Diabetic Medicine*, **25**, 597–605.

Salazar-Martinez, E., Willett, W. C., Ascherio, A., Manson, J. E., Leitzmann, M. F., *et al.* (2004) Coffee consumption and risk for type 2 diabetes mellitus. *Ann Intern Med*, **140**, 1–8.

Salmeron, J., Ascherio, A., Rimm, E. B., Colditz, G. A., Spiegelman, D., *et al.* (1997a) Dietary fiber, glycemic load, and risk of NIDDM in men. *Diabetes Care*, **20**, 545–50.

Salmeron, J., Hu, F. B., Manson, J. E., Stampfer, M. J., Colditz, G. A., *et al.* (2001) Dietary fat intake and risk of type 2 diabetes in women. *Am J Clin Nutr*, **73**, 1019–26.

Salmeron, J., Manson, J. E., Stampfer, M. J., Colditz, G. A., Wing, A. L. and Willett, W. C. (1997b) Dietary fiber, glycemic load, and risk of non-insulin-dependent diabetes mellitus in women. *JAMA*, **277**, 472–7.

Sargeant, L. A., Khaw, K. T., Bingham, S., Day, N. E., Luben, R. N., *et al.* (2001) Fruit and vegetable intake and population glycosylated haemoglobin levels: the EPIC-Norfolk Study. *Eur J Clin Nutr*, **55**, 342–8.

Sarkkinen, E., Schwab, U., Niskanen, L., Hannuksela, M., Savolainen, M., *et al.* (1996) The effects of monounsaturated-fat enriched diet and polyunsaturated-fat enriched diet on lipid and glucose metabolism in subjects with impaired glucose tolerance. *Eur J Clin Nutr*, **50**, 592–8.

Schulze, M. B., Liu, S., Rimm, E. B., Manson, J. E., Willett, W. C. and Hu, F. B. (2004a) Glycemic index, glycemic load, and dietary fiber intake and incidence of type 2 diabetes in younger and middle-aged women. *Am J Clin Nutr*, **80**, 348–56.

Schulze, M. B., Manson, J. E., Ludwig, D. S., Colditz, G. A., Stampfer, M. J., *et al.* (2004b) Sugar-sweetened beverages, weight gain, and incidence of type 2 diabetes in young and middle-aged women. *JAMA*, **292**, 927–34.

Somersalo, O. (1954) Studies of childhood diabetes. I. Incidence in Finland. *Ann Paediatr Fenn*, **1**, 239–49.

Song, Y., Manson, J. E., Buring, J. E. and Liu, S. (2004a) Dietary magnesium intake in relation to plasma insulin levels and risk of type 2 diabetes in women. *Diabetes Care*, **27**, 59–65.

Song, Y., Manson, J. E., Buring, J. E. and Liu, S. (2004b) A prospective study of red meat consumption and type 2 diabetes in middle-aged and elderly women: the women's health study. *Diabetes Care*, **27**, 2108–15.

Stampfer, M., Colditz, G., Willet, W., Manson, J., Arky, R., *et al.* (1988) A prospective study of moderate alcohol drinking and risk of diabetes in women. *Am J Epid*, **128**, 549–58.

Stene, L. C., Hongve, D., Magnus, P., Ronningen, K. S. and Joner, G. (2002) Acidic drinking water and risk of childhood-onset type 1 diabetes. *Diabetes Care*, **25**, 1534–8.

Stene, L. C. and Joner, G. (2003) Use of cod liver oil during the first year of life is associated with lower risk of childhood-onset type 1 diabetes: a large, population-based, case-control study. *Am J Clin Nutr*, **78**, 1128–34.

Stevens, J., Ahn, K., Juhaeri, J. Houston, D., Steffan, L. and Couper, D. (2002) Dietary fiber intake and glycemic index and incidence of diabetes in African-American and white adults: the ARIC study. *Diabetes Care*, **25**, 1715–21.

Storlien, L. H., Pan, D. A., Kriketos, A. D., O'connor, J., Caterson, I. D., *et al.* (1996) Skeletal muscle membrane lipids and insulin resistance. *Lipids*, **31** (Suppl), S261–5.

The Diabetes Prevention Program Research Group (2002) Reduction in the incidence of type 2 diabetes with lifestyle intervention or metformin. *N Engl J Med*, **346**, 393–403.

The Eurodiab Substudy 2 Study Group (1999) Vitamin D supplement in early childhood and risk for Type I (insulin-dependent) diabetes mellitus. *Diabetologia*, **42**, 51–4.

The Teddy Study Group (2007) The Environmental Determinants of Diabetes in the Young (TEDDY) study: study design. *Pediatr Diabetes*, **8**, 286–98.

The Trigr Study Group (2007) Study design of the Trial to Reduce IDDM in the Genetically at Risk (TRIGR). *Pediatr Diabetes*, **8**, 117–37.

Tuomilehto, J., Hu, G., Bidel, S., Lindström, J. and Jousilahti, P. (2004) Coffee consumption and risk of type 2 diabetes mellitus among middle-aged Finnish men and women. *JAMA*, **291**, 1213–19.

Tuomilehto, J., Lindström, J., Eriksson, J. G., Valle, T. T., Hämäläinen, H., *et al.* (2001) Prevention of type 2 diabetes mellitus by changes in lifestyle among subjects with impaired glucose tolerance. *N Engl J Med*, **344**, 1343–50.

Uusitalo, L., Kenward, M. G., Virtanen, S. M., Uusitalo, U., Nevalainen, J., *et al.* (2008a) Intake of antioxidant vitamins and trace elements during pregnancy and risk of advanced beta cell autoimmunity in the child. *Am J Clin Nutr*, **88**, 458–64.

Uusitalo, L., Knip, M., Kenward, M. G., Alfthan, G., Sundvall, J., *et al.* (2005) Serum alpha-tocopherol concentrations and risk of type 1 diabetes mellitus: a cohort study in siblings of affected children. *J Pediatr Endocrinol Metab*, **18**, 1409–16.

Uusitalo, L., Nevalainen, J., Niinisto, S., Alfthan, G., Sundvall, J., *et al.* (2008b) Serum alpha- and gamma-tocopherol concentrations and risk of advanced beta cell autoimmunity in children with HLA-conferred susceptibility to type 1 diabetes mellitus. *Diabetologia*, **51**, 773–80.

Valle, T., Tuomilehto, J. and Eriksson, J. (1997) Epidemiology of type 2 diabetes in Europids. In Alberti, K., Zimmet, P., Defronzo, R. and Keen, H. (eds) *International Textbook of Diabetes Mellitus*, 2nd edn, John Wiley and Sons Ltd.

van Dam, R. M., Rimm, E. B., Willett, W. C., Stampfer, M. J. and Hu, F. B. (2002a) Dietary patterns and risk for type 2 diabetes mellitus in U.S. Men. *Ann Intern Med*, **136**, 201–9.

van Dam, R. M., Willett, W. C., Manson, J. E. and Hu, F. B. (2006) Coffee, caffeine, and risk of type 2 diabetes: a prospective cohort study in younger and middle-aged U.S. women. *Diabetes Care*, **29**, 398–403.

van Dam, R. M., Willett, W. C., Rimm, E. B., Stampfer, M. J. and Hu, F. B. (2002b) Dietary fat and meat intake in relation to risk of type 2 diabetes in men. *Diabetes Care*, **25**, 417–24.

van De Vijver, L. P., Kardinaal, A. F., Couet, C., Aro, A., Kafatos, A., *et al.* (2000) Association between trans fatty acid intake and cardiovascular risk factors in Europe: the TRANSFAIR study. *Eur J Clin Nutr*, **54**, 126–35.

Verge, C. F., Howard, N. J., Irwig, L., Simpson, J. M., Mackerras, D. and Silink, M. (1994) Environmental factors in childhood IDDM. A population-based, case-control study. *Diabetes Care*, **17**, 1381–9.

Vessby, B., Uusitupa, M., Hermansen, K., Riccardi, G., Rivellese, A. A., *et al.* (2001) Substituting dietary saturated for monounsaturated fat impairs insulin sensitivity in healthy men and women: The KANWU Study. *Diabetologia*, **44**, 312–19.

Villegas, R., Gao, Y. T., Yang, G., Li, H. L., Elasy, T. A., *et al.* (2008a) Legume and soy food intake and the incidence of type 2 diabetes in the Shanghai Women's Health Study. *Am J Clin Nutr*, **87**, 162–7.

Villegas, R., Shu, X. O., Gao, Y. T., Yang, G., Elasy, T., *et al.* (2008b) Vegetable but not fruit consumption reduces the risk of type 2 diabetes in Chinese women. *J Nutr*, **138**, 574–80.

Virtanen, S. M., Hypponen, E., Laara, E., Vahasalo, P., Kulmala, P., *et al.* (1998) Cow's milk consumption, disease-associated autoantibodies and type 1 diabetes mellitus: a follow-up study in siblings of diabetic children. Childhood Diabetes in Finland Study Group. *Diabet Med*, **15**, 730–8.

Virtanen, S. M., Jaakkola, L., Rasanen, L., Ylonen, K., Aro, A., *et al.* (1994) Nitrate and nitrite intake and the risk for type 1 diabetes in Finnish children. Childhood Diabetes in Finland Study Group. *Diabet Med*, **11**, 656–62.

Virtanen, S. M., Kenward, M. G., Erkkola, M., Kautiainen, S., Kronberg-Kippila, C., *et al.* (2006) Age at introduction of new foods and advanced beta cell autoimmunity in young children with HLA-conferred susceptibility to type 1 diabetes. *Diabetologia*, **49**, 1512–21.

Virtanen, S. M. and Knip, M. (2003) Nutritional risk predictors of beta cell autoimmunity and type 1 diabetes at a young age. *Am J Clin Nutr*, **78**, 1053–67.

Virtanen, S. M., Laara, E., Hypponen, E., Reijonen, H., Rasanen, L., *et al.* (2000) Cow's milk consumption, HLA-DQB1 genotype, and type 1 diabetes: a nested case-control study of siblings of children with diabetes. Childhood diabetes in Finland study group. *Diabetes*, **49**, 912–17.

Virtanen, S. M., Rasanen, L., Aro, A., Lindström, J., Sippola, H., *et al.* (1991) Infant feeding in Finnish children less than 7 yr of age with newly diagnosed IDDM. Childhood Diabetes in Finland Study Group. *Diabetes Care*, **14**, 415–17.

Virtanen, S. M., Roivainen, M., Andersson, M. A., Ylipaasto, P., Hoornstra, D., *et al.* (2008) In vitro toxicity of cereulide on porcine pancreatic Langerhans islets. *Toxicon*, **51**, 1029–37.

Virtanen, S. M., Uusitalo, L., Kenward, M. G., Nevalainen, J., Uusitalo, U., *et al.* (in press) Maternal food consumptionduring pregnancy and risk of advanced beta-cell autoimmunityin the offspring. *Pediatr Diabetes*.

Weickert, M. O., Mohlig, M., Koebnick, C., Holst, J. J., Namsolleck, P., *et al.* (2005) Impact of cereal fibre on glucose-regulating factors. *Diabetologia*, **48**, 2343–53.

Weickert, M. O., Mohlig, M., Schofl, C., Arafat, A. M., Otto, B., *et al.* (2006) Cereal fiber improves whole-body insulin sensitivity in overweight and obese women. *Diabetes Care*, **29**, 775–80.

Wilkin, T. J. (2001) The accelerator hypothesis: weight gain as the missing link between Type I and Type II diabetes. Diabetologia, **44**, 914–22.

Wolever, T. M. and Mehling, C. (2002) High-carbohydrate-low-glycaemic index dietary advice improves glucose disposition index in subjects with impaired glucose tolerance. *Br J Nutr*, **87**, 477–87.

Wolever, T. M., Nguyen, P. M., Chiasson, J. L., Hunt, J. A., Josse, R. G., *et al.* (1994) Determinants of diet glycemic index calculated retrospectively from diet records of 342 individuals with non-insulin-dependent diabetes mellitus. *Am J Clin Nutr*, **59**, 1265–9.

World Health Organization (2003) Diet, nutrition and the prevenion of chronic diseases. Report of a joint FAO/WHO consultation. Geneva, World Health Organization.

Ziegler, A. G., Schmid, S., Huber, D., Hummel, M. and Bonifacio, E. (2003) Early infant feeding and risk of developing type 1 diabetes-associated autoantibodies. *Jama*, **290**, 1721–8.

12

Functional foods and cognition

A. Scholey, D. Camfield, L. Owen, A. Pipingas and C. Stough, Swinburne University, Australia

Abstract: Many people take nutraceuticals and supplements in the belief that they improve alertness or offset cognitive decline. Over the past decade or so there has been a large increase in the amount of research examining the links between diet, nutraceuticals and psychological function. This has revealed cognitive benefits from a number of sources. For example glucose administration improves cognitive functioning, and the mechanisms underlying this effect are increasingly understood. The glycaemic index (GI) of a food can also influence mental performance. There is also good evidence that certain dietary supplements have cognition-enhancing properties. These include endogenous substances which support neural structure and function (amino acids and polyunsaturated fatty acids). Other substances which improve cognitive function appear to do so by increasing energy availability to the brain either directly (e.g. creatine) or via improving cardiovascular functioning (e.g. CoQ10). Additionally certain herbal extracts can improve mood and cognitive function (in this chapter we use sage and lemon balm as examples). These effects are probably mediated by multiple actions including direct neurotransmitter modulation. Interestingly in the case of herbs, the behavioural effects are often in keeping with their usage in traditional medicine systems. There are numerous challenges in understanding the effects of nutraceuticals on cognition. As well as the issue of standardisation, there is the problem of understanding the mechanisms and underlying effects which involve multiple processes. These challenges are increasingly being met by new technologies which enhance our understanding of brain functioning.

Key words: cognition, memory, attention, ageing, glucose, herbal extract.

12.1 Introduction

'Cognitive functions' is a term used to describe brain functions which allow us to perceive, evaluate, store, manipulate, and use information from external sources (i.e. our environment) and internal sources (experience, memory, concepts, thoughts), and to respond to this information. Cognitive functions can be clustered into several main domains, including executive functions, memory, attention, perception,

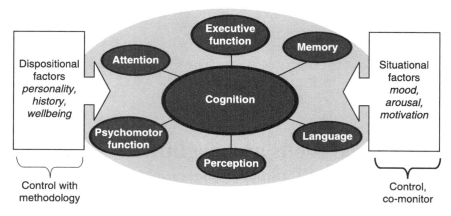

Fig. 12.1   An example taxonomy of measurable cognitive functions with some influences.

psychomotor functions and language (see Fig. 12.1). Each of the cognitive domains can be further divided in a number of more specified functions. Memory, for example, can be subdivided in numerous ways, including into working memory and episodic memory. Phases of memory processing include encoding, storage and retrieval. Further differentiation is made with regard to the sensory modality or type of information that is processed (auditory, visual, verbal, spatial, abstract, procedural). Attention can be subdivided in selective, focused, divided and sustained attention functions, whereas executive functions encompass more complex processes such as reasoning, planning, inhibition, concept formation, evaluation and strategic thinking.

It is important to note that despite their classification in separate cognitive functions, these various processes are often interlinked. Cognitive psychologists describe tasks as being more or less 'domain pure', but in reality this is unusual, efficient functioning of one cognitive process is often dependent on the integrity of others. For example, efficient storage of new information in long-term memory cannot occur without proper attention to the relevant information, adequate perceptual processing, and the use of executive learning strategies. By evaluating cognitive performance over a wide area of cognitive domains it is often possible to gain insight into the relative contribution of the separate domains. This is particularly important at the early stages of behavioural assessment of new compounds, ingredients or extracts.

12.2   Modulators of cognitive functions

Cognitive functioning is also mediated by a number of other factors, which are not themselves considered to be cognitive functions. These can be divided in two broad categories of 'dispositional' factors which include influences on an individual's demeanour, including their personality, developmental history and their current state of health (including psychological health and well-being). The other important mediators of cognitive function comprise 'situational' factors which can modulate cognition – these include an individual's mood, motivation or level of arousal. Both sets of factors present methodological challenges but these are not insurmountable and can be controlled and/or co-monitored with the appropriate methodology.

Mood state is also known to directly and indirectly modulate cognitive function as well as motivation. In addition, physical discomfort can adversely influence cognition. Again, these factors can influence each other. One key mediator of cognitive performance is the level of central arousal, a psychological concept that is used to describe performance changes due to mental fatigue or activation, sedation or stimulation. It is thought that the relationship between the level of arousal and task performance follows an inverted U-curve where performance is best at an optimal level of arousal and relative decrements can occur due to under- and over-arousal. The optimal level of arousal level is thought to be inversely related to task complexity. Mood state and physical well-being can be assessed using validated self-rating scales (visual analogue scales and questionnaires). Currently, no objective mood assessment methods are available, but changes in responses to stimuli with emotional valence in neuropsychological tests can provide some indication of mood states and changes therein.

Several compound measures that provide information on overall cognitive ability are also available. These typically consist of a (limited) selection of neuropsychological tests and/or questionnaires yielding a single, composite outcome measure. A well known example of this type of measure is IQ (intelligence quotient). Another example is the MMSE (Mini Mental State Examination) for dementia. These measures are often designed and validated as tools for comparative measures or clinical diagnosis of specific cognitive disorders, and although they are sometimes used in an experimental setting, their sensitivity to relatively subtle changes due to short-term nutritional interventions is limited.

Cognitive performance can vary considerably. Age, health, level of education and life events may affect cognitive performance between individuals. The performance level of an individual may also fluctuate due to factors such as fatigue, motivation, mood, hunger, thirst, adverse effects, stress, familiarity or hormonal status. Cognition can also be influenced by environmental factors, such as noise and ambient temperature. Controlling these factors as much as possible is essential to reduce variability and thus enhance study sensitivity. Using clear screening criteria, standardisation of the volunteers' condition by imposing living instructions dietary rules, restricting alcohol/drug intake, ensuring sufficient sleep, etc., and standardisation of the testing conditions (procedure, timing, instructions, appropriate facilities) helps reduce variability in test results.

12.3   Selection of appropriate cognitive outcome measures

Careful selection of the tests and other measurements is also essential. The test battery must be tailored to the nutritional manipulation. The cognitive domains that are most likely to be affected by the manipulation should be identified based on the best scientific data and the tests must be sensitive to the expected effect size. Furthermore the tests should be at the correct level of difficulty for the study population, thereby avoiding floor and ceiling effects. The test battery should assess multiple cognitive domains to determine the specificity of the effect. Mood changes and adverse effects of the manipulation should be incorporated in the test battery to assess their potential influence. Finally, the timing and duration of the assessments must be compatible with the onset and duration of the psychopharmacological effect of the manipulation. A lengthy task battery induces fatigue and may diminish motivation. When using a repeated-measures design, the use of matched, parallel versions of the cognitive tests is essential to avoid learning effects. It is well known that cognitive test performance may change with repeated assessments. Practice effects can manifest themselves as either a decline or improvement in performance (for example due to fatigue or improving skills respectively).

Understanding the way in which neural activity is translated into behaviour remains one of the biggest challenges to modern science. As well as possessing a unique information-processing capacity, the brain is also governed by the same biological processes and is subject to the same influences as other tissue. It follows that there are a number of ways of modulating brain activity and behaviour. Many of these processes can be modulated by dietary components.

12.4 Nutraceuticals and cognitive function

There are a number of reasons why one might expect foods to impact on cognitive function. First, the brain is the most metabolically active organ in the human body and is reliant on a constant supply of glucose in the bloodstream to function effectively. Secondly, some foods may have properties which optimise this high energy utilisation (e.g. through an effective glycaemic index). Thirdly, some nutraceuticals may influence the action of neurotransmitters which act as chemical signalling molecules in the brain. Finally, the high energy utilisation of the brain is not without costs and means that neural tissue is particularly susceptible to the damage from oxidative stress and related processes – some nutritional interventions may protect against such damage.

In terms of enhancing cognition there are numerous developmental stages which may be more or less susceptible to cognition enhancement. It is beyond the scope of this chapter to detail every nutraceutical with potential nootropic (cognition-enhancing) properties. Instead we will concentrate on selected examples in relation to cognitive enhancement in healthy children and young adults, and the prevention of cognitive decline in ageing.

12.5 Effects of ageing on cognition and brain biology

Declines in a range of cognitive abilities, including processing speed, episodic memory, spatial ability and reasoning have all been found to be associated with normal ageing (Hedden and Gabrieli, 2004). On the basis of longitudinal and cross-sectional brain imaging studies, these declines have been correlated most strongly with decreases in the volume of the prefrontal cortex (PFC) of the brain, occurring at a rate of around 5% per decade after the age of 20 (compared with around 2–3% per decade in other areas (Hedden and Gabrieli, 2004).

Reactive oxygen species (ROS) are ions or molecules, including free radicals and peroxides, that contain unpaired electrons making them highly reactive (Riley, 1994). ROS are found in the environment and are also produced in the body as a by-product of normal metabolism. While they are necessary for certain biological processes, excessive levels do considerable cellular damage, especially to brain tissue (Halliwell, 1992). According to the free radical theory of ageing (Harman, 1957), organisms age because of the accumulation of damage by these highly reactive molecules over time. Mitochondrial DNA, RNA and proteins are common targets of this damage (Cadenas and Davies, 2000). ROS that are commonly implicated in damage to neurons include superoxide, hydrogen peroxide and the hydroxyl radical. The reactive nitrogen species (RNS) peroxynitrite is also frequently implicated. The human brain, which consumes 20% of the body's total oxygen and contains a large proportion of polyunsaturated fatty acids in its neurons, is particularly vulnerable to damage by ROS (Halliwell, 1992). In a process known as lipid peroxidation, ROS sequester electrons from cell membranes, causing oxidative damage to the neurons.

A number of endogenous antioxidants such as glutathione (GSH) and superoxide dismutase (SOD) are produced by the body in order to counteract the effects of excess ROS and RNS (Rossi et al., 2008). However, compared with other tissue, the brain produces relatively low levels of antioxidant enzymes (Floyd, 1999), and as the brain ages it becomes increasingly vulnerable to oxidative damage (Gracy et al., 1999). Reasons for this increased susceptibility include an accumulation of transition metals such as iron and copper which catalyse hydroxyl radical production (Halliwell and Gutteridge, 1990; Zecca et al., 2004), as well as a decreased ability to modify genes involved in the production of antioxidant enzymes (Lu et al., 2004).

The brain's inflammatory response to oxidative stress is another important factor in both normal ageing and cognitive decline. Advanced age is essentially associated with a chronic low-level inflammation (Sarkar and Fisher, 2006) which may play a causative role in cognitive decline. Systemic inflammation has also been found to be associated with an increased risk of dementia (Gelinas et al., 2004).

The high energy requirements of the mammalian brain mean that it has a relatively high number of mitochondria per cell (Veltri et al., 2005). While mitochondria are essential for meeting the energy requirements of the cell, they are also major contributors to ROS production. A large turnover of molecular oxygen is required by mitochondria in order to provide energy in the form of adenosine triphosphate (ATP). However as the mitochondria process oxygen a certain proportion of ROS are generated due to electron leakage. Over time, oxidative damage to the mitochondria accumulates, rendering them less efficient at producing energy. Additionally oxidative damage to DNA can cause mutations in both mitochondrial and, to a lesser extent, cellular DNA. The end result of damage to DNA, together with damage to antioxidant enzymes and protein repair mechanisms themselves, is eventual cell death (Kidd, 2005). For these reasons, any substance that may act as an antioxidant in the mitochondria, or aid in enhancing its efficiency will play an important neuroprotective role. Alpha-lipoic acid, acetyl-L-carnitine and coenzyme Q10 are three substances that play an important role in mitochondria function and will be discussed later in the chapter.

12.6   Effects of glucose and carbohydrates

As the primary 'fuel' for brain function glucose has received a great deal of attention as a potential cognition enhancer. In general the finding is that following glucose loading in the form of administration of a drink containing 25 or 50 g, cognitive performance improves compared to drinking a sensorily matched control drink (containing saccharine or aspartame). The effect is most marked after an overnight fast, though is also observed within a few hours of a meal (Sünram-Lea *et al.*, 2001). It has also been suggested that glucose enhancement of cognition is most marked for more 'heavily loaded' tasks – i.e. those which require more mental effort to perform (Scholey, 2001; Scholey *et al.*, 2001, 2006, 2009).

The phenomenon has attracted attention for a number of reasons. First, glucose is the primary substrate for brain metabolism so the delineation of any differential effects on cognitive function might aid understanding of fundamental brain-behaviour relationships – for example whether certain cognitive functions are prioritised or limited by glucose availability. Secondly, processing emotional information leads to better memory and a release in blood glucose (Ford *et al.*, 2002). While this may indicate that glucose release underlies improved memory for emotional material, it has also been shown that the two processes can be dissociated (Parent, 2006; Scholey *et al.*, 2006). Thirdly, as an effect resulting from the ingestion of a simple carbohydrate, glucose enhancement of cognitive function offers a useful prototype to develop paradigms for studying the effects of more complex nutritional and nutrition-like interventions. Finally, poor glucose metabolism is a feature of a number of processes and psychopathologies which co-present with difficulties in cognitive performance including ageing, Down's syndrome, Alzheimer's disease, schizophrenia and others. Understanding the effects of glucose on cognitive performance may offer some insight into this aspect of the diseases. The hippocampus is rich in insulin receptors (Park 2001; Messier 2004) whose role in the brain, like other tissues, includes the promotion of cellular glucose uptake (e.g. Watson and Craft, 2008). As in other tissue, glucose enters the brain using facilitative transport via GLUT transporters, which are capable of plastic changes in response to region-specific task demands (Choeri *et al.*, 2004). Brain glucose is likely to be involved in metabolism rather than glycogen storage. Certain glucose transporters, including the insulin-sensitive GLUT4, are enriched in the hippocampus but appear to be more abundant in the cerebellum (Messari *et al.*, 2002; McEwen and Regen, 2004) where they may be implicated in the psychomotor deficits observed in diabetes (Ryan and Williams, 1993; Zhao *et al.*, 2004). Thus insulin-dependent glucose transport may underlie the preferential effects of glucose on psychomotor tracking over memory performance (Scholey *et al.*, 2009).

Although glucose loading provides useful information regarding the potential of foods to improve cognitive performance, it is neither practical nor desirable to use glucose drinks as cognitive enhancers in a real-world setting. Research has therefore concentrated on the effects of meals with differing GIs on cognitive function. In children, it has been shown that skipping breakfast leads to impaired cognitive function in the subsequent hours (Wesnes *et al.*, 2003). Furthermore comparing breakfasts with differing GIs showed that children's memory and attention was better following a lower than a higher GI breakfast (Ingwersen *et al.*, 2007). This result confirms earlier data in adults where a lower GI food was associated with better memory compared with a higher GI food (Benton *et al.*, 2003). Interestingly this paper showed that the difference in memory scores did not coincide with significant differences in blood glucose levels, suggesting that some other mechanism underlies the cognition enhancing effects. One possibility is that insulin production may be critically involved (Watson and Craft, 2004).

12.7   Nutraceuticals for cognitive enhancement

12.7.1   Phosphatidylserine

Phosphatidylserine (PS) is a naturally occurring membrane phospholipid that is found in high concentrations in brain tissue, where it comprises 10–20% of the total phospholipid pool (Pepeu *et al.*, 1996). PS plays an important role in a host of cellular functions including mitochondrial membrane integrity, presynaptic neurotransmitter release, postsynaptic receptor activity and activation of protein kinase C in memory formation (Kidd, 2008). Under normal conditions PS is contained within the inner leaflet of the plasma membrane, however in cases of cell death, apoptosis, it becomes exposed on the surface of the cell. With PS exposed, phagocytes recognise the cell as apoptotic and engulf it. Following this, anti-inflammatory cytokines are released by macrophages and microglia (Hashioka *et al.*, 2007). Phosphatidylserine is not easily obtained through dietary sources other than brain; however, exogenous PS can be manufactured from both bovine and vegetarian, soy bean, sources. Due to the risk of infectious encephalopathies, the vegetarian source of PS is currently favoured. Across a number of studies, the effects of the two forms of PS have been found to be equivalent (Osella *et al.*, 2008).

Being the main phospholipid of the plasma membrane PS plays a key role in the biosynthesis and release of neurotransmitters, with PS administration being found to enhance acetylcholine release (Vannucchi and Pepeu, 1987; Vannucchi *et al.*, 1990), as well as norepinephrine (Zanotti *et al.*, 1989), serotonin and dopamine (Argentiero and Tavolato, 1980). PS may also elevate glucose metabolism (Bruni *et al.*, 1976). In relation to the cholinergic system, PS has been found to restore age-related decreases in choline-acetyltransferase-positive neurons (Milan *et al.*, 1988) as well as densities of muscarinic and NMDA receptors (Nunzi *et al.*, 1989; Gelbmann and Muller, 1992). As the brain ages there is a reduction in the density of cell-surface receptors for nerve growth factor (NGF) which promotes neuronal differentiation and neuroplasticity. Animal research suggests that PS supplementation brings about increases in NGF-receptor density, with aged animals displaying associated increases in nueron numbers as well as size (Nunzi *et al.*, 1992) as a result. PS administration has also been found to provide protection from neuron death (Suzuki *et al.*, 1999), a finding that has been attributed to the ability of PS to increase membrane fluidity (Calderini *et al.*, 1985). It has also been found to display anti-inflammatory and antioxidant properties, inhibiting microglial activation as well as superoxide and nitric oxide production associated with amyloid-β protein (Hashioka *et al.*, 2007).

In six double-blind randomised trials PS has been found to be effective in ameliorating symptoms of Alzheimer's disease (AD). Clinical global impressions of change and activities of daily living have been found to be improved with daily doses of 200–300 mg for up to six months. In milder cases of AD, significant improvements to concentration, learning and memory for names, locations and recent events have also been observed (Kidd, 2008). In the largest of these studies using 494 elderly patients with moderate to severe AD, Cenacchi and colleagues (Cenacchi *et al.*, 1993) reported improvements to memory and learning following 300 mg PS/day for 6 months.

In relation to studies of PS supplementation in normal ageing, Crook and colleagues (Crook *et al.*, 1991) administered 300 mg/day PS to 149 elderly patients (aged 50–75 years) with age-associated memory impairment for 12 weeks, and observed significant improvements in performance tests of learning and recall abilities such as name-face matching. In a multi-centre trial by Villardita and colleagues (Villardita *et al.*, 1987), 300 mg/day PS vs placebo was administered to 170 aged patients for 90 days. Significant improvements in attention, concentration and short-term memory were found for those receiving PS.

There is an impressive amount of research pointing to the efficacy of PS as a neuroprotective agent which enhances both cholinergic function and neuroplasticity. However, the majority of clinical research to date has been restricted to investigations of the chronic use of PS in elderly populations with cognitive decline and dementia. It is yet to be established whether there is an acute nootropic (cognition enhancing) effect associated with PS, and whether supplementation in young healthy adults results in improvements to cognitive function.

12.7.2   Taurine

Taurine, 2-aminoethanesulfonic acid, is a naturally occurring sulfonic acid derived from cysteine which is the most abundant intracellular amino acid in the human body. Taurine is distributed throughout the body either free or in simple peptides, such as glutaurine in the brain. Higher concentrations are found in tissues that are excitable and prone to oxidative stress and in the adult brain, taurine content is second only to glutamate. Taurine is understood to play an important role in cellular membrane protection, either by reducing toxic substances or by acting as an osmoregulator (Jacobsen and Smith, 1968; Bergstrom *et al.*, 1974; Schaffer *et al.*, 2000). The human body possesses a limited ability to synthesise taurine from the precursors methionine and cysteine, occuring mainly in the liver and the brain. For this reason it has been described as a semi-essential amino acid. Average daily endogenous synthesis in adults ranges between 50–125 mg/day (Lourenco and Camilo, 2002) while average dietary intake of taurine in omnivores is around 123 mg/day, predominantly obtained through seafood and meat (Stapleton *et al.*, 1997). Taurine is commonly found in commercially available 'energy' drinks, such as the popular 'Red Bull' drink which contains 1000 mg of taurine per can (Alford *et al.*, 2001).

Peak plasma levels (t_{max}) of taurine following intraperitoneal injection have been found to occur at around 15–20 minutes. An exact half-life could not be found in the literature, although it was mentioned that plasma taurine values return to baseline again after about four hours. Taurine crosses the blood brain barrier freely through an active transport mechanism, with this process becoming saturated at higher concentrations (Korang *et al.*, 1996; Lallemand and De Witte, 2004).

Taurine levels have been found to be decreased in various brain regions in aged rodents (Banay-Schwartz *et al.*, 1989), while dietary supplementation with taurine has been found to partially restore tissue levels relative to age-matched controls (Eppler and Dawson, 2001). It has been suggested that taurine may augment cognitive function by enhancing inhibitory processes; acting as an agonist at both $GABA_A$ and glycine receptors (Del Olmo *et al.*, 2000; El Idrissi and Trenkner, 2004; Wu *et al.*, 2008). Taurine has also been found to cause long-lasting potentiation of synaptic transmission due to increasing presynaptic fiber excitability and synaptic efficacy through a hypothesised intracellular effect on Na+ channels (Galarreta *et al.*, 1996). Taurine has been found to counteract glutamate-induced mitochondrial damage and cell death through regulation of calcium homeostasis in neurons (El Idrissi and Trenkner, 2004). Under stressful conditions, taurine levels in the brain have been found to increase significantly, which suggests that it may play an important role in neuroprotection (Wu *et al.*, 1998).

So far there is not strong evidence to suggest that taurine has an acute effect on cognitive function in humans. A study by Bichler and colleagues (Bichler *et al.*, 2006) failed to find any significant improvement in short-term memory when taurine was administered concurrently with caffeine pills. Warburton and colleagues (Warburton *et al.*, 2001) investigated the cognitive effects of acute administration of a caffeinated, taurine-containing beverage vs placebo in 42 volunteers, controlling for sugar content. Significant improvements in attention and verbal reasoning were found for those receiving the taurine-containing beverage, although no effects on memory were observed. Similarly, in a study of the performance effects of Red Bull Energy Drink (containing 1000 mg taurine per drink as well as 80 mg caffeine and 600 mg glucuronolactone), Alford and colleagues (Alford et al., 2001) reported a significant improvement in mental performance including choice reaction time, concentration and immediate recall in participants receiving Red Bull in comparison to a control drink. An obvious limitation of these studies is that it is difficult to differentiate the cognitive effects of taurine in comparison to caffeine and other substances.

The experimental and preclinical research suggests that chronic taurine supplementation may be useful as a neuroprotective agent, particularly under stressful conditions or in aged populations where taurine levels are decreased. The clinical human research to date is very limited, with most studies confounding caffeine administration with taurine, and no investigation as to the chronic effects in humans appears in the literature. Further clinical trials are warranted, yet at present there is weak evidence in support of nootropic effects associated with acute or chronic taurine supplementation in humans.

12.7.3   Creatine

Creatine is a naturally occurring nitrogenous organic acid that is found in vertebrates, with around 95% of total human creatine found in skeletal muscle. Creatine can be formed endogenously from the amino acids arginine, glycine and methionine, and can also be obtained through dietary sources. Since creatine is concentrated in muscle tissue, the highest levels of creatine are found in fish and red meat. Following intestinal absorption, creatine is delivered to body tissues including the heart and smooth muscles, brain and testes. Creatine is metabolised and broken down in the muscles to the degradation product creatinine, which is eventually excreted in urine. The creatine store of an average-sized adult (70 kg) is approximately 120 g, with a daily turnover to creatinine being around 1.6% of the total (Balsom et al., 1995). It has been estimated that the typical omnivore consumes between 0.25–1 g of creatine per day. The creatine levels of vegetarian or vegan individuals are typically much lower than for omnivores (Conway and Clark, 1996).

The absorption of creatine has been found to demonstrate non-linear kinetics due to creatine transporter uptake in the gastrointestinal tract. For oral doses less than 10 g, peak plasma levels (t_{max}) have been found to occur in less than 2 hours, while for doses greater than 10 g t_{max} increases to >3 hours, while a 20 g dose displays a steady-state-like plateau due to saturation of gastrointestinal transporters. The elimination half-life ($t_{1/2}$) for creatine has been estimated to be between 0.68 and 2.1 hours (Persky et al., 2003). Creatine has been found to be safe and well-tolerated in chronic administration. A review in 2000 (Poortmans and Francaux, 2000) concluded that there was no evidence for adverse effects of creatine supplementation in healthy individuals. Occasional anecdotal reports of gastrointestinal disturbances and muscle cramps have been reported in the literature (Poortmans and Francaux, 2000).

Creatine is stored in the form of phosphocreatine, also known as creatine phosphate (PCr). In times of high energy demand, PCr is converted back to creatine in order to regenerate ATP from ammonium dihydrogen phosphate (ADP) (aerobically). In times of excess ATP when energy expenditure is low, creatine is converted back to PCr by donating a phosphate group back to form ADP. These reactions are catalysed by creatine kinases. Due to the role that creatine and PCr play in adjusting cellular metabolism to energy demands, they provide a temporal buffer of ATP concentration. PCr plays a particularly important role in tissues that have high, fluctuating energy demands such as muscle and brain. During times of increased brain activity, brain PCr decreases rapidly in order to maintain constant ATP levels (Sappey-Marinier *et al.*, 1992; Rango *et al.*, 1997). Through the use of nuclear magnetic resonance spectroscopy (NMRS) it has been demonstrated that creatine and PCr can be increased in the brains of healthy adults following creatine supplementation (Dechent *et al.*, 1999; Lyoo *et al.*, 2003).

There are relatively few studies assessing the effects of creatine on cognitive performance in humans, and of these only chronic effects have been reported. A study by McMorris and colleagues (McMorris *et al.*, 2006) assessed the effect of supplementation with 20 g creatine per day over seven days following 24 hours of sleep deprivation. Individuals receiving creatine supplementation demonstrated significantly reduced decrements in choice reaction time following sleep deprivation. In a further study, individuals receiving creatine supplementation demonstrated improved performance on a random number generation test of executive function following 36 hours of sleep deprivation (McMorris *et al.*, 2007a). In a further study by McMorris and colleagues (McMorris *et al.*, 2007b) supplementation with 20 g of creatine per day for seven days to elderly participants resulted in improved performance on random number generation, forward and backward number and spatial recall, and long-term memory tasks but no effect on backward recall performance. Using near infrared spectroscopy, Watanabe and colleagues (Watanabe *et al.*, 2002) reported that five days of 8 g/day creatine supplementation in healthy young participants was associated with task-evoked increases in cerebral oxygenated hemoglobin when repeatedly performing a simple mathematical calculation. On the basis of these results, the authors suggest that creatine may be useful in conditions of mental fatigue. In a study by Rawson and colleagues (Rawson *et al.*, 2008) in young adults under normal conditions (i.e. not fatigued), 0.03 g/kg creatine supplementation for six weeks was not found to be associated with any improvements on a cognitive test battery. However, chronic supplementation with 5 g/day creatine monohydrate over a six-week period in a vegetarian sample was found to have a significantly positive effect on both working memory (backward digit span) and general intelligence (Raven's Advanced Progressive Matrices).

The preclinical evidence suggests that creatine may be effective as a neuroprotective agent. The clinical evidence to date suggests that chronic supplementation with creatine may be effective in enhancing cognitive function under conditions of mental fatigue or sleep deprivation in young healthy individuals. There is also evidence to suggest that chronic creatine supplementation may be effective in enhancing cognitive function in elderly populations as well as vegetarians who may be deficient in creatine. However, further large scale clinical trials are needed in order to further assess the efficacy of creatine as a nootropic agent in populations of different ages.

12.7.4 *Melissa officinalis*

Melissa officinalis (lemon balm) is a perennial herb from the Lamiaceae family that is native to southern Europe and the Mediterranean and has a history of use dating back over 2000 years. Traditionally it was used as a mild sedative and anxiolytic, however early records from the middle ages indicate that it has also been long recognised for its positive effects on memory (Kennedy *et al.*, 2002). The putative biologically active compounds in *M. officinalis* include monoterpenoid aldehydes (including citronellal, neral and geranial), flavonoids and polyphenolic compounds such as rosmarinic acid and monoterpene glycosides (Mulkens *et al.*, 1985; Carnat *et al.*, 1998; Sadraei *et al.*, 2003).

There is evidence to suggest that *M. officinalis* enhances cholinergic transmission, based on the fact that it binds to both nicotinic and muscarinic acetylcholine receptors within the central nervous system (Perry *et al.*, 1996; Wake *et al.*, 2000). However, large variation in receptor binding affinities have been noted between varying strains and preparations of *M. officinalis*, with the more reliable action of the plant across samples being its calming effects (Kennedy *et al.*, 2003). The anxiolytic effects of *M. officinalis* are most likely due to a non-cholinergic mechanism that is yet to be identified. There is also evidence to suggest that *M. officinalis* acts as a moderately effective free radical scavenger, which can be attributed to its flavonoid content (Hohmann *et al.*, 1999; Mantle *et al.*, 2000).

A number of studies have investigated the anxiolytic effects of *M. officinalis*, however a discussion of these findings is beyond the scope of the current report. In relation to cognitive effects, two recent studies by Kennedy and colleagues (Kennedy *et al.*, 2002, 2003) have investigated the effects of acute administration. In the first of these studies 20 healthy young participants received single doses of 200, 600 and 900 mg *M. officinalis* ethanolic extract vs placebo in a randomised, double-blind, crossover design. At 1, 2.5, 4 and 6 hours following dosing their cognitive performance was assessed using the Cognitive Drug Research (CDR) test battery together with serial subtraction tasks. Accuracy at attention was found to be significantly improved following the middle dose of 600 mg of *M. officinalis*, however at the highest dose (900 mg) decrements in memory performance together with reduced alertness were observed.

In vitro analysis of the extract revealed low binding affinity for nicotinic and muscarinic receptors, prompting Kennedy and colleagues to conduct a further study using an extract with greater cholinergic activity. In the second study, eight samples of *M. officinalis* were screened using *in vitro* analysis, and the extract with the highest binding affinity for both muscarinic and nicotinic receptors. Following a similar crossover design to the previous study, 600 mg, 1000 mg and 1600 mg *M. officinalis* extract vs placebo was then administered to 20 healthy young participants. At the highest dosage level of 1600 mg performance on the

Quality of Memory factor of the CDR was found to be significantly improved at both 3 and 6 hours post-dose. At the lowest dose (600 mg) performance decrements were noted for the same timed memory tasks used in the previous study, together with a newly introduced task of rapid visual information processing (RVIP). These effects were found to decrease as the dose was increased, with the authors speculating that two distinct mechanisms of action could explain the results. Presumably the cholinergic effect associated with the extract was responsible for the improvements to cognition, an effect which only counteracted a sedative effect at the higher dosage levels (>1000 mg).

In relation to the chronic effects of *M. officinalis*, a study by Akhondzadeh and colleagues (Akhondzadeh *et al.*, 2003a) investigated the efficacy of 60 drops/day tincture vs placebo over a four-month period in 35 patients with mild to moderate AD, aged 65 and 80 years. Cognitive function, as measured by the ADAS-Cog and clinical dementia rating scale, was found to be significantly improved in comparison to placebo at four months.

Regarding *M. officinalis* it appears that there are other nutraceutical compounds with more well established cholinergic effects. The primary effect for this substance appears to be one of mood modulation, rather than cognitive enhancement. While careful selection of an extract which demonstrates higher binding affinity for nicotinic and muscarinic receptors may improve its efficacy, it appears that there are more potent nootropic agents to choose from.

12.7.5 *Salvia officinalis*

Salvia officinalis is part of the Salvia genus in the Labiatae family, containing over 700 species of plants. It has been used over several millennia across a number of different cultures including Ayurvedic medicine, as well as early Greek and Chinese civilisations as a treatment for the amelioration

The proposed mechanisms of action for *S. officinalis* include acetylcholinesterase inhibition (ChEI), butyrylcholinesterase inhibition (BuChe), antioxidant, anti-inflammmatory and oestrogenic effects (Perry *et al.*, 1999; Kennedy and Scholey, 2006).

To date two randomised controlled trials have been conducted to assess the acute memory enhancing effects of *S. officinalis*. A study by Kennedy and colleagues (2006) examined the acute effects of *S. officinalis* on cognition in 30 healthy participants, who completed a test battery at baseline as well as 1 hour and 4 hours post dose on three separate testing occasions. On each occasion they received a different treatment, either placebo, 300 or 600 mg of dried sage leaf. The higher dose was found to be associated with improved performance on the Stroop test as well as an aggregate score obtained from a battery of tests including tasks of mathematical processing and memory search tasks at both post-dose time points.

In a more recent study by Scholey and colleagues (2008), the acute effects of *S. officinalis* on memory was examined using 20 elderly volunteers (over 65) administered 167, 333, 666 and 1332 mg of dried sage and tested 1, 2.5, 4 and

6 hours post-dose. Significant improvements in secondary memory performance (aggregate percentage accuracy in word recognition, picture recognition, immediate word recall and delayed word call from the CDR battery) were noted for the 333 mg dose in comparison to placebo at all post-dose time points. The extracts used in the study were subjected to *in vitro* analysis, confirming cholinesterase-inhibiting properties in comparison to an ethanol control sample. These findings have been corroborated by investigations into the acute effects of *Salvia lavandulaefolia* essential oil, another ChEI of the Sage family containing similar components to *S. officinalis*. A study by Tildesley and colleagues (2003) reported a significant improvement in immediate and delayed word recall post-dose using a 50 μl dose of the oil in 20 young healthy volunteers. A second study by Tildesley and colleagues (2005) using the CDR battery reported an improvement in secondary memory performance at 1 hour post-dose and Speed of Memory at 2.5 hours post-dose using 25 μl of *S. lavandulaefolia*. Improvements in speed of memory at 4 and 6 hours post-dose were also reported with the higher dose of 50 μl.

In regard to studies of the chronic effects of *S. officinalis* among the clinical population, a study by Akhondzadeh and colleagues (2003b) examined the effects of *S. officinalis* on memory in 39 AD patients. Significantly improved scores on the ADAS-Cog were reported for those in the *S. officinalis* group in comparison to placebo at 16 weeks. However, this study was not without criticism, with reviewers drawing attention to the unexpectedly large effect size, an ill-defined herb extract and no description of the placebo (Kennedy and Scholey, 2006). However, an open label trial using the *S. lavandulaefolia* essential oil from the Sage family by Perry and colleagues (2003) also reported a significant improvement in the accuracy of performing a vigilance task at the six-week end point amongst 11 AD patients.

To date the findings from the relatively few studies that have been conducted using *S. officinalis* and *S. lavandulaefolia* are promising, suggesting efficacy associated with both acute and chronic supplementation. Further randomised control trials (RCT)s, as well as longitudinal studies, using larger samples from both the non-clinical population as well as mild cognitive impairment (MCI) and AD patients are warranted in order to properly establish the efficacy of these nutraceuticals as nootropics.

12.7.6   Alpha-lipoic acid (ALA)

Alpha-lipoic acid (also referred to as lipoic acid) is a coenzyme involved in mitochondrial metabolism. Once it has crossed the blood brain barrier it is reduced to dihydrolipoic acid which is a powerful mitochondrial antioxidant reacting with oxidants such as superoxide radicals, hydroxyl radicals, hypochlorous acid, peroxyl radicals and singlet oxygen (Liu, 2008).

Peak plasma levels of alpha-lipoic acid have been found to occur between 10 to 45 minutes following oral administration. The elimination half-life ($t_{1/2}$) for alpha-lipoic acid has been reported to be 0.56 hours (Teichert *et al.*, 2003).

There is evidence to suggest multiple mechanisms of action with this compound including increased ACh production by activation of choline acetyltransferase, increased glucose uptake, chelation of redox-active transition metals, scavenging of ROS reducing inflammatory cytokine levels, scavenging of lipid peroxidation products and induction of enzymes required for glutathione synthesis (Maczurek *et al.*, 2008).

The use of LA as a treatment for dementia was discovered serendipitously in 1997 due to a case study featuring an elderly patient with mild AD concurrently receiving LA for treatment of diabetic polyneuropathy. LA has been used as a treatment for diabetic polyneuropathy in Germany for over 30 years. The patient received 600 mg LA on a daily basis in conjunction with a standard course of ChEI for AD. Over the following years neuropsychological tests revealed an unusually slow progress of cognitive impairment, and the diagnosis of mild AD was reassessed several times (Maczurek *et al.*, 2008). On the basis of this case study the first open pilot study of LA in the treatment of dementia was conducted in 2001. Hager and colleagues (2001) administered 600 mg LA daily to nine elderly patients with probable AD in conjunction with their standard ChEI treatment over a period of 337 ± 80 days. Treatment with LA was found to stabilise previously declining scores in cognitive function, as measured by MMSE and ADAS-Cog for approaching 12 months.

A follow-up study was conducted by Hager and colleagues (2007), in which the analysis was extended to 43 patients receiving the same 600 mg daily dose of LA over a 48-month period. In patients with mild dementia the disease was found to progress extremely slowly, while for patients with moderate dementia it progressed at around twice the rate. The authors reported that the rate of cognitive decline was dramatically lower than that reported for untreated patients or patients on standard ChEI treatments in the second year of long-term studies. While these preliminary findings are promising it is important to note that this trial was not randomised or double-blinded and patients were only diagnosed with probable AD, and for these reasons a larger scale Phase II RCT is needed in order to gain stronger evidence of efficacy of LA in the treatment of AD.

These sentiments were echoed by the Cochrane review (Klugman *et al.*, 2004), in which no current randomised double-blind trials were discovered. Two recently completed clinical trials that have combined lipoic acid with other interventions are yet to be published. Shinto (2004) has presented an abstract from an RCT using omega-3 fatty acid in conjunction with lipoic acid for 39 participants with probable AD, with findings suggesting advantages over placebo in MMSE and activities of daily living. Galasko (2005) conducted an RCT using vitamins C and E in conjunction with lipoic acid in a sample of 75 participants with probable AD, however the findings are yet to be released. At present no other ongoing trials for lipoic acid have been found.

Preclinical studies have provided strong evidence for the neuroprotective properties of alpha-lipoic acid. There is also promising clinical evidence to suggest that alpha-lipoic acid may be effective in slowing down the progression of cognitive decline and dementia in elderly participants. However, to date little is known of the acute cognitive effects, or its efficacy as a chronic supplementation strategy for cognitive enhancement in young and healthy populations.

12.7.7   Acetyl-L-carnitine (ALCAR)

Acetyl-L-carnitine (ALCAR) is an endogenous mitochondrial membrane compound involved in the maintenance of mitochondrial function as well as the production of acetylcholine in cholinergic neurons.

Peak plasma levels (t_{max}) of ALCAR have been found to occur at around 3.1 ± 0.2 hours following oral administration of a 500 mg tablet. Subsequent to oral administration, ALCAR easily crosses the blood-brain barrier. The elimination half-life ($t_{1/2}$) for ALCAR has been reported to be 4.2 ± 1.6 hours (Kwon and Youn, 2004). Oral supplementation using ALCAR 2 g/day has been found to increase circulating ALCAR content by 43% (Rebouche, 2004).

ALCAR facilitates the transport of long chain fatty acids from the cytoplasm to the mitochondria, where they can be used as substrates for the oxidative phosphorylation process that produces ATP (Pettegrew et al., 2000). ALCAR also aids in protecting mitochrondria from oxidative damage and boosts the production of ATP (Beal et al., 2003; Mazzio et al., 2003).

It has been found that ALCAR has a beneficial effect in AD by reducing amyloid β (Aβ) formation, via the stimulation of α-secretase activity and cleaving APP to block Aβ from forming (Epis et al., 2008). It has also been found that ALCAR up-regulates levels of the endogenous antioxidant glutathione as well as heat shock proteins which have a neuroprotective effect against Aβ toxicity (Abdul et al., 2006).

In an early study by Pettegrew and colleagues (1995) ALCAR was administered to seven probably AD patients, in comparison to five placebo-treated probably AD patients and 21 healthy age-matched controls over a 12-month period. MRS scans were taken at baseline and at follow-up, together with MMSE and ADAS tests. Brain measures of membrane phospholipid and high-energy phosphate metabolism revealed by MRS were found to be normalised at follow-up compared to baseline in the ALCAR group in comparison to the placebo group. This corresponded with significantly less deterioration in MMS and ADAS scores in the ALCAR group in comparison to the placebo group.

In a meta-analysis of the efficacy of ALCAR in the treatment of MCI and mild AD using RCTs of 3–12 months in duration and 1.5–3.0 g/day ALCAR dose, Montgomery and colleagues (2003) concluded that ALCAR had a clear benefit over placebo in slowing the rate of cognitive decline from three months onwards. However, a more recent Cochrane's review (Hudson and Tabet, 2003) of 16 studies ranging from 3 months to 1 year using 30–431 participants given 1–3 g ALCAR for the treatment of AD concluded that there was no evidence to recommend its routine use in clinical practice. Interestingly, a statistically significant treatment effect for MMSE was observed at 24 weeks, while it was not present at 52 weeks. Similarly, clinical global impression of change was found to be significantly higher for the ALCAR treatment in comparison to placebo at 12 and 24 weeks when treated as a dichotomous variable.

While the authors attribute these findings to statistical chance, it appears that ALCAR may require further investigation. Hudson and Tabet (2003) also draw attention to the fact that there is limited pharmacokinetic data available regarding ALCAR metabolism in humans. For this reason, there may exist large inter-individual variability in ALCAR plasma levels across patients in these studies. It is foreseeable that more consistent results may appear if the dose selection was determined using pharmacokinetic analysis. Since the time of the Cochrane's review no further RCTs have appeared in the literature, although a clinical trial is currently underway amongst MCI patients as part of the Memory XL study, where ALCAR is administered together with a range of other vitamins.

The experimental and preclinical data demonstrates that ALCAR is a neuroprotective agent that is useful in ameliorating neurodegenerative symptoms. There is also evidence to suggest that chronic ALCAR supplementation is effective in slowing the rate of cognitive decline and dementia in clinical samples. However, further research into both the acute and chronic effects of ALCAR supplementation in healthy populations is required to in order to assess its efficacy as a nootropic for general consumption.

12.7.8   Co-enzyme Q10 (ubiquinone)

Co-enzyme Q10 (CoQ10) is a lipid soluble antioxidant that has been found to up-regulate mitochondrial function and facilitate the synthesis of ATP. A deficiency in CoQ10 is detrimental to brain function, associated with both an increase in oxidative stress as well as a reduction in ATP synthesis (Quinzii et al., 2008).

The intestinal absorption of exogenous CoQ10 is limited and slow due to its hydrophobicity and large molecular weight (Zhang et al., 1995). For this reason, many commercially available CoQ10 capsules are combined with oil suspensions or administered in more water-soluble forms in order to aid absorption. Bioavailability is typically as low as 3%, but can be increased up to 15% when combined with another substance such as a water-soluble form of vitamin E (Nishimura et al., 2009). Using a standard gel-cap formulation at a dosage level of 200 mg/kg in rats, peak plasma levels (t_{max}) of CoQ10 have been estimated to occur at around 4.1 ± 0.7 hours following oral administration. The elimination half-life ($t_{1/2}$) for CoQ10 has been estimated to be 2.4 ± 0.7 hours (Li et al., 2008b).

CoQ10 plays a crucial role in oxidative phosphorylation, passing electrons from complexes I and II to complex III, while also providing antioxidant protection for the inner membrane of the mitochondria (Alberts et al., 2002). It has also been implicated in the production of α-tocopherol (vitamin E), with α-tocopherol acting as a direct scavenger of radicals to form tocopheroxyl radical, and the reduced form of ubiquinone, ubiquinol, reacting with tocopheroxyl radical to convert it back into α-tocopherol (McDonald et al., 2005). CoQ10 exerts neuroprotective effects by activation of mitochondrial uncoupling proteins, resulting in reduction of mitochondrial free radical generation (Chaturvedi and Beal, 2008) and has also been found to have a wide-reaching effect on the pattern of gene expression, affecting the expression of hundereds of human genes involved in cell signalling, metabolism and nutrient transport (Groneberg *et al.*, 2005). With particular relevance to neurodegenerative diseases, CoQ10 has been found to exert anti-inflammatory properties via modulation of gene expression controlling tumor necrosis factor alpha (TNF-α) secretion (Schmelzer *et al.*, 2008).

Sohal and colleagues (2006) reviewed the results of a series of studies investigating CoQ10 supplementation in healthy mammals. They demonstrated that CoQ10 administration via food to young adult mice or rats resulted in augmentation of CoQ10 levels in plasma as well as in homogenates and mitochondria of liver, heart and skeletal muscle. An increase was also observed in mitochondria of the brain, but of a lesser magnitude. Greater increases in CoQ10 were observed in mitochondria in comparison to homogenate across all tissues. It was also found that the longer the period of CoQ10 administration, the greater the augmentation of CoQ10 levels in the body. However, despite the resulting increase in CoQ10 levels due to dietary supplementation, no evidence has been found to suggest that supplementation affects levels of oxidative stress and mitochondrial respiratory function in healthy mammals. Sohal and colleagues (2006) found that long-term CoQ10 intake lasting 2.5 up to 25 months in mice had no effect on either mitochondrial respiratory capacity, levels of oxidative stress or long-term survival. It was concluded that while CoQ10 acts as an antioxidant *in vitro*, it has no discernable *in vivo* effects on levels of oxidative stress or mitochondrial respiratory functions.

There is evidence to suggest that CoQ10 has a neuroprotective effect on cholinergic neurons, with enhanced performance with CoQ10 supplementation observed in rats completing the Morris water maze who sustained oxidative damage to the hippocampus and cerebral cortex (Ishrat *et al.*, 2006). There is also evidence to suggest that CoQ10 provides protection against loss of dopamine in Parkinson's Disease (PD). The MPTP neurotoxin has been used as a model of PD because it produces neuropathologic changes in human and non-human primates analogous to those observed in PD (Beal, 2001). Cleren and colleagues (2008) found that both CoQ10 and its reduced form ubiquinol were effective in providing neuroprotection against MPTP-induced loss of dopamine (DA) in mice. When MPTP was administered chronically for one month, CoQ10 was also found to be neuroprotective against DA depletion. Similar findings have been reported in regards to the neuroprotective effect of CoQ10 against striatal lesions in rats produced by aminoxyacetic acid and the mitochondrial toxin malonate and 3-NP (Chaturvedi and Beal, 2008).

Evidence for the potential of CoQ10 in the treatment of AD has been provided by transgenic mice models of AD. Li and colleagues (2008a) administered CoQ10 to double transgenic amyloid precursor protein (APP)/presenilin 1 (PS1) mice, as well as single transgenic APP and PS1 mice for 60 days. MRI scans revealed that significantly less atrophy in hemisphere and hippocampi occurred in those treated with CoQ10 in comparison to placebo. The neuroprotective effect was greater in the APP/PS1 mice compared to the APP and PS1 mice. Recent research has also found decreased Aβ42 levels, decreased β-amyloid plaque area and number, as well as improvements to cognitive performance following CoQ10 treatment in the Tg19959 transgenic mouse model of AD (Chaturvedi and Beal, 2008). Research by Ono and colleagues (2003) have provided findings suggesting that CoQ10 exerts its anti-amyloidogenic effect by destablising preformed β-amyloid fibrils *in vitro*.

A common trend is yet to emerge from the literature in regards to age-related changes in CoQ10 levels in humans (Sohal and Forster, 2007). There is a widespread assumption that CoQ10 levels decline over the course of the lifespan (Ernster and Dallner, 1995), however there is currently little evidence to support this view. Analysis of differences in blood plasma levels of both ubiquinone and ubiquinol in young compared to older adults has revealed that these levels are largely unchanged (Miles *et al.*, 2003, 2004). However, there is evidence to suggest that the redox status of CoQ10 (%CoQ10), ubiquinone/(ubiquinone + ubiquinol) $\times$ 100, is greater in older people, presumably due to the increased oxidation of ubiquinol back to ubiquinone associated with enhanced oxidative stress in the elderly. For this reason it has been proposed as a potential biomarker of ageing (Wada *et al.*, 2007).

The evidence for differences in tissue homogenates is also non-conclusive. An oft-cited earlier study by Kalen and colleagues (1989), reported that CoQ10 in human tissue homogenates from various organs was lower in older compared to younger people. However, a study by Beyer and colleagues (1985) reported no age-related changes in CoQ10 levels in homogenates of rat brain and lungs and decreases for heart, kidney and skeletal muscles. Sohal and colleagues (Sohal *et al.*, 2006) reported no age-related losses in CoQ10 content in tissue homogenates of mouse liver, heart, kidney, skeletal muscle or brain. A review by Sohal and Forster (2007) concluded that age-associated changes in CoQ10 content were most evident in mitochondria rather than tissue homogenates (Lass *et al.*, 1999; Kamzalov and Sohal, 2004), which is in line with the current understanding that there is a preferential cellular uptake of CoQ10 into the mitochrondria (Saito *et al.*, 2009). However, there is insufficient evidence to suggest that this pattern occurs throughout the body, as so far age-related declines in mitochondrial CoQ10 levels have only been observed in certain tissues.

Despite the intensive research focus that CoQ10 has received using animals, there have been relatively few RCTs conducted in clinical patients. Of the trials that have been conducted, the majority have been in relation to PD. In a Phase II clinical trial in 20 early PD patients, Shults and colleagues (2002) administered 300, 600 and 1200 mg/day of CoQ10 together with vitamin E at 2000 IU/day over a 16 month period. A significant dose-dependent Unified Parkinson's Disease Rating Scale score reduction was observed in patients administered CoQ10 in comparison to placebo. A subsequent dose escalation study up to 3600 mg/day revealed that plasma CoQ10 levels reach a plateau at 2400 mg/day (Shults *et al.*, 2004). Currently, no RCTs of CoQ10 in AD have been conducted, although a few RCT have been conducted in AD patients using the synthetic, shorter chained CoQ derivative Idebenone. A double-blind, placebo-controlled multi-centre study of 300 AD patients receiving Idebenone revealed a significant improvement in ADAS score after six months, as part of a two-year study (Weyer *et al.*, 1997). Two subsequent trials reported similar improvements with Idebenone treatment slowing the progression of cognitive deficits in AD patients (Gutzmann and Hadler, 1998; Gutzmann *et al.*, 2002). To date, no clinical trials examining the cognitive effects of CoQ10 in healthy adult populations have been conducted, and as such the role of CoQ10 in the prevention of dementia is unclear.

A lesser known function of CoQ10 is its role as a lipid-soluble carrier of electrons across the cellular membrane. External quinine oxidases, known as ENOX proteins, drive plasma membrane oxidoreductases (PMOR) activity that is used in glycolysis. Of these proteins, the age-related ENOX protein (arNOX) is located on the outside of the cell membrane and generates superoxide at the cell surface. The superoxide can then form H_2O_2 and other ROS that spread to adjacent cells and tissues. Before the age of 30 years arNOX proteins are barely detectable, and then steadily increase with age until 60–70 years. CoQ10 has been found to inhibit the formation of arNOX by binding to a site that is unique to arNOX (Morre and Morre, 2003, 2006). A study by Morre and colleagues (2008) investigated the effect of CoQ10 supplementation on the activity of the NADH oxidase (arNOX) protein in 25 healthy female participants between the ages of 45 and 65 years. Using a 3×60 mg daily dose of CoQ10, arNOX activity was found to be reduced between 25 and 30% overall, and approaching 40% for ages 51 to 65 years compared to all participants.

In regards to the acute effects of CoQ10 administration, to date no study has explicitly investigated nootropic effects, yet a small number of studies have investigated the effects of CoQ10 on myocardial function. Of these, one study used an oral form of CoQ10 and collected data on biomarkers of oxidative stress in athletes. Cooke and colleagues (Cooke *et al.*, 2008) administered a fast-melt form of CoQ10 to healthy trained and untrained athletes, and found that biomarkers of oxidative stress were decreased and muscle concentrations of CoQ10 were increased at 60 minutes post-dose. A single dose of CoQ10 was found to be associated with a trend towards lower serum SOD, whereas malondialdehyde tended to be significantly higher. Plasma CoQ10 levels were also found to be significantly correlated with muscle CoQ10 levels.

The experimental and preclinical data provides strong evidence for CoQ10 as a neuroprotective agent. There is also limited clinical evidence to suggest that CoQ10 and the synthetic form idebenone are effective in ameliorating symptoms associated with Huntington's and AD. However, despite the widespread commercial sale of CoQ10 as a nootropic dietary supplement, there is inconclusive evidence in support its efficacy in healthy individuals. Further research is also required in order to establish if significant age-related declines in CoQ10 occur. Improvements in CoQ10 capsule formulation will aid in improving bioavailability, which may result in greater efficacy especially in regards to acute effects. At this stage, further large scale clinical trials are needed in order to establish the efficacy of CoQ10 as a nootropic for general consumption.

12.7.9   Docosahexaenoic acid (DHA)

Docosahexaenoic acid (DHA) is a polyunsaturated omega-3 fatty acid commonly found in fish oils and constitutes more than 30% of the total phospholipid composition of plasma membranes in the brain (Gomez-Pinilla, 2008). The human body is inefficient in synthesising DHA itself, and for this reason we are largely reliant on dietary sources (Plourde and Cunnane, 2007). Epidemilogical studies have linked dietary deficiency of DHA to an increased risk of several disorders including ADHD, dyslexia, mood disorders and dementia (Freeman *et al.*, 2006).

Omega-3 fatty acid ethyl esters are well absorbed from the intestine, with DHA taken up predominantly into triacylglicerols rather than cholesteryl esters. In a multiple dose study, where 1-g capsules containing omega-3 fatty acid ethyl esters containing 45% DHA were administered every 8 hours, peak plasma levels (t_{max}) of DHA were found to occur on average at 5.96 ± 2.24 hours following oral administration. After 24 days of continues administration, DHA levels were found to be on average double compared to baseline (Rusca *et al.*, 2009).

DHA plays an important role in supporting neural plasticity and cognition, stimulating hippocampal levels of brain-derived neurotrophic factor (BDNF) which facilitates synaptic transmission and long term potentiation required for memory and learning (Gomez-Pinilla, 2008). BDNF is found to be depleted in AD hippocampus and has been implicated in the positive effects of exercise on cognition (Neeper *et al.*, 1995). DHA has also been found to stimulate mitochondrial function and glucose utilisation and transport, resulting in reduced oxidative stress in the brain (Wu *et al.*, 2004; Pifferi *et al.*, 2007). Further, a lipoxygenase metabolite of DHA, neuroprotectin D1 (NPD1), plays an important neuroprotective role by up-regulating anti-apoptotic and down-regulating pro-apoptotic mediators of cell death (Bazan, 2005).

In 2005 the US Department of Health and Human Services requested a meta-analysis of research into omega-3 fatty acid and dementia. On the basis of this review it was concluded that there was sufficient evidence to warrant clinical trials for the treatment and prevention of AD using omega-3 fatty acids (Maclean *et al.*, 2005). However, to date few randomised controlled trials (RCTs) with DHA have been conducted, and of those that have been conducted, no clear benefit of DHA supplementation on cognitive function is yet to emerge. Cunnane and colleagues (2009) recently conducted an extensive review assessing the current status of DHA in the treatment and prevention of dementia, comparing evidence from epidemiological studies, RCTs and animal research. They concluded that future RCTs need greater focus in addressing specific mechanisms of action by which DHA may exert a neuroprotective effect and that at this stage there is greater evidence for DHA playing a preventative role in AD, rather than being an effective treatment.

Cole and colleagues (2009) argue strongly for the use of antioxidants in combination with DHA supplementation, particularly in cases of late stage AD. They base this argument on the fact that Aβ increases oxidative damage to the brain, and considering that DHA is readily oxidised, antioxidants such as vitamin E and C are necessary in order to stop toxic oxidised forms of DHA from forming. Their argument is in line with the findings from previous independent clinical trials by Freund-Levi *et al.* (2006), Kotani (2006) and Chiu (2008) in which DHA was found to stabilise MMSE scores in cases of MCI but not once AD was established.

Another factor that appears to play an important role in the efficacy of DHA for cognitive improvement is polymorphisms in apolipoprotein E (ApoE). It has been estimated that 23% of the Caucasian population carries the $\varepsilon 4$ allele of ApoE, which is the genetic risk factor most associated with late-onset AD (Jofre-Monseny et al., 2008). A recent study provides evidence to indicate that higher fish intake is not associated with the same benefit in dementia risk for carriers of the ApoE4 allele in comparison to non-carriers (Huang et al., 2005). Cunnane and colleagues (2009) have provided preliminary findings to indicate that the ApoE4 genotype influences the metabolism of DHA, with DHA not being incorporated into plasma lipids to the same extent for carriers of the $\varepsilon 4$ allele in comparison to non-carriers.

At present, further trials are required in order to assess the nootropic efficacy of DHA supplementation in non-clinical samples. However, one recent study by van de Rest and colleagues (van de rest et al., 2008) investigated the effect of eicosapentaenoic acid (EPA) and docosahexaenoic acid (DHA) supplementation on cognitive performance in 302 cognitively healthy individuals aged 65 years or older. Participants were randomly assigned to either a high dose fish oil group (1800 mg/d EPA-DHA), or a low dose fish oil group (400 mg/d EPA-DHA), or placebo group for 26 weeks. Plasma concentrations of EPA-DHA increased by 238% in the high-dose and 51% in the low-dose fish oil group compared with placebo over the course of the trial. However, no significant between-group differences were found after 26 weeks in *any* cognitive domains, including attention, sensorimotor speed, memory, and executive function.

While it is apparent that DHA is an important substance for brain function, there is currently inconclusive evidence to suggest that supplementation beyond the normal dietary range has any benefit for cognitive function in clinical and non-clinical samples alike. The epidemiological evidence in support of the neuroprotective effects associated with high fish consumption are strong, yet these findings are yet to be corroborated in randomised controlled trials. A possible explanation is that there are other components in fish that may be responsible for the beneficial cognitive effects, or perhaps there is an interaction according to ApoE polymorphism. Currently, further trials are required in order to clarify whether DHA supplementation is effective for enhancing cognitive function in healthy individuals without an existing deficiency in DHA.

12.8   Conclusions

We have outlined above a number of nutraceutical interventions which are known to improve cognitive function or are promising candidates. The list is by no means exhaustive and discussion of nutraceuticals with a long history of research such as caffeine are beyond the scope of this chapter. For many of the substances there has been a period of development involving extensive preclinical work. For others their use as functional foods has stemmed from traditional use. In all cases there is a need for systematic trials which include co-monitoring relevant biomarkers in order to examine the relationships between cognitive ageing-sensitive changes and neurocognitive changes. Such markers should include oxidative stress, inflammation, hormonal changes, insulin resistance and cardiovascular measures as well as increasingly sophisticated brain imaging techniques including functional magnetic resonance imaging (fMRI), electroencephalography (EEG) and magnetoencephalography (MEG). Additionally there are several psychological processes which can impinge on cognitive function, these include sleep, stress and anxiety as well as overall mood. The interactions between these in the context of nutraceutical interventions for enhancing cognition will provide valuable information for future research. In addition to this there are numerous supplements and herbal extracts which through anecdote and traditional use have positive mood and cognitive effects. Many of these have not yet been subject to empirical investigation. Likewise technology is emerging which will allow foods to be tailored to enrich certain psychoactives (in much the same way as marijuana is now grown with much higher levels of tetrahydrocannabinol (THC) the major psychoactive ingredient. The notion of foods being developed to enhance cognition raises important ethical issues as well as offering exciting research opportunities.

12.9   Sources of further information and advice

- http://faculty.washington.edu/chudler/ehc.html – The home pages of Eric Chudler, a good place to start learning about brain function including nutrition and the brain.
- http://www.erowid.org – The Vaults of Erowid, for information on all things mind-altering (including nutraceuticals).
- http://www.alz.org – Alzheimer's Association, a good starting point for understanding cognitive decline and AD.

12.10   References

Abdul, H. M., Calabrese, V., Calvani, M. and Butterfield, D. A. (2006) Acetyl-L-carnitine-induced up-regulation of heat shock proteins protects cortical neurons against amyloid-beta peptide 1-42-mediated oxidative stress and neurotoxicity: Implications for Alzheimer's disease. *Journal of Neuroscience Research*, **84**, 398–408.

Akhondzadeh, S., Noroozian, M., Mohammadi, M., Ohadinia, S., Jamshidi, A. H. and Khani, M. (2003a) Melissa officinalis extract in the treatment of patients with mild to moderate Alzheimer's disease: A double blind, randomised, placebo controlled trial. *Journal of Neurology Neurosurgery and Psychiatry*, **74**, 863–866.

Akhondzadeh, S., Noroozian, M., Mohammadi, M., Ohadinia, S., Jamshidi, A. H. and Khani, M. (2003b) Salvia officinalis extract in the treatment of patients with mild to moderate Alzheimer's disease: A double blind, randomized and placebo-controlled trial. *Journal of Clinical Pharmacy and Therapeutics*, **28**, 53–59.

Alberts, B., Johnson, A., Lewis, J. and Al., E. (2002) *Molecular Biology of the Cell*, New York, Garland Science/Taylor and Francis.

Alford, C., Cox, H. and Wescott, R. (2001) The effects of Red Bull Energy Drink on human performance and mood. *Amino Acids*, **21**, 139–150.

Argentiero, V. and Tavolato, B. (1980) Dopamine (DA) and serotonin metabolic levels in the cerebrospinal fluid (CSF) in Alzheimer's presenile dementia under basic conditions and after stimulation with cerebral cortex phospholipids (BC-PL). *Journal of Neurology*, **224**, 53–58.

Balsom, P., Soderlund, K., Sjodin, B. and Ekblom, B. (1995) Skeletal muscle metabolism during short duration high-intensity exercise: influence of creatine supplementation. *Acta Physiologica Scandinavica*, **154**, 303–310.

Banay-Schwartz, M., Lajtha, A. and Palkovits, M. (1989) Changes with aging in the levels of amino acids in rat CNS structural elements. II. Taurine and small neutral amino acids. *Neurochemical Research*, **14**, 563–570.

Bazan, N. G. (2005) Neuroprotectin D1 (NPD1): A DHA-derived mediator that protects brain and retina against cell injury-induced oxidative stress. *Brain Pathology*, **15**, 159–166.

Beal, M. F. (2001) Experimental models of Parkinson's disease. *Nature Reviews Neuroscience*, **2**, 325–332.

Beal, M. F., Rascol, Marek, Olanow, Kordower, Isacson, Stocchi, Schapira and Tatton (2003) Bioenergetic approaches for neuroprotection in Parkinson's disease. *Annals of Neurology*, **53**, S39–47.

Benton, D., Ruffin, M., Lassel, T., Nabb, S., Messaoudi, M., Vinoy, S., Desor, D. and Lang, V. (2003) The delivery rate of dietary carbohydrates affects cognitive performance in both rats and humans. *Psychopharmacology*, **166**, 86–90.

Bergstrom, J., Furst, P., Noree, L. O. and Vinnars, E. (1974) Intracellular free amino acid concentration in human muscle tissue. *Journal of Applied Physiology*, **36**, 693–697.

Beyer, R. E., Burnett, B. A. and Cartwright, K. J. (1985) Tissue coenzyme Q (ubiquinone) and protein concentrations over the life span of the laboratory rat. *Mechanisms of Ageing and Development*, **32**, 267–281.

Bichler, A., Swenson, A. and Harris, M. A. (2006) A combination of caffeine and taurine has no effect on short term memory but induces changes in heart rate and mean arterial blood pressure. *Amino Acids*, **31**, 471–476.

Bruni, A., Toffano, G., Leon, A. and Boarato, E. (1976) Pharmacological effects of phosphatidylserine liposomes. *Nature*, **260**, 331–333.

Cadenas, E. and Davies, K. J. A. (2000) Mitochondrial free radical generation, oxidative stress, and aging. *Free Radical Biology and Medicine*, **29**, 222–230.

Calderini, G., Aporti, F. and Bonetti, A. C. (1985) Pharmacological effect of phosphatidylserine on age-dependent memory dysfunction. *Annals of the New York Academy of Sciences*, **444**, 504–506.

Carnat, A. P., Carnat, A., Fraisse, D. and Lamaison, J. L. (1998) The aromatic and polyphenolic composition of lemon balm (Melissa officinalis L. subsp. officinalis) tea. *Pharmaceutica Acta Helvetiae*, **72**, 301–305.

Cenacchi, T., Bertoldin, T., Farina, C., Fiori, M. G., Crepaldi, G., *et al.* (1993) Cognitive decline in the elderly: A double-blind, placebo-controlled multicenter study on efficacy of phosphatidylserine administration. *Aging – Clinical and Experimental Research*, **5**, 123–133.

Chaturvedi, R. K. and Beal, M. F. (2008) Mitochondrial approaches for neuroprotection. In Gibson, G. E., Ratan, R. R. and Beal, M. F. (eds) *Annals of the New York Academy of Sciences*, 395–412.

Chiu, C. C., Su, K. P., Cheng, T. C., Liu, H. C., Chang, C. J., *et al.* (2008) The effects of omega-3 fatty acids monotherapy in Alzheimer's disease and mild cognitive impairment: A preliminary randomized double-blind placebo-controlled study. *Progress in Neuro-Psychopharmacology and Biological Psychiatry*, **32**, 1538–1544.

Choeiria, C., Staines, W., Mikic, T., Seinoc, S. and Messier, C. (2005) Glucose transporter plasticity during memory processing. *Neuroscience*, **130**, 591–600.

Cleren, C., Yang, L., Lorenzo, B., Calingasan, N. Y., Schomer, A., *et al.* (2008) Therapeutic effects of coenzyme Q10 (CoQ10) and reduced CoQ10 in the MPTP model of Parkinsonism. *Journal of Neurochemistry*, **104**, 1613–1621.

Cole, G. M., Ma, Q. L. and Frautschy, S. A. (2009) Omega-3 fatty acids and dementia. *Prostaglandins Leukotrienes and Essential Fatty Acids*, **81**(2–3): 213–21.

Conway, M. and Clark, J. (1996) *Creatine and Creatine Phosphate: Scientific and Clinical Perspectives*, Academic Press, San Diego.

Cooke, M., Iosia, M., Buford, T., Shelmadine, B., Hudson, G., *et al.* (2008) Effects of acute and 14-day coenzyme Q10 supplementation on exercise performance in both trained and untrained individuals. *Journal of the International Society of Sports Nutrition*, **5**, doi:10.1186/1550-2783-5-8 (open access).

Crook III, T. H., Tinklenberg, J., Yesavage, J., Petrie, W., Nunzi, M. G. and Massari, D. C. (1991) Effects of phosphatidylserine in age-associated memory impairment. *Neurology*, **41**, 644–649.

Cunnane, S. C., Plourde, M., Pifferi, F., Bégin, M., Féart, C. and Barberger-Gateau, P. (2009) Fish, docosahexaenoic acid and Alzheimer's disease. *Progress in Lipid Research*, **48**, 239–256.

Dechent, P., Pouwels, P., Wilken, B., Hanefeld, F. and Frahm, J. (1999) Increase of total creatine in human brain after oral supplementation of creatine-monohydrate. *American Journal of Physiology- Regulatory, Integrative and Comparative Physiology*, **277**, 698–704.

Del Olmo, N., Bustamante, J., Del Río, R. M. and Solís, J. M. (2000) Taurine activates GABAA but not GABAB receptors in rat hippocampal CA1 area. *Brain Research*, **864**, 298–307.

El Idrissi, A. and Trenkner, E. (2004) Taurine as a modulator of excitatory and inhibitory neurotransmission. *Neurochemical Research*, **29**, 189–197.

Epis, R., Marcello, E., Gardoni, F., Longhi, A., Calvani, M., *et al.* (2008) Modulatory effect of acetyl-l-carnitine on amyloid precursor protein metabolism in hippocampal neurons. *European Journal of Pharmacology*, **597**, 51–56.

Eppler, B. and Dawson Jr, R. (2001) Dietary taurine manipulations in aged male Fischer 344 rat tissue: Taurine concentration, taurine biosynthesis, and oxidative markers. *Biochemical Pharmacology*, **62**, 29–39.

Ernster, L. and Dallner, G. (1995) Biochemical, physiological and medical aspects of ubiquinone function. *Biochimica et Biophysica Acta – Molecular Basis of Disease*, **1271**, 195–204.

Floyd, R. A. (1999) Antioxidants, oxidative stress, and degenerative neurological disorders. *Proceedings of the Society for Experimental Biology and Medicine*, **222**, 236–245.

Ford, C., Scholey, A., Ayre, G. and Wesnes, K. A. (2002) The effect of glucose administration and the emotional content of words on heart rate and memory. *J Psychopharmacol*, **16**, 241–244.

Freeman, M. P., Hibbeln, J. R., Wisner, K. L., Davis, J. M., Mischoulon, D., *et al.* (2006) Omega-3 fatty acids: Evidence basis for treatment and future research in psychiatry. *Journal of Clinical Psychiatry*, **67**, 1954–1967.

Freund-Levi, Y., Eriksdotter-Jönhagen, M., Cederholm, T., Basun, H., Faxén-Irving, G., *et al.* (2006) ω-3 fatty acid treatment in 174 patients with mild to moderate Alzheimer disease: OmegAD study – A randomized double-blind trial. *Archives of Neurology*, **63**, 1402–1408.

Galarreta, M., Bustamante, J., Del Río, R. M. and Solís, J. M. (1996) A new neuromodulatory action of taurine: Long-lasting increase of synaptic potentials. *Advances in Experimental Medicine and Biology*, **403**, 463–471.

Galasko, D. (2005) Evaluation of the safety, tolerability and impact on biomarkers of anti-oxidant treatment of mild to moderate Alzheimer's disease. http://www.Alzheimers.org/Clinicaltrials.

Gelbmann, C. M. and Muller, W. E. (1992) Chronic treatment with phosphatidylserine restores muscarinic cholinergic receptor deficits in the aged mouse brain. *Neurobiology of Aging*, **13**, 45–50.

Gelinas, D. S., Dasilva, K., Fenili, D., St. George-Hyslop, P. and Mclaurin, J. (2004) Immunotherapy for Alzheimer's disease. *Proceedings of the National Academy of Sciences of the United States of America*, **101**, 14657–14662.

Gomez-Pinilla, F. (2008) Brain foods: The effects of nutrients on brain function. *Nature Reviews Neuroscience*, **9**, 568–578.

Gore, J. B., Krebs, D. L., Parent, M. B. (2006) Changes in blood glucose and salivary cortisol are not necessary for arousal to enhance memory in young or older adults. *Psychoneuroendocrinology*, **31**, 589–600.

Gracy, R. W., Talent, J. M., Kong, Y. and Conrad, C. C. (1999) Reactive oxygen species: The unavoidable environmental insult? *Mutation Research – Fundamental and Molecular Mechanisms of Mutagenesis*, **428**, 17–22.

Groneberg, D. A., Kindermann, B., Althammer, M., Klapper, M., Vormann, J., Littarru, G. P. and Döring, F. (2005) Coenzyme Q10 affects expression of genes involved in cell signalling, metabolism and transport in human CaCo-2 cells. *International Journal of Biochemistry and Cell Biology*, **37**, 1208–1218.

Gutzmann, H. and Hadler, D. (1998) Sustained efficacy and safety of idebenone in the treatment of Alzheimer's disease: Update on a 2-year double-blind multicentre study. *Journal of Neural Transmission, Supplement*, **54**, 301–310.

Gutzmann, H., Kühl, K. P., Hadler, D. and Rapp, M. A. (2002) Safety and efficacy of idebenone versus tacrine in patients with Alzheimer's disease: Results of a randomized, double-blind, parallel-group multicenter study. *Pharmacopsychiatry*, **35**, 12–18.

Hager, K., Kenklies, M., Mcafoose, J., Engel, J. and Münch, G. (2007) Alpha-lipoic acid as a new treatment option for Alzheimer's disease – a 48 months follow-up analysis. *Journal of Neural Transmission*, **72**, (Supple), 189–193.

Hager, K., Marahrens, A., Kenklies, M., Riederer, P. and Münch, G. (2001) Alpha-lipoic acid as a new treatment option for Alzheimer type dementia. *Archives of Gerontology and Geriatrics*, **32**, 275–282.

Halliwell, B. (1992) Reactive oxygen species and the central nervous system. *Journal of Neurochemistry*, **59**, 1609–1623.

Halliwell, B. and Gutteridge, J. M. C. (1990) Role of free radicals and catalytic metal ions in human disease: An overview. *Methods in Enzymology*, **186**, 1–85.

Harman, D. (1957) Aging: A theory based on free radical and radiation chemistry. *Journal of Gerentology*, **2**, 298–300.

Hashioka, S., Han, Y. H., Fujii, S., Kato, T., Monji, A., *et al.* (2007) Phosphatidylserine and phosphatidylcholine-containing liposomes inhibit amyloid beta and interferon-gamma-induced microglial activation. *Free Radical Biology and Medicine*, **42**, 945–954.

Hedden, T. and Gabrieli, J. D. E. (2004) Insights into the ageing mind: A view from cognitive neuroscience. *Nature Reviews Neuroscience*, **5**, 87–96.

Hohmann, J., Zupkó, I., Rédei, D., Csányi, M., Falkay, G., *et al.* (1999) Protective effects of the aerial parts of Salvia officinalis, Melissa officinalis and Lavandula angustifolia and their constituents against enzyme- dependent and enzyme-independent lipid peroxidation. *Planta Medica*, **65**, 576–578.

Huang, T. L., Zandi, P. P., Tucker, K. L., Fitzpatrick, A. L., Kuller, L. H., *et al.* (2005) Benefits of fatty fish on dementia risk are stronger for those without APOE β4. *Neurology*, **65**, 1409–1414.

Hudson, S. and Tabet, N. (2003) Acetyl-L-carnitine for dementia. *Cochrane database of systematic reviews (Online)*.

Ingwersen, J., Defeyter, M., Kennedy, D., Wesnes, K. and Scholey, A. (2007) A low glycaemic index breakfast cereal preferentially prevents children's cognitive performance from declining throughout the morning. *Appetite*, **49**, 240–244.

Ishrat, T., Khan, M. B., Hoda, M. N., Yousuf, S., Ahmad, M., *et al.* (2006) Coenzyme Q10 modulates cognitive impairment against intracerebroventricular injection of streptozotocin in rats. *Behavioural Brain Research*, **171**, 9–16.

Jacobsen, J. G. and Smith, L. H. (1968) Biochemistry and physiology of taurine and taurine derivatives. *Physiological Reviews*, **48**, 424–511.

Jofre-Monseny, L., Minihane, A. M. and Rimbach, G. (2008) Impact of apoE genotype on oxidative stress, inflammation and disease risk. *Molecular Nutrition and Food Research*, **52**, 131–145.

Kalen, A., Appelkvist, E. L. and Dallner, G. (1989) Age-related changes in the lipid compositions of rat and human tissues. *Lipids*, **24**, 579–584.

Kamzalov, S. and Sohal, R. S. (2004) Effect of age and caloric restriction on coenzyme Q and α-tocopherol levels in the rat. *Experimental Gerontology*, **39**, 1199–1205.

Kennedy, D. O., Pace, S., Haskell, C., Okello, E. J., Milne, A. and Scholey, A. B. (2006) Effects of cholinesterase inhibiting sage (Salvia officinalis) on mood, anxiety and performance on a psychological stressor battery. *Neuropsychopharmacology*, **31**, 845–852.

Kennedy, D. O. and Scholey, A. B. (2006) The psychopharmacology of European herbs with cognition-enhancing properties. *Current Pharmaceutical Design*, **12**, 4613–4623.

Kennedy, D. O., Scholey, A. B., Tildesley, N. T. J., Perry, E. K. and Wesnes, K. A. (2002) Modulation of mood and cognitive performance following acute administration of Melissa officinalis (lemon balm). *Pharmacology Biochemistry and Behavior*, **72**, 953–964.

Kennedy, D. O., Wake, G., Savelev, S., Tildesley, N. T. J., Perry, E. K., *et al.* (2003) Modulation of mood and cognitive performance following acute administration of single doses of Melissa officinalis (Lemon balm) with human CNS nicotinic and muscarinic receptor-binding properties. *Neuropsychopharmacology*, **28**, 1871–1881.

Kidd, P. M. (2005) Neurodegeneration from mitochondrial insufficiency: Nutrients, stem cells, growth factors, and prospects for brain rebuilding using integrative management. *Alternative Medicine Review*, **10**, 268–293.

Kidd, P. M. (2008) Alzheimer's disease, amnestic mild cognitive impairment, and age-associated memory impairment: Current understanding and progress toward integrative prevention. *Alternative Medicine Review*, **13**, 85–115.

Klugman, A., Sauer, J., Tabet, N. and Howard, R. (2004) Alpha lipoic acid for dementia. *Cochrane database of systematic reviews (Online: Update Software)*.

Korang, K., Milakofsky, L., Hare, T. A., Hofford, J. M. and Vogel, W. H. (1996) Levels of taurine, amino acids and related compounds in plasma, vena cava, aorta and heart of rats after taurine administration. *Pharmacology*, **52**, 263–270.

Kotani, S., Sakaguchi, E., Warashina, S., Matsukawa, N., Ishikura, Y., *et al.* (2006) Dietary supplementation of arachidonic and docosahexaenoic acids improves cognitive dysfunction. *Neuroscience Research*, **56**, 159–164.

Kwon, O. S. and Youn, B. C. (2004) HPLC determination and pharmacokinetics of endogenous acetyl-L-carnitine (ALC) in human volunteers orally administered a single dose of ALC. *Archives of Pharmacal Research*, **27**, 676–681.

Lallemand, F. and De Witte, P. (2004) Taurine concentration in the brain and in the plasma following intraperitoneal injections. *Amino Acids*, **26**, 111–116.

Lass, A., Kwong, L. and Sohal, R. S. (1999) Mitochondrial coenzyme Q content and aging. *BioFactors*, **9**, 199–205.

Li, G., Jack, C. R., Yang, X. F. and Yang, E. S. (2008a) Diet supplement CoQ10 delays brain atrophy in aged transgenic mice with mutations in the amyloid precursor protein: An in vivo volume MRI study. *BioFactors*, **32**, 169–178.

Li, L., Pabbisetty, D., Carvalho, P., Avery, M. A. and Avery, B. A. (2008b) Analysis of CoQ10 in rat serum by ultra-performance liquid chromatography mass spectrometry after oral administration. *Journal of Pharmaceutical and Biomedical Analysis*, **46**, 137–142.

Liu, J. (2008) The effects and mechanisms of mitochondrial nutrient α-lipoic acid on improving age-associated mitochondrial and cognitive dysfunction: An overview. *Neurochemical Research*, **33**, 194–203.

Lourenco, R. and Camilo, M. E. (2002) Taurine: A conditionally essential amino acid in humans? An overview in health and disease. *Nutricion Hospitalaria*, **17**, 262–270.

Lu, T., Pan, Y., Kao, S. Y., Li, C., Kohane, I., et al. (2004) Gene regulation and DNA damage in the ageing human brain. *Nature*, **429**, 883–891.

Lyoo, I., Kong, S., Sung, S., Hirashima, F., Parow, A., et al. (2003) Multinuclear magnetic resonance spectroscopy of high-energy phosphate metabolites in human brain following oral supplementation of creatine-monohydrate. *Psychiatry Research: Neuroimaging*, **123**, 87–100.

Maclean, C. H., Issa, A. M., Newberry, S. J., Mojica, W. A., Morton, S. C., et al. (2005) Effects of omega-3 fatty acids on cognitive function with aging, dementia, and neurological diseases. *Evidence report/technology assessment (Summary)*, 1–3.

Maczurek, A., Hager, K., Kenklies, M., Sharman, M., Martins, R., et al. (2008) Lipoic acid as an anti-inflammatory and neuroprotective treatment for Alzheimer's disease. *Advanced Drug Delivery Reviews*, **60**, 1463–1470.

Mantle, D., Pickering, A. T. and Perry, E. K. (2000) Medicinal plant extracts for the treatment of dementia: A review of their pharmacology, efficacy and tolerability. *CNS Drugs*, **13**, 201–213.

Mazzio, E., Yoon, K. J. and Soliman, K. F. A. (2003) Acetyl-L-carnitine cytoprotection against 1-methyl-4-phenylpyridinium toxicity in neuroblastoma cells. *Biochemical Pharmacology*, **66**, 297–306.

McDonald, S. R., Sohal, R. S. and Forster, M. J. (2005) Concurrent administration of coenzyme Q10 and α-tocopherol improves learning in aged mice. *Free Radical Biology and Medicine*, **38**, 729–736.

McEwen, B. S. and Reagan, L. P. (2004) Glucose transporter expression in the central nervous system: relationship to synaptic function. *European Journal of Pharmacology*, **490**, 13–24.

McMorris, T., Harris, R., Howard, A., Langridge, G., Hall, B., et al. (2007a) Creatine supplementation, sleep deprivation, cortisol, melatonin and behavior. *Physiology & Behavior*, **90**, 21–28.

McMorris, T., Harris, R., Swain, J., Corbett, J., Collard, K., et al. (2006) Effect of creatine supplementation and sleep deprivation, with mild exercise, on cognitive and psychomotor performance, mood state, and plasma concentrations of catecholamines and cortisol. *Psychopharmacology*, **185**, 93–103.

McMorris, T., Mielcarz, G., Harris, R., Swain, J. and Howard, A. (2007b) Creatine supplementation and cognitive performance in elderly individuals. *Aging, Neuropsychology, and Cognition*, **14**, 517–528.

Messari, S. E., LeLoup, C., Quignon, M., Brisorgueil, M.-J., Penicaud, L. and Arluison, M. (1998) Immunocytochemical localization of the insulin responsive glucose transporter 4 (Glut4) in the rat central nervous system. *Journal of Comparative Neurology*, **399**, 492–512.

Messier, C. (2004) Glucose improvement of memory: a review. *European Journal of Pharmacology*, **490**, 33–57.

Milan, F., Guidolin, D. and Polato, P. (1988) Structural changes of basal forebrain cholinergic neurons in the aged rat. Effect of phosphatidylserine administration. In Pepeu, G., Tomlinson, B. and Wischik, C. M. (eds) *New Trends in Aging Research*. Padova, Italy, Liviana Press 221–231.

Miles, M. V., Horn, P. S., Morrison, J. A., Tang, P. H., Degrauw, T. and Pesce, A. J. (2003) Plasma coenzyme Q10 reference intervals, but not redox status, are affected by gender and race in self-reported healthy adults. *Clinica Chimica Acta*, **332**, 123–132.

Miles, M. V., Horn, P. S., Tang, P. H., Morrison, J. A., Miles, L., *et al.* (2004) Age-related changes in plasma coenzyme Q10 concentrations and redox state in apparently healthy children and adults. *Clinica Chimica Acta*, **347**, 139–144.

Montgomery, S. A., Thal, L. J. and Amrein, R. (2003) Meta-analysis of double blind randomized controlled clinical trials of acetyl-L-carnitine versus placebo in the treatment of mild cognitive impairment and mild Alzheimer's disease. *International Clinical Psychopharmacology*, **18**, 61–71.

Morre, D. J. and Morre, D. M. (2003) Cell surface NADH oxidases (ECTO-NOX proteins) with roles in cancer, cellular time-keeping, growth, aging and neurodegenerative diseases. *Free Radical Research*, **37**, 795–808.

Morre, D. M. and Morre, D. J. (2006) Role of membrane redox in aging-related diseases. *Acta Biologica Szegediensis*, **50**, 67–69.

Morre, D. M., Morre, D. J., Rehmus, W. and Kern, D. (2008) Supplementation with CoQ10 lowers age-related (ar) NOX levels in healthy subjects. *BioFactors*, **32**, 221–230.

Mulkens, A., Stephanou, E. and Kapetanidis, I. (1985) Glycosides with volatile genins in leaves of Melissa officinalis. *Heterosides a genines volatiles dans les feuilles de melissa officinalis l. (lamiaceae)*, **60**, 276–278.

Neeper, S. A., Gomez-Pinilla, F., Choi, J. and Cotman, C. (1995) Exercise and brain neurotrophins. *Nature*, **373**, 109.

Nishimura, A., Yanagawa, H., Fujikawa, N., Kiriyama, A. and Shibata, N. (2009) Pharmacokinetic profiles of coenzyme Q10: Absorption of three different oral formulations in rats. *Journal of Health Science*, **55**, 540–548.

Nunzi, M. G., Guidolin, D., Petrelli, L., Polato, P. and Zanotti, A. (1992) Behavioral and morpho-functional correlates of brain aging: A preclinical study with phosphatidylserine. *Advances in Experimental Medicine and Biology*, **318**, 393–398.

Nunzi, M. G., Milan, F., Guidolin, D., Polato, P. and Toffano, G. (1989) Effects of phosphatidylserine administration on age-related structural changes in the rat hippocampus and septal complex. *Pharmacopsychiatry, Supplement*, **22**, 125–128.

Ono, K., Yoshiike, Y., Takashima, A., Hasegawa, K., Naiki, H. and Yamada, M. (2003) Potent anti-amyloidogenic and fibril-destabilizing effects of polyphenols in vitro: Implications for the prevention and therapeutics of Alzheimer's disease. *Journal of Neurochemistry*, **87**, 172–181.

Osella, M. C., Re, G., Badino, P., Bergamasco, L. and Miolo, A. (2008) Phosphatidylserine (PS) as a potential nutraceutical for canine brain aging: A review. *Journal of Veterinary Behavior: Clinical Applications and Research*, **3**, 41–51.

Park, C. R. (2001) Cognitive effects of insulin in the central nervous system. *Neuroscience & Biobehavioral Reviews*, **25**, 311–323.

Pepeu, G., Pepeu, I. M. and Amaducci, L. (1996) A review of phosphatidylserine pharmacological and clinical effects. Is phosphatidylserine a drug for the ageing brain? *Pharmacological Research*, **33**, 73–80.

Perry, E. K., Pickering, A. T., Wang, W. W., Houghton, P. J. and Perry, N. S. L. (1999) Medicinal plants and Alzheimer's disease: From ethnobotany to phytotherapy. *Journal of Pharmacy and Pharmacology*, **51**, 527–534.

Perry, N., Court, G., Bidet, N., Court, J. and Perry, E. (1996) European herbs with cholinergic activities: Potential in dementia therapy. *International Journal of Geriatric Psychiatry*, **11**, 1063–1069.

Perry, N. S. L., Bollen, C., Perry, E. K. and Ballard, C. (2003) Salvia for dementia therapy: Review of pharmacological activity and pilot tolerability clinical trial. *Pharmacology Biochemistry and Behavior*, **75**, 651–659.

Persky, A. M., Brazeau, G. A. and Hochhaus, G. (2003) Pharmacokinetics of the dietary supplement creatine. *Clinical Pharmacokinetics*, **42**, 557–574.

Pettegrew, J. W., Klunk, W. E., Panchalingam, K., Kanfer, J. N. and Mcclure, R. J. (1995) Clinical and neurochemical effects of acetyl-L-carnitine in Alzheimer's disease. *Neurobiology of Aging*, **16**, 1–4.

Pettegrew, J. W., Levine, J. and Mcclure, R. J. (2000) Acetyl-L-carnitine physical-chemical, metabolic, and therapeutic properties: Relevance for its mode of action in Alzheimer's disease and geriatric depression. *Molecular Psychiatry*, **5**, 616–632.

Pifferi, F., Jouin, M., Alessandri, J. M., Haedke, U., Roux, F., *et al.* (2007) n-3 Fatty acids modulate brain glucose transport in endothelial cells of the blood-brain barrier. *Prostaglandins Leukotrienes and Essential Fatty Acids*, **77**, 279–286.

Plourde, M. and Cunnane, S. C. (2007) Extremely limited synthesis of long chain polyunsaturates in adults: Implications for their dietary essentiality and use as supplements. *Applied Physiology, Nutrition and Metabolism*, **32**, 619–634.

Poortmans, J. and Francaux, M. (2000) Adverse effects of creatine supplementation: fact or fiction? *Sports Medicine*, **30**, 155.

Quinzii, C. M., López, L. C., Von-Moltke, J., Naini, A., Krishna, S., *et al.* (2008) Respiratory chain dysfunction and oxidative stress correlate with severity of primary CoQ10 deficiency. *FASEB Journal*, **22**, 1874–1885.

Rango, M., Castelli, A. and Scarlato, G. (1997) Energetics of 3.5 s neural activation in humans: a 31P MR spectroscopy study. *Magnetic Resonance in Medicine*, **38**, 878–883.

Rawson, E., Lieberman, H., Walsh, T., Zuber, S., Harhart, J. and Matthews, T. (2008) Creatine supplementation does not improve cognitive function in young adults. *Physiology & Behavior*, **95**, 130–134.

Rebouche, C. J. (2004) Kinetics, pharmacokinetics, and regulation of L-Carnitine and acetyl-L-carnitine metabolism. *Annals of the New York Academy of Sciences*, **1033**, 30–41.

Riley, P. A. (1994) Free radicals in biology: Oxidative stress and the effects of ionizing radiation. *International Journal of Radiation Biology*, **65**, 27–33.

Rossi, L., Mazzitelli, S., Arciello, M., Capo, C. R. and Rotilio, G. (2008) Benefits from dietary polyphenols for brain aging and Alzheimer's disease. *Neurochemical Research*, **33**, 2390–2400.

Rusca, A., Di Stefano, A. F. D., Doig, M. V., Scarsi, C. and Perucca, E. (2009) Relative bioavailability and pharmacokinetics of two oral formulations of docosahexaenoic acid/eicosapentaenoic acid after multiple-dose administration in healthy volunteers. *European Journal of Clinical Pharmacology*, **65**, 503–510.

Ryan, C. M., Williams, T. M. (1993) Effects of insulin-dependent diabetes on learning and memory efficiency in adults. *Journal of Clinical and Experimental Neuropsychology*, **15**, 685–700.

Sadraei, H., Ghannadi, A. and Malekshahi, K. (2003) Relaxant effect of essential oil of Melissa officinalis and citral on rat ileum contractions. *Fitoterapia*, **74**, 445–452.

Saito, Y., Fukuhara, A., Nishio, K., Hayakawa, M., Ogawa, Y., *et al.* (2009) Characterization of cellular uptake and distribution of coenzyme Q10 and vitamin E in PC12 cells. *Journal of Nutritional Biochemistry*, **20**, 350–357.

Sappey-Marinier, D., Calabrese, G., Fein, G., Hugg, J., Biggins, C. and Weiner, M. (1992) Effect of photic stimulation on human visual cortex lactate and phosphates using 1H and 31P magnetic resonance spectroscopy. *Journal of Cerebral Blood Flow and Metabolism*, **12**, 584.

Sarkar, D. and Fisher, P. B. (2006) Molecular mechanisms of aging-associated inflammation. *Cancer Letters*, **236**, 13–23.

Schaffer, S., Takahashi, K. and Azuma, J. (2000) Role of osmoregulation in the actions of taurine. *Amino Acids*, **19**, 527–546.

Schmelzer, C., Lindner, I., Rimbach, G., Niklowitz, P., Menke, T. and Döring, F. (2008) Functions of coenzyme Q10 in inflammation and gene expression. *BioFactors*, **32**, 179–183.

Scholey, A. (2001) Food for thought. *Psychologist* **14**, 196–201.

Scholey, A., Sünram-Lea, S., Greer, J., Elliott, J. and Kennedy, D. (2009) Glucose administration prior to a divided attention task improves tracking performance but not word recognition: evidence against differential memory enhancement? *Psychopharmacology*, **202**, 549–558.

Scholey, A. B., Harper, S. and Kennedy, D. O. (2001) Cognitive demand and blood glucose. *Physiology & Behavior*, **73**, 585–592.

Scholey, A. B., Laing, S. and Kennedy, D. O. (2006) Blood glucose changes and memory: Effects of manipulating emotionality and mental effort. *Biological Psychology*, **71**, 12–19.

Scholey, A. B., Tildesley, N. T. J., Ballard, C. G., Wesnes, K. A., Tasker, A., *et al.* (2008) An extract of Salvia (sage) with anticholinesterase properties improves memory and attention in healthy older volunteers. *Psychopharmacology*, **198**, 127–139.

Shinto, L. H. (2004) Fish oil and alpha lipoic acid in mild Alzheimer's disease. http://www.clinicaltrials.gov/ct/sho/NCT00090402.

Shults, C. W., Beal, M. F., Song, D. and Fontaine, D. (2004) Pilot trial of high dosages of coenzyme Q10 in patients with Parkinson's disease. *Experimental Neurology*, **188**, 491–494.

Shults, C. W., Oakes, D., Kieburtz, K., Flint Beal, M., Haas, R., *et al.* (2002) Effects of coenzyme Q10 in early Parkinson disease: Evidence of slowing of the functional decline. *Archives of Neurology*, **59**, 1541–1550.

Sohal, R. S. and Forster, M. J. (2007) Coenzyme Q, oxidative stress and aging. *Mitochondrion*, **7**, S103–111.

Sohal, R. S., Kamzalov, S., Sumien, N., Ferguson, M., Rebrin, I., *et al.* (2006) Effect of coenzyme Q10 intake on endogenous coenzyme Q content, mitochondrial electron transport chain, antioxidative defenses, and life span of mice. *Free Radical Biology and Medicine*, **40**, 480–487.

Stapleton, P. P., Charles, R. P., Redmond, H. P. and Bouchier-Hayes, D. J. (1997) Taurine and human nutrition. *Clinical Nutrition*, **16**, 103–108.

Sünram-Lea, S., Foster, J., Durlach, P. and Perez, C. (2001) Glucose facilitation of cognitive performance in healthy young adults: examination of the influence of fast-duration, time of day and pre-consumption plasma glucose levels. *Psychopharmacology*, **157**, 46.

Suzuki, S., Furushiro, M., Takahashi, M., Sakai, M. and Kudo, S. (1999) Oral administration of soybean lecithin transphosphatidylated phosphatidylserine (SB-tPS) reduces ischemic damage in the gerbil hippocampus. *Japanese Journal of Pharmacology*, **81**, 237–239.

Teichert, J., Hermann, R., Ruus, P. and Preiss, R. (2003) Plasma kinetics, metabolism, and urinary excretion of alpha-lipoic acid following oral administration in healthy volunteers. *Journal of Clinical Pharmacology*, **43**, 1257–1267.

Tildesley, N. T. J., Kennedy, D. O., Perry, E. K., Ballard, C. G., Savelev, S., *et al.* (2003) Salvia lavandulaefolia (Spanish Sage) enhances memory in healthy young volunteers. *Pharmacology Biochemistry and Behavior*, **75**, 669–674.

Tildesley, N. T. J., Kennedy, D. O., Perry, E. K., Ballard, C. G., Wesnes, K. A. and Scholey, A. B. (2005) Positive modulation of mood and cognitive performance following administration of acute doses of Salvia lavandulaefolia essential oil to healthy young volunteers. *Physiology and Behavior*, **83**, 699–709.

van de Rest, O., Geleijnse, J. M., Kok, F. J., Van Staveren, W. A., Dullemeijer, C., *et al.* (2008) Effect of fish oil on cognitive performance in older subjects: A randomized, controlled trial. *Neurology*, **71**, 430–438.

Vannucchi, M. G., Casmenti, F. and Pepeu, G. (1990) Decrease of acetylcholine release from cortical slices in aged rats: Investigations into its reversal by phosphatidylserine. *Journal of Neurochemistry*, **55**, 819–825.

Vannucchi, M. G. and Pepeu, G. (1987) Effect of phosphatidylserine on acetylcholine release and content in cortical slices from aging rats. *Neurobiology of Aging*, **8**, 403–407.

Veltri, K., Espiritu, M. and Singh, G. (2005) Distinct genomic copy number in mitochondria of different mammalian organs. *Journal of Cellular Physiology*, **143**, 160–164.

Villardita, C., Grioli, S. and Salmeri, G. (1987) Multicentre clinical trial of brain phosphatidylserine in elderly patients with intellectual deterioration. *Clinical Trials Journal*, **24**, 84–93.

Wada, H., Goto, H., Hagiwara, S. I. and Yamamoto, Y. (2007) Redox status of coenzyme Q10 is associated with chronological age [3]. *Journal of the American Geriatrics Society*, **55**, 1141–1142.

Wake, G., Court, J., Pickering, A., Lewis, R., Wilkins, R. and Perry, E. (2000) CNS acetylcholine receptor activity in European medicinal plants traditionally used to improve failing memory. *Journal of Ethnopharmacology*, **69**, 105–114.

Warburton, D. M., Bersellini, E. and Sweeney, E. (2001) An evaluation of a caffeinated taurine drink on mood, memory and information processing in healthy volunteers without caffeine abstinence. *Psychopharmacology*, **158**, 322–328.

Watanabe, A., Kato, N. and Kato, T. (2002) Effects of creatine on mental fatigue and cerebral hemoglobin oxygenation. *Neuroscience research*, **42**, 279–285.

Watson, G. and Craft, S. (2004) Modulation of memory by insulin and glucose: neuropsychological observations in Alzheimer's disease. *European Journal of Pharmacology*, **490**, 97–113.

Watson, G. S., Craft, S. (2008) Insulin Resistance Alzheimer's Disease: Pathophysiology and Treatment. *Progress in Neurotherapeutics and Neuropsychopharmacology*, **3**, 85–110.

Wesnes, K., Pincock, C., Richardson, D., Helm, G. and Hails, S. (2003) Breakfast reduces declines in attention and memory over the morning in schoolchildren. *Appetite*, **41**, 329–331.

Weyer, G., Babej-Dolle, R. M., Hadler, D., Hofmann, S. and Herrmann, W. M. (1997) A controlled study of 2 doses of idebenone in the treatment of Alzheimer's disease. *Neuropsychobiology*, **36**, 73–82.

Wu, A., Ying, Z. and Gomez-Pinilla, F. (2004) Dietary omega-3 fatty acids normalize BDNF levels, reduce oxidative damage, and counteract learning disability after traumatic brain injury in rats. *Journal of Neurotrauma*, **21**, 1457–1467.

Wu, J., Kohno, T., Georgiev, S. K., Ikoma, M., Ishii, H., et al. (2008) Taurine activates glycine and Gamma-aminobutyric acid a receptors in rat substantia gelatinosa neurons. *NeuroReport*, **19**, 333–337.

Wu, J. Y., Tang, X. W., Schloss, J. V. and Faiman, M. D. (1998) Regulation of taurine biosynthesis and its physiological significance in the brain. *Advances in Experimental Medicine and Biology*, **442**, 339–345.

Zanotti, A., Valzelli, L. and Toffano, G. (1989) Chronic phosphatidylserine treatment improves spatial memory and passive avoidance in aged rats. *Psychopharmacology*, **99**, 316–321.

Zecca, L., Youdim, M. B. H., Riederer, P., Connor, J. R. and Crichton, R. R. (2004) Iron, brain ageing and neurodegenerative disorders. *Nature Reviews Neuroscience*, **5**, 863–873.

Zhang, Y., Aberg, F., Appelkvist, E. L., Dallner, G. and Ernster, L. (1995) Uptake of dietary coenzyme Q supplement is limited in rats. *Journal of Nutrition*, **125**, 446–453.

Zhao, W.-Q., Chen, H., Quon, M. J., Alkon, D. J. (2004) Insulin and the insulin receptor in experimental models of learning and memory. **490**, 71–81.

13

Functional foods and bone health

S. J. Whiting and H. Vatanparast, University of Saskatchewan, Canada

Abstract: There are many nutrients required for optimal bone health throughout the lifecycle. Bone is a living tissue and needs all the nutrients that other tissues require. In addition, bone has extraordinary requirements for calcium, phosphorus and protein, as these make up its major structural components. Other nutrients such as vitamin D, vitamin K, and dietary factors such as soy isoflavones and milk basic protein (MBP) have been shown to promote optimal bone health. In several case studies of functional foods provided in Canada that are intended to promote bone health, we show that there can be a combination of bone-enhancing factors in 'familiar' foods that will appeal to different target populations.

Key words: calcium, vitamin D, phosphorus, protein, soy, isoflavones, vitamin D, vitamin K, milk basic protein.

13.1   Introduction

Osteoporosis is a major public health problem and a costly disease worldwide. As the average age of the world's population shifts upward, the incidence and prevalence of osteoporosis and its economic burden on society will increase further. It is defined as 'a systemic skeletal disease characterized by low bone mass and micro-architectural deterioration of bone tissue, leading to enhanced bone fragility and a consequent increase in fracture risk' (NIH Consensus Development Panel on Osteoporosis, 2001). Osteoporotic fractures contributed to 0.83% of the global burden of non-communicable diseases, and estimates indicate that the number of osteoporotic hip fractures occurring in the world each year will rise from 1.66 million to 6.29 million by the year 2050 (Cole *et al.*, 2008, Johnell and Kanis, 2006). All osteoporotic fractures are associated with increased morbidity; fractures of the hip and vertebrae are also linked with significant mortality.

There are three stages in bone growth and maintenance where nutrition is of critical concern: development of peak bone mass, postmenopausal bone loss, and age-related bone loss (Fig. 13.1). Development of peak bone mass is thought to be a major determinant of vulnerability to osteoporosis. Almost all of an adult's bone mineral is achieved by the end of adolescence. As bone loss is a normal consequence of aging, those who acquire a greater bone mass during the first two decades of life should be at reduced risk for related skeletal health problems later in life (Heaney *et al.*, 2000a). However, early bone mass acquisition may not persist to late adulthood (Gafni and Baron, 2007) so nutritional and other influences continue to be important throughout the lifespan. These other influences include: genetic determinants, sex hormones, endocrine factors, mechanical forces, and exposure to risk factors (Chevalley *et al.*, 2009). Although genetic factors play an important role, it is also well established that peak bone mass is influenced by multiple lifestyle factors (Rizzoli, 2008). Therefore most preventive strategies attempt to reduce or reverse bone loss through dietary intakes in addition to exercise.

Aging bone loss is negative calcium balance at the sites of bone remodeling where the rate of calcium release is higher than deposition of calcium in bony tissue calcium. There is progressive erosion of skeletal architecture characterized by cortical thinning and increased porosity, trabecular thinning, and loss of bone connectivity. In Fig. 13.1, postmenopausal bone loss is considered separately from aging loss as bone loss occurs at an accelerated rate over a relatively short period of time (United States Department of Health and Human Services, 2004).

Osteoporosis is a skeletal disorder characterized by low bone mass and microarchitectural deterioration of bone tissue with a consequent increase in the fragility of bone and hence susceptibility to fracture, as shown in Fig. 13.1. Bone is a living tissue and needs all the nutrients that other tissues require. In addition, bone has extraordinary requirements for the nutrients calcium, phosphorus and

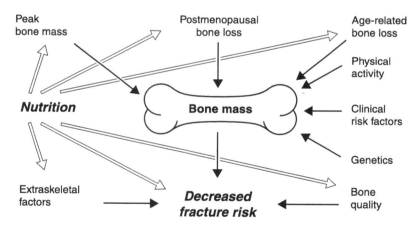

Fig. 13.1   Many factors affect bone mass. Appropriate nutrition is one important strategy for maximizing bone growth (achieving peak bone mass) and achieving bone maintenance (forestalling postmenopausal and age-related bone loss). Nutrition improves bone mass as well as reducing falls through extraskeletal actions, thus reducing the risk of osteoporosis. Modified from Rizzoli (2008).

protein, as these are the main structural components. Approximately 80–90% of bone mineral content is comprised of calcium and phosphorus in the form of hydroxyapatite [$Ca_{10}(PO_4)_6(OH)_2$] (Institute of Medicine, 1997). Vitamin D is necessary for active absorption of calcium and phosphorus. In addition, vitamin D is a transcription factor that functions within all cells of the body and is thus required for all tissue growth and maintenance including bone. Growth and maintenance are under hormonal control. During childhood, bone undergoes growth (i.e., bone formation) and breakdown (i.e., bone resorption) separately while in adults bone is remodelled, during which time formation and resorption are programmed to be cyclical in nature (US Department of Health and Human Services, 2004).

While calcium, phosphorus (and the vitamin D needed for absorption) and protein are directly involved in bone acquisition as substrates, there are also many nutrients which have a more indirect function on bone (Ilich and Kerstetter, 2000). In this regard there are vitamin cofactors such as vitamin C, required for collagen synthesis, and vitamin K required for synthesis of osteocalcin and bone matrix protein. Further, the elements magnesium and potassium as well as the B-vitamins and the micro-elements (zinc, copper, iron, etc) are involved in bone growth and maintenance. When diets are not healthy, i.e., following the food guides of the respective country, some nutrients can be limiting. For example, in diets that are low in vegetables and fruit (a typical failing in Canada and the USA), magnesium, potassium, vitamin K, and vitamin C are difficult to obtain. To illustrate how a nutrient can be implicated in bone health, we have chosen vitamin K as an example, as this nutrient, while not assessed in national surveys, is thought to be limiting in the diet due to low intake of green leafy vegetables in the typical western diet (Booth and Suttie, 1998). Recent developments in nutrition research have demonstrated that active compounds have bone-promoting and/or bone-sparing qualities. Most research has been conducted on soy isoflavones. A relatively new active ingredient added to foods for the purpose of slowing bone loss is milk basic protein (MBP).

Functional food sources of bone nutrients are needed as it has become apparent from dietary studies that the amounts of bone-specific nutrients are limited in the natural diet of persons in North America and Europe (Bonjour et al., 2009). Further, many of the dietary factors such as MBP and soy isoflavones are not in typical North American or European foods in sufficient quantity to be of value to bone health unless either added to foods. It is important to provide nutrients and dietary factors proven to be efficacious in a form that is readily accepted by consumers.

13.2   Overview of bone growth and maintenance

An individual's bone is formed during the prenatal period through two different processes: bone growth between embryonic membrane identified as intra-membranous bone formation, and endochondral process that is bone formation from cartilage (Yang, 2009). There are three types of bone cells. Osteoblast, the bone-forming cell, is of mesenchymal origin and its main function is to produce new bone matrix, osteoid, and to mineralize it. When an osteoblast is entrapped in the bone matrix, it becomes an osteocyte, and takes on new roles (Verborgt *et al.*, 2002). Bone resorption is carried out by osteoclasts, which originate from the hematopoetic-macrophage lineage (Rubinacci *et al.*, 1999).

There are two types of bones, cortical and trabecular (Malina *et al.*, 2004). In a healthy adult, cortical contributes approximately 80% of total bone mass, and is most abundant in the shafts of long bones. It has a high mineral content (approximately 70%), and its function is principally mechanical. Trabecular bone is composed of a network of fine bone plates filled with haemopoetic marrow, fat-containing marrow, or blood vessels. Trabecular bone is located in vertebral bodies, flat bones and in the epiphyses of adult long bones. Trabecular bone serves to reduce skeletal weight without compromising strength, and its multiple surfaces are important sites of bone remodelling, the process that is meanly responsible for replacing old bone by new bone. Approximately 30% of bone mass is remodelled in a year (Malina *et al.*, 2004). Bone tissue is under constant reconstruction which is necessary for normal skeletal maintenance particularly during adulthood (Rubinacci *et al.*, 1998).

In the growing individual a positive relationship between bone mass and age reflects rapid bone deposition (Malina *et al.*, 2004). In young and middle-aged adults, rates of bone deposition and bone resorption are typically in balance. However during late adulthood, there is a negative association between age and bone mass in such a way that as age increases bone mass decreases reflecting more rapid rate of bone resorption compared to bone deposition (Malina *et al.*, 2004). During menopause, women lose approximately 3% of the total body bone mineral mass per year followed by around 1% per year bone loss after the age 65 in both females and males (Dawson-Hughes *et al.*, 1997). This condition results in microarchitectural deterioration of bone tissue and consequently loss of bone strength, thus making bone more fragile and easily susceptible to fracture. These characteristics explain osteoporosis (Brown and Josse, 2002).

13.3   How key nutrients and dietary factors impact bone health

In this section we present a brief overview of nutrients and dietary factors that are important for bone health that would be target dietary factors for functional foods designed for bone health. The nutrients, calcium, vitamin D and vitamin K, are also of interest because they are not plentiful in the diet. The dietary factors are soy isoflavones and milk basic proteins. One exception is phosphorus, for which an important role is noted yet current intakes of Americans and Canadians suggest that this nutrient need not be enhanced in foods. In Table 13.1, these selected nutrients and dietary factors needed for optimal bone health are listed along with estimated or calculated amounts needed for optimal bone health.

Table 13.1 Nutrients and dietary factors needed for optimal bone health with estimated or calculated amounts

Nutrient/dietary factor	Recommendation or estimated requirement for bone health	References
Calcium	1000–1500 mg/day	Kanis et al., 2008
		Brown and Josse, 2002
Phosphorus	700 mg/day	Institute of Medicine, 1997
Vitamin D	800–1000 IU/day	International Osteoporosis Foundation (IOF), 2009
		Brown and Josse, 2002
Protein	1.0 g/kg body weight per day	Kanis et al., 2008
Vitamin K	1000–5000 µg/day	Cockayne et al., 2006
		Cheung et al., 2008
Soy isoflavone	120 mg/day	Wong et al., 2009; Alekel et al., 2010
	Ipriflavone (synthetic isoflavone) 200 mg three times a day	Brown and Josse, 2002
Milk basic protein	40 mg	Aoe et al., 2001; Yamamura et al., 2002; Uenishi et al., 2007

Values provided are recommended or estimated for adult men and women.

13.3.1 Calcium

Calcium is the most common mineral in the human body; along with phosphorus it comprises approximately 80–90% of bone mineral content which is hydroxyapatite $[Ca_{10}(PO_4)_6(OH)_2]$ (Institute of Medicine, 1997). Calcium is needed throughout the lifespan, but the high velocity of bone mineral accumulation during puberty is illustrative of mechanisms when dietary calcium needs are high. During this time, an increase in plasma 1,25-dihydroxyvitamin D, the active form of vitamin D which increases intestinal absorption, and the stimulation of the renal tubular reabsorption of calcium, are two adaptive mechanisms to cope with increased demand for calcium during pubertal growth spurt. In adults, calcium requirements are set to maintain calcium balance or to minimize calcium losses (Institute of Medicine, 1997).

Although 99% of calcium is located in bones and teeth, it is the small ionized fraction of serum calcium that performs the numerous regulatory functions of calcium, including neuromuscular transmission of chemical and electrical stimuli, cellular secretion, blood clotting, oxygen transport, and enzymatic activity. Because of this regulatory role, the normal range for total serum calcium is narrow, maintained hormonally at three sites: the intestine, the kidney, and bone. Calcium absorption increases with increasing dietary calcium, reflecting passive absorption. Active absorption increases when there is a need for calcium, due to stimulation of circulating 1,25-dihydroxyvitamin D production (described below). Typically, in adults consuming mixed North American diets containing ~800 mg or more calcium per day, absorption of calcium approximates 30%, but in periods of severe dietary deficiency, fractional intestinal calcium excretion may increase to 75% (Institute of Medicine, 1997). Plasma calcium is filtered by the kidney; reabsorption occurs along the length of the nephron and is controlled by the parathyroid hormone. As described previously, bone is resorbed and formed continuously throughout life in a process called bone turnover. An average adult contains over 1000 grams of calcium in his or her skeleton, and approximately 1.5 grams of this is exchanged between bones and body fluid daily (Lemann *et al.*, 1979). Bone acts as a vast reservoir of calcium ions, and it acts as the first source of calcium used to raise low serum calcium levels. With time, this loss of calcium from bone can lead to osteoporosis if dietary calcium is not adequate to replace bone mineral calcium. This can occur in men as well as women (Daly *et al.*, 2006).

Recent systematic reviews have indicated that calcium is needed for bone growth and maintenance (e.g., Vatanparast and Whiting, 2006; Tang *et al.*, 2007). As many trials, especially in older adults, provided both calcium and vitamin D, and likely both nutrients are needed (Dawson-Hughes *et al.*, 1997). Current dietary recommendations for calcium for adults over 50 years are shown in Table 13.1. The values are derived from the Institute of Medicine's recommendation set in 1997 (Otten *et al.*, 2006), wherein values for adults were based on minimizing bone losses as measured using calcium balance techniques.

13.3.2   Phosphorus

Phosphorus, as phosphate is found in the bone mineral hydroxyapatite $[Ca_{10}(PO_4)_6(OH)_2]$ (Institute of Medicine, 1997). Its metabolism closely mirrors that of calcium but there are important distinctions. While both minerals are released from bone in times of need, when calcium is low (hypocalcemia) triggering parathyroid hormone release (PTH), urinary excretion of calcium is minimized but urinary excretion of phosphorus (as phosphate) is increased. While phosphorus is required for bone mineral formation, when calcium intake is low, excessive dietary phosphorus intake can be deleterious to bone as PTH secretion remains elevated, thus contributing to increased calcium bone resorption (Calvo and Carpenter, 2003). Phosphorus is found in many natural food sources (as shown in Table 13.2); however, with food processing and packaged foods, phosphate is a common food additive and thus dietary intakes in western countries is well above recommended intake, whereas calcium intake fails to meet recommendations (Vatanparast *et al.*, 2009). An improvement in this situation can be achieved through minimizing phosphate use as well as by improving calcium intake (Kemi *et al.*, 2006). As improving phosphorus intake of persons eating a Western diet is not a concern, consideration of phosphorus for use in functional foods that are targeted to bone health is not appropriate.

13.3.3   Vitamin D

Vitamin D is synthesized in the skin through the action of ultra-violet light or is obtained from dietary sources. In the skin, there is 7-dehydrocholesterol which reacts, in the presence of UVB radiation to form previtamin D_3. Previtamin D_3 forms rapidly; however, skin pigmentation (melanin) competes with 7-dehydrocholesterol for the UVB photons, and therefore reduces the amount of UVB that can act on 7-dehydrocholesterol to form previtamin D_3. Should more UVB photons reached the epidermis and dermis, previtamin D_3 is converted to inactive compounds with no vitamin D activity. Thus excess exposure to UVB does not result in excess vitamin D production. Skin synthesis of vitamin D can be limited by lack of UVB radiation during winter, clothing, being indoors or behind glass, sunscreen use, to name the most common. In these situations, the population is reliant on limited dietary sources (Whiting *et al.*, 2008).

Vitamin D_3 (also called cholecalciferol) and vitamin D_2 (ergocalciferol) in the diet are absorbed, and intestinal absorption is not known to be a limiting factor except when there is fat malabsorption (e.g., cystic fibrosis, Crohn's disease). Generally, fat-soluble vitamins are better absorbed with dietary fat, but vitamin D_3 added to orange juice is well absorbed (Tangpricha *et al.*, 2003). There are two steps leading to the active form of vitamin D, which is 1,25-dihydroxyvitamin D (also called calcitriol). The first step is converting vitamin D to the major circulating form, 25-hydroxyvitamin D (25(OH)D) in the liver. The amount of 25(OH)D that circulates is determined by the availability of the parent compound, thus diet is important when skin synthesis is lacking. It is important to appreciate that 25(OH)D is the key metabolite indicating vitamin D status. It is not the metabolically most active form but it is the form that most accurately reflects deficiency or excess and is therefore used as a measure of vitamin D nutritional status. The molecule 25(OH)D has a half-life of two weeks, however, due to contribution from stores in adipose and muscle, the amount in blood has an effective half-life of 2 months (Whiting *et al.*, 2008).

There are two pathways for conversion of 25(OH)D to 1,25-dihydroxyvitamin D. The better known pathway, now referred to as the endocrine pathway. 1,25-dihydroxyvitamin D is synthesized in the kidney but circulates to other tissues. A rise in parathyroid hormone (which itself is stimulated by a low circulating plasma calcium level) or a fall in intracellular phosphate levels are major stimulators of 1,25-dihydroxyvitamin D synthesis and release into blood. The main action of circulating 1,25-dihydroxyvitamin D is to increase calcium (and phosphate) active transport in the small intestine and therefore absorption. A second important action of circulating 1,25-dihydroxyvitamin D is to promote synthesis of mature osteoclasts, which are responsible for bone resorption. The net result is release of calcium and phosphate into circulation. Thus, having been made in the kidney in response to a need for calcium or phosphate, 1,25-dihydroxyvitamin D's actions in the intestine and bone have resulted in an increase into the blood of both of these compounds. The other pathway for conversion of 25(OH)D to 1,25-dihydroxyvitamin D is called the paracrine/autocrine pathway because these terms denote that the molecule is used locally in adjacent cells or used in the same cell in which it is made, respectively. Vitamin D receptors are present in most tissues. Extra-renal 1,25-dihydroxyvitamin D production is not regulated by serum calcium, phosphate or parathyroid. It functions as a transcription factor and its actions in the cell are highly regulated. With respect to bone metabolism, vitamin D's actions are required for optimal calcium and phosphate metabolism, including absorption and excretion, and for regulation of osteoblast and osteoclast synthesis (Whiting *et al.*, 2008).

13.3.4   Vitamin K

Vitamin K is best known for its functioning in the blood clotting system. However, knowledge that it plays a role in synthesis of at least one protein involved in bone formation has made it a nutrient of interest in bone health. Two types of vitamin K occur naturally: vitamin K_1 which is the major dietary form of the vitamin, also called phylloquinone; and vitamin K_2 which is a family of compounds called menaquinones. The latter has many different forms, of which MK-4 is distinct in being formed from vitamin K1 *in vivo*. Vitamin K has a role in bone biology as there are vitamin K-dependent proteins in bone and cartilage including osteocalcin, matrix Gla protein, protein S, Gas6 and periostin (Bonjour *et al.*, 2009; Bugel *et al.*, 2003).

There is mounting evidence that dietary vitamin K at doses higher than current recommendations may be beneficial in postmenopausal osteoporosis, the major benefit being fracture prevention. High levels of dietary vitamin K are associated with lower risk of hip fracture, and vitamin K levels in circulation are lower in patients with hip fractures compared to controls (Bonjour *et al.*, 2009; Bugel *et al.*, 2003). Vitamin K may be efficient in slowing bone loss in postmenopausal women with osteoporosis; however, its bone protective effect has not been shown to be superior to calcium and vitamin D. In 2006, a meta-analysis of intervention trials with vitamin K found a strong association of a specific vitamin K_2, called menatetrenone (MK-4) and reduced fracture incidence as well as reduced bone loss (Cockayne *et al.*, 2006). Another vitamin K_2 form, menatetrenone, has been reported to have positive bone effects (Iwamoto *et al.*, 2006). In one study the combination of high dose vitamin K1 (1000 µg), vitamin D and calcium slowed bone loss at the femoral neck better than any of these nutrients taken singly (Cockayne *et al.*, 2006). In 2008, a four year clinical trial in which 5000 µg vitamin K1 was given to postmenopausal women with osteopenia, showed no effect on the age-related decline in bone mineral density but appeared to protect against fractures (Cheung *et al.*, 2008). The dose of menatetrenone has also been high, starting at 30 mg/kg body weight (Iwamoto *et al.*, 2006). These doses suggest that vitamin K must be provided in pharmacologic amounts; therefore, while we acknowledge the vitamin K content in one of our functional food examples, it may not be contributing to bone health (Booth, 2009).

13.3.5   Soy

Soy-derived foods provide many nutrients that may influence bone health. The positive association between soy products intake and bone health was seen first in cross-sectional studies (Mei *et al.*, 2001; Somekawa *et al.*, 2001; Kim *et al.*, 2002;

Kritz-Silverstein and Goodman-Gruen, 2002), and this encouraged further research to examine the cause and effect relationship between different components and bone health. The exact mechanisms of the effect of soy products on bone are not clear. The estrogens-like effect of soy isoflavones, as well as enhancement of calcium economy and an anabolic effect on bone through promoting insulin-like growth factors due to soy protein are mechanisms proposed by researchers (Mei *et al.*, 2001; Arjmandi *et al.*, 2003).

Soy foods are high in protein, and protein is an important factor in bone health. Increasing protein intake among those who have inadequate dietary protein reduces the risk of hip fracture in men and women (Brown and Josse, 2002; Darling *et al.*, 2009). In a systematic review of randomized placebo-controlled trials, Darling *et al.* (2009) found a positive effect of protein supplementation on lumbar spine bone mineral density that supports the positive association between protein intake and bone health found in cross-sectional surveys. However, there does not appear to be a specific effect of soy protein alone on maintenance of bone mineral content, which means it is the protein itself that is important. A recent randomized controlled trial (Kenny *et al.*, 2009) examining the long-term effect of soy protein on skeletal health in late healthy postmenopausal women found no significant effect of soy protein intake on bone mineral density at various skeletal sites.

Soy isoflavones are phytoestrogens, compounds that are structurally or functionally related to ovarian or placental estrogens and their active metabolites. The beneficial effect of phytoestrogens on bone in postmenopausal women might be better explained by a hormone replacement effect. While there are other phytoestrogens found in plants, such as lignans in flax seed and coumestans in bean sprouts, most research has been conducted using soy isoflavones. Populations with high phytoestrogens intake such as Asians in Asia have lower rates of hip fracture than North Americans (Scheiber and Rebar, 1999). Soybean isoflavones appeared to reduce bone resorption in postmenopausal women, but the early studies (e.g., Morabito *et al.*, 2002; Uesugi *et al.*, 2002; Atkinson *et al.*, 2004) indicated the need for determining long-term effects. However, even longer studies remain inconsistent. While, soy isoflavones reduce bone resorption biomarkers, they have not convincingly increased bone mineral density at hip and lumbar spine in recent studies (Brink *et al.*, 2008; Kenny *et al.*, 2009; Liu *et al.*, 2009). The high inter-individual variability in bioavailability and metabolism of phytoestrogens may compromise their biological effects (Rowland *et al.*, 2003; Nettleton *et al.*, 2005), as it has been hypothesized that the ability to produce equol (an active metabolite of soy isoflavone with greater estrogenic effect) after ingestion of soy isoflavones is a major determinant of any beneficial effect of soy isoflavones on bone (Vatanparast and Chilibeck, 2007). As Kenny and coworkers (2009), in their randomized controlled trial, found no effect of soy isoflavones on BMD among equol producers and non-producers in their sample of postmenopausal women, the role equol production on bone health in postmenopausal women needs further investigation (Vatanparast and Chilibeck, 2007; Chilibeck and Cornish, 2008).

Two recent studies, two-year randomized controlled trials, found modest bone-sparing effects in post-menopausal women using a dose of 120 mg isoflavones on top of adequate calcium and vitamin D (Wong *et al.*, 2009; Alekel *et al.*, 2010). It is unlikely this dose would be recommended for treatment but it still may have some protective effects.

The beneficial effect of a synthetic phytoestrogen isoflavone, Ipriflavone, on bone mineral density and biomarkers has been investigated in various studies among post menopausal women. However, due to differences in measuring techniques and bone sites, results are not thoroughly comparable (Brown and Josse, 2002). In a recent randomized controlled trial of 60 osteoporotic postmenopausal women, there were a decrease in bone resorption biomarkers and an increase in bone formation biomarkers (Zhang *et al.*, 2009). While evidence suggests that 200 mg Ipriflavone, three times a day, maintains bone mineral density in lumbar spine of postmenopausal women (Kovacs, 1994; Gambacciani *et al.*, 1997), this is not sufficient enough to prevent fracture. Whether Ipriflavone affects the estrogen sensitive tissues such as breast and uterus also needs to be clarified. Further, no information is available on the effect of Ipriflavone in men and premenopausal women. Currently, in Canada, because of inconclusive data on the effect of Ipriflavone on bone in postmenopausal women and long-term safety concerns, it was recommended for the treatment of postmenopausal osteoporosis, but only as second-line therapy (Brown and Josse, 2002), and no further statements regarding its use have been forthcoming.

13.3.6   Milk basic proteins

Cow's milk naturally contains two types of protein, casein, which can precipitate especially in the presence of the enzyme rennin, and lactalbumin, which is soluble. Both have high biological value. Having sufficient dietary protein itself is beneficial for bone growth and maintenance of bone mineral content (Darling *et al.*, 2009). In vitro studies initially demonstrated that milk whey proteins and more specifically its basic fraction (milk basic protein or MBP) stimulate the proliferation and differentiation of osteoblastic cells and suppress the osteoclast-mediated bone resorption and osteoclast cell formation (Takada *et al.*, 1996, 1997a). Furthermore, the same researchers found that the oral administration of milk whey proteins had no effect on calcium absorption but enhanced bone strength and hydroxyproline content in young ovariectomized rats (Takada *et al.*, 1997b). Active components from MBP have been found to be a bone formation promoter (increasing proliferation of osteoblasts) (Yamamura *et al.*, 2000) and the bone resorption inhibitor cystatin C, which promotes osteoclastic inhibition (Matsuoka *et al.*, 2002). Animal studies have demonstrated these bone protective properties (Takada *et al.*, 1996, 1997a; Yamamura *et al.*, 2000).

Intervention trials with MBP have been done in premenopausal women, postmenopausal women and men. When young healthy women were randomly assigned to receive, once-a-day, a beverage containing 40 mg of MBP or placebo for six months (matched for bone mineral density and other criteria), bone mineral density gain of the calcaneus (a trabecular bone), and the bone mineral density of the radius (a cortical bone) was significantly higher in the MBP group (Aoe *et al.*, 2001). Biochemical markers of bone resorption were significantly reduced in the MBP group. Similar findings were reported by Yamamura *et al.* (2002) and Uenishi *et al.* (2007). MBP, again 40 mg per day, was also tested in healthy postmenopausal women. Analysing only those who completed the six-month trial successfully, investigators found per cent changes in lumbar spine were higher after MBP (Aoe *et al.*, 2001, 2005). Beverages containing 300 mg of MBP were administered daily for 16 days in young adult men, and a marker of bone formation was increased while a marker of bone resorption decreased with MBP (Toba *et al.*, 2001).

As a food supplement, 40 mg MBP daily would be beneficial for bone health in pre- and postmenopausal women and could be considered based on the current scientific literature. However, all published studies from cell cultures, to animal and human clinical studies have been produced and reported by a single research group in collaboration with a Japanese dairy company. Thus it is recognized that the overall literature is small and limited to studies conducted in Japanese populations.

13.4   Dietary sources of nutrients and dietary factors related to bone health, and safety considerations

In this section, food sources of selected nutrients and dietary factors that illustrate nutrition considerations for bone health and for which functional foods exist, are described. For each factor, natural sources and their likely consumption are provided. In countries such as Canada, some foods are now fortified with these factors, and two of these will be described. As fortification could lead to concerns of safety, aspects of safety considerations are discussed for these nutrients and dietary factors. In Table 13.2, examples of natural food sources are shown to indicate why these bone health nutrients and factors are needed in amounts not commonly consumed from many foods or food groups.

13.4.1   Calcium

Naturally calcium-rich foods such as dairy products and green vegetables are not only good sources of calcium, but also sources of a variety of other nutrients which are necessary for bone health (Ilich and Kerstetter, 2000). Milk products are the main source of calcium in the Canadian (Vatanparast *et al.*, 2009) and American (Forshee *et al.*, 2006) diet. They also contain other nutrients beneficial for bone growth including protein, phosphorus, magnesium, zinc, and a range of other nutrients (Cadogan *et al.*, 1997; Dawson-Hughes 2003; Huncharek *et al.*, 2008). Alternate sources of calcium include calcium-fortified soy, rice beverages and juices. In a sample of Canadian adolescents, milk products were the major source of dietary calcium (61%), followed by grain products (9%), vegetables and fruit (7%), meat and alternatives (2%) and other foods (21%) which is close to data from the United States (Iuliano-Burns *et al.*, 1999). While fluid milk is the

Table 13.2 Natural sources of nutrients and active factors for bone health from different food groups (healthy food examples providing low energy and high protein), illustrating the difficulty in meeting key bone nutrients and dietary factors requirements from food

Food groups and food examples, 100 g	Energy (kcal)	Protein (g)	Vitamin D (IU)	Calcium (mg)	Phosphorus (mg)	Vitamin K (µg)	Soy isoflavones (mg)	Milk basic protein (mg)
Milk products								
Fluid low fat milk	50	3.3	1	120	92	0.2	0	5
Natural yogurt low fat	63	5.3	1	183	144	0.2	0	10
Grain products								
Whole grain bread	265	13.4	0	103	228	1.4	0.01	0
Cooked brown rice	111	2.6	0	10	83	0.6	0.02	0
Vegetables and fruit								
Raw dark green lettuce	17	1.2	0	33	30	102.5	0	0
Cooked sweet potato	76	1.4	0	27	27	2.1	0	0
Raw oranges	47	0.9	0	40	14	0	0	0
Meat								
Cooked lean beef	238	31.1	28	13	235	–	0	0
Cooked wild Atlantic salmon	182	25.4	328	15	256	–	0	0
Protein alternatives								
Cooked white beans	139	9.7	0	90	113	3.5	0	0
Cooked tempeh	196	18.2	0	96	253	–	38	0
Range	17–265	1–31	0–328	10–183	14–256	0–102	0–38	0–10
(approximate values)	kcal	g	IU	mg	mg	µg	mg	mg

Note: values taken from the United States Department of Agriculture (USDA) National Nutrient Database for Standard Reference, release 22 online (http://www.ars.usda.gov/main/site_main.htm?modecode=12-35-45-00) except milk basic protein (values from references in section 13.4.4) and vitamin D in beef and salmon (Canadian Nutrient File http://webprod.hc-sc.gc.ca/cnf-fce/index-eng.jsp).

main source of dietary calcium in Canada and the USA, other beverages such as carbonated and non-carbonated soft drinks and fruit juice are replacing this food (Whiting *et al.*, 2001). As intake of milk is declining, there has been an effort to increase calcium content, through calcium fortification of high quality beverages such as orange juice or plant-based drinks such as soy beverages. Intake data suggest that for certain segments of the population, current levels of fortification of nondairy foods has not resulted in an significant increase in calcium intakes in Canada (Vatanparast *et al.*, 2009) and the USA (Forshee *et al.*, 2006).

There are safety concerns about dietary calcium. As part of the 1997 Dietary Reference Intake process, a daily tolerable upper intake level (UL) for calcium was set at 2500 mg (Otten *et al.*, 2006). The UL is defined as a safe level of intake, but risk for adverse effects increases with increasing intakes above this value. Excess calcium intake is associated with hypercalcemia leading to milk-alkali syndrome, a potentially lethal condition of calcification of soft tissues resulting in kidney failure. As well, excessive calcium intake has been linked to renal stone formation and to inhibition of micromineral absorption (Institute of Medicine, 1997). Thus, adding calcium to foods must be done judiciously, targeting those who need additional dietary calcium (e.g., young and older women) while avoiding consumption by young men for whom dietary calcium may be already adequate (Vatanparast *et al.*, 2009).

13.4.2   Vitamin D

Dietary intake of vitamin D is a concern as many people do not frequently consume the few foods that are naturally high in vitamin D such as fatty fish (Table 13.2) or irradiated mushrooms (Calvo and Whiting, 2010). Other natural food sources include meats and eggs (where the vitamin D is made through skin synthesis by the animal or it has been added to feed). In some countries there is no fortification with vitamin D. Canada is an example of a country with mandatory fortification of milk and margarine, and some discretionary (i.e., permitted) fortification of fruit juice, meal replacements and liquid nutrition supplements (Calvo *et al.*, 2004). Because of these fortification practices, milk products are the main source of dietary vitamin D of Canadians, especially children under nine years of age (Vatanparast *et al.*, 2010). However, there still is a large gap in availability of vitamin D in foods compared to requirements. is not consistent with current healthy eating guidelines to recommend increased consumption of oily fish, and increased consumption of other sources such as liver.

It is important to recognize that vitamin D_2 and D_3 are different molecules. There is some debate as to whether they are equivalent (Whiting *et al.*, 2008). If a large, infrequent bolus of Vitamin D is the protocol, the vitamin D_3 is preferred over vitamin D_2 as more of vitamin D_2 may be required to increase and then maintain levels of 25(OH)D. However, if vitamin D_2 is taken daily, there appears to be no difference in response between it and vitamin D_3 (Holick *et al.*, 2008; Calvo and Whiting, 2010). Vitamin D_2 is from non-animal sources, primarily UV-irradiated yeasts and mushrooms, so it is appropriate for vegetarian diets.

Canadians and Americans are largely dependent on fortified foods and dietary supplements to meet their vitamin D needs because foods that are naturally rich in vitamin D are less frequently consumed (Calvo and Whiting, 2010) The Canadian approach has been one of mandatory fortification of food staples. Milk and milk alternatives and margarine are required to be fortified in Canada. There are a few instances where other foods for which vitamin D additions are permitted – meal replacements, nutritional supplements, and formulated liquid diets. In the United States, there are more foods to which vitamin D may be added, e.g., breakfast cereal, cheese and yogurt, bread products. In most cases these are discretionary additions, with fluid fortified milk being the exception. Despite these attempts to fortify the food supply, dietary intakes of Canadians and Americans are higher than in countries where fortification has not occurred, but still remain less than optimal (Calvo *et al.*, 2005; Whiting *et al.*, 2007).

In 1997, a UL for vitamin D of 50 µg (2000 IU) was established for persons aged one year and older, in order to discourage potentially dangerous self-medication. For infants 0–1 year of age, the UL was set at 25 µg (1000 IU). A recent risk assessment for vitamin D used newer data to derive what could be a revised to 10 000 UL in adults (Hathcock *et al.*, 2007). The primary adverse effect that is expected at very high levels of vitamin D is hypercalcemia, which can lead, over time, to calcification of soft tissues such as arteries (arteriosclerosis) and kidney (nephrocalcinosis) (Otten *et al.*, 2006). In contrast to calcium, there is less concern about vitamin D added to foods, except for infants and very young children.

13.4.3   Soy isoflavones

Numerous soy food and beverage items are available in the US food market (USDA, 2008). Dietary sources of soy isoflavones in North America include traditional soy foods (e.g. tofu, tempeh, miso food), manufactured soy foods/beverages such as vegetable soy burger, soy cheese and soy milk, and supplements (e.g. isoflavone pills and liquid nutrition drinks). Among 20 dietary sources of soy isoflavones found in grocery stores in the early 2000s, the top five items contributing to total isoflavone intake were cooked soybeans or green soy beans, pills containing soy isoflavones, tofu, soy milk and soy protein powders (Frankenfeld, 2003). A recent pharmacokinetic study among 12 healthy adults reported that the serum concentration of isoflavones after eating soy foods containing 96 mg isoflavones was higher than that from an isoflavone supplement, suggesting higher bioavailability of isoflavone from food than from supplements (Gardner *et al.*, 2009).

Considerable attention has been given to soy products in regard to breast cancer, both for decreasing and increasing its risk. The anti-breast cancer activity of soy products may be mediated by antioxidant actions, while, estrogen-like effects may increase the risk for cancer. However, most cell culture, animal and human studies support the opposite, that is, an overall anti-breast cancer activity of soy products (Atkinson *et al.*, 2002; Valachovicova *et al.*, 2004; Dave *et al.*, 2005). Animal and in vitro studies suggest that the isoflavone 'genistein' enhances the proliferation of breast cancer cells and estrogen-dependent mammary tumor growth (Helferich *et al.*, 2008; Taylor *et al.*, 2009). Further, reported both synergic and antagonistic interaction between soy isoflavones and tamoxifen, a selective estergen receptor modulator used for breast cancer treatment, is another area of uncertainty (Taylor *et al.*, 2009). A recent population-based prospective study among over 5000 breast cancer survivors with a median follow-up of 3.9 years reported that soy food intake is safe among breast cancer patients and was associated with lower rates of mortality and reduced recurrence (Shu *et al.*, 2009). Most recent randomized controlled trials reported that soy isoflavones and soy protein did not modify breast density in postmenopausal women (Verheus *et al.*, 2008; Maskarinec *et al.*, 2009). There is, however, remaining concern about high doses of purified isoflavones which cannot be recommended in individuals who might be at risk of breast cancer (Helferich *et al.*, 2008).

13.4.4   Milk basic protein

Milk basic protein (MBP) is extracted from milk with a yield of approximately 40 mg of MBP for 800 mL of skim milk (Uenishi *et al.*, 2007). It is available commercially in Japan in several derived dairy products (Snow Brand Milk Products Company). The amount of MBP in milk can be estimated, but whether it survives processing in other dairy foods is not known. In terms of safety, there are animal as well as human studies. In rats, levels up to 2 g/kg body weight have been tested in rats. In total, acute oral toxicity tests, teratology studies, subchronic oral toxicity studies, and reverse mutation assays have revealed no treatment related adverse events (Kruger *et al.*, 2007). In Japan, and now in Canada, MBP at a dose of 40 mg per serving has been evaluated as an ingredient in food and concluded to be safe for its intended use.

13.5   Case studies of functional foods designed to improve intake of bone health factors

Two functional foods, presented in Table 13.3, are currently available in Canada. They illustrate functional foods that resemble familiar foods, yet have nutrients and dietary factors that promote bone health. The yogurt product, available in Canada as Yoplait Asana, contains twice as much calcium as regular yogurt, has as much vitamin D as is allowable in Canada at this time (i.e., this yogurt is made using fortified milk), and contains added milk basic proteins. As well, yogurt contains protein that is important for bone health, is a natural source of vitamin K, and has other nutrients which would benefit bone. Yogurt is familiar in the marketplace. Secondly, we show a soy beverage, for which there are numerous commercial examples. Soy foods, as previously described, may function in bone health in many ways, provided they are fortified with calcium and vitamin D in amounts similar to cow's milk, as is common in Canada and the USA. They can provide soy isoflavones at the approximate level of 20 mg per 250 mL serving

Table 13.3 Case studies of fortified foods available in Canada where nutrients and/or dietary factors important for bone health have been enhanced and/or added

Functional food	Active ingredients (+ indicates added) per serving	Target market
Fortified soy beverage*, serving size 250 mL	24 mg soy isoflavone 308 mg calcium (+) 85 IU vitamin D$_2$ (+)	Milk-like beverage containing protein that appeals to people who do not drink cows' milk yet want a similar beverage
Yogurt with added calcium, vitamin D and milk basic protein (MBP), serving size 100 g	200 mg calcium (#,+) 37 IU vitamin D$_2$ (+) 0.2 μg vitamin K 40 mg MBP (+)	Yogurt is already a bone-healthy food but this product doubles the calcium, has added vitamin D (to levels currently allowed in Canada)

* Data from http://www.yoplait.ca and USDA, 2008; # indicates natural source; + indicates added as fortification.

(USDA, 2008). In addition they are also a good source of protein and other nutrients. Soy beverages are familiar in the marketplace in that they resemble cow's milk in appearance and may be used in place of cow's milk in cooking and food preparation.

In adding nutrients to foods, it has been necessary to prove bioavailability and effectiveness. With respect to calcium, this is a challenge as calcium available is highly variable from foods (Weaver and Plawecki, 1994) and from supplemental sources (Whiting and Pluhator, 1992). Availability of calcium was a challenging problem for soy beverages. When these products were initially available on the marketplace, soy beverages were fortified with calcium as calcium triphosphate, but this insoluble form proved to be undesirable. When tested, calcium absorption from these calcium-fortified soy beverages was not equivalent to the absorption of calcium from cow's milk, averaging about 75% (Heaney *et al.*, 2000b). Examining some plant-based milk-like beverages in an *in vitro* system, they were scored only between 60–70% relative to cow's milk (Heaney *et al.*, 2005a, 2005b). Further, these values were obtained only when resuspension of calcium sediments was ensured by thoroughly shaking the original container prior to consuming. However, when calcium was added as calcium carbonate, products showed equivalent bioavailability as calcium from cow's milk (Zhao *et al.*, 2005). Now that current fortification of plant-based beverages in Canada and the United States is with calcium carbonate, availability concerns are less.

When fortification of fruit beverages with vitamin D was initially proposed, it was necessary to evaluate bioavailability. In a 12-week study, Tangpricha *et al.* (2003) found that orange juice was a suitable vehicle, despite being a low fat food. A recent review concluded that intake of different fortified sources of vitamin D – fluid milk, milk powder, wheat bread, rye bread and orange juice – increased vitamin D status (O'Donnell *et al.*, 2008).

13.6   Future trends

Nutrition recommendations have not differed much between those for prevention and treatments. While the latter condition requires more serious attention to diet, to promote nutrition for prevention of later bone loss would likely reduce the incidence of osteoporosis. For treatment, several groups have made specific recommendations. The European Society for Clinical and Economic Aspects of Osteoporosis and Osteoarthritis recommends that general management include the maintenance of mobility, avoidance of falls and correction of nutritional deficiencies, particularly of calcium, vitamin D and protein. Intakes of at least 1000 mg/day of calcium, 800 IU of vitamin D and of 1 g/kg body weight of protein are recommended (Kanis *et al.*, 2008). These values are similar to those recommended by Osteoporosis Canada (Brown and Josse, 2002).

However, more is known about the effect of nutrition in treatment (Fig. 13.2). In contrast, less is known about prevention. Currently, recommendations stress improvement of the overall diet. For example, the International Osteoporosis Foundation makes these recommendations: ensure an adequate dietary calcium intake, appropriate for stage of life; maintain a sufficient supply of vitamin D through safe sun exposure, diet, or if required, supplements; enjoy a nutritious diet including adequate protein; and a balanced diet will provide magnesium, vitamin K and phosphorus for healthy bones. As we illustrate in Table 13.2, it is not easy to obtain bone-healthy nutrients in natural food sources.

13.6.1   What are the nutrition needs of established nutrients for bone health?

There is a clear consensus that calcium and vitamin D are required for bone health throughout the lifespan (International Osteoporosis Federation, 2009). Further, when examining intakes of these two nutrients, there are reasons to be concerned about adequacy. For calcium, the need is especially urgent for adolescent and adult females in Canada (Vatanparast *et al.*, 2009) and in the United States (Forshee *et al.*, 2006). Current vitamin D fortification practices may not be sufficient to prevent poor vitamin D status during winter (Calvo *et al.*, 2004). There are few natural food sources of vitamin D (Table 13.2). Since those foods are not commonly consumed, in North America most of the intake of vitamin D from food comes from fortified food items (Calvo *et al.*, 2004).

13.6.2   What are the nutrition needs of other dietary factors for bone health?

Generally practice guidelines for osteoprosis include only a few nutrients, usually just calcium and vitamin D (e.g. Dawson-Hughes, 2008) as these nutrients have the best evidence for fracture prevention (Brown and Josse, 2002; Bischoff-Ferrari *et al.*, 2009). However, other nutrients and dietary factors are emerging as promoting bone formation or preventing bone loss. We chose soy isoflavones and

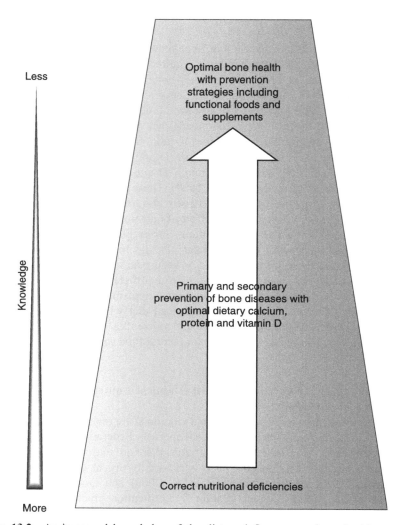

Fig. 13.2 As improved knowledge of the dietary influences on bone health emerges through research, recommendations for bone health will expand beyond treating deficiencies through to ensuring adequacy of key nutrients to encompassing nutrients and dietary factors that promote bone formation and/or inhibit bone resorption (modified from Institute of Medicine (2008)).

milk basic protein to illustrate that these other factors may be added to a functional food. What is not known whether all dietary factors and nutrient effects are additive in their actions toward bone. For example, one would expect a bone formation inducer to be additive with a bone resorption inhibitor, but not many combinations have been studied.

13.7   Issues related to product targeting and consumer acceptance of bone-healthy functional foods

The case studies of two functional foods that are currently available in Canada (Table 13.3) are examples of bone healthy foods that resemble traditional foods. This is the most appropriate way to introduce functional foods with bone healthy ingredients. Further, it is important that these foods are capable of being fortified with calcium, as ensuring appropriate bioavailability of this nutrient can be a challenging (Heaney *et al.*, 2000b). One of these case studies is in a dairy food, which has good availability; the other was described as having had challenges with respect to calcium availability but these are overcome. In terms of vitamin D, the form (whether vitamin D_2 and D_3) is no longer considered a concern (Holick *et al.*, 2008). For vegetarians, vitamin D_2 is the preferred form. That these functional foods contain a good source of protein is also important (Darling *et al.*, 2009). Nutrients and dietary factors, whether naturally found (e. g., vitamin K, or isoflavones) or added to increase dosage to an effective level (e.g., milk basic protein), may also be in these foods.

Factors that may affect the nature of functional foods for bone health include the following: age, sex, dietary preferences (e.g., vegetarianism) and cultural preferences. In Table 13.3, we gave two examples. A fortified soy beverage could appeal to young and old, as it can be used to replace milk, a common beverage for all age groups. Similarly yogurt is a food that most age groups are familiar with, but it may appeal more to older adults who wish to consume a dairy product but who may not drink milk. More research is needed to examine consumer preferences. Wansink (2005) has described five approaches to improve consumer use of healthy food choices such as offered through functional foods. These five approaches, which have been tested for effectiveness, include: increase the availability and accessibility to achieve consumer awareness; increase substitutability to achieve acceptance; choose appropriate frames of reference such as emphasizing a person's loss at not consuming the food; use commitment of influential social groups; and position functional foods as socially acceptable products. The examples in Table 13.3 illustrate these approaches, in part by being enhanced traditional or substitute foods.

Finally, it is important to stay abreast of recent developments in understanding bone growth and development. Societies that provide information on bone health and osteoporosis are listed in Table 13.4. These societies also provide evidence-based dietary recommendations for bone health that are posted at their websites. As countries have unique foods and may have different fortification policies, it is necessary to consider local food composition data; locations of these are found in Table 13.4.

In conclusion, in this chapter we focused on nutrients which in addition to being necessary for bone health are also nutrients which are limiting in the diet of those living in Western countries such as Canada, USA and Europe, i.e. calcium, and its major influencer, vitamin D. Some nutrients needed for bone health, such as phosphorus, are not limiting in the diet and therefore need not be added to

Table 13.4   Resources and further information on nutrition and bone health

Topic	Reference
General information on bone health and osteoporosis	Osteoporosis Canada website includes most up-to-date practice guideline information http://www.osteoporosis.ca/ The National Institutes of Health Osteoporosis and Related Bone Diseases National Resource Center http://www.niams.nih.gov/Health_Info/Bone/ *The Introduction to Clinical Osteoporosis* slide set, International Bone and Mineral Society (IBMS) http://www.bonekey-ibms.org/
Bone health and osteoporosis guidelines having nutrition recommendations	International Osteoporosis Foundation (IOF) 'Good Nutrition for healthy Bones' http://www.iofbonehealth.org/download/osteofound/filemanager/publications/pdf/good_nutrition_for_healthy_bones.pdf (accessed December 30, 2009). Brown J P and Josse R G (2002) Clinical practice guidelines for the diagnosis and management of osteoporosis in Canada', *Can Med Assoc J*, **167**, S1–34. Dawson-Hughes B (2008) 'National Osteoporosis Foundation Guide Committee. A revised clinician's guide to the prevention and treatment of osteoporosis in postmenopausal women', *J Clin Endocrinol Metab* **93**(7), 2463–2465. http://www.nof.org/professionals/NOF_Clinicians_Guide.pdf Kanis J A, Burlet N, Cooper C (2008), 'European Society for Clinical and Economic Aspects of Osteoporosis and Osteoarthritis (ESCEO) Osteoporosis guidelines', *Osteoporos Int* **19**, 399–428.
Information on food composition for different countries around the world	FAO, The international network of Food Data Systems http://www.fao.org/infoods/data_en.stm Health Canada's Canadian Nutrient File site http://webprod.hc-sc.gc.ca/cnf-fce/index-eng.jsp USA, USDA Nutrition Data laboratory http://www.nal.usda.gov/fnic/foodcomp/search/ Europe, EuroFIR, Food Composition database http://www.eurofir.net/public.asp?id=4210 Asia, Food Composition Tables http://www.fao.org/infoods/tables_asia_en.stm

foods. We also focused on dietary factors that illustrate how research is shaping functional foods that are not in the marketplace.

13.8   References

Alekel D L, Van Loan M D, Koehler K J *et al.* (2010) 'The Soy Isoflavones for Reducing Bone Loss (SIRBL) Study: a 3-y randomized controlled trial in postmenopausal women', *Am J Clin Nutr*, **91**, 218–230.

Aoe S, Toba Y, Yamamura J *et al.* (2001) 'Controlled trial of the effects of milk basic protein (MBP) supplementation on bone metabolism in healthy adult women', *Biosci Biotechnol Biochem*, **65**, 913–918.

Aoe S, Koyama T, Toba Y, Itabashi A and Takada Y. (2005) 'A controlled trial of the effect of milk basic protein (MBP) supplementation on bone metabolism in healthy menopausal women', *Osteoporos Int*, **16**, 2123–2128.

Arjmandi B H, Khalil DA, Smith B J *et al.* (2003) 'Soy protein has a greater effect on bone in postmenopausal women not on hormone replacement therapy, as evidenced by reducing bone resorption and urinary calcium excretion', *J Clin Endocrinol Metab*, **88**, 1048–1054.

Atkinson C, Bingham S A (2002) 'Mammographic breast density as a biomarker of effects of isoflavones on the female breast', *Breast Cancer Res*, **4**, 1–4.

Atkinson C, Compston J E, Day N E *et al.* (2004) 'The effects of phytoestrogen isoflavones on bone density in women, a double-blind, randomized, placebo-controlled trial', *Am J Clin Nutr*, **79**, 326–333.

Bischoff-Ferrari H A, Willett W C, Wong J B *et al.* (2009) 'Prevention of nonvertebral fractures with oral vitamin D and dose dependency: a meta-analysis of randomized controlled trials', *Arch Int Med*, **169**, 551–561.

Bonjour J P, Gueguen L, Palacios C, Shreaer M J and Weaver C M (2009) 'Minerals and vitamins in bone health, the potential value of dietary enhancement', *Br J Nutr*, **101**, 1581–1596.

Booth S L (2009) 'Roles for vitamin K beyond coagulation', *Annu Rev Nutr*, **29**, 89–110.

Booth S L and Suttie J W (1998) 'Dietary intake and adequacy of vitamin K', *J Nutr*, **128**, 785–788.

Brink E, Coxam V, Robins S, Wahala K, Cassidy A and Branca F (2008) 'Long-term consumption of isoflavone-enriched foods does not affect bone mineral density, bone metabolism, or hormonal status in early postmenopausal women, a randomized, double-blind, placebo controlled study', *Am J Clin Nutr*, **87**, 761–770.

Brown J P and Josse R G (2002) 'Clinical practice guidelines for the diagnosis and management of osteoporosis in Canada', *Can Med Assoc J*, **167**, S1–34.

Bugel S (2003) 'Vitamin K and bone health', *Proc Nutr Soc*, **62**, 839–843.

Cadogan J, Eastell R, Jones N, and Barker M E (1997) 'Milk intake and bone mineral acquisition in adolescent girls: randomised, controlled intervention trial', *BMJ*, **15**, 1255–1260.

Calvo M S and Carpenter T O (2003) 'Influence of phosphorus on the skeleton'. In *Nutritional Aspects of Bone Health*, 1st edition, Susan New and Jean-Philippe Bonjour (eds.), Royal Chemistry Society, Cambridge, UK, pp. 229–265.

Calvo M S, Barton C N and Whiting S J (2004) 'Vitamin D fortification in the US and Canada: current status and data needs', *Am J Clin Nutr*, **80**, S1710–1716.

Calvo M S, Whiting S J and Barton C N (2005) 'Vitamin D intake: A global perspective of current status', *J Nutr*, **135**, 310–316.

Calvo M S, and Whiting S J (2010) 'Determinants of vitamin D intake'. In M Holick (ed.) *Vitamin D: Physiology, Molecular Biology, and Clinical Application*, Humana (Springer), New York, pp. 361–382.

Cheung A M, Tile L and Lee Y (2008) 'Vitamin K supplementation in postmenopausal women with osteopenia (ECKO Trial), a randomized controlled trial', *PLoS Med*, **5**, 1–12.

Chevalley T, Bonjour JP, Ferrari S and Rizzoli R (2009) 'The influence of pubertal timing on bone mass acquisition: a predetermined trajectory detectable five years before menarche', *J Clin Endocrinol Metab*, **94**, 3424–3431.

Chilibeck P D and Cornish S M (2008) 'Effect of estrogenic compounds (estrogen or phytoestrogens) combined with exercise on bone and muscle mass in older individuals', *Appl Physiol Nutr Metab*, **33**, 200–212.

Cockayne S, Adamson J, Lanham-New S, Shearer M J, Gilbody S and Torgerson D J (2006) 'Vitamin K and the prevention of fractures, systematic review and meta-analysis of randomized controlled trials', *Arch Intern Med*, **166**, 1256–1261.

Cole Z A, Dennison E M and Cooper C (2008) 'Osteoporosis epidemiology update', *Curr Rheumatol Rep*, **10**, 92–96.

Daly R M, Brown M, Bass S, Kukuljian S and Nowson C (2006) 'Calcium- and vitamin D3-fortified milk reduces bone loss at clinically relevant skeletal sites in older men: a 2-year randomized controlled trial', *J Bone Miner Res*, **21**, 397–405.

Darling A L, Millward D J, Torgerson D J, Hewitt C E and Lanham-New S (2009) 'Dietary protein and bone health: a systematic review and meta-analysis', *Am J Clin Nutr*, **90**, 1674–1692.

Dave B, Eason R R, Till S R, Geng Y, Velarde M C *et al.* (2005) 'The soy isoflavone genistein promotes apoptosis in mammary epithelial cells by inducing the tumor suppressor PTEN', *Carcinogenesis*, **26**, 1793–1803.

Dawson-Hughes B, Harris S S, Krall E A *et al.* (1997) 'Effect of calcium and vitamin D supplementation on bone density in men and women 65 years of age or older', *N Engl J Med*, **337**, 670–676.

Dawson-Hughes B (2003) 'Role of calcium in reducing postmenopausal bone loss and in fracture prevention'. In S New and JP Bonjour (eds) *Nutritional Aspects of Bone Health*, Cambridge, UK, The Royal Society of Chemistry, pp. 145–156.

Dawson-Hughes B (2008) 'National Osteoporosis Foundation Guide Committee. A revised clinician's guide to the prevention and treatment of osteoporosis in postmenopausal women', *J Clin Endocrinol Metab* **93**, 2463–2465.

Forshee R A, Anderson P A and Storey M L (2006) 'Changes in calcium intake and association with beverage consumption and demographics: comparing data from CSFII 1994–1996, 1998 and NHANES 1999–2002', *J Am Coll Nutr*, **25**, 108–116.

Frankenfeld C L, Patterson R E, Horner N K *et al.* (2003) 'Validation of a soy food-frequency questionnaire and evaluation of correlates of plasma isoflavone concentrations in postmenopausal women', *Am J Clin Nutr*, **77**, 674–680.

Gafni R I and Baron J (2007) 'Childhood bone mass acquisition and peak bone mass may not be important determinants of bone mass in late adulthood', *Pediatrics*, **119**, S131–136.

Gambacciani M, Ciaponi M, Cappagli B, Piaggesi L and Genazzani AR (1997) 'Effects of combined low dose of the isoflavone derivative ipriflavone and estrogen replacement on bone mineral density and metabolism in postmenopausal women', *Maturitas*, **28**, 75–81.

Gardner C D, Chatterjee L M and Franke AA (2009) 'Effects of isoflavone supplements vs. soy foods on blood concentrations of genistein and daidzein in adults', *J Nutr Biochem*, **20**, 227–234.

Hathcock J N, Shao A, Vieth R and Heaney R P (2007) 'Risk assessment for vitamin D', *Am J Clin Nutr*, **85**, 6–18.

Heaney R P, Abrams S, Dawson-Hughes B *et al.* (2000a) 'Peak bone mass', *Osteoporos Int*, **11**, 985–1009.

Heaney R P, Dowell M S, Rafferty K *et al.* (2000b) 'Bioavailability of the calcium in fortified soy imitation milk, with some observations on method', *Am J Clin Nutr*, **71**, 1166–1169.

Heaney R, Rafferty K and Bierman J (2005a) 'Not all calcium-fortified beverages are equal', *Nutri Today*, **40**, 39–44.

Heaney R P, Rafferty K, Dowell M S and Bierman J (2005b) 'Calcium fortification systems differ in bioavailability', *J Am Diet Assoc*, **105**, 807–809.

Helferich W G, Andrade J E and Hoagland M S (2008) 'Phytoestrogens and breast cancer: a complex story', *Inflammopharmacol*, **16**, 219–226.

Holick M F, Biancuzzo R M, Chen T C *et al.* (2008) 'Vitamin D2 is as effective as vitamin D3 in maintaining circulating concentrations of 25-hydroxyvitamin D', *J Clin Endocrinol Metab*, **93**, 677–681.

Huncharek M, Muscat J and Kupelinick B (2008) 'Impact of dairy products and dietary calcium on bone-mineral content in children, results of a meta-analysis', *Bone*, **43**, 312–321.

Ilich J Z and Kerstetter J E (2000) 'Nutrition in bone health revisited: A story beyond calcium', *J Am Coll Nutr*, **19**, 715–737.

Institute of Medicine (1997) *Dietary Reference Intakes for Calcium Phosphorus, Magnesium, Vitamin D and Fluoride*, National Academy Press, Washington DC.

Institute of Medicine (2008) *The Development of DRIs 1994–2004. Lessons Learned and New Challenges*. National Academy Press, Washington DC.

International Osteoporosis Federation (IOF) (2009) 'Good nutrition for healthy bones', http://www.iofbonehealth.org/download/osteofound/filemanager/publications/pdf/good_nutrition_for_healthy_bones.pdf (accessed 30 December 2009).

Iuliano-Burns S, Whiting S J, Faulkner R A and Bailey D A (1999) 'Levels, sources, and seasonality of dietary calcium intake in children and adolescents enrolled in the University of Saskatchewan Pediatric Bone Mineral Accrual Study', *Nutr Res*, **19**, 1471–1483.

Iwamoto J, Takeda T and Sato Y (2006) 'Enatetrenone (vitamin K2) and bone quality in the treatment of postmenopausal osteoporosis', *Nutr Rev*, **64**, 509–517.

Johnell O and Kanis J A (2006) 'An estimate of the worldwide prevalence and disability associated with osteoporotic fractures', *Osteoporos Int*, **17**, 1726–1733.

Kanis J A, Burlet N and Cooper C (2008) 'European Society for Clinical and Economic Aspects of Osteoporosis and Osteoarthritis (ESCEO) Osteoporosis guidelines', *Osteoporos Int*, **19**, 399–428.

Kemi V E, Karkkainen M U and Lamberg-Allardt C J (2006) 'High phosphorus intakes acutely and negatively affect Ca and bone metabolism in a dose-dependent manner in healthy young females', *Br J Nutr*, **96**, 545–552.

Kenny A M, Mangano K M, Abourizk R H *et al.* (2009) 'Soy proteins and isoflavones affect bone mineral density in older women, a randomized controlled trial', *Am J Clin Nutr*, **90**, 234–242.

Kim M K, Chung B C, Yu V Y *et al.* (2002) 'Relationships of urinary phytoestrogen excretion to BMD in postmenopausal women', *Clin Endocrinol (Oxf)*, **56**, 321–328.

Kovacs A B (1994) 'Efficacy of ipriflavone in the prevention and treatment of postmenopausal osteoporosis', *Agents Actions*, **41**, 86–87.

Kritz-Silverstein D and Goodman-Gruen D L (2002) 'Usual dietary isoflavone intake, bone mineral density, and bone metabolism in postmenopausal women', *J Womens Health Gend Based Med*, **11**, 69–78.

Kruger C, Marano K, Morita Y *et al.* (2007) 'Safety evaluation of a milk basic protein fraction', *Food Chem Toxicol*, **45**, 1301–1307.

Lemann J, Adams N D and Gray R W (1979) 'Urinary calcium excretion in human beings', *N Engl J Med*, **301**, 535–541.

Liu J, Ho S C, Su Y X *et al.* (2009) 'Effect of long-term intervention of soy isoflavones on bone mineral density in women, a meta-analysis of randomized controlled trials', *Bone*, **44**, 948–953.

Malina R M, Bouchard C and Bar-Or O (2004) *Growth, Maturation, and Physical Activity*, Champaign, IL: Human Kinetics.

Maskarinec G, Verheus M, Steinberg F M *et al.* (2009) 'Various doses of soy isoflavones do not modify mammographic density in postmenopausal women', *J Nutr*, **139**, 981–986.

Matsuoka Y, Serizawa A, Yoshioka T *et al.* (2002) 'Cystatin C in milk basic protein (MBP) and its inhibitory effect on bone resorption *in vitro*', *Biosci Biotechnol Biochem*, **66**, 2531–2536.

Mei J, Yeung S S and Kung A W (2001) 'High dietary phytoestrogen intake is associated with higher bone mineral density in postmenopausal but not premenopausal women', *J Clin Endocrinol Metab*, **86**, 5217–5221.

Morabito N, Crisafulli A, Vergara C *et al.* (2002) 'Effects of genistein and hormone-replacement therapy on bone loss in early postmenopausal women, a randomized double-blind placebo-controlled study', *J Bone Miner Res*, **17**, 1904–1912.

Nettleton J A, Greany K A, Thomas W, Wangen K E, Adlercreutz H and Kurzer M S (2005) 'The effect of soy consumption on the urinary 2:16-hydroxyestrone ratio in postmenopausal women depends on equol production status but is not influenced by probiotic consumption', *J Nutr*, **135**, 603–608.

NIH Consensus Development Panel on Osteoporosis (2001) *JAMA*, **285**, 785–795.

O'Donnell S, Cranney A, Horsley T *et al.* (2008) 'Efficacy of food fortification on serum 25-hydroxyvitamin D concentrations: systematic review', *Am J Clin Nutr*, **88**, 1528–1534.

Otten J J, Hellwig J P and Meyers L D (2006) *Dietary Reference Intakes: The Essential Guide to Nutrient Requirements*. Washington, DC: National Academies Press.

Rizzoli R (2008) 'Nutrition: its role in bone health', *Best Pract & Res Clin Endocrinol Metab*, **22**, 813–829.

Rowland I, Faughnan M, Hoey L, Wähälä K, Williamson G and Cassidy A (2003) 'Bioavailability of phyto-oestrogens', *Br J Nutr*, **89**, S45–58.

Rubinacci A, Melzi R., Zampino M, Soldarini A and Villa, I (1999) 'Total and free deoxypyridinoline after acute osteoclast activity inhibition', *Clin Chem*, **45**, 1510–1516.

Scheiber M D and Rebar R W (1999) 'Isoflavones and postmenopausal bone health: a viable alternative to estrogen therapy?', *Menopause*, **6**, 233–241.

Shu X O, Zheng Y, Cai H, Gu K, Chen Z *et al.* (2009) 'Soy food intake and breast cancer survival', *JAMA*, **302**, 2437–2443.

Somekawa Y, Chiguchi M, Ishibashi T and Aso T (2001) 'Soy intake related to menopausal symptoms, serum lipids, and bone mineral density in postmenopausal Japanese women', *Obstet Gynecol*, **97**, 109–115.

Takada Y, Aoe S and Kumegawa M (1996) Whey protein stimulates the proliferation and differentiation of osteoblastic MC3T3-E1 cells. *Biochem Biophys Res Commun*, **223**, 445–449.

Takada Y, Kobayashi N, Matsuyama H *et al.* (1997a) 'Whey protein suppresses the osteoclast-mediated bone resorption and osteoclast cell formation', *Int Dairy J*, **7**, 821–825.

Takada Y, Matsuyama H, Kato K *et al.* (1997b) 'Milk whey protein enhances the bone breaking force in ovariectomized rats', *Nutr Res*, **17**, 1709–1720.

Tang B M, Eslick G D, Nowson C, Smith C, Bensoussan A (2007) 'Use of calcium or calcium in combination with vitamin D supplementation to prevent fractures and bone loss in people aged 50 years and older: a meta-analysis', *Lancet*, **370**, 657–666.

Tangpricha V, Koutkia P, Rieke S M, Chen T C, Perez A A and Holick M F (2003) 'Fortification of orange juice with vitamin D: a novel approach for enhancing vitamin D nutritional health', *Am J Clin Nutr*, **77**, 1478–1483

Taylor C K, Levy R M, Elliott J C and Burnett B P (2009) 'The effect of genistein aglycone on cancer and cancer risk: a review of in vitro, preclinical, and clinical studies', *Nutr Rev*, **67**, 398–415.

Toba Y, Takada Y, Matsuoka Y *et al.* (2001) 'Milk basic protein promotes bone formation and suppresses bone resorption in healthy adult men', *Biosci Biotechnol Biochem*, **65**, 1353–1357.

Uenishi K, Ishida H, Toba Y, Aoe S, Itabashi A and Takada Y (2007) 'Milk basic protein increases bone mineral density and improves bone metabolism in healthy young women', *Osteoporos Int*, **18**, 385–390.

Uesugi T, Fukui Y and Yamori Y (2002) 'Beneficial effects of soybean isoflavone supplementation on bone metabolism and serum lipids in postmenopausal Japanese women, a four-week study', *J Am Coll Nutr*, **21**, 97–102.

United States Department of Health and Human Services (2004) *Bone Health and Osteoporosis: A Report of the Surgeon General*, Rockville, MD: US Department of Health and Human Services, Office of the Surgeon General.

USDA (United States Department of Agriculture) (2008) *Database for the Isoflavone Content of Selected Foods*, Release 2.0. Available at http://www.ars.usda.gov/Services/docs.htm?docid=6382.

Valachovicova T, Slivova V, Bergman H, Shuherk J and Sliva D (2004) 'Soy isoflavones suppress invasiveness of breast cancer cells by the inhibition of NF-kappaB/AP-1-dependent and -independent pathways', *Int J Oncol*, **25**, 1389–1395.

Vatanparast H and Whiting S J (2006) 'Calcium supplementation trials and bone mass development in children, adolescents and young adults', *Nutr Rev*, **64**, 204–209.

Vatanparast H and Chilibeck P D (2007) 'Does the effect of soy phytoestrogens on bone in postmenopausal women depend on the equol-producing phenotype?', *Nutr Rev*, **65**, 294–299.

Vatanparast H, Dolega-Cieszowski J and Whiting S J (2009) 'Adult Canadians are not meeting current calcium recommendations from food and supplement intake', *Appl Physiol Nutr Metabol*, **34**, 191–196.

Vatanparast H, Green T, Calvo M and Whiting S J (2010) Despite Mandatory fortification of staple foods, vitamin D Intakes of Canadian children and adults are inadequate. *J Steroid Biochem Molec Biol*, **121**, 301–303.

Verborgt O, Tatton N A, Majeska R J and Schaffler M B (2002) 'Spatial distribution of Bax and Bcl-2 in osteocytes after bone fatigue: complementary roles in bone remodeling regulation?', *J Bone Miner Res*, **17**, 907–914.

Verheus M, van Gils CH, Kreijkamp-Kaspers S *et al.* (2008) 'Soy protein containing isoflavones and mammographic density in a randomized controlled trial in postmenopausal women', *Cancer Epidemiol Biomarkers Prev*, **17**, 2632–2638.

Wansink B (2005) *Marketing Nutrition: Soy, Functional Foods, Biotechnology, and Obesity*. University of Illinois Press, Urbana and Chicago.

Weaver C M and Plawecki K L (1994) 'Dietary calcium: adequacy of a vegetarian diet', *Am J Clin Nutr*, **59**, S1238–1241.

Whiting S J and Pluhator M M (1992) 'Comparison of in vitro and in vivo tests for determination of availability of calcium from calcium carbonate tablets', *J Am Coll Nutr*, **5**, 553–560.

Whiting S J, Healey A, Psiak S, Mirwald R, Kowalski K and Bailey D A (2001) 'Relationship between carbonated drinks and other low nutrient dense beverages and bone mineral content of adolescents', *Nutr Res*, **21**, 1107–1115.

Whiting S J, Green T J and Calvo M S (2007) 'Vitamin D intakes in North America and Asia-Pacific countries are not sufficient to prevent vitamin D insufficiency', *J Steroid Biochem Molec Biol*, **103**, 626–630.

Whiting S J, Calvo M S and Stephensen C (2008) 'Current Understanding of Vitamin D Metabolism, Nutritional Status and Role in Disease Prevention', in A Coulston and C J Boushey, *Nutrition in the Prevention & Treatment of Disease*, Elsevier, Inc., Chapter 43.

Wong W W, Lewis R D, Steinberg F M *et al.* (2009) 'Soy isoflavone supplementation and bone mineral density in menopausal women: a 2-y multicenter clinical trial', *Am J Clin Nutr*, **90**, 1433–1143.

Yang Y (2009) 'Skeletal morphogenesis during embryonic development', *Crit Rev Eukaryot Gene Expr*, **19**, 197–218.

Yamamura J, Takada Y, Goto M, Kumegawa M and Aoe S (2000) 'Bovine milk kininogen fragment 1•2 promotes the proliferation of osetoblastic MC3T3-E1 cells', *Biochem Biophys Res Commun*, **269**, 628–632.

Yamamura J, Aoe S, Toba Y *et al.* (2002) 'Milk basic protein (MBP) increases radial bone mineral density in healthy adult women', *Biosci Biotechnol Biochem*, **66**, 702–704.

Zhang X, Li S W, Wu J F *et al.* (2009) 'Effects of ipriflavone on postmenopausal syndrome and osteoporosis', *Gynecol Endocrinol*, **11**, 1–5.

Zhao Y, Martin B R and Weaver C M (2005) 'Calcium bioavailability of calcium carbonate fortified soymilk is equivalent to cow's milk in young women', *J Nutr*, **135**, 2379–2382.

Part III

Developing functional food products

14

Maximising the functional benefits of plant foods

D. G. Lindsay, Euroscience Perspectives, Spain

Abstract: Plant foods are a source of essential vitamins and minerals, fibre, health-promoting phytochemicals and fatty acids. All healthy eating guidelines propose the consumption of a plant-rich diet, but firm scientific evidence to justify the enhancement of the levels of any one component (above those found in a balanced diet) is often lacking. Food production, distribution and processing techniques should be applied that help conserve these components or make them more readily bioavailable. The situation in the developing world is very different. Populations heavily dependent on a single, basic plant food can suffer from diseases related to nutritional deficiencies. There is a strong argument for the improvement of nutritional quality of these crops by selective breeding and genetic manipulation.

Key words: nutritional enhancement, genetic manipulation, micronutrients, health protective factors, plant lipids, fruit and vegetables, food processing.

14.1   Introduction

Plant foods are rich sources of nutrients and of lower caloric density than animal-derived foods. Plants contain 17 mineral nutrients, 13 vitamins and numerous phytochemicals. They are particularly good sources of certain vitamins (provitamin A carotenoids, vitamin C and folate), and minerals (potassium, selenium). The only nutrients not available in plant foods are vitamins B_{12} and D. In addition fruit and vegetables have high amounts of fibre and phytochemicals that are increasingly being shown to play a major role in the health benefits associated with a plant-rich diet. The non-nutritional compounds in fruits and vegetables consist of terpenoids (carotenoids, phytosterols, etc.) sulphur derivatives (glucosinolates, diallyl sulphides, etc.) and polyphenols (flavonoids, hydroxybenzoic acid derivatives, etc.).

The potential health benefits of a plant-rich diet have led to an explosion of research in identifying the likely benefits of specific compounds and to better understand their mechanism of action *in vivo*. There is a belief, not substantiated in every case by hard evidence, that any increase in the intake of certain vitamins and minerals or phytochemicals from plants, naturally absorbed through ingestion, will bring health benefits to all.

The diet is implicated as an important risk factor in the initiation or progression of those diseases that are the greatest contributors to ill health in the developed countries, namely cardiovascular disease and cancer. It has also been implicated as an important factor in determining the rate of progress of other diseases where environment influences the outcome of the disease such as maturity-onset diabetes. The World Health Organisation recommends that the intakes of fruits and vegetables, legumes, whole grains and nuts are increased in order to reduce the risk of disease (WHO, 2004). This particular recommendation clearly emphasises the importance of plant-derived foods in meeting dietary goals.

The unwillingness to regularly consume fresh fruit and vegetables is an issue that continues to be unsolved, especially among certain cultures and social classes. The current solution is to resort to the fortification of basic foods or to the use of nutritional supplements. A scientific understanding of what specific compositional traits of plant foods contribute to a healthy diet is growing. But it still remains the case that for those people who eat a healthy and varied diet the need for changing the composition of any one plant food is not yet overwhelming.

14.2   The concept of functionality

It can be argued that since plant foods are known to reduce the risk of the development of chronic disease, the only action that is required is to encourage greater consumption of these foods. Under such circumstances the need to consider any specific enhancement of their functional benefits is reduced in importance. This argument ignores the fact that:

- Consumer choice in the developed world will depend on socio-economic and cultural constraints. Changes are more probable if plant foods are available that are enjoyable, convenient, affordable, as well as nutritionally balanced. Frequently the manufactured versions of these foods are more readily available and cheaper.
- Plant composition is constantly changing as new varieties are marketed. The consumption of commercial varieties of plant foods may not provide optimal protection against the risk of disease. Too many plant varieties have been developed for agronomic and storage benefits and not for taste and enjoyment and for optimal nutrition.

As it is still not proven what are the exact health protective mechanisms induced by eating fruit and vegetables (Matteson and Cheng, 2006; Hirshi, 2009), it is not possible to link composition to specific functional mechanisms. At present there are no criteria that can be applied to the development of plant varieties, in terms of their composition, other than that they remain the same. This is an unsatisfactory basis on which to base the future of the plant breeding industry. Phytochemicals or vitamins vary by an order of magnitude or more in the gene pool. It could help in the prevention of disease to know in which direction this pool should be altered, and with what likely consequences. For this reason there needs to be a systematic examination of those bioactive, protective phytochemicals (including nutrients) that will:

- improve knowledge about their uptake, metabolism and their localisation in tissues and cells, as well as understanding the basis of their activity;
- define the steps that determine their biosynthesis in the plant and their turnover;
- enable the intakes to be determined that will maximise their protective effects without causing toxicity;
- above all ensure that the varieties that naturally contain high levels of phytochemicals are acceptable to consumers since the possibility exists that adverse organoleptic effects might result from varieties with high levels of certain phytochemicals.

Nutritional adequacy is not only determined by the nutrient content of a food but the amount of the food consumed on average. Generally cereals are a major component of the diet. Increasingly fats from plant-derived sources are the most important sources of fat-soluble vitamins and essential fatty acids. Nonetheless there are major processing steps involved before these raw materials enter the diet and these steps must be considered before any strategy is adopted. Plant breeders working in this field must collaborate closely with nutritionists, toxicologists, food technologists and consumer scientists to ensure a successful outcome. In the past this has rarely occurred.

14.3   The situation in the developing world

In contrast to the needs of the developed world there are 40–50% of the world's population who will suffer at some time or other from a deficiency of essential minerals and vitamins (WHO, 1995, FAO, 2006). Infants and pregnant women in the developing world are particularly susceptible. One hundred million children worldwide are vitamin A deficient and improving the vitamin A content of their food could prevent as many as two million deaths annually (WHO, 1995). This is apart from the deficiencies in iodine intake, resulting in goitre, and in iron-deficient anaemia which are estimated to affect millions in the developing world. There is also an important need to improve the amino acid content of legume proteins that are deficient in essential sulphur amino acids and the scientific evidence that improvement of one or more nutritional factor in their basic diets will bring substantial health benefits is overwhelming. Nutritional deficiencies can lead to a reduction in immune responsiveness, rather than a specific attributable disorder, making it difficult to clearly establish how many people are suffering from malnutrition (Calder and Jackson, 2000).

Another worldwide problem is with spina bifida and other birth defects caused by an insufficient intake of green leafy vegetables during pregnancy (Rush, 2000;

Sifakis and Pharmakides, 2000). Currently, some Western countries make fortification of grain products with synthetic folic acid mandatory to help their populations reach the recommended dietary allowance, which is 400 µg/day for adults and 600 µg/day for pregnant women (Bailey and Gregory, 1999). However, food fortification is difficult to implement in developing countries due to recurrent costs, distribution inequities, and lack of an industrial food system. In these areas folate deficiency causes at least 200 000 severe birth defects every year (Adamson, 2004). Although folate deficiency in pregnant women in developed countries has been shown to cause severe malformations in the foetus (Rush, 2000; Sifakis and Pharmakides, 2000), the consequences of folate deficiency in developing countries make the issue of even greater importance.

This target population requires a very different strategy for research and one where the need for immediate policy action is very compelling. However, strategies that fail to take into account social constraints, cultural traditions, feasibility and cost could result in the research failing to achieve the desired impact.

14.4   The priorities for nutritional enhancement

14.4.1   For the developed world

Although it is known that the distribution and processing of food can lead to a significant loss in nutritional quality, there are few instances today where present evidence suggests there is a need to change current practices, apart from ensuring that the beneficial compounds present in a plant are not significantly reduced, or less available, through harvesting, storage, distribution and manufacturing. There is very little evidence for nutritional deficiencies. In those cases where public health authorities have such evidence they have resorted to basic food supplementation with nutrients. The use of nutritional supplements is now widespread and the public health priority is not in ensuring adequate nutrient intake but in targeting food over consumption and excessive caloric intake.

Dietary Reference Intakes (DRI) have been set for many essential vitamins and minerals and these obviously provide a yardstick for setting relevant goals for plant breeders (Food and Nutrition Board, 2003). Targets for markets where the diet is varied raise the difficulty that the objective is to maximise the organism's response to external challenges, e.g. immunological defence. In such cases is it not known what are the optimal intakes of a vitamin, or trace element, which will minimise the risks of suffering from long-term disease (Verkerk and Hickey, 2010). Research is needed to define optimal intakes for generalised health responses before being able to more precisely determine a strategy for plant breeding.

Far less is known about the long-term benefits of the other complex constituents of a specific plant food. The very complexity of the numerous secondary metabolites in plant foods does pose real challenges in determining which, if any, should be changed. While the focus of current interest is on the need to consider nutrients and other phytochemicals as protective against the development of disease in later life, the levels of intake that may be necessary to optimise protection are far from resolved at the present time.

14.4.2   For the developing world

In the case where a plant forms a major component of the diet in subsistence economies the need for nutritional enhancement is significantly greater. In such situations it is unquestionably important to ensure that the dietary staple provides the basic nutritional requirements for healthy growth. Rice, wheat, cassava and maize, which are the basic foods most frequently consumed by at-risk populations, contain insufficient levels of several individual micronutrients to meet minimum daily requirements.

International agricultural research centres have generated improved varieties of rice and wheat. Progress is also being made with maize, sorghum, millet, potatoes and groundnuts. The increased food production from improved varieties has contributed significantly to a steady decline in macronutrient nutritional deficiencies, from 40% in 1970 to 20% in 1990. The result has been the growth of food supply but this has not provided the much-needed micronutrients, which are still a nutritional challenge (Toenniessen, 2002; Graham *et al.*, 2001).

14.5   Strategies for nutritional enhancement

There is no single approach to achieving an improvement in the nutritional quality of plant foods since there are many factors influencing the approaches that should be adopted, depending on the plant and its importance in the diet and the target population. These approaches include:

- the application of traditional breeding methods to select for varieties with an increased level of the bioactive compound;
- biofortification using genetic engineering to produce varieties with improved nutritional characteristics;
- a reduction in the content of anti-nutritional factors;
- the use of post-harvest abiotic stress;
- improvements in handling, storage and food processing technologies.

Each of these approaches may have a role to play. For some crops, nature has not provided – or plant breeders have not yet found – mutant lines with a high enough level of essential nutrients to meet daily requirements for the developing world's challenges. This is the case with β-carotene (the vitamin A precursor) in non-photosynthetic edible tissues. The biosynthetic pathways that provide for sufficient quantities of these essential vitamins in the endosperm of cereals are often absent, truncated or inhibited in some way.

The challenge is to raise overall nutritional quality whilst maintaining the other favorable characteristics of the varieties commonly grown and to do so in such a way that the process is price-competitive and acceptable to the consumer.

Biofortification faces many obstacles not least because the enhancement of one micronutrient is not likely to overcome the overall health problems associated with malnutrition. But at the least it is a step in the right direction. Nonetheless fierce debate exists on the application of genetically engineered crops and the relevance of the approach to the developing world's nutritional problems (Grain, 2000).

Studying and engineering secondary metabolism in plants can be compromised by the sheer complexity of the pathways, which may have multiple branches, multifunctional enzymes, cell type-specific and compartmentalised enzymes, and complex feedback mechanisms. The complex inter-relationships between biosynthetic pathways make it difficult to predict the outcome on other compositional factors of changing one factor. Selection for one attribute may lead to a reduction of levels for another. It is not an easy challenge to maintain important agronomic traits and improve nutritional quality as well.

For some plant foods where the focus might be on improving the content of bioactive secondary metabolites there is the complication that they may not exert a specific effect, but rather contribute to a pleiotropic effect, where the benefit derives from more than one factor in the specific plant or other plants present in the diet. The evidence is growing that a combination of plant phytochemicals present in a varied diet can act through common mechanisms to reduce the occurrence of degenerative diseases.

As mentioned above processing greatly affects the nutritional composition and the bioavailability of many plant trace elements, nutrients and secondary metabolites with beneficial characteristics. All these data must be evaluated before any major programme of plant breeding is considered.

14.5.1   Application of 'traditional' engineering methods

There are wide natural variations that can be found in the gene pool of crop plants that can be exploited to improve nutritional quality (Dorais and Ehret, 2008).

Variations in the micronutrient content of genotypes have been published. The range is not that great however varying between two and 20-fold (Quintana *et al.*, 1996; Schonhof and Krumbein, 1996; Wang and Goldman, 1996; IFPRI, 1999; Kushad *et al.*, 1999). In the case of broccoli it has been possible to develop advanced broccoli breeding with high glucosinolates by introgressing three genomic segments of *Brassica villosa* into a standard broccoli variety. *B. villosa* is believed to have a non-functional gene that gives rise to higher glucoraphanin levels (Faulkner *et al.*, 1998).

For pro-vitamin A carotenoids plants provide highly variable amounts depending on their colour. There is a large natural diversity found in different species and cultivated varieties. Varieties of sweet potato may contain levels varying from 0.13 mg to 11.3 mg g^{-1} dry weight of ß-carotene (Solomons and Bulux, 1997). Similar variations in levels can be found in carrots and cassava. A successful breeding programme at USDA has obtained many lines of tomatoes with almost 25 times the levels of β-carotene found in conventional varieties

(Stommel *et al.*, 2005) while a tomato line has recently been released from the Asian Vegetable Research and Development Centre with a ten-fold increase β-carotene compared with conventional varieties (Yang *et al.*, 2007)

In the case of the tomato genes have been identified that are associated with high and low lycopene content with cherry tomatoes containing the highest amounts (Leonardi *et al.*, 2000). Incorporation of genes that increase lycopene content, and or elimination of genes that decrease the lycopene content, can be done by pedigree selection and backcross programmes. Such techniques have produced hybrids with a three or four-fold content of lycopene in tomato fruits.

As there are over 10 000 individual polyphenols known in plants it is really important to know primarily what the specific objective of the breeding programme is going to be. The genetic diversity is vast with a large pool of species and cultivars to utilise. The genotypes of important berry crops like *Vaccinium, Rubus, Ribes* and *Fragaria* have been exploited to breed new varieties with increased anthocyanin content. The development of a cultivar of strawberry with 40% more ellagic acid and proanthocyanidins than most cultivars is an example of what can be achieved (Khanizadeh *et al.*, 2006). A cranberry cultivar 'High Red' has high flavonoid content and has shown to lower cholesterol by 21% over a five week period in pigs (Zeldin *et al.*, 2007).

Biofortification programmes based on conventional breeding have met with only marginal success in grains. For example, four polymorphisms at the *lycopene epsilon cyclase (lcyE)* locus in corn were recently shown to alter the flux between the β-carotene and α-carotene branches of the carotenoid pathway, potentially allowing breeding for enhanced β-carotene levels (Harjes *et al.*, 2008). Selection of favorable *lcyE* alleles with inexpensive molecular markers will enable developing-country breeders to more effectively produce maize grain with higher provitamin A levels. However, such a quantitative trait locus (QTL)-based approach will require years of conventional breeding to achieve significant enhancement in locally adapted varieties grown by subsistence farmers in the developing world.

14.5.2   Application of genetic engineering

Genetic engineering is being applied to enhance levels of functional compounds in food crops. Indeed for some purposes it will be the only approach feasible especially where there are widespread deficiency diseases and the population is dependent on staple crops which are not sources of the nutrient required. There are many examples where the technology has been applied with success although there are no products which have yet reached the marketing stage where nutritional benefits have been the main focus.

Potential strategies for the enhancement of specific metabolites could target on:

1. Over-expression of enzymes that control the final steps in the biosynthesis of a metabolite.
2. Over-expression of rate-limiting enzymes.

3. Silencing of genes whose expression causes the metabolite to be degraded.
4. Increased expression of genes that are not subject to metabolic feedback control.
5. Increasing the number of plastids in a plant.
6. Increasing metabolic flux into the pathway of interest.
7. Expression in storage organs using site-specific promoters.

In practice if a substantial increase in the concentration of a metabolite is required, the use of specific promoters directing the synthesis to a particular organelle normally used for storage purposes, or where the plant normally synthesises the metabolite, is essential. Failure to do so could cause toxicity in the plant by interfering with the production or function of other essential metabolites. However this strategy presupposes the metabolite of interest is the final one in a particular pathway.

The accumulation of sequence data of both chromosomal DNA and expressed sequence tags of plants and other species is providing rapid advances in knowledge of the genetic make-up and functions of several plants and it is expected that these other possibilities will soon be feasible. So far there are only a few strategies where multiple gene insertions have been introduced to produce the metabolite(s) of interest.

There are a number of successful and notable examples where nutritional engineering that has been achieved and reviewed (Davies, 2007). These include rice and potato with enhanced β-carotene levels, lysine-rich corn, iron-rich lettuce, and lycopene-enhanced tomatoes.

Significant progress has been made in biofortification of vitamin E and provitamin A in plants both of which are important micronutrients that are lacking in subsistence diets (Dellapenna and Pogson, 2006).

Vitamin E consists of a mixture of tocopherols but α-tocopherol is the most important for health and has the highest vitamin activity. In the USA the adult recommended allowance for vitamin E is 8–10 mg (α-tocopherol) based on an avoidance of vitamin deficiency diseases. However, current evidence suggests that an intake of 100–250 mg α-tocopherol is required if long-term disease risks are to be avoided. This is not feasible from unsupplemented diets if general nutritional guidelines are followed.

A significant increase in the α-tocopherol levels in plants has been achieved through the over-expression of γ-tocopherol methyltransferase (γ-TMT), the final stage in the biosynthetic pathway. The fact that many oilseeds contain high levels of γ-tocopherol suggests that the final step of the biosynthetic pathway is rate limited by the activity of γ-TMT (see Fig. 14.1).

The manipulation of carotenoid levels in plants well illustrates the nature of the challenges faced by plant biotechnologists. A simplified version of the pathways leading to the synthesis of the carotenoids principally found in food plants is shown in Fig. 14.2.

A crucial enzyme involved in their synthesis is phytoene synthase (PSY1) which converts geranylgeranylphosphate (GGDP) into phytoene. Inhibition of PSY1 through the use of antisense gene-silencing techniques resulted in a 90%

HO
H
CH3
CH3
γ-Tocopherol
SAM
γ-TMT
α-Tocopherol

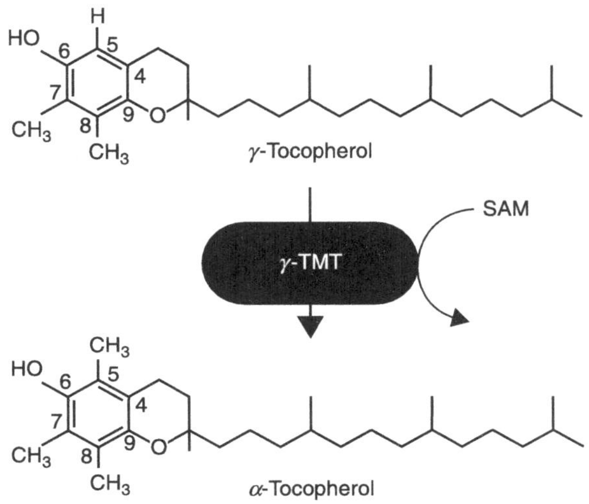

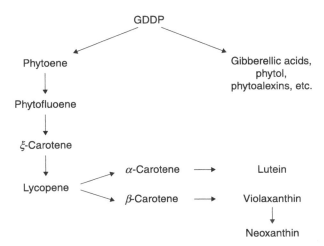

Fig. 14.1 Biosynthesis of α-tocopherol from γ-tocopherol; SAM = S-adenosyl methionine.

reduction in carotenoid levels compared with wild type in the tomato (Brown *et al.*, 1991). Over-expression of PSY1 results in dwarfed tomato plants (Fray and Grierson, 1994). This has been explained by the increased flow of metabolites into the carotenoid branch of the isoprenoid pathway leading to a reduction in the metabolites available for gibberellin synthesis. The general, isoprenoid pathway is utilised by plants for the synthesis of many important products including sterol, chlorophyll, quinone and phytoalexin production, as well as for the gibberellins.

GDDP
Phytoene
Gibberellic acids, phytol, phytoalexins, etc.
Phytofluoene
ξ-Carotene
Lycopene
α-Carotene
Lutein
β-Carotene
Violaxanthin
Neoxanthin

Fig. 14.2 Biosynthesis of carotenoids from GGDP.

It illustrates the complex interactions that are occurring and the potential lack of benefits arising from the manipulation of the level of any one enzyme.

Improvements in the process can be made by ensuring that genes are expressed in a tissue-specific manner through the insertion of specific promoters. This has been achieved for rice where carotenoid levels have been increased significantly through the use of the daffodil *psy* gene (Burkhardt *et al.*, 1997). In the case of tomato, a twofold increase in total carotenoid levels occurs using this *psy* transformant which is significantly lower than for rice. In rice the daffodil *psy* cDNA insertion is under the control of an endosperm-specific promoter. The choice of promoter will very much affect the timing and tissue-specific expression of a gene.

It has been possible to induce xanthophyll accumulation in potato tubers that do not normally contain *β*-carotene (Brown *et al.*, 1989). The use of bacterial *psy* genes instead of the daffodil *psy* gene in tomatoes produces a sevenfold increase in *β*-carotene levels but this is at the expense of the ripening pigment lycopene which is the predominant carotenoid in tomato.

A major development has been in the enhancement of folate, one of the most important of the B vitamins (Diaz de la Garza *et al.*, 2007). Plant foods are the primary source of folate in the human diet. Folate enhancement in plants presents a major challenge since it is assembled from three different molecular components: pteridine, *para*-amino benzoic acid (PABA), and glutamate. The pteridine moiety is synthesized in the plant cytosol, PABA is synthesised in the chloroplast, and folates are synthesised from these two precursors in the plant mitochondria (Fig. 14.3). In addition to biosynthetic enzymes, membrane-bound transporters for folates and various pathway intermediates must be present.

In tomato fruit engineered for guanosine triphosphate cyclohydrolase-1 (GCH1) over-expression PABA levels were depleted. This led to the hypothesis that PABA synthesis might limit folate levels. Consistent with this hypothesis it was found that folate levels were substantially increased when PABA was added to tomato fruit over-expressing GCH1. Over expression of the nuclear encoded, chloroplast-targeted enzyme aminodeoxychorismate synthase (ADCS) accumulated PABA in tomato fruit at levels nearly 20-fold higher than controls, although folate levels were still unchanged relative to controls (Diaz de la Garza *et al.*, 2007). When the ADCS over-expressing lines were crossed to previously characterised GCH1 over-expressing lines the total folate level of fruit was increased up to 25-fold relative to controls. This resulted in a level of folate several times higher than those found in green leafy vegetables which are considered some of the best sources of folate in the diet. The level of folate accumulated in these transgenic tomatoes is more than sufficient to provide for the entire daily allowance of folate for a pregnant woman (600 μg per day). The information gathered from these experiments has thrown substantial light on how folate levels can be increased without leading to the accumulation of other intermediates in the biosynthetic chain.

Changes in more than one nutrient in a specific crop presents a major challenge but one that must be overcome for the production of crops that are able to meet the needs of the developing world. This will require the manipulation of complex metabolic pathways which can have multiple branches, multifunctional enzymes,

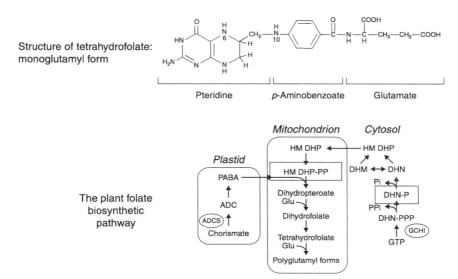

Structure of tetrahydrofolate: monoglutamyl form

Pteridine   p-Aminobenzoate   Glutamate

The plant folate biosynthetic pathway

Fig. 14.3 Biosynthesis of folates. The two enzymes (GCHI and ADCS) are the ones engineered by Diaz de la Garza *et al.* (2007) (redrawn from Diaz de la Garza *et al.*, 2007); PABA = p-aminobenzoic acid, DHM = dihydromonopterin, HMOHP = hydroxymethyldihydropterin, ADC = aminodeoxychovismate, GCHI = GTP cyclohydrolase I, ADCS = ADC synthase, DHN = dihydroneopterin, -P = monophosphate, -PP = pyrophosphate, -PPP = triphosphate.

cell-specific and compartmentalised enzymes, and complex feedback mechanisms. It is also essential to ensure that the transgenes are stable.

The chances of failure for at least one of the transgenes increases with the number of genes introduced, requiring the generation of very large populations to ensure that the pathway has been completely reconstructed. Alternative approaches, such as individual transformation followed by crossing to 'stack' transgenes, are unworkable for large numbers of genes because of the time taken to stack all transgenes in one line and the likelihood that unlinked genes will segregate in later generations.

A strategy to simplify the process of metabolic analysis and engineering in plants has been developed based on combinatorial nuclear transformation to create metabolically diverse transgenic libraries. Multiple transgenes were introduced randomly into a variety of white corn (Zhu *et al.*, 2008). The principle developed was that the population could be screened for metabolic variants, reflecting the expression of different combinations of transgenes. Some plants contained and expressed all input genes and recapitulated the entire pathway under investigation, whereas others expressed subsets of transgenes and displayed corresponding metabolic profiles.

A white corn variety was transformed by bombarding immature zygotic embryos with metal particles coated with five constructs (consisting of the selectable marker *bar* and 4 genes/cDNAs encoding enzymes in the metabolic pathways for the vitamins β-carotene, ascorbate, and folate.

To increase β-carotene levels, corn phytoene synthase (*psy1*) cDNA was introduced under the control of the wheat low molecular weight glutenin promoter and the *Pantoea ananatis crtI* gene (encoding carotene desaturase) under the control of the barley D-hordein promoter.

To increase ascorbate levels rice dehydroascorbate reductase (*dhar*) cDNA was introduced. Folate levels were increased using the *E. coli folE* gene encoding GCH1; both of these genes were introduced under the control of the barley D-hordein promoter.

These manipulations achieved significantly improved levels of different carotenoids, exceeding the best levels achieved by conventional breeding with 36-fold more β-carotene, a 20–30% increase in lutein, a greater than four-fold increase in zeaxanthin, and the accumulation of a large amount (23 µg/g) of lycopene. 100–200 g of grain provide the full RDI of β-carotene (as a sole source of vitamin A), an adequate intake of folate, and approximately 20% of the RDI of ascorbate.

More recently, Carlson *et al.* (2007) constructed a minichromosome vector that remains autonomous from the plant's chromosomes and stably replicates when introduced into maize cells. This work makes it possible to design minichromosomes that carry cassettes of genes, enhancing the ability to engineer plant processes such as the production of complex biochemicals.

Whilst genetic engineering offers many opportunities to selectively introduce or activate genes that are absent or repressed in certain plant endosperms, the technology has provoked widespread concern, especially in Europe, that has severely limited its application. The concerns over potentially adverse health effects have generated an enormous amount of scientific research but none of this has so far demonstrated any measurable risks associated with the application of the technology for human health. Genetically-modified plant foods are now being grown widely around the world. No adverse health effects have been reported from their use.

Reduction in anti-nutritional factors
Many plants contain natural substances that have evolved as defensive mechanisms and inhibit nutrient uptake in various ways or are toxic to humans. They may interfere with intestinal cell function, reduce the ability to breakdown complex molecules such as proteins and starch, or may be toxic if consumed in sufficient quantity. Some of these substances are rendered harmless with cooking or processing, but others are resistant to digestion, heat treatment, or other forms of processing.

The biotechnological interest in reducing anti-nutritional factors in plants has been predominately focused around improving the nutritional value of feedingstuffs. Phytates are present in many plant seeds and limit phosphorous uptake as well as other elements. Lines of corn, barley, rice, and soybean with slightly different phytic acid characteristics have been used to develop varieties with reduced seed phytic acid (Raboy *et al.*, 2001). Reduction in phytate in the range of 50% to 66%

has been achieved with these mutant lines. In soybeans and corn, 80% reduction has been achieved. However, several hybrids developed with the mutant strains exhibited lower yields. It has been shown that these low phytate mutants are linked to the reduced expression of the enzyme myoinositol phosphate synthase, the first enzyme in the synthesis pathway for phytic acid.

The potential for introducing a phytase gene into feedingstuffs has been explored (Pen *et al.*, 1993; Chier *et al.*, 2004). These genetically engineered low phytate crops have not been commercialised as animal feeds.

Phytase is inactivated above 60° and is of limited use as a strategy for human nutrition. Thioredoxin is thought to be an activator of the germination process in seeds (Pen *et al.*, 1993). It is able to activate proteins to degradation by proteolysis and results in improved digestability (Lozano *et al.*, 1996). It also has the potential advantage of being able to reduce allergenicity presumably because of its capacity to break disulphide bonds by the action of the reduced thiol groups in the molecule and ensure the tertiary structure of the protein is accessible to degradation by proteases (Lozano *et al.*, 1996). The insertion of the wheat thioredoxin gene into barley has produced a transgenic plant where thioredoxin accounts for 7% of the total protein content in the barley and is a good source of sulphur amino acids (Buchanan *et al.*, 1997).

Post-harvest abiotic stress
Plants can respond to adverse environmental conditions through genetically determined adaptation or resistance. Both biotic and abiotic factors can induce stress which activate defence responses in the plants that affects both the anabolic and the catabolic pathways of secondary plant metabolites. Research has been undertaken into how to illicit responses that add health value to a plant food (Espín de Gea, 2008).

Of particular interest has been the inducement of the phytoalexin stilbenes such as resveratrol and piceid that are found in grapes and specifically in wine. Lesser amounts of resveratrol are found in groundnuts and *Vaccinium* berries. This interest was stimulated by studies that revealed resveratrol had anti-carcinogenic properties (Jang *et al.*, 1997).

The most promising controlled, post-harvest treatments that can give reproducible induction responses are the techniques of UV-irradiation, ozone, and anoxic atmospheres. Post-harvest UV-C radiation has the potential to increase the level of stilbenes in grapes. An average concentration of 2–3 mg/100 mg FW has been achieved which provides sources of exposure for those people who cannot take alcohol (Cantos *et al.*, 2003). Ozone gives similar results but effects on sensory characteristics can result at exposure levels and times necessary to cause similar levels of resveratrol to those produced by UV-C.

In general the usefulness of abiotic stress treatment appears limited to a very few compounds since other phytoalexins are produced in very low amounts and at levels where in vivo effects are probably very limited. Some inducers cause off flavours which is the case with the phytoalexin coumarin methoxymellein, induced in carrots on storage, slicing or chopping (De Girolamo *et al.*, 2004).

14.6   Improvements in handling, storage and food processing technologies

Unfavourable conditions during harvesting and storage have a considerable effect on the overall quality of fruit and vegetables which include their nutritional quality. Storage conditions are particularly important for preserving the quality of fruit and vegetables and the use of chilled and modified atmosphere packaging is now widespread. Vitamin C is slowly degraded even under optimal storage conditions whereas other beneficial factors are mostly stable (Breene, 1994). In general the stronger the processing conditions, the greater the degradation of specific nutrients and phytochemicals. However there are some compounds that are remarkably stable and survive quite severe cooking conditions either in the factory or the home. In addition after processing the concentration of bioactive phytochemicals is quite stable on storage whereas vitamin C levels decline further.

14.6.1   Processing of oils

The initial stages of refining of crude vegetable oils use water or steam to de-gum, followed by centrifugation. Physical or chemical refining procedures can then be used. Physical methods involve steam treatment to volatilise free fatty acids and bleaching is normally adopted. This removes any carotenoids but without this step the oils are less stable. A compromise has to be adopted to remove materials producing instability and the preservation of some antioxidants. Chemical methods involve saponification with sodium hydroxide, followed by centrifugation.

There are considerable benefits in retaining high levels of antioxidants throughout the processing stages to improve overall product quality and avoid rancidity. However, the processes to produce high quality oils, i.e. oils acceptable to users, require them to be low in flavour and cloudiness, and light in colour. These demands can lead to oils that are much lower in antioxidant content than the oilseeds from which they are derived.

Given the fact that energy costs of edible oil production are high, and that the nutritional quality is an added value, other processes, such as membrane separation, are being considered. The preservation of antioxidants in oils is best achieved through the use of stainless steel equipment since metal ions encourage the auto-oxidation of lipids. In addition, air must be removed at temperatures below 100 °C before the oil is heated to the final stripping temperature.

Virgin oils are also susceptible to oxidation, even though they have a high antioxidant content. It is essential to keep the peroxide value of these oils low in order to avoid rancidity and the loss of antioxidants since, once oxidation occurs, the process is auto-catalytic. Oil extraction using a two-phase centrifugal decanter yields olive oil with improved quality when compared with those that use the conventional three-phase equipment. The oils produced by the two-phase technology have a higher content of polyphenols, ortho-diphenols, hydroxytyrosol and tocopherols and a higher stability (Lindley, 1998).

14.6.2   Processing of fruits and vegetables

A very significant part of the fruit and vegetable products consumed in the developed world are in the form of minimally processed or manufactured products. It is important to understand what effects these processes are having on overall nutritional quality or on beneficial factors they contain. Some of the compounds are remarkably stable to heat. Others are severely depleted following harvesting, long periods of storage and cooking (Howard, 2008).

Cellular localisation and structure of plant phytochemicals often influence their retention during processing. Water soluble compounds such as phenolics and flavonoids are leached into water during blanching or canning, as a result of membrane destruction, whilst cell wall bound phenolics resist leaching and may be more easily extracted or bioavailable after processing due to tissue softening.

Lipid-soluble compounds such as the carotenoids are retained in blanching although losses are possible through thermal degradation and oxidation. But many processed vegetables have higher levels of carotenoids than the raw material or in a more bioavailable form (Dewanto et al., 2002). Mechanical destruction of the food matrix and heating enhances the release of carotenoids from foods. As a consequence ingestion of tomato paste showed a 2.5 higher concentration of lycopene in human plasma compared with the equivalent consumption of fresh tomato (Gartner et al., 1997).

Removal of skins and seeds during processing can result in a considerable loss in phytochemicals in the final product. 98% of the flavonols in tomatoes are located in the skin (Stewart et al., 2000). At the same time as waste products they can be a rich source of phytochemicals for exploitation as novel food ingredients, supplements and raw materials for pharmaceutical use.

High-temperature short-time processing favours the retention of anthocyanins (Jackman et al., 1987) and carotenoids (Lin and Chen, 2005). While the folate content of fruits and vegetables is affected during storage, processing and cooking, it has been found that pasteurisation at low temperatures did not cause folate levels to be reduced in the preparation of tomato puree (Perez-Conesa et al., 2009).

High-pressure processing (HPP) studies on the preparation of juices, purees and soups have generally shown that the antioxidant or phytochemical content of fruit and vegetables are retained. In studies on HPP treatments some studies indicate an improvement in the extractability of carotenoids whilst others did not observe this. However there is generally no loss unless higher pressures are utilised (Howard, 2008).

There still remains the need to examine of the effects of processing on the levels and chemical composition of many bioactive phytochemicals in plant foods. The information that is available is mostly confined to the effects on nutrients, carotenoids and some phenolic components of plant foods. Even so there is incomplete information on the effects of particular processes on the overall nutritive value of fruits and vegetables

Although the levels of nutrients and phytochemicals can be greatly influenced by agronomic practices, optimal processes for maintaining the content of antioxidant vitamins in fruit and vegetables start from post-harvest handling

(Kadler, 2002). Careful attention to temperature in harvesting and minimisation of light and oxygen help reduce loss. Loss of vitamins in fresh vegetables is invariably associated with wilting. The cold storage of vegetables with appropriate humidity helps to preserve vitamin content. Some vegetables, such as broccoli, are more sensitive than others, e.g. green beans, to refrigerated storage. On the other hand, the vitamin content of fresh fruits is not stable for long periods of time in the refrigerator. Inactivation of polyphenol oxidase also helps to maintain antioxidant status (Lindley, 1998; Tomás-Barberán and Espín, 2001).

Modified atmosphere packaging is widely used in fruit and vegetable marketing. While the removal of oxygen and the use of plastics with low gas permeability membranes might be expected to lead to the stability of nutrients, carbon dioxide accumulation occurs, leading to anoxia and loss of quality. Active packaging offers the possibility to overcome these problems from the use of oxygen-scavenging materials such as vitamins C or E into the film. However, this is not happening at the moment. The vitamin A content of sweet potato is maintained after four months' storage if it is stored in an impermeable plastic material with an oxygen scavenger in the packaging material, compared with a retention of only 45% in permeable plastic, 62% in impermeable material with air in the head space, and 73% in vacuum-sealed impermeable plastics (Solomons and Bulux, 1997). Cutting of fruit and vegetables prior to modified atmosphere packaging can affect the overall quality including nutritional quality (Gil and Kader, 2008).

Dehydration of fruits and vegetables invariably leads to a loss in nutrients other than trace elements due to the greater surface area and exposure to oxygen and light. Beta carotene levels are reasonably stable on processing provided that oxygen is rigidly excluded from the process. A decrease of only 30–55% in levels occurs following canning because of the anoxic environment. Freeze-drying does not significantly alter total carotenoid levels. Freezing generally preserves carotenoids, whereas sun or solar drying leads to considerable losses. In developing countries sufficient amounts may remain, however, to provide vitamin A requirements (Rodriguez-Amaya, 1997). The problem of vitamin A deficiency is often attributable to the seasonable variations in availability of pro-vitamin A rich foods.

Processing of plant foods rich in phenolic compounds can result in increased levels of some of the phenols after processing. Raspberry juice, prepared by a diffusion extraction process where the juice is held at high temperatures (65°C) for a long period, results in an increased content of ellagic acid. Jam making also increases levels of this compound. Anthocyanins appear to survive the jam-making process but conversion to other compounds occurs – probably chalcones – and these compounds are not characterised. These changes are possibly due to the release of ellagic acid from the cell walls by hydrolysis of ellagitanins (Rommel and Wrolstad, 1993). However, the changes in phenolic content can vary widely, depending on the process and compound. Technological processes in juice and wine production can have a marked effect. Skin fermentation of wines results in a higher content of phenols in the product but in general the levels of total phenols in wine are less than found in juices (Auw *et al.*, 1996; Schlesier *et al.*, 1997).

Very complex changes occur to the anthocyanins when wine is produced. Cooking of onions and tomatoes leads to a marked reduction in the levels of quercitin (Crozier *et al.*, 1997). The phenolic compounds in olives are transformed depending on the method used in their curing. It is clear that the characterisation of the effects of processing on the concentration of phenolics in plants will need investigating at the level of the individual process and compound since some compounds will increase, others decrease, and a considerable number will be transformed. The biological significance of these changes is going to be extremely complex to unravel. The focus will have to be on those compounds that are consumed in the greatest amounts.

Apart from effects on the overall levels in foods, processing can affect the chemical composition of the food which may have biological consequences. The carotenoids have been studied in most detail in this regard. Processing can lead to significant losses of epoxicarotenoids (e.g. lutein-5-6-epoxide, neoxanthin and violaxanthin, lutein) and to a lesser extent the carotenes where trans to cis isomerisation occurs (e.g. 5-cis-lycopene and 13-cis-3-carotene), as well as to different carotenoid by-products. The extent of these changes is dependent upon the type of vegetable, the method of cooking, and the temperature and time conditions. The higher the temperature, and the longer the period of cooking, the greater the change (Nguyen and Swartz, 1998).

New processing techniques, such as high electric pulse fields, or high pressure processing, especially of fruit juices, help to maintain vitamin levels (Knorr *et al.*, 2002).

14.7   Future trends

Most nutritional deficiencies that have been observed in the developed world have been dealt with through supplementation of staple foods with nutrients, or are treated through the use of nutritional supplements. The benefits of increasing levels of nutrients and phytochemicals though conventional plant breeding or through the use of biotechnology above those normally present will require careful thought before the research is undertaken. The application of biotechnological methods will always run the risk of not necessarily being successful in the marketplace unless the product is able to make a strong health claim. The potential risks include consumers reaction to the product, including organoleptic effects. Priority research will need to be targeted on ensuring that increases in levels of one or a group of plant constituents are significant in terms of the food as consumed and will have measurable health benefits. This will require multi-disciplinary research.

Recent advances in the biotechnology of plant genomes have shown that there is a real possibility of producing food plants that have can meet a number of nutritional deficiencies in a single crop. This makes it possible to develop basic crops for many deprived regions of the world that will be nutritionally complete. The feasibility of making such technologies available to the developing world, and in a form that enables these crops to be produced economically, is a major challenge but one that will remain the major thrust for plant biotechnologists.

14.8   Sources of further information and advice

Henry C J K and Chapman C (2002), *The Nutrition Handbook for Food Processors*, Boca Raton, London, New York, Washington DC: CRC.

Liu Q and Chen Y-Q (2010) A new mechanism in plant engineering: The potential roles of microRNAs in molecular breeding for crop improvement, *Biotechnology Advances*, **22**, 301–307.

Sands D C, Morris C E, Dratz E A and Pilgeram A L (2009), Elevating optimal human nutrition to a central goal of plant breeding and production of plant-based foods, *Plant Science* **177**, 377–389.

14.9   References

Adamson P (2004) UNICEF, The Micronutrient Initiative in Vitamin & Mineral Deficiency (P&LA, Oxfordshire, UK), pp. 20–40.

Auw J M, Blanc V, O'Keefe, S F and Sims C A (1996), Effect of processing on the phenolics and color of Cabernet Sauvignon, Chambourcin, and Noble wines and juices, *Am J Enol Vitic* **47**, 279–286.

Bailey L B and Gregory J F (1999), Folate metabolism and requirements *Journal of Nutrition*, **129**, 779–782.

Breene W M (1994) Healthfulness and nutritional quality of fresh versus processed fruit and vegetables: a review. *J Foodservice Systems* **8**, 1–45.

Brown C R, Edwards C G, Yang, C P, *et al.* (1989), Orange flesh trait in potato – inheritance and carotenoid content, *J Am Soc Hort Sci*, **118**, 145–150.

Brown C R, Ray J A, Fletcher J D, *et al.* (1991), Using antisense RNA to study gene function – inhibition of carotenoid biosynthesis in transgenic tomatoes, *Biotechnology*, **9**, 635–639.

Buchanan B B, Adamidi C, Lozano RM, Yee BC, Momma M, *et al.* (1997), Thioredoxin-linked mitigation of wheat allergies, *Proc Natl Acad Sci USA*, **94**, 5372–5377.

Burkhardt P K, Beyer P, Wunn J, *et al.* (1997) Transgenic rice (*Oryza sativa*) endosperm expressing daffodil (*Narcissus pseudonarcissus*) phytoene synthase, accumulates phytoene a key intermediate in pro-vitamin A synthesis, *Plant J*, **11**, 1071–1078.

Calder PC and Jackson AA (2000) Undernutrition, infection and immune function, *Nutrn Res Rev*, **13**, 3–29.

Cantos E, Tomás-Barberán FA Martínez A and Espín J C (2003) Differential stilbene induction susceptibility of seven red wine grape varieties upon postharvest UV-*C* irradiation, *Eur Food Res Technol*, **217**, 253–258.

Carlson S R, Rudgers G W, Zieler H, Mach J M, Luo S, *et al.* (2007) Meiotic transformation of an in-vitro autonomous maize minichromosome, *PLoS Genet*, **3**, 1965–1974.

Chier J M, Finer J J and Grabau E A (2004) Ectopic expression of a soybean phytase in developing seeds of Glycine max to improve phosphorus availability, *Plant Mol Biol*, **56**, 895–904.

Crozier A, Lean M E J, McDonald M S and Black C (1997) Quantitative analysis of the flavonoid content of commercial tomatoes, onions, lettuce and celery, *J Ag Food Chem*, **45**, 590–595.

Davies KM (2007) Genetic modification of plant metabolism for human health benefits. *Mutat Res*, **622**, 122–137.

De Girolamo A, Solfrizzo M, Vitti C and Visconti A (2004) Occurrence of 6-methoxymellein in fresh and processed carrots and relevant effect of storage and processing, *J Agric Food Chem*, **52**, 6478–6484.

Dellapenna D and Pogson B (2006), Vitamin synthesis in plants:tocopherols and carotenoids, *Annu Rev Plant Biol*, **57**, 711–738.

Dewanto V, Wu X, Adom K and Liu R H (2002) Processed sweet corn has higher antioxidant capacity, *J Agric Food Chem*, **50**, 4959–4964.

Diaz de la Garza R I, Gregory J F III and Hanson A D (2007) Folate biofortification of tomato fruit, *Proc Natl Acad Sci USA*, **10**, 4218–4222.

Dorais M and Ehret D L (2008) 'Agronomy and the nutritional quality of fruit', in Tomás-Barberán F A and Gil M I (eds), *Improving the Health-promoting Effects of Fruit and Vegetable Products*, Boca Raton, London, New York, Washington DC, CRC Press, 346–391.

Espín de Gea J C (2008) 'Postharvest enhancement of bioactive compounds in fresh produce using abiotic stress', in Tomás-Barberán F A and Gil M I (eds), *Improving the Health-promoting Effects of Fruit and Vegetable Products*, Boca Raton, London, New York, Washington DC, CRC Press, 431–448.

Faulkner K, Mithen R, and Williamson G (1998) Selective increase of the potential anticarcinogen 4-methylsulphinylbutyl glucosinolate in broccoli, *Carcinogenesis*, **19**, 605–609.

Food and Agriculture Organization of the United Nations (2006) State of Food Insecurity in the World, Food and Agriculture Organization of the United Nations. Available at www.fao.org

Food & Nutrition Board (2003) Dietary Reference Intakes: Guiding Principles for Nutrition Labelling & Fortification. Institute of Medicine, US National Academies Press.

Fray D and Grierson D (1994), Molecular genetics of tomato fruit ripening, *Trends Genet*, **9**, 438–443.

Gartner C, Stahl W and Siess, H (1997) Lycopene is more bioavailable from tomato paste than fresh tomato, *Am J Clin Nutr*, **66**, 116–122.

Gil M I and Kader A A (2008) 'Fresh-cut fruit and vegetables', in Tomás-Barberán F A and Gil M I (eds), *Improving the Health-promoting Effects of Fruit and Vegetable Products*, Boca Raton, London, New York, Washington DC, CRC Press, 475–504.

Graham R D, Welch R M, and Bouis H E (2001) Assessing micronutrient malnutrition through enhancing the nutritional quality of staple foods: Principles, perspectives and knowledge gaps, *Adv Agron*, **70**, 77–142.

Grain (2000). Engineering solutions to malnutrition. http://www.grain.org

Harjes C E, Rocheford T R, Bai L, Brutnell T P, Kandianis C B, *et al.* (2008) Natural genetic variation in lycopene epsilon cyclase tapped for maize biofortification, *Science*, **319**, 330–333.

Hirshi K D (2009) Nutrient biofortification of food crops, *Annual Rev. Nutrition*, **29**, 401–421.

Howard L (2008) 'Processing techniques and their effect on fruit and vegetables', in Tomás-Barberán F A and Gil M I (eds), *Improving the Health-promoting Effects of Fruit and Vegetable Products*, Boca Raton, London, New York, Washington DC, CRC Press, 449–471.

IFPRI (1999), International Food Policy Research Institute, 'Agricultural strategies for micronutrients'. http://www.cgair.org/ifpri/themes/grp06.htm

Jackman R L, Yada R Y, Tung M A and Speers R A (1987) Anthocyanins as food colorants – a review, *J Food Biochem*, **11**, 201–247.

Jang MS, Cai E N, Udeani G O, Slowing K V, Thomas CF, *et al.* (1997) Cancer chemopreventive activity of resveratrol, a natural product derived from grapes, *Science*, **275**, 218–220.

Kadler A A (2002) 'Quality parameters of fresh-cut fruit and vegetables', in Lamiikanra O (ed.), *Fresh-cut Fruits and Vegetables Science, Technology and Market*, Boca Raton, London, New York, Washington DC, CRC Press, 11–20.

Khanizadeh S, Ehsani-Moghadda B and Levasseur A (2006) Antioxidant capacity in June-bearing and day-neutral strawberry, *Can J Plant Sci*, **86**, 1387–1390.

Knorr D, Ade-Omowaye B I O and Heinz V (2002) Nutritional improvement of plant foods by non-thermal processing, *Proc Nutr Soc*, **61**, 311–318.

Kushad MM, Brown AF, Kurilich AC, Juvik JA, Klein BP, *et al.* (1999) Variation of glucosinolates in vegetable crops of *Brassica oleracea, J Agric Food Chem*, **47**, 1541–1548.

Leonardi C, Ambrosino P, Esposito F and Fogliano V (2000) Antioxidative activity and carotenoid and tomatine contents in different typologies of fresh consumption tomatoes, *J Agric Food Chem*, **48**, 4723–4727.

Lin C H and Chen B H (2005) Stability of carotenoids during processing, *Eur Food Res Tech*, **221**, 274–280.

Lindley M G (1998) The impact of food processing on antioxidants in vegetable oils, fruits and vegetables, *Trends in Fd Sci & Tech*, **9**, 336–340.

Lozano R M, Wong J H, Yee B C, Peters A, Kobrehel K and Buchanan B B, (1996) New evidence for a role for thioredoxin h in seedling development and germination, *Planta*, **200**, 100–106.

Luo J, Butelli E, Hill L, Parr A, Niggeweg R, *et al.* (2008) AtMYB12 regulates caffeoyl quinic acid and flavonol synthesis in tomato: expression in fruit results in very high levels of both types of polyphenol, *The Plant Journal*, **56**, 316–326.

Matteson A P and Cheng A (2006) Neurohormetic phytochemicals: low-dose toxins that induce adaptive neuronal stress responses, *Trends in Neurosciences*, **29**, 632–639.

Nyugen ML and Swartz SJ (1998) Lycopene stability during food processing, *Proc Exp Biol Med*, **218**, 101–105.

Pen J, Verwoerd T C, Van Paridon P A, Beudecker RF, van den Elzen P J M, *et al.* (1993) Phytase-containing transgenic seeds as a novel feed additive for improved phosphorous utilisation, *Biotechnology*, **11**, 811–814.

Pérez-Conesa D, García-Alonso J, García-Valverde V, Iniesta M-D, Jacob K, *et al.* (2009) Changes in bioactive compounds and antioxidant activity during homogenisation and thermal processing of tomato puree, *Innov Food Sci Emerg Technol*, **10**, 179–188.

Quintana JM, Harrison HC, Nienhuis J, Palta JP and Grusak MA, (1996) Variation in calcium concentration among sixty S1 families and four cultivars of snap bean (Phaseolus vulgaris L.), *J. Amer Soc Hort Sci*, **121**, 789–793.

Raboy V, Young K A, Dorsch J A and Cook A (2001) Genetics and breeding of seed phosphorus and phytic acid, *J Plant Physiol*, **158**, 489–497.

Rodriguez-Amaya D B (1997) Carotenoids and food preparation: the retention of pro-vitamin A carotenoids in prepared, processed and stored foods, USAID, OMNI Project.

Rommel A and Wrolstad R E (1993) Ellagic acid content of red raspberry juice as influenced by cultivar, processing, and environmental factors, *J Agric Food Chem*, **41**, 1951–1960.

Rush D (2000) Nutrition and maternal mortality in the developing world, *Am J Clin Nutr*, **72**, S212–240.

Schlesier K, Shahrzad S, Bitsch, I and Dietrich H (1997) Actively anticarcinogenic phenolcarboxylic acids in fruit juices and wines from the same batch of fruit, *Zeitschrift für Ernährungswissenschaft*, **36**, 79–80.

Schonhof I and Krumbein A (1996) Gehalt an wertgebenden Inhaltsstoffen verschiedener Brokkolitypen (Brassica oleracea var italica Plenck), *Gartenbauwissenschaft*, **61**, 281–288.

Sifakis S and Pharmakides G (2000) Anemia in pregnancy, *Ann NY Acad Sci*, **900**, 125–136.

Solomons NW, and Bulux J (1997) Identification of local carotene-rich foods to combat vitamin A malnutrition, *Eur J Clin Nutrn*, **51**, (Suppl.), S39–45.

Stewart A J, Bozzonet S, Mullen W, Jenkins G I, Lean M J and Crozier A (2000) Occurrence of flavonols in tomatoes and tomato-based products, *J Agric Food Chem*, **48**, 2663–2669.

Stommel J R, Abbot J A and Saftner RA (2005) USDA 02L1058 and 02L1059: Cherry tomato breeding lines with high fruit beta-carotene content, *HortScience*, **40**, 1569–1570.

Toenniessen G H (2002) Crop genetic improvement for enhanced nutrition, *J Nutr*, **132**, S2493–2946.

Tomás-Barbarán F A and Espín J C (2001) Phenolic compounds and related enzymes as determinants of quality in fruits and vegetables, *J Sci Food Agric*, **81**, 853–876.

Verkerk R H J and Hickey S A (2010) Critique of prevailing approaches to nutrient risk analysis pertaining to food supplements with specific reference to the European Union. *Toxicology* doi:10.1016/j.tox.2009.12.017

Wang M and Goldman I L (1996) Phenotypic variation in free folic acid content among F1 hybrids and open-pollenated cultivars of red beets, *J Am Soc Hortic Sci*, **121**, 1040–1042.

World Health Organisation (1995) Global prevalence of vitamin A deficiencies. Micronutrient deficiency information systems, Working Paper No 2, WHO Geneva.

World Health Organisation (2004) Global Strategy on Diet, Physical Activity & Health, WHO Geneva, ISBN 92 4 159222 2.

Yang RY, Hanson PM and Lumpkin TA (2007) Better health through horticulture – AVRDC's approach to improved nutrition for the poor, *Acta Hortic*, **744**, 71–77.

Zeldin E L, McCown B H, Krueger C G and Reed J D (2007) Biochemical characterization and breeding of American cranberry for increased health benefits, *Acta Hortic*, **744**, 253–258.

Zhu C, *et al.* (2008) Combinatorial genetic transformation generates a library of metabolic phenotypes for the carotenoid pathway in maize, *Proc Natl Acad Sci USA*, **105**, 18232–18237

15

Developing functional ingredients: a case study of pea protein

A.-S. Sandberg, Chalmers University of Technology, Sweden

Abstract: Legumes, such as peas, are suitable for human consumption, and especially for the development of novel protein foods, which could be used as meat replacement. This chapter discusses the nutritional value and anti-nutritional factors of pea protein and processing issues to improve pea protein. The chapter then describes adding pea protein to food products and a case study of evaluating the nutritional, functional and sensory properties of improved pea protein products.

Key words: pea protein concentrate, pea protein isolate, nutritional value, anti-nutritional factors, functional properties.

15.1 Introduction: the nutritional properties of peas

Legumes include peas, beans, lentils, peanuts and other podded plants that are used as food. Legumes are rich sources of food proteins from plants and have provided a protein source for humans and animals since the earliest of civilisations. Peas (*Pisum sativum*) are known to have been cultivated since 6000 BC in the Near East[1] and at least 4000 years ago in the New World.[2] Legumes were traditionally an important component of the human diet as protein source and there are numerous traditional recipes in European countries that are based on legumes. Nevertheless, their consumption has declined steadily since the end of World War II, partly due to their image as the so-called 'food for the poor' and partly due to undesirable gastrointestinal effects associated with the consumption of legumes. The recent interest towards sustainable production of protein rich foods may however change this trend. Novel protein foods (NPFs) from plants are a promising alternative to meat production that can reduce the disturbing impact of food production on the environment. Legumes, such as peas, are suitable for production of proteins for human consumption, and especially for the development of NPFs, which could be used as meat replacement.[3,4] The use of such proteins in foods as functional ingredients to improve the stability, texture and nutritional value of the product or for economic reasons is very extended.[5] Processing conditions should be controlled to minimise unwanted compounds that interfere with the nutritional value, sensorial characteristics or functional properties of the final product.

Peas are consumed both as fresh immature seeds as well as dry seeds. The latter are mostly consumed as whole seeds after cooking. Pea flour can be used to make a large variety of savouries, e.g. used as the basis for many soups and curries. The green pea has become an important green vegetable, being consumed as a fresh or processed product, either canned or frozen.

Nowadays there is a consumer trend towards more natural and 'healthy' foods and the food industry is constantly searching for ways to meet the demand for healthy wholefoods and food ingredients. The pea has an image of a traditional, natural foodstuff and pea protein products may fulfil these requirements. Pea seeds contain high levels of protein and digestible carbohydrates, relatively high concentrations of insoluble dietary fibre and low concentrations of fat. The average starch and crude protein content is about 440 (214–486) and 225 g per kg dry matter respectively.[6,7]

The average protein content in *Pisum sativum* is reported to be 25% with a wide variation between plants, cultivars and varieties. Selections of a high protein content and high yield in field peas are major goals of plant breeders. Pea protein is a good source of essential amino acids with a high content of lysine and threonine, but like other legumes, it is deficient in sulphur-containing amino acids. Globulins account for 65 to 80% of the proteins in peas.[8] The digestibility of pea protein is between 83% and 93% as assessed by rat assays.

Dietary fibre constitutes about 63 g per kg dry matter in whole peas, and the content of total free sugars, raffinose, stachyose and verbascose is about 125; 12, 32 and 19 g per kg dry matter respectively.[9] The range of fat content is 10–24 g per kg dry matter and oleic and linoleic acid are the predominating fatty acids.[6,10] Peas are good sources of minerals and water-soluble vitamins and are particularly rich in B-group vitamins.

Recently, the nutritional interest for peas and other legumes has increased because of the markedly attenuating effect on blood sugar and insulin response and thereby their potential use for prevention and control of diabetes.[11,12] The digestibility of starch in legumes is restricted due to intact cell walls,[13] which enclose the starch granules and limit interaction with amylotic enzymes.[14] However, other mechanisms may also be involved; phytic acid polyphenols (tannic acid) and lectins can inhibit α-amylase activity *in vitro*, suggesting that an interaction with starch digestion also could occur *in vivo*.[15] *In vitro* studies have also indicated that the protein matrix in legume products limits the accessibility of starch to amylase.[16] A reduced rate of starch digestion attenuates the blood glucose and insulin response after a meal.

Foods containing carbohydrates which are slow to digest and absorb are of importance in the dietary management of diabetic patients. However, diets

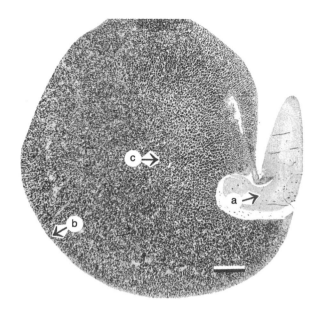

Fig. 15.1   Cross-section of pea seed: a, germ; b, outer cotyledon; c, inner cotyledon. The scale bar corresponds to a length of 1 mm (from Dr Karin Autio, VTT, Finland).

characterised by such foods have also been found to improve glucose tolerance in healthy subjects. In fact, dietary carbohydrates that cause a rapid rise in post-prandial insulin levels are extensively discussed as a risk factor for development of metabolic diseases.[17] The goal of diabetes therapy is to achieve normal glycemia and to prevent late complications. The development of vascular complications in diabetes has been related to the metabolic aberrations of uncontrolled diabetes.[18] In a recent review it was concluded that there is strong evidence to suggest that eating a variety of whole grain foods and legumes is beneficial in the prevention and management of diabetes type II.[19]

A dietary fibre content of 63 g per kg with 34% soluble fibre has been reported in light-hulled peas.[20] Generally, cell wall polysaccharides of seeds from such plants are dominated by pectic substances, cellulose, xyloglucans and glycoproteins.[21] Viscous soluble polysaccharides, such as pectic substances, are considered to have beneficial effects on carbohydrate and lipid metabolism in humans[22–25] by improving glucose tolerance, increasing ileal fat and bile acids excretion and decreasing blood lipids.[26] Pea fibre was shown to lower fasting and post-prandial blood triglyceride concentrations in humans,[27] one of the established risk factors for the development of cardiovascular disease. Except for prevention of non-insulin-dependent diabetes, pea fibre therefore has a potential use in the prevention of cardiovascular disease.

Anti-nutritional factors lower the nutritional value of a food by lowering the digestibility or bioavailability of nutrients. Peas contain a number of anti-nutritive and anti-physiological factors, which may be controlled by suitable processing and breeding programmes. However, the level of anti-nutritional factors is generally lower than in soy and other grain legumes. The anti-nutritional factors present in pea protein include proteinase inhibitors (e.g. trypsin inhibitors and chymotrypsin inhibitors) and lectins. Non-protein components recognised as anti-nutritional factors in peas include saponins, polyphenols, phytate and raffinose oligosaccharides. All commercial varieties of field peas are considered not to contain polyphenols. The utilisation of peas is restricted due to the presence of these anti-nutritional factors. Trypsin inhibitors decrease the protein digestibility and availability. Lectins are proteins, or glycoproteins, with the unique ability to bind to specific carbohydrate containing molecules on the surface of cells. Lectins have the ability to agglutinate red blood cells[28] and to bind to the intestinal epithelium, resulting in disruption of the brush border[29] atrophy of the microvilli[30] and reduced viability of the epithelial cells,[31] resulting in impaired nutrient transport. Thus, lectins can reduce the uptake of glucose and cause damage to the intestinal mucosal layer, but as these proteins are high in sulphur-containing amino acids (and are of importance for the yield and resistance to plant disease), inactivation of the inhibitors by processing should be preferred to genetic selection of cultivars with low inhibitor levels. Phytate present in peas and their protein products may negatively affect the digestibility of pea proteins. The mineral content of legumes is generally high, but the bioavailability is poor, due to the presence of phytate.[32] Phytate and some of its degradation products form complexes with certain essential dietary minerals (Fe, Zn, Ca), thereby impairing their absorption.[33]

Saponins adhere to proteins and have a bitter taste, generally considered unpleasant. Moreover, saponins may deteriorate the intestinal wall through a detergent effect.[34] Saponins increase the permeability of intestinal mucosal cells, thereby facilitating the uptake of substances to which the mucosa is normally impermeable.[48] This may lead to uptake of antigens, causing allergic reactions.[49] Like trypsin inhibitors, selection of these anti-nutritional factors may have an impact on resistance to plant disease. Therefore, development of processing methods that inactivate the anti-nutritional factors post-harvest is preferable. Flatulence is associated with consumption of legume seeds including peas and causes some individuals to avoid these foods. Some indigestible oligosaccharides including raffinose, stachyose and verbascose are responsible for at least some of the flatulence of legume seeds through their fermentation by gut bacteria. Pea protein isolate, prepared by wet processing, contains much less of these oligosaccharides than the concentrated form.[35]

Like other legume proteins, pea proteins may be a potential allergen. The antigenicity of pea proteins is expected to be comparable to that of soy proteins. Reports indicate that around 15% of infants who have developed allergy to cow milk protein and switched to soy formula will also be sensitised against soy protein.[36]

One of the most valuable ingredients extracted from pea is its protein fraction, which can be extensively purified as a protein concentrate or a protein isolate (Fig. 15.2). Up until now the major outlet for protein isolate is its use as a

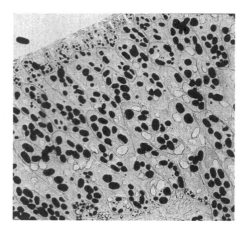

Fig. 15.2   Microscopic image of embedded section of cotyledon of pea. Starch is stained black and protein is stained in a lighter colour (from Dr Karin Autio, VTT, Finland).

functional ingredient, such as an emulsifier, thickener or foaming agent. The pea protein isolate is a valuable protein source, which has a potential to replace soy protein and enhance the nutritional value of foods. Furthermore the primary structures of pea protein are peptide sequences that can potentially be used in the formulation of therapeutic products for the treatment and prevention of human diseases. Enzymatic treatment can be used to convert inactive pea proteins into bioactive peptides with potential antimicrobial, antihypertensive, antioxidant and immunomodulatory activity.[37]

15.2   Improving pea protein

The digestibility of pea protein is between 83% and 93%.[8] Phytic acid present in peas is accumulated in the pea protein fraction and may negatively affect digestibility of the pea protein. Heating may improve the nutritional quality of pea protein materials by increasing protein digestibility or by inactivating anti-nutritional factors such as trypsin inhibitors or lectin. The nutritional quality of pea protein using the protein efficiency ratio (PER) method was found to increase slightly when cooked (boiled for one hour).[38] Deo *et al.*[39] demonstrated that cooking destroyed the trypsin inhibitor of all the peas evaluated and an improved digestibility was found. The mode of action of chymotrypsin inhibition was expected to be very similar to that of trypsin inhibitors. The effect of heat treatment on chymotrypsin inhibitors in peas was similar to that for trypsin inhibitors.[40]

Lectins are also heat labile. The activity was completely eliminated by autoclaving of peas at 121°C for five minutes.[41] Removal of 65% of activity after soaking the peas for 18 h was also reported by Bender.[42] Heating can also improve palatability.

Biological food processing techniques increasing the endogenous enzyme activity or adding enzymes can produce an additional and substantial reduction of the anti-nutritional factors. Furthermore, positive effects on carbohydrate and lipid metabolism in humans as a result of fermentation of cereals and legumes have been found. Controlled degradation of phytate by fermentation or by the addition of phytase has been demonstrated to increase the absorption of iron and zinc in meals based on cereals or soy.[43–45]

The pre-digestion of protein and formation of amino acids during fermentation was found to increase the nutritional value of protein and improve the amino acid composition of cereals and legumes. The fermentation process also has the potential to degrade saponins and oligosaccharides. Tempeh fermentation of peas and other legumes by *Rhizopus oligosporus* was found to degrade the oligosaccharides of the raffinose family.[46]

Pea protein is a potential allergen.[47] Experience with soy proteins show that steam heating does not reduce this antigenicity substantially, whereas other treatments such as proteolytic cleavage does. The fermentation of pea protein might be a possible means of reducing the antigenicity by hydrolysing protein and degrading the saponins.

The raffinose family of oligosaccharides, causing flatulence, tend to concentrate in the protein fraction of air-classified pea concentrate.[50] Pea protein isolate, prepared by wet processing, contains much less of these oligosaccharides than pea protein concentrate because some of the carbohydrates are washed away in the effluent.[35] Removal of these compounds can be performed by ultrafiltration, addition of α-galactosidase enzymes or fermentation by microorganisms producing α-galactosidase.

Selection of cultivars with high protein and high amino acid content, particularly methionine, is of great importance. Development of processing methods, which inactivate or degrade anti-nutritional factors post-harvest, would significantly improve the nutritional quality of pea protein.

15.3   Processing issues in improving pea protein

15.3.1   Standard procedures for preparation of pea protein

One of the most valuable ingredients extracted from pea is its protein fraction. The preparation of pea protein could be an alternative to the well-established versatile soy protein products that dominate the food protein market. Soy protein products are used to extend or replace animal protein such as meat. It is also used as a protein source in infant formulas. Soy milk is used for replacement of cow's milk by vegetarians and persons with intolerance to milk protein. Depending on the low fat content of peas, the need for an oil extraction stage is eliminated and furthermore the relatively low content of anti-nutritive substances compared to soy is an advantage. Pea protein can be prepared in three forms: pea flour, pea protein concentrate and pea isolate. Pea flour is prepared by dry milling of dehulled peas. Pea protein concentrate is usually prepared by dry separation methods, while pea protein isolate is produced by wet processing methods. The advantage of dry over wet separation techniques are lower costs and the absence of effluents. On the other hand the dry process gives a lower yield and a lower protein content.[4] Processing conditions should be chosen to avoid unwanted reactions such as lipid oxidation, polyphenol oxidation and protein denaturation.

Dry process (pea flour, pea protein concentrate)
Pea protein and starches can be efficiently fractionated by dry milling and air classification. By fine grinding, flours containing populations of particles are differentiated by size and density. Air classification of these flours separates the protein (fine fraction) from the starch (coarse fraction).[51] Whole or dehulled peas are, by this dry process, milled to very fine flour. During milling the starch granules remain relatively intact, while the protein matrix is broken down to fine particles. There is, however, a risk for damage of the starch granules during milling. Air classification of the pea flour is performed in a spiral air stream into a fine fraction containing around 75% of the protein, and a coarse fraction containing most of the starch granules. After milling, some starch is still embedded in the protein matrix and some protein bodies still adhere to starch granules. By repeated milling and air classification, the separation of starch and protein can be improved.[51] It was also found that the percentage protein in air-classified pea fractions positively correlates with the protein content of the original pea flour.[52] Moreover, the percentage of starch recovered in the starch fraction as well as the percentage of protein recovered in the protein fractions both increase with increasing protein content of the pea.[53] Furthermore, air classifying at low speed increases protein content of the protein fractions but also starch fractions with higher levels of protein. Air classification provides a lower cost, effluent-free process for preparing pea protein concentrate, but not as pure fractions as aqueous extraction.

Wet processes (pea protein isolate, pea protein concentrate)
Protein isolates (highly concentrated protein fractions) and protein concentrates from pea can be produced by wet processing. The protein separation is based on solubilisation of protein followed by an isoelectric process or an ultrafiltration process[54] for subsequent recovery. Other processes include 'hydrophobic-out' or 'salting-out'.[8]

Variations of the isoelectric precipitation process and the ultrafiltration process are used commercially. The different steps in the isoelectric process for pea protein isolate are milling of the peas, solubilisation of the proteins in water, alkali, or acid; then centrifugation to remove insoluble components. Then the solubilised proteins are precipitated at their isoelectric pH, and collected by centrifugation, or sieving, and dried as such or neutralised and dried.

The yield of the protein isolate prepared by isoelectric precipitation is influenced by several factors such as particle size of the flour, the kind of solubilising agent, as well as pH of solubilisation and precipitation. Furthermore, the isolate composition is affected by the solubilising and precipitating pH. Isolates precipitated below 5.3

have been found to be lower in protein content and to have higher lipid content than those precipitated at pH 5.3.[55]

Ultrafiltration with non-cellulosic membranes can be used to isolate protein from wet slurries.[55] These membrane systems are stable over a wide range of pH values and elevated temperature and thus offer an alternative to the conventional acid precipitation methods. Ultrafiltration using a hollow fibre system can give protein recoveries of 90–94%. An advantage is that low molecular weight compounds such as oligosaccharides are removed by ultrafiltration.

15.3.2   Possible modifications of the procedure

Possible means to remove anti-nutritional factors in the process for preparation of pea protein include increasing the endogenous enzyme activity by soaking the peas, and fermentation by addition of certain starter cultures or addition of enzymes. This kind of modification can be performed in the wet process for preparation of isolates or the pea flour. Fermentation using lactic acid bacteria, fungi or yeast, is traditionally used in Asian food manufacturing of soybean based products (e.g. soy sauce, miso, tempeh). The effect of fermentation of peas has so far mainly been studied in relation to protein quality, while systematic studies of the possibility to optimise the reduction of anti-nutritional factors of pea products and, in particular, pea protein for human consumption through biological processing techniques are lacking.

The functional properties of pea proteins suggest that pea proteins have a high potential for use in food products. The type of process used for the preparation of pea concentrate or pea protein isolate affects functional properties of the product. Different combinations of thermal treatment and pH should be evaluated in order to understand the relation between process conditions and functionality.

15.3.3   Pea protein hydrolysates

Protein hydrolysates are of interest for the food industry because of their beneficial effects for the food products and for human health. Enzymatic hydrolysis is preferred because they are milder and the nature and extent of the treatment can be controlled due to inherent specificity of various proteases.[56] The possibility of production of pea protein hydrolysates with desirable nutritional properties and a low bitterness threshold has recently been evaluated. Selecting papain and alfa-chymotrypsin for enzymatic hydrolysis were found desirable for producing high quality pea protein hydrolysates with low bitterness and good physiochemical and physiological functional properties (antimicrobial, antihypertensive, antioxidative, immunomodulatory).[57]

15.4   Adding improved protein to food products

Effective utilisation of pea proteins in foods for human consumption depends to a large extent on consumer acceptance. Some studies have been conducted on the potentiality of applications of pea products in food; in addition or in substitution to flour (in bread or pasta) or to meat (in patties, hamburgers), in textured products, soups, snacks, and in substitution to milk. The addition of pea products influences the cooking time and texture. As such, modifications of the formulae were sometimes necessary to have acceptable organoleptic properties. Pea protein concentrates have been found useful for producing non-fat dry milk replacements for the baking industry. A non-dairy frozen dessert was developed utilising pea protein isolate with good organoleptic characteristics. In some applications pea proteins could replace soy proteins. It would be of interest to develop tailored pea proteins for specific applications.

Pea materials sometimes have unacceptable flavours but a pea protein isolate with a bland flavour can also be produced. The functional requirements for a plant protein to be useful as a meat extender include good fat and water absorption, emulsification capacity and stability, gelation texturisability and sensory properties. Pea protein isolate has a high solubility, water and fat binding capacity and emulsifying and foaming capacity to give desired texture and stability. Possible applications are meat and fish products, biscuits and pastry making, desserts, prepared dishes, soups and sauces, dietary, health and baby food. For use of plant protein in infant formulas a high bioavailability of minerals, a high nutritive value of the protein and a low antigenicity are desired.

15.4.1   Cereal and bakery products

The nutritional quality of wheat protein has been improved by addition of pea flour or pea protein concentrate[58] to wheat flour. Replacing 20% of the wheat flour with pea flour gives bread with excellent protein quality. However, at this level of supplementation the bread had decreased in volume and had a relatively poor crumb structure[59,60] and the acceptance of the supplemented bread was limited due to poor sensory properties.[61] Also, it was found that addition of pea flour to yeast breads significantly affects the texture. Protein enrichment of pasta product with pea protein has also been performed. Supplemented pasta has a better protein quality, cooks faster and is slightly firmer.[62] The flavour was, however, found to be somewhat inferior to that of unsupplemented wheat pasta. For the application of pea protein in biscuits a series of experiments were first performed to choose process type (creaming or crumbling) and formula (partial substitution of flour or substitution of milk powder). The creaming process was found to be the most suitable process. Colour was found to depend on protein source but was not influenced by fat, sugar and protein content. Biscuits containing milk powder were darker than biscuits made with pea proteins. Hardness was influenced by protein source. Biscuits made with milk proteins were harder than those made with pea protein. A higher percentage of protein also increased hardness, an effect that also was found with increasing sugar content, though not as extensive. Crispiness decreased with high amount of fat and tended to increase with the level of sugar.[63]

15.4.2   Meat products

The requirement for plant proteins to be used as extenders in meat products include good fat and water absorption, emulsification capacity and stability, gelation texturisability and sensory attributes. High solubility is not a determinant of the usefulness of a plant protein in meat systems; in some cases proteins of low solubility are engineered for use in meat systems. The use of pea protein in meat products has mainly been in meat patties,[64] hamburgers and sausages. Inferior flavour and aroma as a result of addition of pea protein was found in these products. Sausages extended with pea protein have improved nutritional value compared to unsupplemented products. The optimal sensory concentration was found to be 4–7%; concentrations greater than 10% were found to produce a strong pea flavour.[8]

15.4.3   Milk replacement products

There seems to be some promise in the use of pea protein concentrate as an ingredient for producing non-fat dry milk replacement for the baking industry.[65] Also there have been attempts to produce milk substitutes.[66] Pea milk has a potential use for replacement of cow milk by vegetarians and persons with intolerance and allergy to cow milk and also oral nutritional supplements. Other trials have been carried out to substitute milk powder by pea protein in desserts. The first experiments were made according to a fractional design with five factors: quantity of pea, starch, gum, oil and emulsifier. From the results of the first experiments the most relevant ingredients were then selected, i.e. based upon the quantity of pea protein and starch. These ingredients were then optimised in order to get a dessert close to the commercial form.[63]

15.4.4   Vegetable pâté

The application of pea protein in a vegetable pâté has been investigated. Different quantities of pea protein, gum and starch were tested using a multivate experimental design in order to evaluate the effect of the three factors and to optimise the formula. The main purpose was to get as close as possible to the reference vegetable pâté made with whole egg. Response surface methodology was used to find the optimum formula on physical characteristics with as high an amount of pea protein as possible.

Textural measurements showed only small differences between the reference and the formula. The colour of the vegetable pâté made with pea protein was different from the reference made with whole egg, which also was confirmed in the sensory analysis. Moreover, other characteristics related to appearance (brightness, firmness, straight cut, bubble size) of the pâté were different. For mouth feel the formula was found to be slightly more firm than the reference. Taste of carrot was very close in the samples and the optimal formula was well accepted by the test panel.

The optimisation of vegetable pâté demonstrates, on the one hand, the quality of pea protein as a functional ingredient and, on the other hand, its capability to substitute whole egg. Furthermore, pea protein can reduce the incorporation of other textural agents and has more than 40% less quantity of gum and starch than the reference vegetable pâté.[63,67]

15.5   Evaluating the nutritional, functional and sensory properties of improved pea protein in food products

15.5.1   Evaluating nutritional properties

The genetic variation of peas is considerable. As a first step towards producing an improved pea protein a choice of starting material has to be made. The following criteria are important in the selection of pea raw material:

- high level of protein content in the seed and low level in fat content;
- high level of limiting amino acids (methionine, cysteine, trypthophan);
- low level of anti-nutritional factors;
- availability of the genotype in sufficient quantities;
- high yield and resistance to plant disease.

Analysis of relevant nutritional parameters such as protein quality, amino acid composition and a number of anti-nutritional factors including oligosaccharides, phytate, proteinase inhibitors, lectins, saponins and polyphenols therefore has to be performed in raw pea seeds and the pea protein products.

Anti-nutritional factors in different starting materials and from modified process for pea protein products

Analyses of protein isolates from a commercial wet process showed that the contents of oligosaccharides and lectins were effectively reduced during the processing and no clear relationship was found between saponins and taste. The trypsin inhibitors were found to be partly inactivated by heat treatment. The major important anti-nutrient in protein isolate was determined to be phytate. Determination of the phytate content in protein isolates showed that the phytate accumulated in the protein isolate. Analyses of the oligosaccharide content in protein isolates from selected pea varieties showed that the contents were lower than in the isolates from the standard process (due to an improvement of the cut-off of the ultrafiltration technique).[68]

The saponin content of the pea seeds was determined to be 2–7 mg/g sample. The content of trypsin inhibitors was found to be 50–100 µg/g sample and lectins 1–2.5 mg/g sample.[69]

Analysis of anti-nutritional factors, in vitro *digestibility and antigenicity*

Addition of exogenous phytase reduced the phytate content in pea protein to very low levels. The use of exogenous phytase was tested on pea flour and two different protein isolates from different steps in the process. The optimal conditions for exogenous phytases were 55 °C and pH 5.5, and the phytate degradation were virtually complete on all substrates tested.[70] The contents of inositol hexaphosphate (phytate) and its degradation products were analysed in dephytinised pea protein isolates and pea protein infant formula. Dephytinised pea protein isolates contained 0.08 µmol/g of phytate and no detectable amounts of lower inositol phosphates. Dephytinised sample incubated with exogenous phytase for one hour instead of two hours, contained 0.5 µmol/g inositol hexaphosphate. Comparison with standard pea protein isolate without enzymatic treatment showed that this sample contained 19.6 µmol/g inositol hexaphosphate. Analysis of pea protein infant formula, produced in the factory scale from dephytinised pea protein isolate, contained only traces of phytate.

The content of proteinase inhibitors (PPI) were much higher in pea flour than in samples incubated at 40% or 70% humidity, both control samples and fermented samples. To investigate the stability of PPI under various conditions a preliminary study was performed. The study showed that only 20% of the original content of PPI were left after 48 hours at 37 °C and 70% humidity.

Lactic acid fermentation of pea flour was found to decrease the saponin content of pea protein isolate. The most effective saponin reduction (90%) was found in a sample fermented with *Lactobacillus plantarum* for 48 hours.

The *in vitro* digestibility was determined by four different methods: reversed phase HPLC, gelfiltration HPLC, sandwich ELISA and SDS-PAGE. The digestibility of dehulled pea seeds, phytase treated pea protein isolate and standard pea protein isolate from the modified process was compared. Analysis by the four methods resulted in a similar outcome for the three investigated products: the pea isolates had an *in vitro* digestibility of 80–90%, whereas the dehulled pea seeds had a much lower digestibility of approximately 40%. The pea protein isolates are thus more digestible than the raw pea.[63]

Bioavailability
The use of pea protein isolate could be an alternative to soy isolate. Soy formulas have been used for a long time period and the nutritional status of infants fed soy formula has been well documented and found to be similar to infants fed cow milk formulas. However, the bioavailability of nutrients, especially minerals, has been reported to be lower than that of milk-based formulas. An important factor contributing to the lower mineral absorption from soy formula is the relatively high concentration of the metal chelator phytic acid, which acts as a dietary inhibitor of the absorption of essential minerals, in particular iron. The negative effect of phytic acid on iron absorption has been shown to be dose dependent.[71] In addition, the soy protein *per se* has recently been demonstrated to inhibit iron absorption.[44] Although the absorption of zinc and calcium may be influenced by the presence of phytic acid, the effect on iron bioavailability is much greater.[33]

The enzymatic degradation of phytate in soy infant formulas was found to improve iron absorption significantly provided that the removal of phytate[74] was virtually complete.[44] The availability of iron and zinc in a dephytinised infant formula based on pea protein was evaluated. Soluble amounts of iron and zinc in the samples were collected during simulated *in vitro* digestion performed in a computer-controlled dynamic gastrointestinal model. Determination of these samples showed that dephytinisation of pea protein increased the amount of iron and zinc potentially available for absorption by 50% and 100%, respectively.[72,73] The iron absorption in humans was increased by more than 50% by dephytinisation.[74]

Antigenicity

A substantial part of the antigens found in pea seeds are still antigenic in fermented pea flour. This was reported by Herian *et al.*[75] who found that soy epitopes can be detected in soy protein isolates as well as fermented soy products. On the other hand, some of the pea antigens have been found to be sensitive to the processing procedures. Monoclonal antibodies can be used to identify these antigens as well as more stable antigens. In contrast to the antigens in general, the inhalation allergen cross-reacting proteins Bet v1 homologue and profilin have been found so labile that they are not only undetectable in the processed protein isolates and fermented samples, but also very reduced in pea flour after incubation at 37°C.[47,63]

15.5.2   Evaluating functional and sensory properties

The required functional properties of the pea protein depend on the desired end product. Research on the functional properties of pea proteins has shown the importance of the preparation treatment of the proteins. Pea proteins are highly soluble at an acidic pH (pH 2), and at alkaline pH 7.3 maximum solubility occurs, the minimum solubility being obtained at pH between 4 and 6. The actual solubility of pea proteins at a given pH in the pH region of 5 to 9 can vary widely.

The following functional and sensorial parameters need to be evaluated in improved pea protein:

- Solubility: These properties enable evaluation of the denaturation state of the protein and are good indicators for evaluating the potential applications of proteins. Good solubility can markedly expand potential utilisation of proteins.
- Dispersibility: Oil and water binding capacity. These take an important place in the quality of meat and charcuterie products, thanks to the binding effect of their components which reduces the loss of water and fat. Water binding capacity (WBC) is useful in food products such as sausages where there is insufficient water for protein to dissolve, but where the hydrated protein imparts structure and viscosity to the food.
- Foaming properties (capacity and stability, texture): These enable the formulation of whipped products. Pea proteins have very high foaming properties in comparison with other vegetable proteins.
- Emulsifying properties (capacity and stability, texture): The emulsifying properties of pea protein can contribute towards the formulation of meat or charcuterie products, which generally have an emulsified structure.
- Gelatinisation and thickening properties: These have an effect on the texture of the different food products.

Such evaluations of pea proteins have been undertaken according to various conditions of use, which are characteristics of the food applications (presence of salt, pH, heat treatment). The properties of the pea proteins developed by bioprocesses have been compared with those of native pea, soy proteins and meat proteins. The potential use of these ingredients and comparison with other ingredients (e.g. meat, other proteins) should then be determined.

Sensory evaluation

A large range of pea protein products have been tested in a food model (sauce) to evaluate sensory characteristics. Different rates of incorporation were tested. Evaluation by an expert panel assessed the main sensory characteristics of the foods: aspect, flavour, mouth feel, texture.

A study has been carried out to evaluate the effect of different functional properties on the selected pea proteins after treatment at various process conditions.[63] It was observed that thermal treatment had a negative effect on solubility. The solubility decreased in the range from 75 °C to 95 °C and then increased again at 120 °C. A further finding was that heat treatment resulted in increased stability of the emulsions. The visco-elastic properties of the medium were different. After treatment at 80 °C for two hours, the firmness of the medium and the viscosity were higher than samples treated at milder conditions. Determination of the functional properties of the modified pea protein showed that the reduction of phytate in the pea protein decreased the solubility and emulsifying and rheological properties.

To study effects of functionality, comparisons have been made between processes without pasteurisation or with pasteurisation at different temperatures (75 °C, 85 °C, 95 °C) or autoclaving at 120 °C. Pea protein isolates produced from the variety Baccara and processed in a pilot plant system using different heat treatments were used to evaluate functional properties. Heating decreased the solubility of the protein and increased the emulsifying stability. The visco-elastic properties of the medium were different: pea protein isolates solidified during heating, remained liquid and exhibited high thickening properties, had different texture compared to lower visco-elastic properties. Gel formation occurred at about 75 °C for one of the pea proteins and was therefore selected for food applications.

15.6 New technologies for improved nutritional and functional value of pea protein (NUTRIPEA)

The work of NUTRIPEA focus on pea protein for human consumption. The general objective of the EU funded project NUTRIPEA (New Technologies for Improved Nutritional and Functional Value of Pea Protein, FAIR CT 95-0193) was to use new technologies to develop improved pea protein products, which are devoid of anti-physiological and anti-nutritional factors. The project concerns a novel research field, which will lead to increased knowledge regarding processing and development of products with increased nutrient availability. The nutritional and functional properties of pea proteins suggest a high potential for use in food products. Therefore, the purpose of the project was to design and develop a technical process to prepare improved pea protein products under pilot plant and factory conditions.

The NUTRIPEA program has verified:

- the technical feasibility of a bioprocess to prepare improved pea protein products;
- the enhancement of nutritional value of the process within one clinical study;
- the legal problems that need to be solved, i.e. development of a phytase 'food grade enzyme' and acceptance of pea protein in European law for infant food;
- that pea protein isolate could be a valuable protein source to replace soy protein isolate.

Additional studies and investments are needed to prove the nutritional benefits and safety of pea protein isolate for infant formula including growth tests and studies in children who are intolerant to cow milk. To reach this main objective the following approach and partial objectives were to be achieved:

- *Task 1* – Evaluation of genetic variation. Starting materials and standard pea protein products were evaluated to set nutritional properties regarding digestibility and some anti-nutritional factors. This task generated information for the selection of suitable starting materials for preparation of pea protein products.
- *Task 2* – To design and develop a technical process to prepare improved pea protein products under pilot plant conditions with two subtasks:

   (a) pilot plant preparation of pea products from the varieties in task 1 and application of different modifications of the standard procedure;
   (b) determination of anti-nutritional factors and antigenicity of pea protein products from the different starting material and from modified process for pea protein products.

The results from these tasks showed that the two anti-nutritional factors, phytate and saponins, were of major importance as the production scheme for pea protein isolate resulted in increased levels of these two anti-nutrients.

- *Task 3* – Bioprocessing of pea protein products to use new technologies to develop improved pea protein products including the following three subtasks:

   (a) preliminary screening of lactic acid bacteria for fermentation processes of pea protein;
   (b) optimisation of the conditions for bioprocessing of pea protein using solid state fermentation and enzymatic treatment;
   (c) evaluation of bioprocessed pea protein regarding contents of anti-nutritional factors, antigenicity, microbiological quality, functional and sensory characteristics.

- *Task 4* – Development of a modified extraction technique at the pilot plant level. This task involved two different processes: the first was developed to reduce the phytate content and the second generated new functional characteristics.

- *Task 5* – Development of test products from pea proteins, infant formulas and pea protein products for adults and evaluation of antigenicity and nutritional and functional value. The abilities of the selected pea proteins developed by food processing were evaluated taking into account technological and sensory aspects. Pea protein infant formulas were produced and evaluated for antigenicity and protein quality in animal models. *In vitro* estimation of iron and zinc bioavailability and iron absorption in humans were also measured.

Determinations of anti-physiological and anti-nutritional factors like oligosaccharides, phytate, proteinase inhibitors, lectins, saponins and tannins have been made in raw pea seeds, pea protein isolates and samples from the production of pea protein isolates. Based on this evaluation, the parameters for the design of a modified process to prepare improved pea protein products were formulated.

The development of pilot plant preparations of pea protein isolates and determination of anti-nutritional factors and antigenicity led to the conclusion that phytate and saponins were the most important anti-nutrients to be reduced, as the production scheme for pea protein isolate resulted in increased levels of both. It was also found that a substantial part of the antigens found in pea seeds were still antigenic in pea protein isolates.

A further task was bioprocessing of pea protein products. The approach of adding exogenous phytase was found to be very effective for reduction of pea protein phytate.[68] Control of the microbiological quality was very important during food processing. Food pathogens and other spoilage organisms such as *Bacillus cereus* originating from peas or the process were found. However, after addition of lactic acid bacteria (LAB) to the soaking water, the growth of spoilage organisms was effectively prevented. Screening of phytase activity of different LAB and fungal strains showed that LAB did not degrade phytate but two food-grade fungi showed phytase activity.[76] Oligosaccharides such as verbascose, stachyose and raffinose were effectively reduced during fermentation with nine selected LAB strains.[63]

The development of a modified extraction technique led to two different modifications of the pilot plant process. The first process was developed in order to reduce the phytate content and the second process was developed to obtain new functionality.

Development of infant pea protein formulas and pea protein products for adults showed that the level of anti-nutritional factors in the final pea protein isolates products were reduced to an acceptable level, i.e. lower than that of soy protein, which is accepted as a protein source in infant feeds. The saponin content of pea protein isolate was compared to soy protein isolate and, although the saponin level in the final pea protein isolate was increased three- to fourfold, this was considerably lower compared to the saponin level in soy protein isolate. This indicated that the pea protein isolate can be regarded as safe for human consumption with regard to saponins. It was also demonstrated that processing steps in the production of pea protein isolates markedly increased the *in vitro* and *in vivo* digestibility of pea protein. Some of the pea antigens were found to be sensitive to the processing procedures but a substantial part of the antigens found in pea seeds were still antigenic in pea protein isolates and fermented pea flour. Evaluation of iron and zinc availability showed a significant increase in the amount of soluble minerals at simulated physiological conditions in a dynamic computer-controlled gastrointestinal model.[72,73] This was also confirmed in a human study, the iron absorption increasing by more than 50% after phytate removal or addition of ascorbic acid to the pea protein infant formula.[63,74]

The following partners were participating in NUTRIPEA (New Technologies for Improved Nutritional and Functional Value of Pea Protein, FAIR CT 95-0193): Chalmers University of Technology, Sweden (co-ordinator), Technical University of Denmark, ETH Zurich, Switzerland, Technical Research Centre of Finland, ADRIA, France, Provital Industries S.A., Belgium, and Semper AB, Sweden.

15.6.1   Conclusions

Bioprocessing of pea protein using addition of exogenous phytase was found to be very effective for the reduction of pea protein phytate. Evaluation of iron and zinc availability also showed a significant increase in the amounts of soluble minerals at simulated physiological conditions.[72,73] Iron absorption increased by more than 50% after phytate removal or addition of ascorbic acid to pea protein infant formulas. Determination of iron absorption using adult women indicated relatively high fractional iron absorption from the bioprocessed pea protein formula, as compared to earlier data on iron absorption from soy formulas in adults.[74] Infant formula based on pea protein could therefore be an alternative to soy isolates.

Control of microbiological quality is very important during food processing. Food pathogens and other spoilage organisms could be controlled by the addition of LAB to the soaking water. This indicates promising possibilities for further developments and up-scaling of the microbicidic soaking and its application in the industrial process.

Screening of phytase activity of different LAB and fungal strains showed that LAB did not degrade phytate but two food-grade fungi exhibited activity. Oligosaccharides such as verbascose, stachyose and raffinose were effectively reduced during fermentation with nine of the selected LAB strains.

15.7   Future trends

Novel protein foods derived from plants are a less expensive and more environmental friendly alternative to meat protein production. Today the major part of European pea production is used for animal feed, but it can be assumed that pea protein in the future have the potential to become an important protein source also for humans. To replace meat in the diet it is essential that the plant protein source can deliver sufficient protein without anti-nutritional factors. Nutritional inadequacy, in particular with regard to iron, occurs in association with vegetarianism. It is presently technically feasible to produce pea products which are low in anti-nutritional factors and have a high nutritional value. Scientific evidence supporting the specific health benefits of consuming pea protein or pea protein hydrolysates (peptides) are still required. To further increase the demand for pea products it is important to perform studies to provide substantiated health claims, such as studies of glycemic index, potential effects on blood lipids, blood pressure and immunomodulatory properties. There is also a need for development of novel products with good sensory properties which are in accordance with consumers wishes.

The 6th European Grain Legumes Conference in Lisbon 2007 defined a strategic vision for legume research which is summarised below:

Legume Research: Perspectives from the European Union
   Tabled and discussed at the 6th European Grain Legumes Conference, Lisbon, November 2007
   Summary:
   This document presents the role of legumes used in agriculture: grains, vegetables, forage legumes and for forestry or coppice and suggests research priorities in crop and model systems.

- Nitrogen fixation by legumes allows them to reduce the energy costs of agriculture and to minimise greenhouse gas production.
- Legumes provide healthy protein sources both for food and livestock feed.
- Legumes contribute to biodiversity in agriculture, in pasture ad in field crop rotations.
- Certain legume shrubs are ideal for land reclamation and others can be the basis of sustainable forestry and biomass production.

The main challenge to legume research is to determine how, once integrated into sustainable farming systems, their profitability can be optimised for the farmer while maintaining their environmental benefit. Two major linked research areas emerge from this challenge:

i. how can these crops best be improved and managed for maximal productivity and minimal environmental impact
ii. how the quality of products: food, feed, fodder, or fuel can be improved or maintained with increasing production efficiency, or be tailored to specific end uses.

15.8   Sources of further information and advice: past and present EU projects, networks and special reports in the field

AEP, the European Association of Grain Legume Research is a European-based but internationally-active network of scientists and end-users concerned with grain legumes (peas, faba beans, lupins, chickpeas, lentils, *Phaseolus* beans, etc).

GL-TTP (Grain Legumes Technology Transfer Platform) is a not-for-profit organisation set up in 2005 to bridge the gap between the research and industry in order to increase the production and quality of grain legumes worldwide.

GLIP (Grain Legumes Integrated Project: New strategies to improve grain legumes for food and feed, 2004–2008) investigates the genetics and biology of legume crops, because these N-fixing plants are under-used in Europe in spite of the fact that they are an ecological source of nitrogen for sustainable agricultural systems.

Past

LINK *Legume Interactive Network* (Concerted Action FAIR-CT-98-3923)

A multidisciplinary scientific network for the benefit of grain legume integrated chain to meet the protein demand of the European end-use industry.

Coordinators: Frédéric Muel, Anne Schneider

PROFETAS

Protein foods, environment, technology and society.

Coordinators: T. van Boekel, H. Verbruggen.

Exploitation of the unique genetic variability of peas in the production of food and non-food ingredients.

Coordinator: H.C. Langelaan.

EFPN

The European field pea network (past)

AMINOPIG

Amino acid true availability in pig.

Coordinator: B. Seve

With the following outline and main objectives:

* to improve scientific knowledge of protein utilisation in pigs;
* to understand better amino acid digestibility, effect of dietary factors on endogenous amino acid losses, metabolic expense for endogenous losses, etc.

PRELEG

Pathogen-resistant grain legumes using gene transfer methods.

Coordinator: G. Ramsay

With the following outline and main objectives:

* selected methods for transformation of grain legumes are developed for routine use to permit the regeneration of the numbers of transformants required;
* effects of each type of gene on selected major pathogens of grain legumes in vivo are explored, using ELISA quantification of pathogen multiplication.

CABINET

Carbohydrate biotechnology network for grain legumes.

Coordinator: C. Hedley

With the following outline and main objective:

* Multidisciplinary approach on legume carbohydrates.

LUPINE
Creation of varieties and technologies for increasing production and utilisation of high quality proteins from white lupin in Europe.
Coordinator: C. Huyghe
With the following outline and main objectives:

- to provide improved genotypes of winter type and determinated lupins;
- to improve cropping management techniques;
- to introduce new technologies (physical and enzymatic treatments) to enhance the use value.

NUTRIPEA. New technologies for improved nutritional and functional value of pea protein.
Coordinator: A.-S. Sandberg
With the following outline and main objectives:

- to use new technologies to develop improved pea protein products that are devoid of anti-physiological and anti-nutritional factors;
- to design and develop a technical process to prepare improved pea protein products under pilot plant and factory conditions;
- to evaluate the functional and sensory properties of improved pea protein products added to a variety of foods for human consumption;
- to screen *in vitro* and in animal models the nutritional properties and antigenicity of the protein products;
- to develop an infant formula based on the improved pea protein products.

UNCLE
Understanding nitrogen and carbohydrate metabolism for legume engineering.
Coordinator: U. Wobus
With the following outline and main objectives:

- to analyse the capacity of selected legume seeds (pea and faba bean) to accumulate storage products (seed sink capacity);
- to analyse the relationship between carbohydrate and storage protein/nitrogen metabolism at the level of gene expression;
- to isolate promoters for temporally and spatially regulated gene expression in seeds;
- to use these promoters, in combination with existing and new gene sequences, to specifically change sink capacity and/or storage product composition in legume seeds, as a prerequisite for quality improvement and engineering into seeds of exogenous high-added-value components.

TRANSLEG
Coordination of a joint approach on grain legume transformation (methods and objectives) to develop commercial applications.
Coordinator: H.-J. Jacobsen
With the following outline and main objectives:

- to establish a network of experts in the European Union sharing the know-how of grain legume transformation;
- to coordinate a ring test to define a widely applicable transformation protocol, to discuss with end-users, such as commercial breeders, about their needs, constraints and priorities regarding commercial applications of transgenic grain legumes;
- to prepare joint research projects on several specific gene transfers.

Increased utilisation of peas in food and feed products by improvement of the protein quality by enzymatic modification.
Coordinator: L. Sijtsma
With the following outline and main objectives:

- improved utilisation of pea proteins;
- improvement of the quality of pea protein;
- design of a model for quality prediction.

EUROPROTEINS 93–96
Development of plant protein-rich products by plant breeding and biotechnology for application in human and animal nutrition.
Coordinator: K. Cherriere
With the following outline and main objectives:

- ruminants: to optimise technological treatments to protect proteins against excessive degradation in the rumen;
- poultry: to determine physical and biological criteria responsible for potential decrease in egg weight and of punctual occurrence in dirty eggs.

Special reports
Give peas a chance – ecoenvironmental analysis in GLIP.
    Echos from Lisboa 2007. European Conference – Grain Legumes. The first outputs from GLIP.

Books
Recent Advances of Research in Antinutritional Factors in Legumes Seeds and Oilseeds, EAAP Scientific Series No 10, Wageningen Academic Publishers 2004.
    Pulses and Human Health. *British Journal of Nutrition*, Volume 88, suppl 3 (December 2002).
    Functional Potential of Legume Proteins. Proceedings of the LINK workshop (Kleinmachnow, 7/8 December 2000). Nahrung/Food Volume 45, No 6 (Wiley-VHC Editor, Germany).

15.9   References

1 Zohary, D. and Hopf, M. (1973) 'Domestication of pulses in the old world', *Science*, **182**, 887–94.

2 Bressani, R. and Elias, L.G. (1974) 'Legumes foods'. In A.M. Altschul (ed.), *New Protein Foods*, pp. 230–97, New York, Academic Press.

3 Linnemann A.R., and Swaving Dijkstra D. (2002) 'Towards sustainable production of protein-rich foods: Aprisal of eight crops for Western Europe. PART I. Analysis of the primary links of the production chain', *Critical Reviews in Food Science and Nutrition*, **42**(4): 377–401.

4 Swaving Dijkstra D., Linnemann A.R., and Van Boekel T.A.J.S. (2003) 'Towards sustainable production of protein-rich foods: Appraisal of eight european crops for Western Europe. PART II: Analysis of the technological aspects of the production chain', *Critical Reviews in Food Science and Nutrition*, **43**(5), 481–506.

5 Makri E., Papalamprou E., and Doxastakis G. (2005) 'Study of functional properties of seed storage proteins from indigenous European legume crops (lupin, pea, broad bean) in admixture with polysaccharides', *Food Hydrocolloids*, **19**: 583–94.

6 Adsule, R.N., Lawande, K.M. and Kadam, S.S. (1989) 'Pea'. In D.K. Salunkhe and S.S. Kadam (eds), *Handbook of World Food Legumes: Nutritional Chemistry, Processing Technology, and Utilization*, pp. 215–51, Boca Raton, FL, CRC Press, 1989.

7 Kadam, S.S., Desphande, S.S. and Jambhale, N.D. (1989) 'Seed structure and composition'. In D.K. Salunkhe and S.S. Kadam (eds), *Handbook of World Food Legumes: Nutritional Chemistry, Processing Technology, and Utilization*, pp. 23–50, Boca Raton, FL, CRC Press.

8 Owusu-Ansah Y.J., and McCurdy S.M. (1991) 'Pea proteins: A review of chemistry, technology of production, and utilization', *Food Rev Int*, **7**, 103–34.

9 Kuo, T.M., Van Middlesworth, J.F. and Wolf, W.J. (1988) Content of raffinose oligosaccharides and sucrose in various plant seeds, *J Agric Food Chem*, **36**, 32–6.

10 Salunkhe, D.K., Sathe, S.K. and Reddy, N.R. (1989) 'Lipids'. In D.K. Salunkhe and S.S. Kadam (eds), *Handbook of World Food Legumes: Nutritional Chemistry, Processing Technology and Utilization*, pp. 99–116, Boca Raton, FL, CRC Press.

11 Jenkins, D.J.A., Wolever, T.M.S., Taylor, R.H., Barker, H.M. and Fielden, M. (1980) Exceptionally low blood glucose response to dried beans: comparison with other carbohydate foods, *Br Med J*, **281**, 578–80.

12 Jenkins, D.J.A., Wolever, T.M.S., Jenkins, A.L. *et al.* (1983) 'The glycaemic index of foods tested in diabetic patients: a new basis for carbohydrate exchange favouring the use of legumes', *Diabetologia*, **24**, 257–64.

13 Wörsch, P., Del Vedovo, S. and Koellreuter, B. (1986) 'Cell structure and starch nature as key determinants of the digestion rate of starch in legumes', *Am J Clin Nutr*, **43**, 25–9.

14 Englyst, H.N. and Cummings, J.H. (1990) 'Non-starch polysaccharides (dietary fiber) and resistant starch'. In I. Furda and C. Brine (eds), *New Developments in Dietary Fiber*, pp. 205–25, New York, Plenum Press.

15 Björck, I. (1996) 'Starch: nutritional aspects'. In A.-C. Eliasson (ed.), *Carbohydrates in Food*, pp. 505–53, New York, Marcel Dekker.

16 Tovar, J., Björck, I.M. and Asp, N.-G. (1990) 'Starch content and alfa-amylosis rate in precooked legume flours', *J Agric Food Chem*, **38**, 1818–23.

17 Ducimetiere, P., Eschwege, E., Papoz, L., Richard, J.L., Claude, J.R. and Rosselin, G. (1980) 'Relationship of plasma insulin levels to the incidence of myocardial infarction and coronary heart disease mortality in a middle-aged population', *Diabetologia*, **19**, 205–10.

18 Wylie-Rosett, J. and Riflein, H. (1985) 'The history of nutrition and diabetes'. In L. Jovanovic and C.M. Peterson (eds), *Nutrition and Diabetes*, pp. 1–13, New York, Alan R. Liss Inc.

19 Venn B.J., and Mann J.I. (2004) 'Cereal grains, legumes and diabetes', *European Journal of Clinical Nutrition*, **58**, 1443–61.

20 Schakel, S., Sievert, Y. and Buzzard, I. (1992) 'Dietary fiber values for common foods'. In G. Spiller (ed.), *Handbook of Dietary Fiber in Human Nutrition*, 2nd edn, Boca Raton, FL, CRC Press, 1992.

21 Selvendran, R.R., Stevens, B.J.H. and Dupont, M.S. (1987) 'Dietary fiber: chemistry, analysis and properties', *Adv Food Res*, **31**, 117–209.

22 Sandberg, A.-S., Ahderinne, R., Andersson, H., Hallgren, B. and Hultén, L. (1983) 'The effect of citrus pectin on the absorption of nutrients in the small intestine', *Hum Nutr: Clin Nutr*, **37C**, 171–83.

23 Bosaeus, I., Andersson, H., Carlsson, N.-G. and Sandberg, A.-S. (1986) 'Effect of wheat bran and pectin on bile salt excretion in ileostomy patients', *Hum Nutr: Clin Nutr*, **40C**, 429–40.

24 Jenkins, D., Wolever, T., Rao, V. *et al.* (1993) 'Effect on blood lipids of very high intakes of fiber in diets low in saturated fat and cholesterol', *N Engl J Med*, **329**, 21–6.

25 Truswell, A.S. and Beynen, A.C. (1992) 'Dietary fibre and plasma lipids: potential for prevention and treatment of hyperlipidaemias'. In T.F. Schweizer and C.A. Edwards (eds), *Dietary Fibre – A Component of Food: Nutritional Function in Health and Disease*, pp. 295–332, London, Springer-Verlag.

26 Jenkins, D., Wolever, T. Collier, G. *et al.* (1987) 'Metabolic effects of a low-glycemic-index diet', *Am J Clin Nutr*, **46**, 968–75.

27 Sandström, B., Trond Hansen, L. and Sörensen, A. (1994) 'Pea fiber lowers fasting and postprandial blood triglyceride concentrations in humans', *J Nutr*, **124**, 2386–96.

28 Liener, I. (1989) 'Control of antinutritional and toxic factors in oilseeds and legumes'. In E. Lusas, D. Erickson and W. Nip (eds), *Food Uses of Whole Oil and Protein Seeds*, pp. 344–71, Champaign, American Oil Chemists' Society.

29 Pusztai, A., Ewen, S., Grant, G. *et al.* (1990) 'Relationship between survival and binding of plant lectins during small intestinal passage and their effectiveness as growth factors', *Digestion*, **46** (Supp. 2), 308–16.

30 Jindahl, S., Soni, G. and Singh, R. (1984) 'Biochemical and histopathological studies in albino rats fed on soybean lectin', *Nutr Rep Int*, **29**, 95–106.

31 Ishiguro, M., Nakashima, H., Tanabe, S. and Sakakibara, R. (1992) 'Interaction of toxic lectin with epithelial cells of rat small intestine in vitro', *Chem Pharm Bull Tokyo*, **40**, 441–5.

32 Sandberg A-S. (2002) 'Bioavailability of minerals in legumes', *Brit J Nutr*, **88**(Suppl 3), S281–85.

33 Rossander-Hulthén, L., Sandberg, A.-S. and Sandström, B. (1992) 'The effect of dietary fibre on mineral absorption and utilization'. In T. Schweizer and C.A. Edwards (eds), *Dietary Fibre – A Component of Food: Nutritional Function in Health and Disease*, pp. 197–216, London, Springer-Verlag.

34 Price, K. and Fenwick, G. (1984) 'Soyasaponin I, a compound possessing undesirable taste characteristics isolated from the dried pea (Pisum sativum L.)', *J Sci Food Agric*, **35**, 887–92.

35 Gueguen, J. (1980) 'Solubility of faba bean (Vicia faba L) and pea (Pisum sativum L.)', *Lebensm Wiss u Technol*, **13**, 156–63.

36 Zeiger, R.S., Sampson, H., Bock, S. *et al.* (1999) 'Soy allergy in infants and children with IgE-associated cow's milk allergy', *J Pediatr*, **134**, 614–22.

37 Aluko R.E. (2008) 'Determination of nutritional and bioactive properties of peptides in enzymatic pea, chickpea, and mung bean protein hydrolysates', *J AOAC Int*, **91**, 947–56.

38 James, K. and Hove, E. (1980) 'The ineffectiveness of supplementary cystine in legume-based rat diets', *J Nutr*, **110**, 1736–44.

39 Deo, S., Savage, G. and Jermyn, W. (1986) 'The effect of cooking on the nutritional quality of New Zealand grown peas', International Food Legume Research Conference on Pea, Lentil, Faba Bean and Chickpea, Washington, DC, Spokane.

40 Griffiths, D. (1984) 'The trypsin and chymotrypsin inhibitor activities of various pea (Pisum spp.) and field bean (Vicia faba) cultivars', *J Sci Food Agr*, **35**, 481–6.

41 Tannous, R. and Ullah, M. (1969) 'Effects of autoclaving on nutritional factors in legume seeds', *Trop Agric*, **46**, 123–9.

42 Bender, A. (1983) 'Haemagglutinins (lectins) in beans', *Food Chem*, **11**, 309–20.
43 Sandberg, A.-S. (1991) 'The effect of food processing on phytate hydrolysis and availability of iron and zinc. Nutritional and Toxicological Consequences of Food Processing. AIN Symposium, Washington 1990', *Adv Exp Med Biol*, **289**, 499–508.
44 Hurrell, R., Juillerat, M.-A., Reddy, M., Lynch, S., Dassenko, S. and Cook, J. (1992) 'Soy protein, phytate, and iron absorption in humans', *Am J Clin Nutr*, **56**, 573–8.
45 Brune, M., Rossander-Hulthén, L., Hallberg, L., Gleerup, A., Sandberg, A.-S. (1992) 'Human iron absorption from bread: inhibiting effects of cereal fiber, phytate and inositol phosphates with different numbers of phosphate groups', *J Nutr*, **122**, 442–9.
46 Nassar A.G., Murabak A.E., and El-Betagy A.E. (2008) 'Nutritional potential and functional properties of tempe produced from mixtures of different legumes. 1: Chemical composition an nitrogenous constituent', *Int J Food Sci Technol*, **43**(10), 1754–58.
47 Barkholt, V., Jörgensen, P., Sörensen, D. *et al.* (1998) 'Protein modification by fermentation: effect of fermentation on the potential allergenicity of pea', *Allergy*, **53**, 106–8.
48 Johnson, I., Gee, J., Price, K., Curl, C., Fenwick, G. (1986) 'Influence of saponins on gut permeability and active nutrient transport in vitro', *J Nutr*, **116**, 2270–7.
49 Gee, J., Price, K., Ridout, C., Wortley, G., Hurrell, R. and Johnson, I. (1993) 'Saponins of quinoa (Chenopodium quinoia): effects of processing on their abundance in quinoa products and their biological effects on intestinal mucosal tissue', *J Sci Food Agric*, **63**, 201–9.
50 Vose, J., Basterrechea, M., Gorin, P., Finlayson, A. and Youngs, C. (1976) 'Air classification of field peas and horsebean flours: chemical studies of starch and protein fractions', *Cereal Chem*, **53**, 928–36.
51 Reichert, R.D. and Youngs, C.G. (1978) 'Nature of the residual protein associated with starch fractions from air-classified field peas', *Cereal Chem*, **55**, 469–80.
52 Tyler, R.T., Youngs, C.G. and Sosulski, F.W. (1981) 'Air classification of legumes. I. Separation efficiency yield, and composition of the starch and protein fractions', *Cereal Chem*, **58**, 144–8.
53 Reichert, R.D. (1982) 'Air classification of peas (Pisum sativum) varying widely in protein content', *J Food Sci*, **47**, 1263–7.
54 Vose, J.R. (1980) 'Production and functionality of starches and protein isolates from legume seeds (field peas and horse beans)', *Cereal Chem*, **57**, 406–10.
55 Gueguen, J. (1983) 'Legume seed protein extraction, processing, and end-product characteristics'. In C.E. Bodwell and L. Petiti (eds), *Plant Proteins for Human Food*, p. 267–303, The Hague, Martinus Nijhoff/Dr W. Junk.
56 Lee J., Lee H., and Lee C. (2001) 'Characterization of hydrolysates produced by mild acid treatment and enzymatic hydrolysis of defatted soybean flour', *Food Res Int*, **34**, 217–22.
57 Humiski L.M., and Aluko R.E. (2007) 'Physiochemical and bitterness properties of enzymatic pea protein hydrolysates', *J Food Sci*, **72**(8), S605–11.
58 Fleming, S.E. and Sosulski, F.W. (1977) 'Nutritive value of bread fortified with concentrated plant proteins and lysine', *Cereal Chem*, **54**, 1238–48.
59 Fleming, S.E. and Sosulski, F.W. (1977) 'Breadmaking properties of four concentrated plant proteins', *Cereal Chem*, **54**, 1124–40.
60 Jeffers, H.C., Rubenthaler, G.L., Finney, P.L., Anderson, P.D. and Bruinsma, B.L. (1978) 'Pea: a highly functional fortifier in wheat flour blends', *Bakers Dig*, **52**, 36.
61 Sosulski, F.W. and Fleming, S.E. (1979) 'Sensory evaluation of bread prepared from composite flours', *Bakers Dig*, **53**, 20–5.
62 Nielsen, M.A., Sumner, A.K. and Whalley, L.L. (1980) 'Fortification of pasta with pea flour and air-classified pea protein concentrate', *Cereal Chem*, **57**, 203–6.
63 EU, New Technologies for Improved Nutritional and Functional Value of Pea Protein: FAIR CT 95-0193, NUTRIPEA C1004-95, Report 1999.

64 Watters, K.H. and Heaton, R.K. (1979) 'Quality characteristics of ground beef patties extended with moist-heated and unheated seed meals', *J Am Oil Chem Soc*, **56**, A86–90.

65 Patel, P.R., Youngs, C.G. and Grant, D.R. (1981) 'Preparation and properties of spray-dried pea protein concentrate-cheese whey blends', *Cereal Chem*, **58**, 249–55.

66 Sosulski, F.W. Chakraborty, P. and Humbert, E.S. (1978) 'Legume-based imitation and blended milk products', *Can Inst Food Sci Technol J*, **3**, 117–23.

67 Dulau, I. and Thebaudin, J.-Y. (1998) 'Functional properties of leguminous protein: applications in food', *Grain Legumes*, **20**, 15–1.

68 Fredrikson, M., Biot, P., Carlsson, N.-G., Alminger-Larsson, M. and Sandberg, A.-S. (2001) 'Production of high quality pea protein isolate, with low content of oligosaccharides and phytate', *J Agric Food Chem*, **49**, 1208–12.

69 Sörensen, A.D., Hansen, A.B., Sörensen, S., Barkholt, V. and Frökier, H. (1998) 'Influence of industrial processing of peas on the content of antinutritional factors and the in vitro digestibility', 3rd European Conference on Grain Legumes, Valladolid, pp. 348–9.

70 Fredrikson, M., Alminger-Larsson, M., Sandberg, A.-S. (2001) 'Phytate content and phytate degradation by endogenous phytase in pea (*Pisum sativum*)', *J Sci Food Agric*, **81**, 1139–44.

71 Hallberg, L., Brune, M. and Rossander, L. (1989) 'Iron absorption in man: ascorbic acid and dose-dependent inhibition by phytate', *Am J Clin Nutr*, **49**, 140–4.

72 Fredrikson, M. (2001) Pea-Protein Products for Food Applications. Methods for improving iron and zinc availability. PhD Thesis. Chalmers University of Technology, Gothenburg, Sweden, pp. 38.

73 Sandberg A-S. (2005) 'Methods and options for in vitro dialyzability; benefits and limitations', *Int J Vit Nutr Res*, **75**, 395–404.

74 Davidsson, L., Dimitriou, T., Walczyk, T. and Hurrell, R.F. (2001) 'Iron absorption from experimental infant formulas based on pea (*Pisum sativum*) protein isolate: the effect of phytic acid and ascorbic acid', *Br J Nutr*, **85**, 59.

75 Herian, A.M., Taylor, S.L. and Bush, R.K. (1993) 'Allergenic reactivity of various soybean products as determined by RAST inhibition', *J Food Sci*, **58**, 385–8.

76 Fredrikson M., Andlid T., Haikara A., and Sandberg A-S. (2002) 'Phytate degradation by microorganisms in synthetic media and pea flour', *J Appl Microbiol*, **93**, 197–204.

16

Functional fats and spreads

A. Turpeinen and P. Merimaa, Valio Ltd, Finland

Abstract: Fats and spreads are consumed daily by most people, thereby providing a good platform for functional ingredients. Products with modified fat content and composition have been available for several decades. During the last two decades, novel technologies have allowed incorporation of a variety of fat-soluble as well as water-soluble functional components into fats and spreads. This chapter gives an overview of some functional ingredients used in these products today: phytosterols, antioxidants, minerals, probiotics and milk peptides.

Key words: fats, spreads, fatty acids, phytosterols, antioxidants, interesterification.

16.1 Introduction

About one-third of the calories consumed by most people in Western countries are provided by fat. In addition to being a concentrated source of energy, fats and spreads contain a variety of compounds with health effects, e.g. specific fatty acids and vitamins. As spreads are consumed daily by most people, they are a good platform for functional ingredients. New technologies allow incorporation of functional components into a wide variety of products.

Replacement of saturated with unsaturated fatty acids has been recommended since the 1950s, which led to the development of spreads containing vegetable oils. Reduced fat spreads were introduced in the late 1960s. As lowering fat intake has been a general trend, reduced fat products have become popular and at present, the fat content in spreads ranges from nearly no fat to 80% fat spreads. During the last two decades, new fat-soluble as well as water-soluble functional ingredients have been added to fats and spreads. This chapter gives an overview of some functional ingredients used in these products today: phytosterols, antioxidants, minerals, probiotics and milk peptides.

16.2   EU legislation on fats and spreads

In Europe, the legislation of foodstuffs is regulated by the European Community with the intention to harmonize rules and regulations throughout all its member states.

Regarding fats and spreads, the main issues are permitted additives, composition, fat content, claims and labelling without forgetting hygiene requirements and contaminants.

Council Regulation (EC) 1234/2007 of 1994 and Comission Regulation (EC) No 445/2007 lay down standards for spreadable fats including functional fats and spreads. They specify fat into different categories: butter, margarines and blends. Spreadable fats are standardized and classified according to their fat content and origin (dairy/non-dairy, vegetable/animal) (Table 16.1). Spreadable fats are products with a fat content of at least 10% but less than 90% by weight and which remain solid at room temperature. Products are mainly water-in-oil emulsions.

The nutrition and health regulation defines the conditions on which foodstuffs may be promoted with nutrition and health claims approved by European Food Safety Authority (EFSA) and determines common rules and approval procedures for the use of claims in all EU countries. Claims used on the labelling, presentation and advertising are regulated by Regulation (EC) 1924/2006 of the European Parliament and the Council, which entered into force on 1 July 2007. An amendment to the previous, Commission Regulation (EU) No 116/2010 of 9 February 2010, includes conditions of use for nutrition claims 'source of' and 'high in' for omega-3 fatty acids, monounsaturated and polyunsaturated fatty acids. It is possible to use the claim 'source of omega-3 fatty acids' if the product contains at least 0.3 g α-linolenic acid per 100 g and per 100 kcal, or at least 40 mg of the sum of eicosapentaenoic acid and docosahexaenoic acid per 100 g and per 100 kcal. The claim 'high omega-3 fatty acids' can be used if the product contains at least 0.6 g α-linolenic acid per 100 g and per 100 kcal, or at least 80 mg of the sum of eicosapentaenoic acid and docosahexaenoic acid per 100 g and per 100 kcal.

The claim 'high monounsaturated fat' may be made where at least 45% of the fatty acids present in the product derive from monounsaturated fat under the

Table 16.1   Classification of spreadable fats

Fat % in product	Butter 100% milk fat	Margarine <3% milk fat	Blend 10–80% milk fat
$80 \leq x < 90$	Butter	Margarine	Blend
$62 < x < 80$	Dairy spread x%	Fat spread x%	Blended spread x%
$60 \leq x \leq 62$	Three-quarter fat butter (butter 60)	Three-quarter fat margarine (margarine 60)	Three-quarter fat blend (fat blend 60)
$41 < x < 60$	Dairy spread x%	Fat spread x%	Blended spread x%
$39 \leq x \leq 41$	Half-fat butter (butter 40)	Half-fat margarine (margarine 40)	Half-fat blend (fat blend 40)
$10 \leq x < 39$	Dairy spread x%	Fat spread x%	Blended spread x%

condition that monounsaturated fat provides more than 20% of energy of the product. The claim 'high polyunsaturated fat' can be used when at least 45% of the fatty acids present in the product derive from polyunsaturated fat under the condition that polyunsaturated fat provides more than 20% of energy of the product. The claim 'high unsaturated fat' may only be made where unsaturated fat provides at least 70% of the fatty acids present in the product.

The European Commission has published a guidance document for the interpretation of the implementation of the claim regulation in order to facilitate practical work. The most important point is that claims cannot be used until the generally accepted scientific evidence for the claim has been approved. The health claims made on foodstuffs as well as certain nutrition labelling will be affected by the Regulation. Nutrition claims shall only be permitted if they are listed in the Annex to the Regulation and are in conformity with the conditions set out in the Regulation.

16.3   Functional ingredients and chronic diseases: applications in fats and spreads

Many ingredients which can be incorporated into fats and spreads have been shown to beneficially affect risk factors of chronic diseases. Table 16.2 summarizes the present evidence on fatty acids, minerals, antioxidants, phytosterols, probiotics and milk peptides, which is described in more detail in the following sections.

Table 16.2   Food components with proposed beneficial effects on risk factors of chronic diseases

Food component	Effect on risk factors of diseases
Fatty acids	
Linoleic acid	Total and LDL cholesterol ⇊
Conjugated linoleic acid	Body fat mass ⇊
α-Linolenic acid	Total and LDL cholesterol ⇊
n-3 fatty acids	Triglycerides ⇊, heart arrhythmias ⇊, blood pressure ⇊
Medium-chain triglycerides	Body fat mass ⇊
Antioxidants	
Vitamin E	Radical scavenging ⇊, lipid peroxidation ⇊
Vitamin A	Radical scavenging ⇊
Polyphenols	Oxidized LDL ⇊, inflammation ⇊, endothelial function ⇑
Phytosterols	Total and LDL cholesterol ⇊
Probiotics	Antibody formation ⇑
Milk peptides	Blood pressure ⇊
Minerals	Blood pressure ⇊, bone mass (calcium) ⇑

⇊ = reduced; ⇑ = increased.

16.3.1   Fatty acids

Fats are a complex mixture of different fatty acids and coexistence of certain fatty acids is typical, thus making it difficult to identify the physiological effects of individual fatty acids. Synthetic pure fatty acids have enabled studying specific fatty acids. The following chapter presents an overview of effects of certain functional fatty acids.

Linoleic acid

Mammals lack delta-12 dehydrogenase and thus the ability to introduce double bonds in fatty acids beyond carbons 9 and 10. Linoleic acid (LA, C18:2 n-6) was identified as an essential fatty acid for humans in the late 1920s (Burr & Burr 1930). Linoleic acid is essential for growth and development, specifically in skin cell membranes. Deficiency has been reported both in premature infants as well as in patients on parenteral feeding and is associated with a variety of metabolic disturbances, dry skin, hair loss and poor wound healing.

Linoleic acid intake between 1 and 2% of energy (en%) prevents deficiency symptoms (Holman 1970) and a dietary intake of 2en% is generally seen as adequate for healthy adults. A higher intake has been proposed based on the hypocholesterolemic effects of LA. Hegstedt *et al.* (1965) published the first equation on the effects of different dietary fatty acids on plasma cholesterol indicating that replacing saturated fatty acids with n-6 PUFA is the most efficient way to decrease total and low-density lipoprotein (LDL) cholesterol. Replacing 1en% saturated fatty acids with polyunsaturated fatty acids decreases total cholesterol by 0.08 mmol/l. A meta-analysis of randomized controlled trials indicated a 10% decrease in coronary heart disease (CHD) risk for a 5en% increase in polyunsaturated fat intake (mainly LA) when replacing saturated fat (Mozaffarian *et al.* 2010).

Yet, there may be disadvantages associated with high LA intake. High LA concentrations may increase the risk of lipid peroxidation (Alexander-North *et al.* 1994). Also, due to competition of n-3 and n-6 fatty acids, increased n-6 polyunsaturated fatty acid (PUFA) intake reduces the incorporation of n-3 PUFA into tissues. As LA is metabolized to arachidonic acid, a precursor for proinflammatory prostanoids, a high LA intake may induce proinflammatory responses. Thus far, an upper limit for LA intake has not been recommended.

The effects of a high LA diet may be partially compensated by increasing intake of n-3 fatty acids. Much discussion has been on the optimal dietary n-6/n-3 ratio. Several national and international agencies have not been able to define an optimal ratio. A ratio of 5:1 has been proposed by the British Nutrition Task Force (1992) and a 5:1–10:1 ratio by the FAO/WHO Expert Committee (1994).

Safflower (78% of fatty acids LA), sunflower (68% LA) and corn oil (59% LA) are rich sources of LA. These oils are widely used in spreads and have increased the intake of n-6 PUFA in western countries.

Alpha-linolenic acid

Alpha-linolenic acid (ALA, C18:3 n-3) cannot be synthesized from saturated fatty acids or converted from n-6 unsaturated fatty acids in humans. A matter of discussion has been whether ALA is essential by itself or due to the fact that it is the precursor for longer-chain n-3 fatty acids eicosapentaenoic acid (EPA) and docosaheaxenoic acid (DHA). Animal experiments have shown that deficiency of ALA results in visual impairment, impaired learning ability and behaviour changes. Also case reports in humans have reported neurological symptoms caused by ALA deficiency in subjects with parenteral nutrition (Bjerve *et al.* 1987; Holman *et al.* 1982).

A 1,4-3 g/day ALA intake has been proposed by various international bodies (see Gebauer *et al.* 2006). Several epidemiological and intervention studies suggest that a high ALA intake may reduce risk of coronary artery disease (Dolecek 1992; de Lorgeril *et al.* 1994; Ascherio *et al.* 1996; Hu *et al.* 1999). In the Health Professionals Follow-Up Study, a 1% increase in ALA intake was associated with a 39% reduction in the risk of myocardial infarction (Ascherio *et al.* 1996). ALA also lowers LDL and total cholesterol – in some studies as efficiently as LA (Chan *et al.* 1991; Valsta *et al.* 1995).

Conversion of ALA to EPA has been estimated to be on average 1% in infants and lower in adults (Brenna *et al.* 2009). In most studies, supplementation with ALA increases EPA levels, but has little effect on plasma DHA concentrations (see Brenna *et al.* 2009). A high dietary LA/ALA ratio decreases the conversion of ALA. Thus, the most effective way to increase conversion efficiency would be a decrease in LA intake and an increase in ALA intake. LA intake greatly exceeds that of ALA in western diets, a typical ratio being from 5:1 to 20:1.

Seed oils are best sources of ALA, especially perilla (58% ALA), linseed (flax seed; 55% ALA), sea buckthorn (32%), rapeseed (canola; 10%) and soybean oils (8%). Spreads containing these oils have a lower n-6:n-3 fatty acid ratio than those based on other vegetable oils.

Trans fatty acids
Trans fatty acids (TFAs) are unsaturated fatty acids that contain at least one double bond in the trans position. Compared to the more typical cis position, the altered configuration affects the chemical and functional properties of the fatty acid. Trans fatty acids have a higher melting point and a more rigid structure than other unsaturated fatty acids. They resemble saturated fatty acids and have traditionally been widely used in manufacturing margarines, bakery products and fried foods, in which semi-solid or solid fat is required. During industrial hydrogenation, trans double bonds are formed in different positions along the fatty acid carbon chain depending on hydrogenation conditions. Typically trans-10 isomers are most abundant.

In addition to hydrogenated oils, dairy products are a dietary source of trans fatty acids. Ruminant fat contains on average 1–3% trans fatty acids, which originate from the action of ruminant bacteria on feed unsaturated fatty acids. The isomeric composition of ruminant trans fatty acids differs from that of industrially hydrogenated fat with vaccenic acid (C18:1 trans-11) predominating.

During the last decade, the health effects of trans fatty acids have been widely studied. Epidemiological studies have reported positive associations between trans fatty acid intake and incidence of coronary heart disease (Mozaffarian *et al.* 2006). In studies which have analysed intake of industrial and ruminant trans fatty acids separately, a clear association has been shown for industrial trans fatty acids, but not for ruminant fat (Willett *et al.* 1993; Pietinen *et al.* 1997).

There is consistent evidence from intervention studies that trans fatty acids negatively affect blood lipids. Industrial trans fatty acids increase LDL cholesterol to a similar degree as saturated fatty acids and also lower high-density lipoprotein (HDL) cholesterol, thus having a more adverse effect than saturated fat (Mozaffarian & Clarke 2009). Proinflammatory effects and endothelial dysfunction have also been reported both in observational and intervention studies (Baer *et al.* 2004; Lopez-Garcia *et al.* 2005). Trans fatty acid intake has also been associated with increased risk of sudden cardiac death and diabetes (Hu *et al.* 2001; Lemaitre *et al.* 2002).

Typical dietary intake of TFA ranges from 1–3 g/day, while in some subgroups consumption may be up to 20 g/day, mainly from industrial sources. As the risk of CHD death has been estimated to increase by 20%, 27% and 32% for a 2en% replacement of saturated, cis-monounsaturated and polyunsaturated fatty acids with trans fatty acids (Mozaffarian *et al.* 2009), efforts to reduce the intake of industrial trans fatty acids have been introduced in several countries. In Denmark, legislation limiting TFA content of foods to 2% of fatty acids came into force in 2003. Inclusion of trans fatty acid on food labels was introduced in the US in 2003 and Canada in 2005. Many US cities have banned use of TFA-containing oils in restaurants. In most European countries, the TFA content of margarines, bakery products and fried foods has markedly decreased during the last decade due to replacement of partial hydrogenation with other hardening methods, e.g. interesterification.

Conjugated linoleic acid
Conjugated linoleic acid (CLA) is a collective term for a group of positional and geometric isomers of linoleic acid (C18:2 n-6) containing conjugated double bonds. The main natural CLA isomer, found in ruminant fat and dairy products, is cis-9, trans-11 CLA. Dietary intake of CLA has been estimated to be a few hundred milligrams (Ritzenthaler *et al.* 2001). CLA is also endogenously formed from trans-vaccenic acid (C18:1 trans-11) in the rumen (Griinari *et al.* 2000) as well as in humans (Turpeinen *et al.* 2002).

Interest in CLA initiated in 1979, when a study by Pariza *et al.* (1979) was published reporting an antimutagenic compound in ground beef. The compound was identified as a conjugated derivative of LA. Thereafter, the anticarcinogenic effects of CLA have been studied in various cancer modes. Most evidence of protective effects exists from rat breast cancer models. CLA decreased the size and incidence of mammary tumors dose-dependently up to 1% (Ip *et al.* 1991) and regardless of the level or type of fat in the diet (Ip *et al.* 1996).

Of the various CLA isomers, thus far the physiological effects of cis-9, trans-11 CLA and trans-10, cis-12 isomers have been studied. In animal models, CLA has also been shown to have antiatherogenic (Nicolosi *et al.* 1997) and antidiabetic effects (Houseknecht *et al.* 1998) as well as effects on body composition (Park *et al.* 1997) and immune function (see O'Shea *et al.* 2004). In clinical studies, effects have generally been modest. In animals, CLA has reduced body fat mass up to 60% in mice (Park *et al.* 1997), while a meta-analysis of clinical studies reported a 0.09 kg/wk reduction in fat mass (Whigham *et al.* 2007). Beneficial effects on parameters of immune function have been reported, but results are controversial (see O'Shea *et al.* 2004). Hypocholesterolemic and antiatherogenic effects seen in rabbits (Lee *et al.* 1994) and hamsters (de Deckere *et al.* 1999) have not been detected in clinical studies (Naumann *et al.* 2006; Tricon *et al.* 2006). Studies in predisposed subjects suggest that the trans-10, cis-12 CLA isomer may induce oxidative stress and insulin resistance (Riserus *et al.* 2002). This isomer is present in synthetic CLA preparations, whereas only in small proportions in natural CLA.

Consumption of butter naturally enriched with CLA did not affect lipid responses or body composition in overweight subjects (Desroches *et al.* 2005). CLA-enriched food products have been introduced in some European countries, but no spread applications are on the market at present.

Long-chain n-3 fatty acids: eicosapentaenoic acid (EPA) and docosahexaenoic acid (DHA)

Eicosapentaenoic acid (EPA; C20:5 n-3) and docosahexaenoic acid (DHA; C22:6 n-3) are the most abundant fatty acids in the brain and the retina. They are essential for brain development and nervous function.

Mammals obtain DHA either directly from the diet or as the precursors ALA or EPA. Fish and sea foods are the richest sources of EPA and DHA, while vegetable fats and oils contain no EPA or DHA. Poultry and eggs contain low amounts, but may be important dietary sources of these fatty acids. Long-chain PUFA intake is highest in countries with high fish consumption, such as Japan, Norway and Iceland, while intake has been reported to be <200 mg/day, e.g. in the USA, France and Australia.

Extensive evidence indicates that LC n-3 PUFA are cardioprotective. Large prospective population studies and well-controlled case-control studies have shown LC n-3 PUFA intake to be associated with reduced risk of cardiovascular events or death from CHD (see Lee *et al.* 2008). Long-chain n-3 fatty acids decrease triglycerides, but have little effect on other lipoproteins. A number of other possible mechanisms have been proposed, including effects on blood pressure, blood clotting, heart arrhythmias and insulin resistance (see Calder 2004).

Governments as well as professional and public health organizations have recommended long-chain n-3 fatty acid intake 400–600 mg/d (ISSFAL 2004; National Health Council of the Netherlands 2006) or two fish meals/week (WHO/FAO 2003, Scientific Advisory Board on Nutrition 2004, Kris-Etherton *et al.* 2002), which equates to 400–500 mg EPA+DHA/day.

The main challenges related to enrichment of products with n-3 fatty acids are associated with sensory quality and shelf life. Microencapsulation, a process where microdroplets of oil are encapsulated, resolves most of the problems. Emulsification and chemical complexing with cyclodextrin are other methods used to stabilize n-3 long-chain PUFA. Currently, a variety of spreads as well as other products enriched with n-3 long-chain PUFA are available.

16.3.2   Medium-chain triglycerides

Medium-chain triglycerides (MCTs) are fatty acid esters of glycerol that contain 6–12 carbons. Coconut oil contains approximately 60–70% MCT. Palm kernel oil also is good source of MCT with approximately 2% C6, 55% C8, 42% C10 and 1% C12 fatty acids.

Traditionally, MCTs have been used in patients with malnutrition or malabsorption syndromes as they do not require energy for absorption, utilization or storage. More recently, the effects of MCTs on weight management have been studied. In several, but not all studies, beneficial effects of MCTs on weight control and body fat mass have been observed (see Marten *et al.* 2006). Glucose and postprandial lipid metabolism may also be affected (see Marten *et al.* 2006). Several studies indicate that moderate doses are better than excessive loads. It needs to be examined, which dose and food matrix offers most benefits, and whether naturally occurring medium chain fatty acids (MCFAs) and MCT oils have the same effect.

According to Marten *et al.* (2006), MCTs reduce fat mass by down-regulation of adipogenic genes as well as peroxisome proliferator activated receptor-gamma (PPAR-γ). Recent studies confirmed the potential of MCFAs to reduce body weight and particularly body fat. This effect was not transient. MCFAs reduce lipoprotein secretion and attenuate postprandial triglyceride response.

MTCs are used in oils, sport drinks, energy bars, meal replacements and also special baby foods. Prosperity Organic Foods has launched a healthy buttery spread in the United States with the claim 'boosts metabolism naturally'. The product is said to be particularly beneficial for hypothyroid sufferers, but should be of interest to all those concerned being overweight or obese.

16.3.3   Phytosterols

Phytosterols are components structurally related to cholesterol, but contain an extra ethyl or methyl group in the side chain. Phytosterols comprise plant sterols and stanols present in vegetable food sources, especially in vegetable oils, nuts and cereals. Sitosterol, campesterol and stigmasterol are the most abundant phytosterols in plants. Stanols, such as sitostanol and campestanol are saturated plant sterols. Phytosterols are not synthesized by the body, an estimated 200–300 mg phytosterols is obtained daily from the diet. Intestinal absorption of phytosterols is low: 0.4–3.5% of plant sterols and <0.5% of plant stanols are absorbed (Ostlund *et al.* 2002). Phytosterols inhibit cholesterol absorption by replacing dietary cholesterol in mixed micelles in the intestine, inhibit the reabsorption of cholesterol from bile acids and increase the activity of hepatic LDL receptors (Child & Kuskis 1986; Plat & Mensink 2002).

Plant sterols and stanols are equally effective in lowering cholesterol. The hypocholesterolemic effect has been demonstrated in tens of clinical studies. LDL cholesterol is reduced on average 5–15%, while HDL cholesterol and triglycerides generally remain unchanged. The effect is evident already at daily intakes of phytosterols <1 g (Hendriks *et al.* 1999). A meta-analysis of 84 clinical studies showed that a 2.15 g/day average intake of plant sterols incorporated into fat-based foods (margarine, butter, mayonnaise) or low-fat foods (milk, yoghurt) lowered LDL cholesterol by 8.8% (Demonty *et al.* 2009) The effect is dose-dependent up to 2 g/day (Demonty *et al.* 2009), with higher intakes providing little additional benefit. Effects have systematically been shown in both genders and in adults as well as children. The EU commission has approved the following health claim for both plant sterols and stanols: 'Plant sterols/stanols have been shown to reduce blood cholesterol. Blood cholesterol lowering may reduce the risk of coronary heart disease.'

Some studies have suggested that phytosterols decrease absorption of fat-soluble vitamins. Plasma concentrations of carotenoids and tocopherols, which are transported by LDL have been reduced, while concentrations of vitamin D or K, which are not transported by lipoproteins have not changed (Gylling *et al.* 1999; Plat & Mensink 2001). When carotenoid and tocopherol concentrations were adjusted for serum lipids, a statistically significant reduction remained for beta-carotene (Noakes *et al.* 2002). The decrease can be prevented by regular consumption of fruits and vegetables, a recommendation added to all products containing plant sterols. An upper limit of 3 g/day is recommended for phytosterols.

Phytosterols are incorporated into food products as esters as esterification of sitostanol and sitosterol was found to enhance their solubility. Phytosterols can also be dispersed in water after emulsification with lecithin. Plant stanol and sterol ester containing spreads were the first products introduced in the 1990s. At present, a wide range of products is available, ranging from fat-based to fat-free products, both solid and liquid.

16.3.4 Antioxidants

Antioxidants protect cells from free radical-induced cell damage, which may contribute to the development of chronic diseases. Antioxidants have been proposed to reduce the risk of cancer, cardiovascular diseases and inflammatory diseases, although results from intervention studies have been somewhat conflicting. The differences between epidemiological data and randomized studies with high supplementary doses of antioxidants may derive from assuming that the benefits of whole foods can be attributed to individual micronutrients (Kritharides & Stocker 2002). At present, a diet rich in antioxidants, but not antioxidant supplementation is recommended.

Vitamin E (tocopherols and tocotrienols) is a fat-soluble antioxidant that protects lipids from oxidation by reducing the production and scavenging reactive oxygen species. Vitamin E is also involved in immune function, cell signalling and regulation of gene expression. Observational studies suggest an inverse association between vitamin E intake and risk of CHD, whereas results from clinical trials are conflicting and in general, do not support the hypothesis that vitamin E supplementation would reduce CHD risk, morbidity or mortality (Kritharides & Stocker 2002). Inconsistent evidence exists also regarding vitamin E and cancer prevention as well as protection against age-related macular degeneration and cataract (Huang *et al.* 2006).

Free-radical damage may be involved in neurogenerative diseases such as Parkinson's and Alzheimer's disease. However, no conclusive evidence of protective effects of vitamin E on cognitive decline in normal ageing or in neurogenerative diseases has been obtained (Isaac *et al.* 2008).

The recommended daily intake of vitamin E for adults is 10 mg. Vegetable oils and spreads containing these oils as well as nuts and seeds are best dietary sources of vitamin E. Spreads with added vitamin E are also available in some countries.

Vitamin A (retinol and carotenoids) plays a role in vision, reproduction, bone growth and cell differentiation. Deficiency is common in developing countries causing blindness and impaired immune function in malnourished children.

Beta-carotene has anticarcinogenic properties in animal studies and epidemiological studies have shown an inverse association between beta-carotene or vitamin A intake and several cancers. Supplementation studies with beta-carotene have, however, not provided evidence of cancer prevention. In fact, beta-carotene supplementation increased lung cancer risk in two large intervention studies (Albanes *et al.* 1995; Redlich *et al.* 1998).

Typically, small amounts of beta-carotene are added to fats and spreads for colour. Vitamin A enriched spreads also exist and are marketed, for example, for maintaining good vision and healthy skin.

Polyphenols may affect several cardiovascular risk factors, e.g. oxidative stress, endothelial function and inflammation. Virgin olive oil is rich in polyphenols, which have been shown to be absorbed in a dose-dependent manner at moderate doses (Miró-Casas *et al.* 2003).

Olive oils with differing phenol content were fed to healthy subjects for three weeks. Linear increases in HDL cholesterol and decreases in oxidized LDL were observed in the low, medium and high phenol olive oil groups (Covas *et al.* 2006). Protective effects related with the phenolic content of the olive oil on circulating oxidized LDL and lipid peroxides were also seen in CHD patients (Fito *et al.* 2005) and on DNA oxidation in postmenopausal women (Salvini *et al.* 2006).

16.3.5 Minerals

Potassium, calcium and magnesium have beneficial effects on blood pressure, especially when combined with a low sodium content. According to a meta-analysis, 3 g/day potassium lowers systolic blood pressure 3 mmHg and diastolic blood pressure 2 mmHg (Whelton *et al.* 1997). Respectively, 1–2 g/day calcium supplementation reduces systolic blood pressure 1.4 mmHg and diastolic pressure 0.8 mmHg (Birkett 1998). Some studies have also shown a small hypotensive for magnesium (Jee *et al.* 2002). Even a small reduction in blood pressure is meaningful: a 2 mmHg decrease in systolic blood pressure has been estimated to reduce the risk of myocardial infarction and stroke by 4% (Selmer *et al.* 2000). Potassium-enriched products for controlling blood pressure are available, however, no spread applications exist thus far.

On the other hand, calcium-enriched spreads are available and are marketed mainly for bone health, i.e. building strong bones, optimizing bone mass and reducing the risk of osteoporosis later in life. Non-dairy calcium-enriched products broaden the variety of dietary sources of calcium and offer alternatives for those who do not consume dairy products.

Minerals in general have adverse effects on taste and texture and thus possess a challenge for product development.

16.3.6   Probiotics

Probiotics are live microorganisms, which when administered in adequate amounts, confer a beneficial health benefit. Effects of probiotics are strain-specific. The most widely researched bacterium is *Lactobacillus rhamnosus* GG (LGG®), which has been shown to decrease the incidence of respiratory infections in children (Hatakka *et al.* 2001), reduce the risk and duration of acute diarrhoea (Szajewska *et al.* 2007), and alleviate symptoms of atopic eczema and intestinal inflammation (Isolauri *et al.* 2000).

Products containing LGG® are sold in nearly 50 countries. The first fat-based product, a low-fat spread containing LGG®, was introduced by Unilever in Sweden and Germany in 2009. Although the variety of food products enriched with probiotic bacteria is large, spreads are a new area of application. The main challenge regarding spreads with living bacteria is to maintain the numbers of viable bacteria until the best before date.

16.3.7   Milk peptides

Biologically active peptide fragments are formed from milk proteins whey and casein during fermentation or by proteolytic enzymes. A variety of different peptides are formed in the process. Certain peptides have been shown to possess physiological effects, e.g. antihypertensive, antimicrobial, immunomodulatory, antioxidative and antithrombotic effects (for review, see Korhonen 2009).

To date, the casein-derived tripeptides isoleucine-proline-proline (IPP) and valine-proline-proline (VPP) have been studied most extensively. The blood pressure-lowering effects of these peptides have been shown in both animal and clinical studies (see Pripp 2008; Xu *et al.* 2008).

Fermented dairy products enriched with these peptides have been available in various countries since the 1990s. The first non-dairy-based, non-fermented product, a low-fat spread was introduced in Finland in 2009 by Valio Ltd. Regarding spreads, peptides pose a challenge both on taste and texture.

16.4   Methods for modifying fats and oils

Fats and oils can be modified with several technological and biological methods to improve chemical, physical and nutritional properties and make them more suitable for end user applications. The trend seems to be to shift from chemical to biological methods.

16.4.1 Interesterification

Interesterification has been used since the 1920s to modify the properties of fat. In this process, fatty acids are moved from one triglyceride molecule to another without altering the fatty acids. The aim of interesterification is to modify the melting point, reduce rancidification, create an oil more suitable for deep frying or to produce raw material for margarines and spreads with good taste and minimize saturated fatty acids and trans fat. It is used for production of triglycerides with specific compositions and nutritional properties. It is also used instead of partial hydrogenation of oils, which produces trans fatty acids, shown to have adverse health effects (see section on 'Trans fatty acids', p. 387).

Interesterification can be done chemically with alkaline catalysts or enzymatically using lipases (Xu *et al.* 2006). Chemical interesterification of fat is used typically to produce margarine ingredients containing less trans fatty acids. It is also used in the production of some special products and solid fats with high content of essential fatty acids. Enzymatic interesterification, in turn, is used for example in the production of cocoa butter equivalents, margarine hardstock and frying fats. The disadvantage of chemical interesterification is that there is no possibility of partial reaction, the catalysts are very reactive and unwanted by-products have to be removed. Enzymatic interesterification is more specific, safe and cost-efficient and will probably be the preferred method in the future.

16.4.2 Animal feeding

Bovine milk fat has one of the most complex compositions of all natural fats and contains also plenty of potential functional components (Mackae *et al.* 2005). Due to the high proportion of hypercholesterolemic fatty acids, the main aim of modifying milk fat has been to reduce C12:0–C16:0 fatty acids.

There are different ways to manipulate the composition and properties of milk fat by feeding. It is possible to soften and modify the nutritional properties of milk fat by feeding cows with vegetable oil or seed expeller from oil seeds (Table 16.3). Rapeseed/canola oil or expeller are the most commonly used methods of manipulating milk fat composition (Givens & Shingfield 2006). Transfer efficiency of feed unsaturated fatty acids into milk is quite low because of extensive rumen

Table 16.3 Milk fat composition (% of total fatty acids) – clover/rapeseed briquette feeding compared to average milk fat composition

	Clover/rapeseed briquette	Average milk fat
Palmitic acid, C 16:0	22.0	27.0
Linolic acid, C 18:2	1.9	1.7
Linolenic acid, C 18:3	1.0	0.5
Conjugated linoleic acid	0.8	0.5
Saturated fatty acids	59.0	65.0

Source: J. Nousiainen, Valio Ltd, unpublished information 2008.

biohydrogenation of unsaturated dietary fatty acids. Nevertheless, using traditional methods in softening of milk fat by dietary manipulation is possible. However, there are limits to how much vegetable fat can be fed to dairy cows without unfavourable influence on feed digestion and metabolism. According to recent results using clover silage, it is possible to improve the transfer efficiency of dietary polyunsaturated fatty acid into bovine milk, especially that of α-linolenic acid.

Researchers of the EU Lipgene project have shown that it is possible to reduce saturated fat in milk from 70% to 55% without significantly altering its shelf-life or sensory qualities. The main focus of the EU Lipgene Agro-Food Technology Program is to alter the microbiota of the rumen to reduce the endogenous trans fats and to use variations in feeding to reduce the endogenous synthesis of saturates and increase the production of monounsaturated fats within the mammary gland.

In 2007, Campina (the Netherlands) launched a butter with a more balanced fatty acid composition produced by using special supplementary feeding together with outdoor grazing. Campina butter contains 20% more unsaturated fatty acids than regular butter. Agral has launched a butter with high α-linolenic acid content, produced using linseed containing feed. The 'Omega-3' butter was launched in Belgium in 2005.

16.5   Future trends

The *New Nutrition Business* trend letter publishes yearly long-term trends in foods, nutrition and health. The ten key trends for years 2008–2010 have been summarized in Table 16.4.

Concerning fats and spreads, the most interesting trends are weight management and natural health. Weight management is linked to the fat content of products,

Table 16.4   Key trends in nutrition and health

2008	2009	2010
Digestive health	Digestive health	Digestive health
Fruit and superfruit	Feel the benefit	Natural health
Naturally healthy	Weight management	A benefit the consumer can feel
Beauty foods	Energy	Energy
Weight management	Naturally healthy	Fruit: the future of functional foods
Mood food	Fruit: the future of functional foods	Antioxidants
Premiumization	Kids' nutrition	Weight management
Snacks	Snacking	Snacking
Kid's nutrition	Target the loyal niches	Packaging and premiumization
Antioxidants	Packaging and premiumization	Bones and movement

Source: Mellentin 2008, 2009, 2010.

but may also include fats and spreads enriched with compounds with potential antiobesity effects (e.g. CLA, MCT). Although the launching of functional spreads seems to level off, so called micro-trends for fats and spreads include cholesterol-lowering, probiotics and omega-3 as functional ingredients.

Consumers look for benefits which are easy to understand and feel. Consumers are moving away from using active health spreads towards more balanced diet management in general and towards using natural ingredients (Brown 2009). Recently, organic and bio spreads based on butter but also low-fat spreads have been launched.

EU legislation on health claims will have an important effect regarding the future of functional foods also in the fats and spreads category.

16.6   Sources of further information and advice

The following sources are recommended for further information on fatty acids and fats:

- Chow CK (ed.) *Fatty Acids in Foods and their Health Implications*, CRC Press 2007: 1298 pp.
- Watson DR (ed.) *Fatty Acids in Health Promotion and Disease Causation*, AOCS Press 2009: 857pp.
- EFSA opinions on health claims: www.efsa.europa.eu
- International Society for the Study of Fatty Acids and Lipids (ISSFAL): http://www.issfal.org.uk
- Lipgene project: http://www.ucd.ie/lipgene/research_program/agro_food_technology.html

16.7   References

Albanes, D., Heinonen, O.P., Taylor, P.R., Virtamo, J., Edwards, B.K. (1995) Effects of alpha-tocopherol and beta-carotene supplements on cancer incidence in the Alpha-Tocopherol Beta-Carotene Cancer Prevention Study. *Am J Clin Nutr* **62**, 1427S–1430S.

Alexander-North, L.S., North, J.A., Kiminyo, K.P., Buettner, G.R., Spector, A.A. (1994) Polyunsaturated fatty acids increase lipid radical formation induced by oxidant stress in endothelial cells. *J Lipid Res* **13**(10), 1773–1785.

Ascherio, A., Rimm, E.B., Giovannucci, E.L., Spiegelman, D., Stampfer, M.J., Willett, W.C. (1996) Dietary fat and risk of coronary heart disease in men: cohort follow up study in the United States. *BMJ* **313**, 84–90.

Baer, D.J., Judd, J.T., Clevidence, B.A., Tracy, R.P. (2004) Dietary fatty acids affect plasma markers of inflammation in healthy men fed controlled diets: a randomised cross-over study. *Am J Clin Nutr* **79**, 969–973.

Birkett, N.J. (1998) Comments on a meta analysis of the relation between dietary calcium intake and blood pressure. *Am J Epidemiol* **148**, 223–238.

Bjerve, K.S., Mostad, I.L., Thoresen, L. (1987) Alpha-linolenic acid deficiency in patients on long-term gastric-tube feeding: estimation of linolenic acid and long-chain unsaturated n-3 fatty acid requirement in man. *Am J Clin Nutr* **45**, 66–77.

Brenna, J.T., Salem, N., Sinclair, A.J., Cunnane, S.C. (2009) α-linolenic acid supplementation and conversion to n-3 long-chain polyunsaturated fatty acids in humans. *Prostagland Leukot Essent Fatty Acids* **80**, 85–91.

British Nutrition Task Force (1992). Unsaturated fatty acids – nutritional and physiological significance: the report of the British Nutrition Foundation's Task Force. The British Nutrition Foundation: London, UK.

Brown, H. (2009) Fat chance. *Food Manufacture* **84**(12), 39–40.

Burr, G.O., Burr, M.M. (1930) On the nature and role of the fatty acids essential in nutrition. *J Biol Chem* **86**, 587–621.

Calder, P. (2004) N-3 Fatty acids and cardiovascular disease: evidence explained and mechanisms explored. *Clin Sci* **107**(1), 1–11.

Chan, J.K., Bruce, V.M., McDonald, B.E. (1991) Dietary α-linoleinic acid is as effective as oleic and linoleic acid in lowering blood cholesterol in normolipidemic men. *Am J Clin Nutr* **53**, 1230–1234.

Child, P., Kuskis, A. (1986) Investigation of the role of micellar phospholipid in the preferential uptake of cholesterol over sitosterol by dispersed rat jejunal villus cells. *Biochem Cell Biol* **64**, 847–853.

Covas, M.I., Nyyssönen, K., Poulsen, H.E., Kaikkonen, J., Zunft, H.J, Kiesewetter, H. *et al.* (2006) The effect of polyphenols in olive oil on heart disease risk factors: a randomized trial. *Ann Intern Med* **145**(5), 333–341.

de Deckere, E.A.M., van Amelsvoort, J.M.M., McNeill, G.P., Jones, P. (1999) Effects of conjugated linoleic acid (CLA) isomers on lipid levels and peroxisome proliferation in the hamster. *Br J Nutr* **82**, 309–317.

Demonty, I., Ras, R.T., van der Knaap, H.C.M., Duchateau, G.S.M.J.E., Meijer, L., *et al.* (2009) Continuous dose-response relationship of the LDL-cholesterol-lowering effect of phytosterol intake. *J Nutr* **139**, 271–284.

Desroches, S., Chouinard, P.Y., Galibois, I., Corneau, L., Delisle, J., *et al.* (2005) Lack of effect of dietary conjugated linoleic acids naturally incorporated into butter on the lipid profile and body composition of overweight and obese men. *Am J Clin Nutr* **82**, 309–316.

Dolecek, T.A. (1992) Epidemiological evidence of relationships between dietary polyunsaturated fatty acids and mortality in the Multiple Risk Factor Intervention Trial. *Proc Soc Exp Biol Med* **200**, 177–182.

FAO/WHO Expert Committee (1994) Fats and oils in human nutrition. FAO: Rome, Haly.

Fitó, M., Cladellas, M., de la Torre, R., Martí, J., Alcántara, M., *et al.* (2005) Antioxidant effect of virgin olive oil in patients with stable coronary heart disease: a randomised, crossover, controlled, clinical trial. *Atherosclerosis* **181**, 149–158.

Gebauer, S.K., Psota, T.L., Harris, W.S., Kris-Etherton, P.M. (2006) n-3 fatty acid dietary recommendations and food sources to achieve essentiality and cardiovascular benefits. *Am J Clin Nutr* **83** (suppl.), 1526S–1535S.

Givens, D.I., Shingfield, K.J. (2006) Optimizing dairy milk fatty acid composition. In: *Improving the Fat Content of Foods*, eds. C. Williams, J. Buttriss. Woodhead Publishing Limited, Cambridge, pp. 252–280.

Griinari, J.M., Corl, B.A., Lacy, S.H., Chouinard, P.Y., Nurmela, K.V.V., Bauman, D.E. (2000) Conjugated linoleic acid is synthesized endogenously in lactating dairy cows by delta-9-desaturase. *J Nutr* **130**, 2285–2291.

Gylling, H., Puska, P., Vartiainen, E., Miettinen, T.A. (1999) Retinol, vitamin D, carotenoids and alpha-tocopherol in serum of a moderately hypercholesterolemic population consuming sitostanol ester margarine. *Atherosclerosis* **145**, 279–285.

Hatakka, K., Savilahti, E., Pönkä, A., Meurman, J.H., Poussa, T., Näse, L. *et al.* (2001) Effect of long term consumption of probiotic milk on infections in attending day care centres: double blind, randomised trial. *BMJ* **322**, 1327–1329.

Health Council of the Netherlands (2006). Guidelines for a healthy diet 2006. Health Council of the Netherlands: Hague, The Netherlands, 2006/21E.

Hegsted, D.M., McGandy, R.B., Myers, M.L., Stare, F.J. (1965) Quantitative effects of dietary fat on serum cholesterol in man. *Am J Clin Nutr* **17**, 281–295.

Hendriks, H.F., Weststrate, J.A., van Meijer, G.W. (1999) Spreads enriched with three different levels of vegetable oil sterols and the degree of cholesterol lowering in normocholesterolaemic and mildly hypercholesterolaemic subjects. *Eur J Clin Nutr* **53**, 319–327.

Holman, R.T. (1970) Biological activities of and requirements for polyunsaturated acids. In: *Progress in the Chemistry of Fats and Other Lipids*, Vol **9**, 607–682, Pergamon Press, New York.

Holman, R.T., Johnson, S.B., Hatch, T.F. (1982) A case of human linolenic acid deficiency involving neurological abnormalities. *Am J Clin Nutr* **35**, 617–623.

Houseknecht, K.L., Van den Heuvel, J.P., Moya-Camarena, S.Y., Portocarrero, C.P., Peck, L.W., *et al.* (1998) Dietary conjugated linoleic acid normalizes impaired glucose tolerance in the Zucker diabetic fatty fa/fa rat. *Biochem Biophys Res Commun* **244**, 678–682.

Hu, F.B., Manson, J.E., Stampfer, M.J., Colditz, G.A., Rosner, B.A. *et al.* (2001) Diet, lifestyle, and the risk of type 2 diabetes mellitus in women. *N Engl J Med* **345**, 790–797.

Hu, F.B., Stampfer, M.J., Morison, J.E. *et al.* (1999) Dietary intake of a-linolenic acid and risk of fatal ischemic heart disease among women. *Am J Clin Nutr* **69**, 890–897.

Huang HY, Caballero B, Chang S. *et al.* (2006) Multivitamin/mineral supplements and prevention of chronic disease. *Evid Rep Technol Assess* **139**, 1–117.

Ip, C., Briggs, S.P., Haegele, A.D., Thompson, H.J., Storkson, J., Scimeca, J.A. (1996) The efficacy of conjugated linoleic acid in mammary cancer prevention is independent of the level or type of fat in the diet. *Carcinogenesis* **17**, 1045–1050.

Ip, C., Chin, S.F., Scimeca, J.A., Pariza, M.W. (1991) Mammary cancer prevention by conjugated dienoic derivative of linoleic acid. *Cancer Res* **51**, 6118–6124.

Isaac, M.G., Quinn, R., Tabet, N. (2008) Vitamin E for Alzheimer's disease and mild cognitive impairment. *Cochrane Database Syst Rev* **16**(3), CD002854.

Isolauri, E., Arvola, T., Sutas, Y., Moilanen, E., Salminen, S. (2000) Probiotics in the management of atopic eczema. *Clin Exp Allergy* **30**, 1604–1610.

ISSFAL (2004). Recommendations for intake of polyunsaturated fatty acids in healthy adults. http://www.issfal.org/index.php?option=com_content&task=view&id=23&lte mid=8

Jee, S.H., Miller, E.R., Singh, G.E., Appel, L.J., Klag, M.J. (2002) The effect of magnesium on blood pressure: a meta-analysis of randomized clinical trials. *Am J Hypertens* **15**(8), 691–696.

Korhonen, H. (2009) Milk-derived bioactive peptides: from science to applications. *J Functional Foods* **1**, 177–187.

Kris-Etherton, P., Harris, W.S., Appel, L.J., for the Nutrition Committee American Heart Association Nutrition Committee (2002). Fish consumption, fish oil, omega-3 fatty acids and cardiovascular disease. *Circulation* **106**, 2747–2757.

Kritharides, L., Stocker, R. (2002) The use of antioxidant supplements in coronary heart disease. *Atherosclerosis* **164**, 211–216.

Lee, J.H., O'Keefe, J.H., Lavie, C.J., Marchioli, R., Harris, W.S. (2008) Omega-3 fatty acids for cardioprotection. *Mayo Clin Proc* **83**(3), 324–332.

Lee, K.N., Kritchevsky, D., Pariza, M.W. (1994) Conjugated linoleic acid and atherosclerosis in rabbits. *Atherosclerosis* **108**, 19–25.

Lemaitre, R.N., King, I.B., Ragunathan, T.E., Pearce, R.M., Weinmann, S., Knopp, R.H. *et al.* (2002) Cell membrane trans fatty acids and the risk of primary cardiac arrest. *Circulation* **105**, 697–701.

Lopez-Garcia, E., Schulze, M.B., Meigs, J.B., Manson, J.E., Rifai, M., Stampfer, M.J. *et al.* (2005) Consumption of trans fatty acids is related to plasma biomarkers of inflammation and endothelial dysfunction. *J Nutr* **135**, 562–566.

de Lorgeril, M., Renaud, S., Mamelle, N., *et al.* (1994) Mediterranean alpha-linolenic acid-rich diet in secondary prevention of coronary heart disease. *Lancet* **343**, 1454–1459.

Mackae, J., O'Reilly, L., Morgan, P. (2005) Desirable characteristics of animal fat from human health perspective. *Livestock Prod Sci* **94**, 95–103.

Marten, B., Pfeuffer, M., Schrezenmeir, J. (2006) Medium-chain triglyserides. *Int Dairy J* **16** (11), 1374–1382.

Mellentin, J. (2007/2008), 10 Key Trends in Food, Nutrition & Health 2008. *New Nutrition Business* **13**(3), 1.

Mellentin, J. (2008/2009), 10 Key Trends in Food, Nutrition & Health 2009. *New Nutrition Business* **14**(3), 1.

Mellentin, J. (2009/2010), 10 Key Trends in Food, Nutrition & Health 2010. *New Nutrition Business* **15**(3), 1.

Miró-Casas, E., Covas, M.I., Fitó, M., Farré-Albadalejo, M., Marrugat, J., de la Torre, R. (2003) Tyrosol and hydroxytyrosol are absorbed from moderate and sustained doses of virgin olive oil in humans. *Eur J Clin Nutr* **57**, 186–190.

Mozaffarian, D., Aro, A., Willett, W.C. (2009) Health effects of trans fatty acids: experimental and observational evidence. *Eur J Clin Nutr* **63**, S5–S21.

Mozaffarian, D., Clarke, R. (2009) Quantitative effects on cardiovascular risk factors and coronary heart disease risk of replacing partially hydrogenated vegetable oils with other fats and oils. *Eur J Clin Nutr* **63**(Suppl. 2), S22–S33.

Mozaffarian, D., Katan, M.B., Ascherio, A., Stampfer, M.J., Willett, W.C. (2006) Trans fatty acids and cardiovascular disease. *N Engl J Med* **354**, 1601–1613.

Mozaffarian, D., Micha, R., Wallace, S. (2010) Effects on coronary heart disease of increasing polyunsaturated fat in place of saturated fat: a systematic review and meta-analysis of randomized controlled trials. *PLoS Med* **7**(3), e1000252.

Naumann, E., Carpentier, Y.A., Saebo, A., Lassel, T.S., Chardigny, J.M., *et al.* (2006) Cis-9, trans-11 and trans-10, cis-12 conjugated linoleic acid (CLA) do not affect the plasma lipoprotein profile in moderately overweight subjects with LDL phenotype B. *Atherosclerosis* **188**, 167–174.

Nicolosi, R.J., Rogers, E.J., Kritchevsky, D., Scimeca, J.A., Huth, P.J. (1997) Dietary conjugated linoleic acid reduces plasma lipoproteins and early atherosclerosis in hypercholesterolemic hamsters. *Artery* **22**, 266–277.

Noakes, M., Clifton, P., Ntanios, F., Shrapnel, W., Record, I., McInerney, J. (2002) An increase in dietary carotenoids when consuming plant sterols or stanols is effective in maintaining plasma carotenoid concentrations. *Am J Clin Nutr* **75**, 79–86.

O'Shea, M., Bassaganya-Riera, J., Mohede, I.C.M. (2004) Immunomodulatory properties of conjugated linoleic acid. *Am J Clin Nutr* **79**, 1199S–1206S.

Ostlund, R.E., McGill, J.B., Zeng, C., Covey, D.F., Stearns, J., *et al.* (2002) Gastrointestinal absorption and plasma kinetics of soy Δ5-phytosterols and phytostanols in humans. *Am J Physiol Endocrinol Metab* **282**, E911–E916.

Pariza, M.W., Ashoor, S.H., Chu, F.S., Lund, D.B. (1979) Effects of temperature and time on mutagen formation in pan-fried hamburger. *Cancer Lett* **7**, 63–69.

Park, Y., Albright, K.J., Liu, W., Storkson, J.M., Cook, M.E., Pariza, M.W. (1997) Effect of conjugated linoleic acid on body composition in mice. *Lipids* **32**, 853–858.

Pietinen, P., Ascherio, A., Korhonen, P., Hartman, A.M., Willett, W.C., *et al.* (1997) Intake of fatty acids and risk of coronary heart disease in a cohort of Finnish men. The Alpha-tocopherol, Beta-carotene Cancer Prevention Study. *Am J Epidemiol* **145**, 876–887.

Plat, J., Mensink, R.P. (2001) Effects of diets enriched with two different plant sterol ester mixtures on plasma ubiquinol-10 and fat-soluble antioxidant concentrations. *Metabolism* **50**, 520–529.

Plat, J., Mensink, R.P. (2002) Effects of plant stanol esters on LDL receptor protein expression and on LDL receptor and HMG-CoA reductase mRNA expression in mononuclear blood cells of healthy men and women. *FASEB J* **16**(2), 258–60.

Pripp, A.H. (2008) Effect of peptides derived from food proteins on blood pressure: a meta-analysis of randomized controlled trials. *Food Nutr Res* **52**, 1–8.

Redlich, C.A., Blaner, W.S., van Bennekum, A.M., Chung, J.S., Clever, S.L., *et al.* (1998) Effect of supplementation with beta-carotene and vitamin A on lung nutrient levels. *Cancer Epidemiol Biomarkers Prev* **7**, 211–214.

Riserus, U., Basu, S., Jovinge, S., Nordin Fredrikson, G., Ärnlöv, J., Vessby, B. (2002) Supplementation with conjugated linoleic acid causes isomer-dependent oxidative stress and elevated c-reactive protein. *Circulation* **106**, 1925–1929.

Ritzenthaler, K.L., McGuire, M.K., Falen, R., Shultz, T.D., Dasgupta, N., McGuire, M.A. (2001) Estimation of conjugated linoleic acid intake be written dietary assessment methodologies underestimated actual intake evaluated by food duplicate methodology. *J Nutr* **131**, 1548–1554.

Salvini, S., Sera, F., Caruso, D., Giovanelli, L., Visioli, F., Saieva, C., *et al.* (2006) Daily consumption of a high-phenol extra-virgin olive oil reduces oxidative DNA damage in postmenopausal women. *Br J Nutr* **95**, 742–751.

Scientific Advisory Committee on Nutrition (2004). Advice to FSA: on the benefits of oily fish and fish oil consumption from SACN. HMSO: London, UK.

Selmer, R.M., Kristiansen, I.S., Haglerod, A., Graff-Iversen, S., Larsen, H.K., *et al.* (2000) Cost and health consequences of reducing the population intake of salt. *J Epidemiol Community Health* **54**, 697–702.

Szajewska, H., Skorka, A., Ruszczynski, M., Gieruszczak-Bialek, D. (2007) Meta-analysis: Lactobacillus GG for treating acute diarrhea in children. *Ailment Pharmacol Ther* **25**, 871–881.

Tricon, S., Burdge, G.C., Jones, E.L., Russell, J.J., El-Khazen, S., *et al.* (2006) Effects of dairy products naturally enriched with cis-9,trans-11 conjugated linoleic acid on the blood lipid profile in healthy middle-aged men. *Am J Clin Nutr* **83**, 744–753.

Turpeinen, A.M., Mutanen, M., Aro, A., Salminen, I., Basu, S., Palmquist, D.L., Griinari, J.M. (2002) Bioconversion of vaccenic acid to conjugated linoleic acid in humans. *Am J Clin Nutr* **76**, 504–510.

Valsta, L.M., Jauhiainen, M., Aro, A., Salminen, I., Mutanen, M. (1995) The effects of serum lipoprotein levels of two monounsaturated fat rich diets differing in their linoleic and a-linolenic acid contents. *Nutr Metab Cardiovasc Dis* **5**, 129–140.

Whelton, P.K., He, J., Cutler, J.A., Brancati, F.L., Appel, L.J., *et al.* (1997) Effects of oral potassium on blood pressure. Meta-analysis of randomised controlled clinical trials. *JAMA* **277**, 1624–1632.

Whigham, L.D., Watras, A.C., Schoeller, D.A. (2007) Efficacy of conjugated linoleic acid for reducing fat mass: a meta-analysis in humans. *Am J Clin Nutr* **85**, 1203–1211.

WHO/FAO Expert Consultation on Diet, Nutrition and the Prevention of Chronic Diseases (2003). WHO technical report series #916. Geneva, Switzerland.

Willett, W.C., Stampfer, M.J., Manson, J.E., Colditz, G.A., Speizer, F.E., *et al.* (1993) Intake of trans fatty acids and risk of coronary heart disease among women. *Lancet* **341**, 581–585.

Xu, J.-Y., Qin, L.-Q., Wang, P.-Y., Li, W., Chang, C. (2008) Effects of milk tripeptides on blood pressure: A meta-analysis of randomized, controlled trials. *Nutrition* **24**, 933–940.

Xu, X., Guo, Z., Zhang, H., Vikbjerg, A.F., Damsrup, M.L. (2006) Chemical and enzymatic interesterification of lipids for use in food. In: *Modifying Lipids in Food*, ed. Gunstone F. D. pp. 234–266.

17

Omega-3 polyunsaturated fatty acids (PUFAs) as food ingredients

C. Jacobsen, National Food Institute, Denmark

Abstract: During the last 30 years there has been an increasing interest in marine omega-3 polyunsaturated fatty acids (PUFAs) for nutritional applications due to their health beneficial effects, which will be briefly summarised. There are different sources of omega-3 PUFAs, but the major source is fish oils. Due to their polyunsaturated nature omega-3 PUFAs are highly susceptible to lipid oxidation, which will lead to formation of undesirable fishy and rancid off-flavours. Such off-flavours can lead to consumer rejection of omega-3 enriched foods. This chapter will summarise our current knowledge about the most important factors affecting lipid oxidation in a range of different omega-3 enriched foods and means to reduce lipid oxidation will also be discussed.

Key words: omega-3 fatty acids, fish oil enrichment, sources of omega-3 PUFA, lipid oxidation, antioxidants.

17.1   Introduction

During the past thirty years there has been an increasing interest in polyunsaturated fatty acids (PUFAs) for food, nutritional and pharmaceutical applications. This is due to the increasing evidence that PUFAs have a wide range of nutritional benefits in the human body. There are two distinct families of PUFAs, namely the omega-3 and the omega-6 families, and these families cannot be interconverted. The terms 'omega-3' and 'omega-6' refer to the position of the first double bond in the carbon chain as counted from the methyl terminus. The health benefits of omega-3 PUFAs have received particular attention during the last decade, and from a nutritional point of view the three most important omega-3 PUFAs are α-linolenic acid (ALA, C18:3 n-3), eicosapentaenoic acid (EPA, C20:5 n-3) and docosahexaenoic acid (DHA, C22:6 n-3). Plant materials such as flaxseed, canola (rape seed) and soybean oil contain relatively high levels of n-3 PUFAs in the form of ALA. However, n-3 and n-6 PUFAs with 18 carbon atoms (ALA and linoleic acid) are competing for the same enzyme systems for conversion of the C18 fatty acids into PUFAs with longer chain length (EPA from ALA and C20:4 n-6 from linoleic acid). Therefore, only a minor part of ALA is converted to EPA and DHA. This is particularly a problem if the intake ratio between n-3/n-6 PUFAs is low. This chapter will therefore mainly focus on EPA and DHA and in the remaining part of this chapter the term n-3 PUFAs refers to EPA plus DHA and not ALA.

The molecular structures of EPA and DHA are shown in Fig. 17.1. The research efforts during the last 30 years have revealed that the potential health effects of EPA and DHA include reduction of cardiovascular disease risk (Harris 1989; Prisco *et al.* 1995; de Leiris 2009), anti-inflammatory effects including reduction of symptoms of rheumatoid arthritis (Broughton *et al.* 1997; Kremer 2000) and Crohns disease (Belluzzi *et al.* 2000). DHA is particularly important in the development of brain and nervous tissue in the infant (van Goor *et al.* 2010). A high intake of EPA and DHA has also been associated with lower risk of developing Alzheimers and depressions (Trautwein 2001; Mischoulon *et al.* 2008). However, there is still a lot to be learned about the effects of omega-3 PUFAs in human health, both with respect to their ability to prevent the development of the above mentioned diseases, but also with respect to their role in weight management and general mental health.

Owing to the increasing number of studies documenting health beneficial effects of omega-3 PUFAs there has been a growing interest in using these healthy lipids in foods. However, due to their polyunsaturated nature omega-3 PUFAs are highly susceptible to lipid oxidation, which will lead to formation of undesirable fishy and rancid off-flavours. Such off-flavours can lead to consumer rejection of omega-3 enriched foods. It is thus crucial that lipid oxidation is prevented if such products are to become successful in the market place. Another important aspect regarding the future for omega-3 PUFA enrichment of food is a stable and adequate supply of omega-3 PUFAs to the food industry. A sustainable source of omega-3 PUFAs is therefore required.

This chapter will give a short summary of the current status on our knowledge about the health beneficial effects of omega-3 PUFAs. Subsequently, the different sources of omega-3 PUFAs will be discussed. The chapter will also summarise the most important factors affecting lipids oxidation in omega-3 enriched foods and will discuss how lipid oxidation can be prevented.

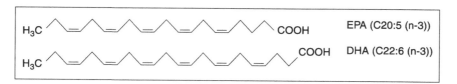

Fig. 17.1   Molecular structure of EPA and DHA n-3 fatty acids.

17.2   Health aspects of omega-3 polyunsaturated fatty acids (PUFAs)

The first evidence regarding the beneficial effects of omega-3 PUFAs came in the 1970s when Dyerberg and Bang (1979) discovered that Greenland inuits had a much lower incidence of cardiovascular diseases than the Danes, who consumed much lower amounts of fish and marine animals than the inuits. Subsequently, several intervention trials have supported the improvement of cardiovascular health associated with intake of omega-3 PUFAs. Several of these trials have demonstrated a beneficial effect of omega-3 PUFAs intake on fatal and nonfatal myocardial infarction (Singh *et al.* 1997; Spiteller 2005).

Moreover, results from epidemiological trials have demonstrated that intake of fish resulted in a lower mortality rate from coronary heart disease probably due to the high content of EPA and DHA in fish (Oomen *et al.* 2000). A large study involving 36 countries showed an association between fish consumption and reduced risk from ischemic heart disease and stroke (Zhang *et al.* 1999). Other studies have found a reduced risk of sudden cardiac death in men (Albert *et al.* 1998), a reduced risk of coronary heart disease in women (Hu *et al.* 2002), a significant reduction in the incidence of certain types of stroke caused by blood clots (Iso *et al.* 2001) and a reduced risk of primary cardiac arrest (Siscovick *et al.* 1995) following consumption of fatty fish rich in omega-3 PUFAs. However, some epidemiological studies have not shown any beneficial effect of fish intake. These conflicting results may for example, be due to different populations examined (high risk versus low risk populations) or to the type of fish consumed (lean versus fatty fish).

Results from clinical studies have indicated that omega-3 PUFAs positively affect coronary disease risk factors by decreasing plasma triacylglycerol (TAG) levels (Harris 1989), improving platelet function (Prisco *et al.*, 1995), lowering blood viscosity (Pauletto *et al.* 1996) and by modulating inflammatory processes as reviewed by Simopoulos (1991). Moreover, omega-3 PUFAs seem to reduce cardiovascular disease risk by decreasing the risk of arrhythmias and the growth rate of atherosclerotic plaque and by lowering blood pressure.

Besides the effects of omega-3 PUFAs in cardiovascular diseases a positive role on immune functions has been demonstrated. For example, patients suffering from rheumatoid arthritis were observed to have a reduced incidence of joint tenderness and morning stiffness during supplementation with fish oil (Kremer 2000). Intake of omega-3 PUFAs also appears to offer some protection against immune-compromised conditions including asthma (Broughton *et al.* 1997), cystic fibrosis (Olveira *et al.* 2010) and Crohn's disease (Belluzzi *et al.* 2000)).

17.3   Sources of omega-3 PUFAs

Currently, the main source of EPA and DHA are fish oils extracted from fatty fish in connection with the production of fish meal. The fish that are processed to produce crude fish oil (and fish meal) can usually be categorised as follows: (1) offal and waste from the edible fisheries, e.g. cutting from filleting industry; (2) fish of a quality that is not high enough to make the fish suitable for human consumption; or (3) fish types that are not considered acceptable or aesthetically pleasing for human consumption. The latter are caught especially for reduction to fish meal and fish oil. In the EU a new hygiene legislation has recently been implemented. This legislation requires that fish oils intended for human consumption must be produced from fish that are fit for human consumption, meaning that some of the raw materials that have previously been used for fish oil production for human consumption can no longer be used. The most important fish species that are caught commercially and processed into fish oil are capelin, herring, mackerel, horse mackerel, sand eel, menhaden, sardine, anchovy and sprat.

The total annual world production of fish oil during the last 10 years has been approximately 1.25 million tonnes (http://www.iffo.org.uk/tech/alaska.htm). The main producers are Japan, Scandinavia, Chile, Peru, USA and Russia. Most of the fish oil is going into salmonid production in Norway, Chile, Canada and in various European countries. Due to the growth in aquaculture it is expected that the demand for fish oil for use in aquaculture may soon exceed the production. However, approximately 25–30 million tonnes of fish are discarded annually. Efforts are being made to increase fish oil production by decreasing the amount of waste and increasing the amount of recycling of the fish waste to fish meal and fish oil production. In addition, efforts are being made to reduce the amount of fish oil used per kg farmed fish produced, e.g. by substituting part of the fish oil with vegetable oil. However, to obtain a satisfactory n-3 PUFA level in farmed fish at the time of slaughtering it may be possible to substitute fish oil with vegetable oil only at the beginning of the feeding period. Fish oil producers can most likely earn a greater profit by up-grading fish oil to a food grade product. Therefore, fish oil may increasingly be produced for enrichment of foods at the expense of being used for aquaculture feeds. Hence, it is expected that fish oils will still be available for food applications in the years to come.

However, there are also other sources of omega-3 PUFAs available. Thus, several micro-organisms are capable of producing omega-3 PUFAs with a chain length above C20, including lower fungi, bacteria and marine micro-algae (Bajpai *et al.* 1991; Kendrick & Ratledge 1992). The most promising micro-organisms for the production of omega-3 PUFAs seem to be the marine micro-algae as they are able to accumulate high amounts of omega-3 PUFAs. The advantage of algae oil compared with fish oil is thus that the oil contains higher levels of, in particular, DHA than fish oil, e.g. up to 52% (Sijtsma 2004). In recent years, production of DHA by heterotrophic marine micro-organisms has received increased commercial attention and today DHA produced this way is used in several infant formula products. Currently, Martek Biosciences uses *Schizochytrium* sp. for the production of DHA, which has been used for DHA-enriched egg and as feed for aquaculture (Sijtsma 2004). The European Commission has approved the use of DHA-rich oil from *Schizochytrium* sp. produced by Martek Biosciences in products such as dairy products, spreads, dressings, breakfast cereals and food supplements (Sijtsma 2004). Martek Biosciences has also patented a process for the production of DHA-rich oil (25–60%) using *Crypthecodinium cohnii* and this DHA-oil is currently used in several infant formula products.

A lot of research efforts are currently devoted to the development of GMO plants that can produce EPA and DHA. Commercial products are not yet on the market, but commercialisation of such oils is expected to occur within the next 5–10 years. One major obstacle seems to be to obtain satisfactory EPA and DHA yields. As a step towards growing plants that can produce EPA and DHA, the biotech company Monsanto has developed a GMO soybean plant that can produce stearidonic acid (SDA; C18:4 n-3). The advantage of this fatty acid is that it has one double bond more than ALA. This means that SDA is more efficiently converted in the human body to EPA than current plant sources (ALA) because it bypasses a step in the conversion process.

17.4 The problems associated with using omega-3 PUFAs in foods

Certain fishing areas are heavily polluted with compounds such as PCBs (polychlorinated biphenyls), dioxins, lead and arsenic. PCB and dioxin are lipid soluble and therefore they will be extracted together with the fish oil during the fish oil manufacturing process. In July 2002, a regulation was imposed in the EU where the limit for dioxin in fish oil was set at 2 pg WHO-PCDD/F-TEQ/g. The legislation was amended in 2006 to include limits for dioxin-like PCBs. Owing to the strict rules, new technologies have been developed to remove dioxin from fish oil. The most common method is to remove the dioxin by activated carbon, but new deodorisation techniques including thin film deodorisation and molecular distillation that efficiently remove these compounds have also been developed. Hence, today PCB's and dioxins have almost been totally removed during the refining and deodorisation process in most commercially available fish oils and such oils can therefore be considered safe for human consumption.

The main technological problem in relation to the use of omega-3 PUFA in both pharmaceutical and food applications is their susceptibility to lipid oxidation, which is due to their highly unsaturated nature. The chemistry behind lipid oxidation is therefore briefly summarised.

17.4.1 Lipid oxidation chemistry
There are three different types of oxidation: autoxidation, photo-oxidation and enzymatic oxidation. Autoxidation is a spontaneous free radical reaction with oxygen and consists of three main stages: initiation, propagation and termination. Photo-oxidation happens only in the presence of light and when the food system contains photosensitisers. Enzymatic oxidation is due to the presence of certain enzymes such as lipoxygenase in plant and animal systems.

Autoxidation and metal catalysis

The autoxidation reaction is initiated by initiators (e.g. metal ions, heat, protein radicals), which causes unsaturated fatty acids (LHs) to form carbon-centred alkyl radicals (L˙) (Fig. 17.2). In the presence of oxygen these radicals will form peroxyl radicals (LOO˙) and later hydroperoxides (LOOH). The hydroperoxides are the primary oxidation products of autoxidation. The free radical chain reaction propagates until two free radicals combine and form a non-radical product to terminate the chain. The hydroperoxides can be decomposed by heat or in the presence of traces of transition metals and thereby alkoxyl and peroxyl radical intermediates (LO˙ and LOO˙) are formed. These radicals propagate the free radical chain reaction. Moreover, these radicals may be further decomposed to form a variety of non-volatile and volatile secondary oxidation products. The latter are termed 'volatiles' and include a wide range of carbonyl compounds (aldehydes, ketones and alcohols), hydrocarbons and furans that are responsible for flavour deterioration (Frankel 2005). In contrast to the volatiles, hydroperoxides are essentially tasteless and odourless.

As already mentioned metal ions are important catalysts of lipid oxidation. They can catalyse the oxidation process by two different mechanisms:

1 By electron transfer:

$$M^{(n+1)+} + RH \rightarrow M^{n+} + R\bullet + H^+ \qquad [17.1]$$

2 By catalysing the decomposition of hydroperoxides

$$M^{n+} + ROOH \rightarrow M^{(n+1)+} + RO\bullet + OH^-$$

$$M^{(n+1)+} + ROOH \rightarrow M^{n+} + ROO\bullet + H^+ \qquad [17.2]$$

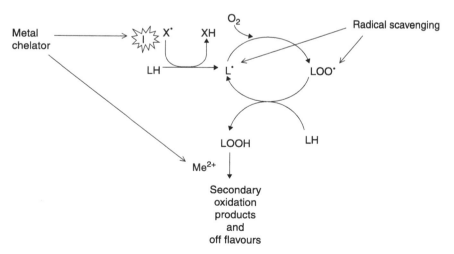

Fig. 17.2 The lipid oxidation process and antioxidant mechanisms, I = initiator.

Fe and Cu are the most active metals, but also Mn, Zn, Co and Ni can act as prooxidants. Ferrous iron (Fe^{2+}) is more effective in decomposing peroxides than the ferric ion (Fe^{3+}) and both ferrous and ferric iron are more effective than copper.

Photooxidation
Photooxidation leads to oxidation of unsaturated fatty acids owing to exposure to light in the presence of photosensitisers. There are two types of photosensitisers, both are activated by absorbing visible or near-UV light. Following activation by light Type I sensitisers react with the substrate, generating substrate radicals, which can react with oxygen. In contrast activated Type II sensitisers react directly with triplet oxygen, transforming it into the short-lived, but highly reactive, high-energy form of singlet oxygen $^1O_2$, which reacts directly with the double bond of unsaturated fatty acids to form hydroperoxides (LOOH) (Frankel 1991, 2005). This is not a free-radical process and will lead to the formation of other lipid hydroperoxides and in turn also to other volatiles than those formed from free radical oxidation. In food systems, chlorophyll, riboflavin or heme proteins, serve as photosensitisers. The hydroperoxides are decomposed by the same reactions as described under autoxidation.

Volatile oxidation products formed from EPA and DHA
Due to the high number of double bonds in EPA and DHA, the oxidation processes may lead to a complex mixture of hydroperoxides and a myriad of volatile, non-volatile and polymeric secondary oxidation products. The structures of some cleavage products are known, but the exact mechanisms for the formation of many of the observed products are not yet completely understood. Omega-3 PUFAs though follow the same cleavage mechanisms as those recognised for linolenic acid. Hence, some of the oxidation products that can be expected from autoxidation of omega-3 PUFAs are propanal, 2-pentenal, 3-hexenal, 4-heptenal, 2,4-heptadienal, 2,6-nonadienal, 2,4,7-decatrienal, as well as 1-penten-3-one and 1,5-octadien-3-one.

Volatile compounds have different sensory threshold values. Importantly, the human sensory apparatus has a particularly low threshold for volatile off-flavours resulting from oxidation of omega-3 PUFAs (Frankel 2005). Thus, 1-penten-3-one as well as (Z)-4-heptenal, (E,Z)-2,6-nonadienal and 2,4,7-decatrienals have been associated with sharp-burnt-fishy off-flavours in oxidised fish oil (Karahadian & Lindsay 1989). However, decatrienals are usually only observed in highly oxidised products and in several studies on fish oil enriched foods this compound was not observed (Hartvigsen *et al.* 2000; Venkateshwarlu *et al.* 2004).

Antioxidant mechanisms
Lipid oxidation may to a certain extent be prevented by the addition of antioxidants. Usually, antioxidants are classified as either primary or secondary antioxidants. Primary antioxidants (AH) are also referred to as free radical scavengers because they act as chain-breaking antioxidants by donating electron/hydrogen to free radicals such as the lipid, peroxyl or the alkoxyl radical (Fig. 17.2). Thereby they

terminate the free radical chain reaction. Primary antioxidants include hindered phenols such as the synthetic antioxidants BHA (butylhydroxyanisole), BHT (butylhydroxytoluene), propyl gallate, naturally occurring compounds such as tocopherol and plant polyphenols such as carnosic acid. The secondary antioxidants act by a number of different mechanisms such as metal chelation, oxygen scavenging and replenishing hydrogen to primary antioxidants. Therefore, the secondary antioxidants often exert synergistic effects together with primary antioxidants.

17.5   Factors affecting lipid oxidation in omega-3 PUFA enriched foods

Many foods to which omega-3 PUFAs are added are oil-in-water (o/w) emulsions such as mayonnaise, milk, dressing or water-in-oil emulsions (w/o) such as spreads. However, omega-3 PUFAs have also been added to other types of foods such as bread, fish pâté, cereals, etc. Although the basic lipid oxidation processes in such foods are the same as described above the factors that can affect the lipid oxidation rate will vary from food system to food system.

Importantly, oxidation generally occurs faster in emulsions than in neat oils (Frankel *et al.* 2002) and it may also be expected to occur faster in most other omega-3 enriched foods than in neat oils. This is due to the mechanical processing that is required for emulsification or mixing, which in some cases necessitates the use of high temperature. It may also be due to other types of heating processes such as baking. Moreover, in many cases, the oil is exposed to air (oxygen) during processing. For emulsions, the increased oxidation rate may also be due to an increased interfacial area as lipid oxidation is thought to be initiated at the interfaces between air, oil and water. Even after refining and deodorisation most fish oils will contain trace levels of peroxides and several food ingredients contain trace levels of metal ions. Therefore, metal catalysed decomposition of peroxides is regarded as the most important driving force for lipid oxidation in many food products.

For the above-mentioned reasons, special precautions have to be taken to avoid oxidative flavor deterioration of omega-3 PUFA enriched foods. In the following the possible means to limit oxidation by choice of ingredients including oil quality and type of emulsifiers, by optimising processing conditions, packaging material and storage conditions, and by addition of antioxidants will be discussed.

17.5.1   The influence of the omega-3 oil quality

The oil quality (i.e. oxidative status of the omega-3 PUFA oil) may significantly influence the oxidative stability of the final omega-3 enriched product and should therefore be evaluated before the oil is used for enrichment. The peroxide value has traditionally been used as a measure of the level of the primary oxidation products (lipid hydroperoxides) in the product. (Let *et al.* 2004, 2005b) showed that the fish oil quality immediately affected oxidative flavour deterioration in fish oil enriched milk. Thus, it was shown that pasteurised milk emulsions based on cod liver oil with a slightly elevated peroxide value (PV) of 1.5 meq/kg oxidised significantly faster than a similar emulsion containing tuna oil with a low PV of 0.1 meq/kg despite the fact that the tuna oil was more unsaturated than the cod liver oil. It was suggested that the slightly elevated level of lipid hydroperoxides in combination with trace metals present in the milk were responsible for the rapid oxidative flavour deterioration of the cod liver oil enriched milk due to the ability of trace metals to decompose lipid hydroperoxides. A subsequent study supported these findings and also showed that a sensory panel was able to distinguish milk emulsions produced with fish oil with a PV of 0.1 meq/kg as being less fishy and rancid as compared to milk produced with fish oil having a PV of 0.5 meq/kg already after one day of storage (Let *et al.* 2005b). Further studies in our laboratory have shown that the quality of the fish oil seems to be less important in yoghurt-like products than in pasteurised milk emulsions (Let *et al.* 2007a). This is most likely due to the fact that yoghurt-like products enriched with omega-3 PUFA seems to be less susceptible to oxidation than omega-3 PUFA enriched milk (Nielsen *et al.* 2007). Recently, we reported that one of the reasons for the high oxidative stability of fish oil enriched yoghurt is that peptides formed during the fermentation of milk have antioxidative properties that are able to reduce the rate at which the omega-3 PUFAs oxidise (Farvin *et al.* 2010a, 2010b).

17.5.2   The influence of emulsifiers and pH

During the emulsification process, emulsifiers are added to promote droplet disruption and stabilise the emulsion. Emulsifiers are surface active molecules with amphiphilic properties, which can interact with the oil-water interface and reduce surface tension. Emulsifiers for food use are either macromolecules, such as proteins unfolding at the interface, or smaller surfactant molecules, such as phospholipids, free fatty acids, monoacylglycerols, diacylglycerols and synthetic surfactants. Due to their ability to interact with other ingredients near the oil-water interface, emulsifiers are able to influence lipid oxidation in different ways. In emulsions stabilised by proteins, pH will generally be either below or above the pI of the protein in order to avoid coalescence of droplets. This results in an either positive or negative surface charge of these droplets. Similarly, charged droplets may also be obtained in emulsions with certain surfactants such as charged phospholipids. The surface charge of emulsion droplets is important for lipid oxidation catalysed by the presence of trace metal ions, such as Fe^{2+}. Negatively charged emulsion droplets will attract trace metals, which are potentially prooxidative, and bring them into closer proximity of the omega-3 PUFA oil and this may promote lipid oxidation. If instead an emulsifier, which creates a positive charge of the droplets, is chosen, trace metals are repelled and oxidation is likely to be reduced (Mei *et al.* 1998). Therefore, the emulsifier should be carefully selected for omega-3 PUFA enriched foods. Practically all food products contain some amount of trace metals and the solubility of trace metals generally increases at decreasing pH (Belitz & Grosch 1999), which potentially can promote oxidation. Therefore, pH of the given food should also be taken into consideration when choosing an appropriate emulsifier for omega-3 PUFA-enriched food emulsions.

Apart from influencing the charge of the emulsifier, pH can also influence oxidation via its ability to affect the emulsifier in other ways. For example, (Jacobsen *et al.* 1999, 2001c) observed that in fish oil enriched mayonnaise lipid oxidation increased when pH was decreased from 6.0 to 3.8. In mayonnaise, egg yolk is used as an emulsifier and egg yolk contains large amounts of iron, which is bound to the protein phosvitin. At the natural pH of egg yolk (pH 6.0), the iron forms cation bridges between phosvitin and other components in egg yolk, namely low density lipoproteins (LDL) and lipovitellin. These components are located at the oil–water interface in mayonnaise. It was therefore hypothesised that when pH is decreased to around 4.0, which is the pH used in mayonnaise, the cation bridges between the before-mentioned egg yolk components are broken and iron becomes dissociated from LDL and lipovitellin. Thereby, iron becomes more active as a catalyst of oxidation (Jacobsen *et al.* 1999, 2001c). Hence, the low pH in combination with the-iron rich egg yolk is the driving force for the rapid oxidation processes in fish oil enriched mayonnaise. It was hypothesised that substitution of egg yolk with a less iron rich emulsifier such as milk protein may reduce oxidation. This strategy was recently evaluated in a light mayonnaise (Sørensen *et al.* 2010a). However, this hypothesis could not be confirmed with the milk protein based emulsifier used in their study. The main reason was suggested to be the low quality of the milk protein based emulsifier, which had 50 times higher lipid hydroperoxide content than the egg yolk. Therefore, it was concluded that not only the iron content, but also the initial oxidative quality of the emulsifier is crucial for the oxidative stability of fish oil enriched mayonnaise. It therefore remains to be proven that the use of a high quality milk protein will have a positive impact on the oxidative stability of fish oil enriched mayonnaise.

17.5.3   Delivery systems

The strategy to reduce oxidation by careful selection of the emulsifier can be taken one step further by using a so-called interfacial engineering strategy. The idea behind this strategy is to design an oxidatively stable simple o/w emulsion by selecting an emulsifier, which will protect the omega-3 PUFA against oxidation and subsequently use this emulsion as a delivery system for omega-3 PUFA. Oxidatively stable o/w emulsions can be obtained by using positively charged proteins as emulsifiers as described by Djordjevic, McClements, and Decker (2004) who evaluated both sodium caseinate and whey protein as emulsifiers. They concluded that whey protein was more suitable as emulsifiers for omega-3 PUFA emulsion delivery systems than sodium caseinate.

The ability of the use of an omega-3 PUFA delivery system to reduce lipid oxidation has been evaluated in different omega-3 enriched food products. (Park *et al.* 2004) used an emulsion based on whey protein isolate as delivery system in omega-3 PUFA enriched surimi. Likewise, Lee *et al.* (2006a) used emulsions with whey protein isolates as emulsifiers as omega-3 delivery systems in turkey and pork patties. The use of an emulsion delivery system was, however, not sufficient to protect the omega-3 oil against oxidation, but addition of an antioxidant mixture containing sodium erythorbate, sodium citrate and rosemary extract could reduce oxidation to the same level as in the control samples without omega-3 oil.

The effect on lipid oxidation of the delivery system for omega-3 PUFAs has also been evaluated in fish oil enriched milk, dressing and yoghurt. Omega-3 PUFAs were thus added either as neat oil or as an oil-in-water emulsion (50% oil) prepared with whey protein as an emulsifier (Let *et al.* 2007). Volatiles and sensory data indicated a better oxidative stability of dressing and yoghurt with neat fish oil compared to the corresponding products with the fish oil-in-water emulsion (Fig. 17.3). So, in these food systems pre-emulsification of the fish oil did not lead to increased oxidative stability. The authors suggested that this finding could be due to increased oxidation in the fish oil-in-water emulsion itself, which was caused by the initial temperature increase (65 °C, 3 min) during homogenisation of this emulsion. They also concluded that addition of antioxidants before homogenisation of the pre-emulsion may be necessary to improve its oxidative stability. However, in the case of milk the use of a delivery system did improve the oxidative stability. A similar positive effect of using a delivery system, either in the form of a microencapsulated powder or a fish oil-in-water emulsion, was observed for fitness bar (Nielsen and Jacobsen 2009). These findings clearly demonstrate that delivery systems may have to be optimised for different products.

17.5.4 Choice of other ingredients than emulsifier

Recently, the effect of fish oil addition on the oxidative stability of fish oil enriched mayonnaise and mayonnaise-based shrimp and tuna salad was reported (Sørensen

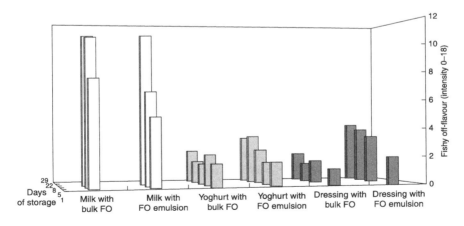

Fig. 17.3 Summarised intensity of fishy odour and flavour of milk, yoghurt and dressing enriched with either neat fish oil (FO) or fish oil-in-water emulsion. Reprinted with permission from Let *et al.* (2007b) (Copyright 2010 American Chemical Society).

et al. 2009). In the same study, the effect on lipid oxidation of the seafood and vegetables added to the salads was also evaluated. Interestingly, the product type and ingredients had a greater influence on lipid oxidation than substitution of 10% of the soya oil with fish oil. A sensory panel could not significantly distinguish the intensity of rancid off-flavour in salads without fish oil from that in salads with fish oil throughout the storage period (57 days) for both salad types, except for tuna salads for which the rancid intensity was higher in the fish oil enriched sample at the very end of the storage period (day 57) only. These results thus indicated that it was possible to add fish oil to these two salad types without compromising the sensory properties if the labelled shelf life was kept below 57 days.

The tuna salads were more oxidised than the shrimp salads, which were more oxidised than the mayonnaise. The higher degree of oxidation in tuna salads compared to mayonnaise and shrimp salads was suggested to be due to the heme content in tuna. Further, it was found that for the shrimp salads, addition of shrimp had a prooxidative effect, whereas asparagus had an antioxidative effect, which was efficient enough to prevent the proxidative effect of the shrimps in this type of salad. For the tuna salad the influence of ingredients herein seemed more complex and it was not possible to draw clear conclusions on the effect of the ingredients. This was suggested to be due to fact that an already high concentration of volatiles in the ingredients might have masked any inhibiting effect on the formation of volatiles, which was used as an important parameter for evaluating oxidation (Sørensen *et al.* 2009).

17.5.5   The effect of the emulsification conditions and droplet size

Preparation of omega-3 enriched food emulsions should be done under optimal conditions to minimise oxidation. One important parameter is the exclusion of air/oxygen. Several studies have shown that a reduction of the access of oxygen during production retards lipid oxidation (Genot *et al.* 2003). Reduction of oxygen can be achieved by processing under vacuum or in a nitrogen atmosphere. This would additionally reduce the amount dissolved or trapped oxygen in the final product, which otherwise would promote oxidation. In the final product, exclusion of headspace oxygen can be obtained by packaging in an air-tight container impermeable to oxygen, and preferably under modified atmosphere. Moreover, both processing and storage temperature should generally be as low as possible.

However, in some cases a low homogenisation temperature will not result in the best oxidative stability. This was recently illustrated in two studies with fish oil enriched milk by (Let *et al.* 2006a; Sorensen *et al.* 2007). In both studies, fish oil was incorporated into milk at different conditions of homogenisation, i.e. different temperatures (50 and 72°C) and pressures (5, 15 and 22.5 MPa). Surprisingly, the highest oxidative stability was obtained at high homogenisation pressure (22.5 MPa) and temperature (72°C), even though the droplet size was smallest under these conditions. A small droplet size and thereby a large interfacial area may in some cases lead to increased oxidation, but this was not the case for omega-3 enriched milk emulsions. It was shown by SDS-PAGE and confocal laser scanning microscopy that a temperature increase from 50°C to 72°C led to an increase in the amount of β-lactoglobulin adsorbed at the oil-water interface and that even more β-lactoglobulin was adsorbed when the pressure was increased from 5 MPa to 22.5 MPa (Sørensen *et al.* 2007) (Table 17.1). In addition, the level of free thiol groups was increased at the high temperature and pressure (72°C and 22.5 MPa), whereas less casein seemed to be present at the oil–water interface with increasing pressure. It was hypothesised that a combination of more β-lactoglobulin and less casein at the oil–water interface was responsible for the increased oxidative stability. Hence, these results demonstrated that the composition of the interface is very important and that thermal oxidation may not necessarily trigger lipid oxidation. Rather, in the case of milk emulsions this high temperature can result in unfolding of the proteins at the interface, which in turn gives the highest protection against oxidation.

As already mentioned the emulsification conditions will affect the droplet size of the emulsion. Usually, a small oil droplet size is preferred in order to increase the physical stability of the emulsions, but this will also result in the formation of a large interfacial area, i.e. a large contact area between the oil and water phase. Initiation of lipid oxidation is suggested to occur at this interface (Frankel 1991), as the oil droplets becomes exposed to the water soluble prooxidants and dissolved oxygen via diffusion through the interfacial membrane. Therefore, in some food emulsions a small droplet size could potentially increase oxidation rate as demonstrated in fish oil enriched mayonnaise (Jacobsen *et al.* 2000b). However, as already mentioned a similar prooxidative effect of the droplet size was not observed in fish oil enriched milk (Let *et al.* 2007b) and this clearly demonstrates that no general recommendation regarding the droplet size can be made.

Table 17.1   Relative quantities of β-lactoglobulin, κ-casein, β-casein, α_{s1}-casein and α_{s2}-casein isolated from the milk fat globule membrane (MFGM) in milk emulsions produced under different homogenisation conditions and from reference milk (without oil added and no further homogenisation)

MFGM sample						
Pressure (MPa)	Temperature (°C)	β-Lactoglobulin	κ-Casein	β-Casein	α_{s1}-Casein	α_{s2}-Casein
5	50	8.01	16.10	5.07	5.94	5.14
	72	10.17	15.94	3.67	4.28	4.09
15	50	9.36	14.97	4.34	5.21	5.08
	72	14.56	14.17	3.65	4.55	4.59
22.5	50	9.45	14.93	5.18	4.56	4.23
	72	13.72	15.86	4.78	3.68	3.74
Reference	No treatment	4.92	17.95	5.74	5.18	4.19

Source: reproduced from Sørensen *et al.* (2007). Copyright 2010 American Chemical Society.

17.6   The effect of antioxidant addition

In this section reported effects of a range of different antioxidants in omega-3 enriched food products will be summarised. Some of the antioxidants are not commercially available, but has been included to illustrate the on-going efforts to search for more efficient and natural antioxidants or antioxidants based on natural compounds.

17.6.1   Effect of tocopherols

Tocopherols have been evaluated in fish oil enriched mayonnaise, salad dressing, milk, milk drink and energy bar. Interestingly, tocopherols did not exert significant antioxidative effects in emulsified n-3 PUFA enriched food emulsions, whereas the opposite was the case in energy bars. A mixture of the tocopherol homologues were thus found either to promote oxidation in mayonnaise when applied in high concentrations (above 16 mg/kg) or to have either no or a weak effect when applied in lower concentrations (Jacobsen *et al.* 2000a, 2001a, 2008). In salad dressing and milk, γ-tocopherol was found to exert some antioxidative effect depending on its concentration, while α-tocopherol was a prooxidant in milk (Let *et al.* 2005a, 2006b; Jacobsen *et al.* 2008). In milk, the highest antioxidative activity of γ-tocopherol was observed at a concentration of 1.65 mg/kg (Let *et al.* 2005a; Jacobsen *et al.* 2008). In addition, γ-tocopherol was found to have a good antioxidative effect in energy bars with the best protective effect observed at a concentration of 33 mg/kg (Fig. 17.4 (c) and (d)) (Horn *et al.* 2009).

The lacking antioxidative effect of the tocopherols in mayonnaise and salad dressing has previously been suggested to be due the finding that in these food systems oxidation is mainly due to metal catalysed break down of peroxides from n-3 PUFA located in the aqueous phase or at the oil–water interface (Jacobsen *et al.* 2008). Therefore, tocopherol can only to a limited extent reduce oxidation by inhibiting deterioration of n-3 PUFA inside the oil droplet. The finding that tocopherol is an efficient antioxidant in energy bars suggests that free radical scavengers can reduce lipid oxidation in this food system, which means that initiation of lipid oxidation by already existing free radicals may be an important factor (Horn *et al.* 2009).

17.6.2   Effect of ascorbic acid and ascorbyl palmitate

Ascorbic acid has been evaluated in mayonnaise and ascorbyl palmitate in mayonnaise, salad dressing, milk, milk drink and energy bar. Interestingly, ascorbic acid and ascorbyl palmitate exerted strong prooxidative activity in mayonnaise (Jacobsen *et al.* 1999, 2001c, 2008) and energy bars (Horn *et al.* 2009), whereas both weak pro- and antioxidative effects were found in salad dressing (Let *et al.* 2006b) and in milk drink (Jacobsen *et al.* 2008) depending on the concentration applied. For energy bars, the strong prooxidative effect was only observed at high concentrations of ascorbyl palmitate, whereas weaker prooxidative effects were observed at the lowest concentration (Fig. 17.4(a)) (Horn *et al.* 2009). In contrast, ascorbyl palmitate efficiently inhibited oxidative flavour deterioration in milk (Let *et al.* 2005b). The prooxidative effect of ascorbic acid and ascorbyl palmitate in mayonnaise, salad dressing and energy bars were suggested to be due to their ability to reduce Fe^{3+} to Fe^{2+} and in the case of mayonnaise also to release protein-bound iron in the egg yolk located at the oil–water interface into the aqueous phase. The antioxidative effect of ascorbyl palmitate was suggested to be due to its ability to regenerate tocopherol naturally present in the oil. The different effects observed in milk drink and milk was explained by the different compositions of the two milk systems (Jacobsen *et al.* 2008). Thus, whereas fish oil enriched milk did not contain any additives, the milk drink contained emulsifiers and stabilisers, which may have reduced the ability of ascorbyl palmitate to regenerate tocopherol. Another possible explanation for the different effects of ascorbyl palmitate in the two systems could be the different antioxidant concentrations applied in milk and milk drink. It cannot be ruled out that ascorbyl palmitate could also have an antioxidative effect in milk drink at lower concentrations and this might also be the case in energy bars.

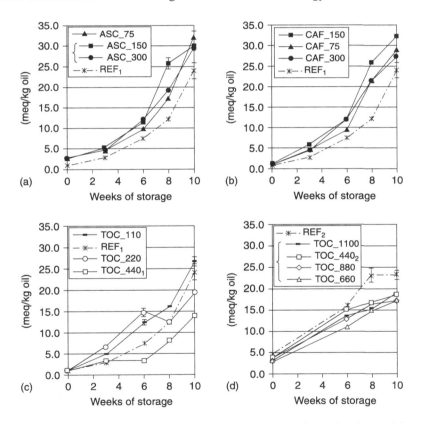

Fig. 17.4 Effect of ascorbyl palmitate (a), caffeic acid (b) and tocopherol (c and d) on formation of lipid hydroperoxides (PV) in fish oil enriched energy bars. ASC = ascorbyl palmitate, CAF = caffeic acid, TOC = γ-tocopherol, REF = reference sample without antioxidants. Numbers after sample indicate concentration of antioxidant in μg/g fish oil. Reprinted with permission from Horn *et al.* (2009) (Copyright 2010 Elsevier).

17.6.3   Effect of lactoferrin

Lactoferrin as an iron-bearing protein present in milk. Lactoferrin has only been evaluated in fish oil enriched mayonnaise and milk drink. In both systems it appeared to exhibit a concentration dependent effect, but even at its optimum level it only exerted a weak antioxidative effect (Nielsen *et al.* 2004; Jacobsen *et al.* 2008). The poor antioxidative effect of lactoferrin may be due to its relatively low binding constant towards Fe^{3+}, which may imply that it is not able to bind iron in an efficient manner. It is also possible that lactoferrin loses its metal chelating properties at the low pH values in mayonnaise (pH 4) or during heating processes as that used to prepare the milk drink.

17.6.4   Effect of phenolic acids

Gallic acid has been evaluated in mayonnaise and in milk drink and caffeic acid in energy bars. Generally, these phenolic compounds could not efficiently retard oxidation in the evaluated food and model systems. Gallic acid promoted oxidation in mayonnaise and did not have any clear antioxidative effect in milk drink (Jacobsen *et al.* 2001b; Timm-Heinrich *et al.* 2003). Caffeic acid strongly promoted oxidative flavour deterioration in energy bars (Fig. 17.4(b)) (Horn *et al.* 2009). Their prooxidative effects were suggested to be due to their ability to reduce Fe^{3+} to Fe^{2+}, which is more active and will then promote oxidation.

Phenolic acids and several other phenolic compounds are polar compounds that to a high degree will be localised in the aqueous phase of emulsions, where they cannot exert their antioxidative activity. It has therefore been suggested that lipophilisation of the compounds by esterification with fatty acids could improve their efficacy. This strategy has recently been evaluated in fish oil enriched emulsion (simple model system) and milk (Sørensen 2010). Two different phenolic compounds were esterified (dihydrocaffeic acid and rutin) with different fatty acids (C8 or C18 and C12 and C16, respectively). In the o/w emulsion, octyl dihydrocaffeate and oleyl dihydrocaffeate were stronger antioxidants than dihydrocaffeic acid, which acted as a prooxidant (Sørensen 2010). Moreover, octyl dihydrocaffeate was more efficient than oleyl dihydrocaffeate and this finding supported a recently reported cut-off effect, which suggested that lipophilisation will only increase antioxidant efficacy in emulsions up to a chain length of 12 carbon atoms in the acyl chain (Laguerre *et al.* 2009). The cut off effect was suggested to be due to formation of micelles when the acyl chain is longer than 12 carbon atoms. In fish oil enriched milk octyl dihydrocaffeate was also more efficient as antioxidant compared to oleyl dihydrocaffeate; however, the differences in their antioxidant efficacy was not as big as observed in the o/w emulsions (Sørensen 2010). Furthermore, rutin esters were stronger antioxidants than rutin in fish oil enriched milk and the same effect of the chain length as observed for dihydrocaffeic acid esters was also observed here (Sørensen 2010) On the basis of the these results it was concluded that the cut-off effect was not only specific for the individual lipophilised phenolic compounds, but also depending on the emulsion system, e.g. simple emulsions and complex food emulsions. However, to be able to further conclude on the optimal acyl chain esterified to dihydrocaffeate and rutin in relation to their strongest antioxidant protection, further research is needed with several different acyl chain lengths and in a range of different emulsion systems.

17.6.5   Effect of synthetic antioxidants and synergism between natural and synthetic antioxidants

Our laboratory has also evaluated the effect of synthetic antioxidants, notably the metal chelator EDTA, in mayonnaise, dressing, milk and milk drink (Jacobsen *et al.* 2008). The results showed that EDTA efficiently prevented oxidation in mayonnaise, salad dressing and milk drink, where it exerted up to 94% reduction in fishy flavour formation in both mayonnaise and milk drink. Moreover, it was found that the antioxidative efficacy of EDTA in salad dressing could be further improved by the simultaneous addition of γ-tocopherol and ascorbyl palmitate (Let *et al.* 2006b). Similar effects may be foreseen in mayonnaise. EDTA did not have a clear antioxidative effect in fish oil enriched milk or in energy bars (Let *et al.* 2003; Nielsen & Jacobsen 2009).

Olsen *et al.* (2006) evaluated the antioxidative effect of addition of citric acid (3300 mg/kg) or EDTA (75 mg/kg) to salmon pâté containing 14% cod liver oil. The fish oil producer had added α-tocopherol (1075 mg/kg), lecithin (1050 mg/kg) and ascorbyl palmitate (375 mg/kg) to the cod liver oil, which was used in this experiment. Analysis of volatiles by gas chromatography–mass spectrometry (GC–MS) as well as sensory analysis suggested that neither citric acid nor EDTA were efficient antioxidants in this food system. In fact, citric acid and EDTA even slightly promoted formation of volatile oxidation products. EDTA had a small positive impact on the sensory perception of the samples, whereas citric acid seemed to slightly increase scores for rancidity. The authors suggested that the poor effect of citric acid was partly due to the fact that addition of citric acid reduced pH, which in some cases has been shown to increase oxidation. Likewise, it was suggested that the increased formation of volatiles in samples with EDTA was due to a too low EDTA concentration.

In another study, the antioxidative effect of EDTA was evaluated in cod surimi enriched with 1.5% algal oil (Park *et al.* 2004). The algal oil was added either as neat oil or as an oil-in-water emulsion. Two different algal oils were evaluated; one without antioxidants added and one with lipid soluble antioxidants (1000 mg/kg tocopherol mixture plus 1000 mg/kg rosemary extract plus 500 mg/kg ascorbyl palmitate). EDTA did not have any effect in cod surimi with neat oil containing lipid soluble antioxidants when evaluated by determination of PV and 2-thiobarbituric acid reactive substances (TBARS). In contrast, an antioxidative effect of EDTA was observed when the algal oil was added to the cod surimi as an emulsion with lipid soluble antioxidants.

Pérez-Mateos *et al.* (2006) also studied the oxidative stability of fish oil enriched surimi in the presence of different antioxidant. In this study, surimi was made from pollock muscle to which menhaden oil or a fish oil concentrate was added, each in two concentrations (7.0 or 11.6% for menhaden oil and 1.7 or 2.8% for the fish oil concentrate). Menhaden oil contained a mixture of tocopherol plus tertiary butyl hydroquinone (TBHQ) added by the fish oil manufacturer, whereas the fish oil concentrate only contained a mixture of tocopherols. Surimi enriched with menhaden oil received better sensory scores than surimi enriched with fish oil concentrate, mainly due to the fact that the latter had a fishy taste. Rosemary (750 mg/kg) or tea extracts (650 mg/kg) were able to partially mask this fishy taste. But both extracts seemed to have weak prooxidative effects in surimi with menhaden oil (Pérez-Mateos et al. 2006).

Lee et al. (2005) evaluated the effect of antioxidant combinations in ground beef patties enriched with 500 mg omega-3 PUFA/110 g meat. The effect of BHA (0.1 mg/kg), a tocopherol mixture (0.3 mg/kg) or rosemary (2 mg/kg) as well as two antioxidant cocktails (1 mg/kg erythorbate + 5 mg/kg citrate + 0.3 mg/kg toco-mix or 1 mg/kg erythorbate + 5 mg/kg citrate + 2 mg/kg rosemary) were evaluated. TBARS decreased in beef patties containing the rosemary extract or BHA, but increased upon addition of the tocopherol mixture. When the antioxidant cocktails were used a decrease in both TBARS and discoloration was observed. Interestingly, control sample without omega-3 PUFA oxidised more than omega-3 PUFA fortified ground beef patties without antioxidants. This finding was suggested to be due to the antioxidative effect of the tocopherols present in the fish oil itself.

Lee et al. (2006a) investigated the effect of an antioxidant cocktail in ground turkey enriched with an algal oil emulsion prepared from: 25% algal oil + 2.5% whey protein isolate + 10 mM sodium citrate + 0.2% potassium sorbate + 500 mg/kg 70% toco-mix + 100 μM EDTA. Ground turkey contained 500 mg omega-3 PUFA/110 g meat. The antioxidant cocktail consisted of 1000 mg/kg sodium erythorbate + 5 mg/kg sodium citrate + 2 mg/kg rosemary extract. Addition of the antioxidant cocktail to the algal oil fortified product lowered TBARS. In fact, no increase in TBARS was seen over time in the product with antioxidants. Further, there was no difference in sensory scores for overall liking between the control samples without omega-3 PUFAs and the ground turkey with omega-3 PUFA and antioxidants. Despite this it was found that the antioxidant cocktail did not prevent a loss of omega-3 PUFAs after frozen storage and cooking of the ground turkey. The omega-3 PUFA level was thus reduced to approximately 65% of the original level present in fresh ground turkey.

The effect of the same antioxidant cocktail was also investigated in restructured hams and pork sausages enriched with the same algal oil emulsion and in the same concentration as above (Lee et al. 2006b). The antioxidant cocktail appeared to be able to control the level of lipid hydroperoxides in the restructured ham. Moreover, nitrite curing of this product delayed lipid oxidation to such an extent that it was no longer possible to determine any effect of the antioxidant treatment when evaluated by TBARS. However, sensory scores for overall liking were lower for the omega-3 enriched product. For pork sausages, the results were quite similar to those of ground turkey. Thus, addition of the antioxidant cocktail resulted in lower and stable TBARS that did not increase over time and there was no difference in the sensory scores for overall liking between the control samples without omega-3 PUFAs and the sausages with omega-3 PUFAs and antioxidants.

17.6.6   Effect of spices and spice extracts

Spices, spice and green tea extracts have been shown to improve the oxidative stability of complex food system such as fish oil enriched tuna salads and milk (Sørensen *et al.* 2010a). Oregano, thyme and rosemary increased the oxidative stability of fish oil enriched tuna salads. Moreover, rosemary and green tea extracts also improved the oxidative stability of fish oil enriched milk. However, the dry spices and rosemary and green tea extracts led to undesirable flavours in the traditional tuna salads and milk. Therefore, they cannot be used for these products, at least not in the concentrations tested.

Valencia *et al.* (2008) investigated antioxidant effects of green tea catechins (200 mg/kg) and green coffee antioxidants (200 mg/kg) in omega-3 enriched pork sausages. In this study, 4.9% fish oil was added in the form of an oil-in-water emulsion prepared with soy protein as emulsifier. Green tea catechins significantly reduced lipid oxidation as evaluated from TBARS, whereas green coffee antioxidants did not have any effect. The authors did not suggest any explanation to the different effects obtained by the green tea catechins and the green coffee antioxidants.

17.7   Future trends

According to several market analyses, it is expected that the growth in the number of new omega-3 PUFA enriched products will continue in the coming years in different food categories. This will require an increasing supply of omega-3 lipids to the food industry. As previously mentioned the supply of fish oils to the food and aquaculture industry cannot be expected to increase. Development of alternative omega-3 PUFA sources will therefore receive increasing attention. Such alternative sources may be oils from micro- and macroalgae, bacteria and GMO plants.

Traditionally, the industry has mainly used free radical chain-breaking synthetic antioxidants for the prevention of oxidation in foods. As mentioned above this strategy seems to be less efficient in preventing lipid oxidation in many food systems enriched with omega-3 PUFAs. With our increased understanding of the important role of trace metals, emulsifiers and processing conditions in lipid oxidation processes, more efforts will be dedicated to use this knowledge to develop alternative strategies to retard lipid oxidation in real foods with omega-3 PUFA oils. One such strategy may be an increased use of both natural metal chelators including plant extracts with both radical scavenging and metal chelating properties. Improvement of antioxidant efficacies by esterification with fatty acids of such compounds can also be expected to receive more attention. Another strategy may be to design oxidatively stable oil-in-water emulsion delivery systems for each particular food system.

17.8   Sources of further information and advice

The Omega-3 Information Network at:
PO Box 24, Tiverton,

Devon EX16 4QQ, UK.
Tel: +44 (0) 1884-257547, Fax: +44 (0) 1884-242757
E-mail: rayrice@eclipse.co.uk

International Fishmeal & Fish Oil Organisation
2 College Yard, Lower Dagnall Street
St. Albans, Hertfordshire AL3 4P4, UK
E-mail: secretariat@iffo.org.uk

Oils and Fats International DMG World Media (UK) Ltd Queensway House,
2 Queensway, Redhill Surrey RH1 1QS, UK Tel: +44 (0) 1737 855068, Fax: +44
(0) 1737 855470 Email: anitarevis@uk.dmgworldmedia.com
The Fish Foundation: http://www.fish-foundation.org.uk/references.htm

Fish Oil. Technology, Nutrition and Marketing. Hamilton, R.J. and Rice, R.D.
(eds) PJ Barnes & Associates, Bucks, UK, 1995.
GOED (Association of the processors, refiners, manufacturers, distributors,
marketers, retailers and supporters of products containing Eicosapentaenoic
Acid (EPA) and Docosahexaenoic Acid (DHA) – Omega-3 Long Chain
Polyunsaturated Fatty Acids (LCPUFAs). http://goedomega3.com.s12.
dotnetpanel.net/

17.9   References

Albert, C. M., Hennekens, C. H., O'Donnell, C. J., Ajani, U. A., Carey, V. J., *et al.* (1998)
    'Fish consumption and risk of sudden cardiac death', *Jama-Journal of the American
    Medical Association*, vol. **279**, no. 1, pp. 23–28.
Bajpai, P., Bajpai, P. K., and Ward, O. P. (1991) 'Production of docosahexaenoic acid by
    thraustochytrium-aureum', *Applied Microbiology and Biotechnology*, vol. **35**, no. 6, pp.
    706–710.
Belitz, H.-D. and Grosch, W. 1999, *Food Chemistry*, 2nd edn, Springer Verlag, Berlin,
    Heidelberg, Germany.
Belluzzi, A., Boschi, S., Brignola, C., Munarini, A., Cariani, G., and Miglio, F. (2000)
    'Polyunsaturated fatty acids and inflammatory bowel disease', *American Journal of
    Clinical Nutrition*, vol. **71**, no. 1, pp. 339S–342S.
Broughton, K. S., Johnson, C. S., Pace, B. K., Liebman, M., and Kleppinger, K. M. (1997)
    'Reduced asthma symptoms with n-3 fatty acid ingestion are related to 5-series
    leukotriene production', *American Journal of Clinical Nutrition*, vol. **65**, no. 4, pp.
    1011–1017.
de Leiris, J., de Lorgeril, M., and Boucher, F. (2009) 'Fish oil and heart health', *Journal of
    Cardiovascular Pharmacology*, vol. **54**, no. 5, pp. 378–384.
Djordjevic, D., McClements, D. J., and Decker, E. A. (2004) 'Oxidative stability of whey
    protein-stabilized oil-in-water emulsions at pH 3: Potential omega-3 fatty acid delivery
    systems (Part B)', *Journal of Food Science*, vol. **69**, no. 5, pp. C356–C362.
Dyerberg, J. and Bang, H. O. (1979) 'Hemostatic function and platelet polyunsaturated
    fatty-acids in eskimos', *Lancet*, vol. **2**, no. 8140, pp. 433–435.
Farvin, K. H. S., Baron, C. P., Nielsen, N. S., Jacobsen, C. (2010a) 'Antioxidant activity of
    yoghurt peptides: Part 1 – *in vitro* assays and evaluation in ω-3 enriched milk', *Food
    Chemistry* (accepted).

Farvin, K. H. S., Baron, C. P., Nielsen, N. S., Jeanette Otte, Jacobsen, C. (2010b) 'Antioxidant activity of yoghurt peptides: Part 2 – characterisation of peptide fractions', *Food Chemistry* (accepted)

Frankel, E. N. (1991) 'Review. Recent advances in lipid oxidation', *J. Sci. Food Agric.*, vol. **54**, pp. 495–511.

Frankel, E. N. (2005) *Lipid Oxidation*, 2nd edn, The Oily Press, Dundee.

Frankel, E. N., Satue-Gracia, T., Meyer, A. S., and German, J. B. (2002) 'Oxidative stability of fish and algae oils containing long- chain polyunsaturated fatty acids in bulk and in oil-in-water emulsions', *Journal of Agricultural and Food Chemistry*, vol. **50**, no. 7, pp. 2094–2099.

Frankel, E. N., Selke, E., Neff, W. E., and Miyashita, K. (1992) 'Autoxidation of polyunsaturated triacylglycerols. 4. Volatile decomposition products from triacylglycerols containing linoleate and linolenate', *Lipids*, vol. **27**, no. 6, pp. 442–446.

Genot, C., Meynier, A., and Riaublanc, A. (2003) 'Lipid oxidation in emulsions', in *Lipid Oxidation Pathways*, A. Kamal-Eldin (ed.), AOCS Press, Champaign, IL, pp. 190–244.

Harris, W. S. (1989) 'Fish oils and plasma-lipid and lipoprotein metabolism in humans – a critical review', *Journal of Lipid Research*, vol. **30**, no. 6, pp. 785–807.

Hartvigsen, K., Lund, P., Hansen, L. F., and Holmer, G. (2000) 'Dynamic headspace gas chromatography/mass spectrometry characterization of volatiles produced in fish oil enriched mayonnaise during storage', *Journal of Agricultural and Food Chemistry*, vol. **48**, no. 10, pp. 4858–4867.

Horn, A. F., Nielsen, N. S., & Jacobsen, C. (2009) 'Addition of caffeic acid, ascorbyl palmitate or γ-tocopherol to fish oil enriched energy bars affects lipid oxidation differently', *Food Chemistry*, vol. **112**, pp. 412–420.

Hu, F. B., Bronner, L., Willett, W. C., Stampfer, M. J., Rexrode, K. M., *et al.* (2002) 'Fish and omega-3 fatty acid intake and risk of coronary heart disease in women', *Jama-Journal of the American Medical Association*, vol. **287**, no. 14, pp. 1815–1821.

Iso, H., Rexrode, K. M., Stampfer, M. J., Manson, J. E., Colditz, G. A., *et al.* (2001) 'Intake of fish and omega-3 fatty acids and risk of stroke in women', *Jama-Journal of the American Medical Association*, vol. **285**, no. 3, pp. 304–312.

Jacobsen, C., Adler-Nissen, J., and Meyer, A. S. (1999) 'Effect of ascorbic acid on iron release from the emulsifier interface and on the oxidative flavor deterioration in fish oil enriched mayonnaise', *Journal of Agricultural and Food Chemistry*, vol. **47**, no. 12, pp. 4917–4926.

Jacobsen, C., Hartvigsen, K., Lund, P., Adler-Nissen, J., Holmer, G., and Meyer, A. S. (2000a) 'Oxidation in fish-oil-enriched mayonnaise 2. Assessment of the efficacy of different tocopherol antioxidant systems by discriminant partial least squares regression analysis', *European Food Research and Technology*, vol. **210**, no. 4, pp. 242–257.

Jacobsen, C., Hartvigsen, K., Lund, P., Thomsen, M. K., Skibsted, L. H., *et al.* (2000b) 'Oxidation in fish oil-enriched mayonnaise 3. Assessment of the influence of the emulsion structure on oxidation by discriminant partial least squares regression analysis', *European Food Research and Technology*, vol. **211**, no. 2, pp. 86–98.

Jacobsen, C., Hartvigsen, K., Lund, P., Thomsen, M. K., Skibsted, L. H., *et al.* (2001a) 'Oxidation in fish oil-enriched mayonnaise: 4. Effect of tocopherol concentration on oxidative deterioration', *European Food Research and Technology*, vol. **212**, no. 3, pp. 308–318.

Jacobsen, C., Hartvigsen, K., Thomsen, M. K., Hansen, L. F., Lund, P., *et al.* (2001b) 'Lipid oxidation in fish oil enriched mayonnaise: Calcium disodium ethylenediaminetetraacetate, but not gallic acid, strongly inhibited oxidative deterioration', *Journal of Agricultural and Food Chemistry*, vol. **49**, no. 2, pp. 1009–1019.

Jacobsen, C., Timm, M., and Meyer, A. S. (2001c) 'Oxidation in fish oil enriched mayonnaise: Ascorbic acid and low pH increase oxidative deterioration', *Journal of Agricultural and Food Chemistry*, vol. **49**, no. 8, pp. 3947–3956.

Jacobsen, C., Let, M. B., Nielsen, N. S., Meyer, A. S. (2008) 'Antioxidant strategies for preventing oxidative flavour deterioration of foods enriched with n-3 polyunsaturated lipids: A comparative evaluation'. *Trends Food Sci. Technol.*, vol. **19/2**, pp. 76–93.

Karahadian, C. and Lindsay, R. C. (1989) 'Evaluation of compounds contributing characterizing fishy flavors in fish oils', *Journal of the American Oil Chemists Society*, vol. **66**, no. 7, pp. 953–960.

Kendrick, A. and Ratledge, C. (1992) 'Lipids of selected molds grown for production of n-3 and n-6 polyunsaturated fatty-acids', *Lipids*, vol. **27**, no. 1, pp. 15–20.

Kremer, J. M. (2000) 'n-3 Fatty acid supplements in rheumatoid arthritis', *American Journal of Clinical Nutrition*, vol. **71**, no. 1, pp. 349S–351S.

Laguerre, M., Giraldo, L. J. L, Lecomte, J., Figueroa-Espinoza, M. C., Barea, B., *et al.* (2009) 'Chain length affects antioxidant properties of chlorogenate esters in emulsion: The cutoff theory behind the polar paradox', *J. Agric. Food Chem.*, vol. **57**, 11335–11342.

Lee, S., Decker, E.A., Faustman, C., Mancini, R.A. (2005) 'The effects of antioxidant combinations on color and lipid oxidation in n-3 oil fortified ground beef patties', *Meat Science*, vol. **70**, pp. 683–689.

Lee, S., Hernandez, P., Djordjevic, D., Faraji, H., Hollender, R., *et al.* (2006a) 'Effect of antioxidants and cooking on stability of n-3 fatty acids in fortified meat products', *Journal of Food Science*, vol. **71**, pp. 233–238.

Lee, S., Faustman, C., Djordjevic, D., Faraji, H., and Decker, E. A. (2006b) 'Effect of antioxidants on stabilization of meat products fortified with n-3 fatty acids', *Meat Science*, vol. **72**, no. 1, pp. 18–24.

Let, M. B., Jacobsen, C., Frankel, E. N., and Meyer, A. S. (2003) 'Oxidative flavour deterioration of fish oil enriched milk', *European Journal of Lipid Science and Technology*, vol. **105**, no. 9, pp. 518–528.

Let, M. B., Jacobsen, C., and Meyer, A. S. (2005b) 'Sensory stability and oxidation of fish oil enriched milk is affected by milk storage temperature and oil quality', *International Dairy Journal*, vol. **15**, pp. 173–182.

Let, M. B., Jacobsen, C., and Meyer, A. S. (2006b) 'Ascorbyl palmitate, gamma-tocopherol, and EDTA affect lipid oxidation in fish oil enriched salad dressing differently', *Journal of Agricultural and Food Chemistry*.

Let, M. B., Jacobsen, C., and Meyer, A. S. (2004) 'Effects of fish oil type, lipid antioxidants and presence of rapeseed oil on oxidative flavour stability of fish oil enriched milk', *European Journal of Lipid Science and Technology*, vol. **106**, no. 3, pp. 170–182.

Let, M. B., Jacobsen, C., and Meyer, A. S. (2007) 'Lipid oxidation in milk, yoghurt, and salad dressing enriched with neat fish oil or pre-emulsified fish oil', *Journal of Agricultural and Food Chemistry*, vol. **55**, no. 19, pp. 7802–7809.

Let, M. B., Jacobsen, C., Pham, K. A., and Meyer, A. S. (2005a) 'Protection against oxidation of fish-oil-enriched milk emulsions through addition of rapeseed oil or antioxidants', *Journal of Agricultural and Food Chemistry*, vol. **53**, no. 13, pp. 5429–5437.

Let, M. B., Jacobsen, C., Sørensen, A. D. S., and Meyer, A. S. (2006a) 'Homogenization conditions affects the oxidative stability of fish oil enriched milk emulsions: Lipid oxidation', *J Agric Food Chem.*

Mei, L., McClements, D. J., Wu, J., and Decker, E. (1997) 'Iron-catalyzed lipid oxidation in emulsion as affected by surfactant, pH and NaCl', *Food Chemistry*, vol. In press.

Mischoulon, D., Best-Popescu, C., Laposata, M., Merens, W., Murakami, J. L., *et al.* (2008) 'A double-blind dose-finding pilot study of docosahexaenoic acid (DHA) for major depressive disorder', *European Neuropsychopharmacology*, vol. **18**, no. 9, pp. 639–645.

Nielsen, N. S., Debnath, D. and Jacobsen, C. (2007) Oxidative stability of fish oil enriched drinking yoghurt. *International Dairy Journal*, vol. **17**, 1478–1485.

Nielsen, N. S., and Jacobsen, C. (2009) Methods for reducing lipid oxidation in fish-oil-enriched energy bars. *Internat J Food Sci Technol.*, vol. **44**, 1536–1546.

Nielsen, N. S., Petersen, A., Meyer, A. S., Timm-Heinrich, M., and Jacobsen, C. (2004) 'Effects of lactoferrin, phytic acid, and EDTA on oxidation in two food emulsions enriched with long-chain polyunsaturated fatty acids', *Journal of Agricultural and Food Chemistry*, vol. **52**, no. 25, pp. 7690–7699.

Olveira, G., Olveira, C., Acosta, E., Espildora, F., Garrido-Sanchez, L., *et al.* (2010) 'Fatty acid supplements improve respiratory, inflammatory and nutritional parameters in adults with cystic fibrosis', *Archivos de Bronconeumologia*, vol. **46**, no. 2, pp. 70–77.

Oomen, C. M., Feskens, E. J. M., Rasanen, L., Fidanza, F., Nissinen, A. M., *et al.* (2000) 'Fish consumption and coronary heart disease mortality in Finland, Italy, and the Netherlands', *American Journal of Epidemiology*, vol. **151**, no. 10, pp. 999–1006.

Olsen, E., Veberg, A., Vogt, G., Tomic, O., Kirkhus, B., *et al.* (2006) 'Analysis of early lipid oxidation in salmon pâté with cod liver oil and antioxidants', *Journal of Food Science*, vol. **71**, pp. 84–292.

Park, Y., Kelleher, S. D., McClements, D. J., and Decker, E. A. (2004) 'Incorporation and stabilization of omega-3 fatty acids in surimi made from cod, Gadus morhua', *Journal of Agricultural and Food Chemistry*, vol. **52**, no. 3, pp. 597–601.

Pauletto, P., Puato, M., Caroli, M. G., Casiglia, E., Munhambo, A. E., *et al.* (1996) 'Blood pressure and atherogenic lipoprotein profiles of fish-diet and vegetarian villagers in Tanzania: The Lugalawa study', *Lancet*, vol. **348**, no. 9030, pp. 784–788.

Pérez-Mateos, M., Lanier, T. C. and Boyd, L. C. (2006) 'Effects of rosemary and green tea extracts on frozen surimi gels fortified with omega-3 fatty acids', *Journal of the Science of Food and Agriculture*, vol. **86**, pp. 558–567.

Prisco, D., Filippini, M., Paniccia, R., Gensini, G. F., and Serneri, G. G. N. (1995) 'Effect of n-3 fatty-acid ethyl-ester supplementation on fatty-acid composition of the single platelet phospholipids and on platelet functions', *Metabolism-Clinical and Experimental*, vol. **44**, no. 5, pp. 562–569.

Simopoulos, A. P. (1991) 'Omega-3-fatty-acids in health and disease and in growth and development', *American Journal of Clinical Nutrition*, vol. **54**, no. 3, pp. 438–463.

Singh, R. B., Niaz, M. A., Sharma, J. P., Kumar, R., Rastogi, V., and Moshiri, M. (1997) 'Randomized, double-blind, placebo-controlled trial of fish oil and mustard oil in patients with suspected acute myocardial infarction: The Indian experiment of infarct survival', *Cardiovascular Drugs and Therapy*, vol. **11**, no. 3, pp. 485–491.

Siscovick, D. S., Raghunathan, T. E., King, I., Weinmann, S., Wicklund, K. G., *et al.* (1995) 'Dietary intake and cell membrane levels of long-chain n-3 polyunsaturated fatty acids and the risk of primary cardiac arrest', *JAMA*, vol. **274**, no. 17, pp. 1363–1367.

Sijtsma, L. (2004) 'Marine micro-organisms as new sources of n-3 polyunsaturated fatty acids (PUFA)' in Arnoldi, A., *Functional Foods, Cardiovascular Disease and Diabetes*, 333–350.

Spiteller, G. (2005) 'Furan fatty acids: Occurrence, synthesis, and reactions. Are furan fatty acids responsible for the card ioprotective effects of a fish diet?', *Lipids*, vol. **40**, no. 8, pp. 755–771.

Sørensen, A. D. M., Baron, C. P., Let, M. B., Bruggemann, D. A., Pedersen, L. R. L., and Jacobsen, C. (2007) 'Homogenization conditions affect the oxidative stability of fish oil enriched milk emulsions: Oxidation linked to changes in protein composition at the oil-water interface', *Journal of Agricultural and Food Chemistry*, vol. **55**, no. 5, pp. 1781–1789.

Sørensen, A.D.M., Nielsen, N.S., Jacobsen, C. (2010a) 'Oxidative stability of fish oil enriched mayonnaise based salads', *Eur. J. Lipid Sci. Technol.* **112**, 476–487.

Sørensen, A. D. M., Nielsen, N.S., Hyldig G., and Jacobsen, C. (2010b) 'The influence of emulsifier type in fish oil enriched light mayonnaise', *Eur. J. Lipid Sci. Technol.* **112**, 1012–1023.

Sørensen, A. D. M. (2010) 'The influence of ingredients or lipophilized antioxidants on oxidation in fish oil enriched food systems', Ph.d. thesis, National Food Institute, Technical University of Denmark.

Timm-Heinrich, M., Xu, X. B., Nielsen, N. S., and Jacobsen, C. (2003) 'Oxidative stability of milk drinks containing structured lipids produced from sunflower oil and caprylic acid', *European Journal of Lipid Science and Technology*, vol. **105**, no. 8, pp. 459–470.

Trautwein, E. A. (2001) 'N-3 Fatty acids – physiological and technical aspects for their use in food', *European Journal of Lipid Science and Technology*, vol. **103**, no. 1, pp. 45–55.

Valencia, I., O'Grady, M.N., Ansorena, D., Astiasarán, I. and Kerry, J.P. (2008) 'Enhancement of the nutritional status and quality of fresh pork sausages following the addition of linseed oil, fish oil and natural antioxidants', *Meat Science*, vol. **80**, pp. 1046–1054.

van Goor, S. A., jck-Brouwer, D. A. J., Doornbos, B., Erwich, J. J. H. M., Schaafsma, A., *et al.* (2010) 'Supplementation of DHA but not DHA with arachidonic acid during pregnancy and lactation influences general movement quality in 12-week-old term infants', *British Journal of Nutrition*, vol. **103**, no. 2, pp. 235–242.

Venkateshwarlu, G., Let, M. B., Meyer, A. S., and Jacobsen, C. (2004) 'Chemical and olfactometric characterization of volatile flavor compounds in a fish oil enriched milk emulsion', *Journal of Agricultural and Food Chemistry*, vol. **52**, no. 2, pp. 311–317.

Zhang, J. J., Sasaki, S., Amano, K., and Kesteloot, H. (1999) 'Fish consumption and mortality from all causes, ischemic heart disease, and stroke: An ecological study', *Preventive Medicine*, vol. **28**, no. 5, pp. 520–529.

18

Probiotic functional foods

M. H. Saarela, VTT Technical Research Centre of Finland, Finland

Abstract: Traditionally probiotics have been added into fermented dairy products. This is due to the fact that dairy-based matrices are good carriers for probiotic bacteria. Currently, probiotics are available for consumers in an increasing variety of foods, especially non-dairy applications. All food matrices have unique characteristics that can either support the viability of probiotics or be detrimental to it. In food applications the factors that need to be considered include raw materials and additives, the process itself, final product and its properties, storage conditions and shelf-life. In fermented milks, several factors such as pH, organic acids, starter microbes, and potential presence of flavouring compounds and various additives (including preservatives) affect the viability of probiotic bacteria. Processing, storage conditions and shelf-lives of fermented milk products vary considerably and all these factors have an impact on the viability and stability of probiotics added into the product. Similarly to dairy-based matrices, cereal-based food matrices may be quite good supporters of probiotic viability and stability. Milk and many cereals have been shown to contain components (e.g. protein, fat, or fibre) that can protect the viability of added microbes. In shelf-stable beverages one of the most important factors affecting probiotic viability is the pH of the product, where values below 4 are typically detrimental to most probiotic strains. Some vegetable-based probiotic applications exist, although these are few in number compared to fruit-based applications.

Key words: probiotic, *Lactobacillus, Bifidobacterium*, dairy, fruit, vegetable, meat, cereal.

18.1 Introduction to probiotics and their health effects

Probiotics are currently defined as 'live microorganisms which when administered in adequate amounts confer a health benefit on the host' (Anonymous 2002). Probiotics are available for the consumers in foods, food supplements and pharmaceutical products. Lactobacilli and bifidobacteria have been most commonly used as probiotics in food applications in Europe whereas some other microbes (e.g. enterococci, *Saccharomyces* yeasts, *Escherichia coli*) are available as supplements or pharmaceutical products.

The typical benefit associated with probiotics is improving digestive health. Since probiotic functional foods still mostly represent fermented milk products, which are traditionally considered as good for digestion, this association is quite natural. However, quite early on the potential of probiotics to alleviate the symptoms of various health conditions was explored. A common feature with these conditions was that they were considered to be somehow linked to gastrointestinal (GI) tract functions in which microbes play an important role. The health effects related to probiotics today are diverse. These include, for example, alleviation of lactose intolerance symptoms, treatment of viral and antibiotic-associated diarrhoea, reduction of symptoms of antibiotic treatment of *Helicobacter pylori*, alleviation of atopic dermatitis symptoms in children and prevention of the risk of allergy in infancy, alleviation of symptoms of IBD (inflammable bowel disease) and IBS (irritable bowel syndrome) and enhancing the immune response (Reid *et al.* 2003; Culligan *et al.* 2009; Lomax & Calder 2009; Wohlgemuth *et al.* 2009). Other potential benefits have been suggested in colon cancer patients, AIDS and in respiratory and urinary tract infections (Kaur *et al.* 2009). Although probiotic health effects and mechanisms of action have been studied actively for a number of years, some effects that are generally accepted can still remain debatable in critical reviews of the published literature. This is reflected in meta-analysis studies, which have sometimes given contradicting conclusions of the probiotic efficacy and may state that there is either inconclusive or promising but still insufficient data of the clinical efficacy (some of the meta-analysis studies and critical reviews are listed in section 18.8). The reason for this situation is the variety of probiotic products/foods (with e.g. different bacterial strains and daily doses), target consumer groups and study designs, and thus the evidence for a specific probiotic strain consumed in a defined manner by a specific consumer group may remain weak. To overcome this situation, high-quality clinical trials, where proper emphasis is given to a good study design, are still needed to support the probiotic health claims. Probiotic health benefits are discussed in more detail in Part II of this book.

18.2   Probiotic food market in Europe and the United States

Although a fair number of potential probiotic strains have been studied for health-benefiting effects over the years the variety of probiotic strains in foods remains quite limited. This is due to the fact that incorporation into foods sets high demands for the technological robustness of the probiotic strains. Thus many strains that show promising properties during the research phase never make it to the larger scale production phase and actual food markets. In studies by Fasoli *et al.* (2003) and Temmerman *et al.* (2003) performed some years ago, *Bifidobacterium animalis* subsp. *lactis* was the only *Bifidobacterium* species detected in probiotic foods regardless of what was claimed on the food product label (the most commonly used strain being Bb-12). Also, in the study of Masco *et al.* (2005) this subspecies was by far the most commonly detected *Bifidobacterium*. The popularity of *B. animalis* subsp. *lactis* is due to its superior technological properties (e.g. tolerance to oxygen and low pH) compared to other *Bifidobacterium* species (Matsumoto *et al.* 2004; Mättö *et al.* 2004). In Europe *Lactobacillus rhamnosus* GG (LGG) is perhaps the most diversely used probiotic bacterium in various foods, both dairy- and non-dairy-based. Other popular probiotics in Europe with more limited food product ranges include, for example, *Lactobacillus casei/paracasei* (Shirota, Immunitas, F19), *Lactobacillus acidophilus* (La-5), *Lactobacillus plantarum* (299 v), and *Lactobacillus reuteri* (ATCC 55730). The same probiotic strains can also be found in probiotic foods in the United States. Enterococci, although traditionally used in fermented dairy products, are not currently actively promoted as probiotics in Europe due to their higher pathogenic potential compared to bifidobacteria and lactobacilli (Vankerckhoven *et al.* 2008).

Although probiotic foods have been available in Europe for well over ten years the market is still increasing. The total EU market for probiotics was $72.9 million (M) (appr. €51 M) in 2008 and it is expected to reach about $162 M (appr. €113 M) in 2015. In Europe, probiotics have traditionally been incorporated into dairy products, mainly fermented ones such as yoghurt, cheese, cultured buttermilk and dairy drink. Other probiotic food products include milk, ice cream, fruit and berry juices and drinks, recovery drinks, cereal-based drinks and snacks. However, in 2008 yoghurt and yoghurt drinks were still the most common probiotic foods consumed (generating appr. three-quarters of the revenues) and non-dairy probiotic foods, especially those in dry form, have remained fairly marginal (Anonymous 2009a). The strong position of fermented probiotic dairy products, especially those of the yoghurt type, originates from the healthy image of yoghurt and the general knowledge that it contains living (friendly) bacteria that are good for your digestion.

European consumers, unlike US consumers, clearly prefer probiotic foods over supplements: approximately only one in ten consumers uses supplements (Anonymous 2009a). This consumer preference has implications to the probiotic industry. Price consciousness plays a large role when food purchase decisions are made, whereas with food supplements the acceptable price range seems to be much wider. However, the food industry has been able to overcome this limitation by launching single/daily dose probiotic food formats (so called 'shots'). These are typically premium-priced products with a high unit price (per L or kg). Some of the key market participants in the European probiotic market include companies such as Chr Hansen A/S, Danisco A/S, Yakult, Danone, Mead Johnson Nutritionals, Nestlé, Probi AB, BioGaia AB, Royal Numico NV, Valio Ltd, Insititut Rosell and Royal DSM N.V. (Anonymous 2009a).

Unlike Europe the probiotic market in the US is still at an emerging state. American consumers are less aware of probiotics and the concept of beneficial bacteria in general, and furthermore they do not have a strong tradition of eating fermented foods. Thus in the US probiotics have been preferably consumed as supplements (representing about 75% of probiotics in digestive health products). The US market for probiotics for digestive health was about $59 M (appr. €41 M) in 2007. Due to the undeveloped nature of the US probiotic dairy food market it is currently dominated by only a few manufacturers, the most important of these currently being the Danone group (Anonymous 2009b).

18.3   Probiotic technology and challenges in the probiotic formulation into foods

Although the market for probiotic foods has expanded and developed substantially the probiotic industry still faces challenges in issues related to probiotic technology. Since the current definition of probiotics still relies on the concept of consuming live microbes, the food industry needs to ensure the stability and viability of probiotic bacteria throughout the food production chain and during storage. For the successful production of high-quality probiotic products a solid knowledge of the characteristics of the probiotic strain is necessary. The properties of probiotic strains can vary substantially, sometimes even among the strains representing the same species. Thus the special characteristics of probiotic strains have to be taken into account during production and formulation.

Viability losses of probiotics occur easily during processing if the microbes encounter stressful situations and conditions. Microbes can become stressed for several reasons; for example they have unique optimal growth conditions and some strains can be very finicky whereas others are more robust and tolerant. Various downstream processing steps of probiotic production (such as harvesting, freezing, drying and other manipulations) unavoidably cause stress to microbes (Kailasapathy & Rybka 1997; Saarela *et al.* 2000; Heller 2001). Encapsulation is often the only option to maintain the viability of very sensitive strains, but unless very small microcapsules that do not affect the sensory properties of the food can be produced, this approach is not feasible for food industry.

During food formulation of probiotics several factors need to be considered such as the raw materials and additives used (potential nutrients and antimicrobials), structure (oxygen permeability, water activity) and pH of the food matrix, possible interactions with starter microbes, and the food process itself (e.g. potential heating, cooling, mixing and aeration steps). Growth of probiotics in non-fermented foods is not desirable (due to possible off-flavour formation), but their growth during the production of fermented foods can lower process costs and enhance the stability of probiotics later on. The starter microbes in fermented foods can sometimes inhibit probiotics but they can also enhance their survival by producing beneficial substances or by lowering the oxygen pressure (Kailasapathy & Rybka 1997; Saxelin *et al.* 1999; Saarela *et al.* 2000; Vinderola *et al.* 2002b). In beverages the most important factor affecting probiotic viability is probably the pH. Shelf-stable beverages typically have pH values below 4.4 to ensure their microbial stability (Eckert & Riker 2007); e.g. fruit juices usually have a pH below 4 or even 3 (Saarela *et al.* 2006b), and these low pH values combined with long shelf life are very demanding for most probiotic strains.

The final step in the production process of probiotic foods is packaging. The packaging material should be a good oxygen barrier (e.g. glass, aluminium foil, some special plastics) to promote the survival of especially anaerobic probiotic bacteria (bifidobacteria) (Saarela *et al.* 2000; Talwalkar & Kailasapathy 2003; Talwalkar *et al.* 2004; Champagne *et al.* 2005). For most probiotic food products transportation and storage at constant refrigerated temperatures are necessary. Storage temperature is an important determinant of the shelf-life; with increasing temperatures viability losses can occur rapidly (Saxelin *et al.* 1999). The effects of various food processing steps on probiotic viability and stability have been discussed in detail in the review of Champagne *et al.* (2005).

18.4   Probiotic food categories

In this context only foods with added and defined probiotic strains are discussed. Especially in the area of fermented foods, the term probiotic is often used loosely to describe products with natural or added starter bacteria but with no actual added probiotic bacteria. These fermented foods (e.g. kefir, sauerkraut, kimchi, miso, natto and tempeh), which are naturally considered to be beneficial to health due the metabolic activities of starter bacteria, are not included in this chapter. Furthermore, only the main food categories (dairy, vegetable/fruit, cereal and meat) relevant for probiotic applications are discussed here. The main factors affecting probiotic stability in various food matrices are listed in Table 18.1.

Table 18.1   Factors affecting the viability and stability of probiotics in food matrices

Food	Main factors affecting probiotic stability
Fermented drinkable milks	• Presence of starter microbes and their metabolites • pH • Storage time
Yoghurt	• Presence of starter microbes and their metabolites • pH • Natural flavourings (berries, fruits), additives • Storage time
Cheese	• Cheese-making process (including salting and ripening process) • Presence of starter microbes and their metabolites • pH, fat content, structure • Ripening and storage time
Fruit and vegetable juices	• Raw materials and their antimicrobial activity • pH and the nature of organic acids present • Storage time and temperature
Sausages	• Sausage-making process • Ingredients and additives (e.g. salt) • Presence of starter microbes and their metabolites • Storage time and temperature

18.4.1   Dairy-based probiotic foods

Today probiotics can be found in a wide variety of commercial dairy products including yoghurt (also drinks), sour and fresh milk, and cheese. Milk is a good carrier for probiotic strains due to its inherent properties and due to the fact that most milk products (notable exception being ice cream and frozen desserts) are stored at refrigerated temperatures. Several *in vitro* studies have shown that milk or milk components can protect lactic acid bacteria and bifidobacteria against low pH and bile (Conway *et al.* 1987; Charteris *et al.* 1998; Fernández *et al.* 2003; Saarela *et al.* 2006a; Gomes da Cruz *et al.* 2009). The protection against low pH is at least partially explained by the buffering effect of milk, but milk components also have additional protective effects. The protective effect of milk has also been shown *in vivo*, when the survival of differently formulated probiotics through the human gastrointestinal (GI) tract has been studied (Saxelin *et al.* 2003).

Probiotic *Lactobacillus* and *Bifidobacterium* strains typically grow poorly in milk due to their low proteolytic activity, inability to utilise lactose, or due to special needs for certain growth factors missing in milk (Kailasapathy & Rybka 1997; Gomes & Malcata 1999; Østlie *et al.* 2003; Roy 2005). During the production of fermented milks the conditions are often non-optimal for probiotics (e.g. low levels of suitable nutrients, low fermentation temperatures, too-high levels of oxygen, potential production of antimicrobial compounds by starter bacteria, and potential presence of antimicrobial flavour compounds). On the other hand probiotic growth can result in the formation of off-flavours (e.g. bifidobacteria produce acetic acid, which gives a vinegar-like taste) (Kailasapathy & Rybka 1997; Gomes & Malcata 1999; Saarela *et al.* 2000; Heller 2001; Østlie *et al.* 2003). Thus the production process of probiotic fermented milks needs careful optimisation to ensure good sensory properties of the final product and viability of high enough numbers of probiotic cells.

Drinkable fresh and fermented milks

There is relative little published information on the survival of probiotics in non-fermented milk compared to fermented milk products such as yoghurt. Typically probiotics, especially bifidobacteria, survive better in non-fermented milk than in fermented milk. This is mainly due to the higher pH values of non-fermented milk compared to fermented ones, but also the presence of starter bacteria and their other metabolites besides organic acids may negatively affect the stability of probiotics (Kailasapathy & Rybka 1997; Heller 2001). If non-fermented probiotic milk is flavoured with, for example, fruits and berries, the effect of these flavour compounds on the probiotic viability and stability has to be considered (Vinderola *et al.* 2002a, b). One of the factors affecting the stability of bifidobacteria in milk is their oxygen sensitivity, which varies between strains (Roy 2005; Bolduc *et al.* 2006). Electrochemical reduction of milk, as well as deaeration or addition of reducing agents (cysteine) into milk have been shown to enhance the survival of oxygen sensitive bifidobacteria in milk during storage at 7°C (Bolduc *et al.* 2006). However, these approaches may not be feasible during the industrial scale production of probiotic milk.

The relatively good, but strain-specific stability during storage at 4°C in fresh milk has been shown for various probiotic bacteria, e.g. *B animalis* subsp. *lactis* Bb-12, *L. acidophilus* La-5, and various other *Bifidobacterium* and *Lactobacillus* strains (Hughes & Hoover 1995; Sanders *et al.* 1996; Saarela *et al.* 2003, 2006a; Martínez-Villaluenga *et al.* 2006). Encapsulation can improve the survival of the probiotic strain in fresh milk but it can also result in the impairment of the sensory properties of milk (Hansen *et al.* 2002). Since probiotic strains vary in their ability to utilise lactose and milk proteins, the inability to grow in milk can be used as a selection criteria for probiotics for fresh milk applications where the bacterial growth would potentially only lead into impairment of the product's sensory properties.

There are limited data on the survival of probiotics in drinkable fermented milks such as cultured buttermilk. However, there are, or have been, many probiotic drinkable fermented drinks on the market with various *Lactobacillus* species and strains and also with some bifidobacteria (Tamime *et al.* 2005). Antunes *et al.* (2007, 2009) reported a good stability (at 8°C for 4 weeks) for *B. animalis* subsp. *lactis* Bb-12 in buttermilk-like fermented milk. Rodas *et al.* (2002) added a *L. reuteri* strain together with starters to produced cultured buttermilk. The viability of *L. reuteri* remained at a reasonable level (above 10^6 colony forming units (CFU)/ml) at the end of cold storage period (10 days). Hernandez-Mendoza *et al.* (2007) used *Bifidobacterium bifidum* and *L. reuteri* strains to ferment reconstituted whey. *B. bifidum* was more stable than *L. reuteri* in the product. However, the levels of both strains were above 10^6 CFU/ml at the end of the storage period (30 days at 4°C).

Yoghurt
Stability and viability of various probiotic strains in yoghurt has been extensively studied during the past 15 years (see e.g. Lourens-Hattingh & Viljoen, 2001). Probiotic strains have shown variable storage stabilities in yoghurt but, although the conditions in yoghurt are more challenging to probiotics compared to many other dairy products, good viability and storage stability have still been achieved with many *Lactobacillus* species and strains (e.g. Shah *et al.* 1995; Nighswonger *et al.* 1996; Schillinger 1999; Gilliland *et al.* 2002; Martín-Diana *et al.* 2003; Donkor *et al.* 2006). However, of various bifidobacteria only *B. animalis* subsp. *lactis*, due to its good acid and oxygen tolerance, shows good survival in yoghurt (Carr & Ibrahim 2005; Jayamanne & Adams 2006; Oliveira *et al.* 2009). Viability of various probiotic strains in yoghurt, as well as the effect of probiotics on biotechnological characteristics of yoghurt, has been extensively reviewed by Sarkar (2008). In yoghurt the low pH and the presence of organic acids produced by the starter bacteria are the most important factors affecting probiotic viability (Vinderola *et al.* 2002b). Also the overall characteristics of the starter bacteria can affect probiotic viability in yoghurts; this interaction probably being species-specific (Dave & Shah 1997b; Shah & Lankaputhra 1997). Addition of fruits in yoghurt may have a negative effect on the viability of probiotics, since fruits and berries have (variable) antimicrobial activities (Kailasapathy *et al.* 2008).

According to Micanel *et al.* (1997) fat content of the yoghurt, on the other hand, does not seem to have a major effect on probiotic stability. Attempts to compensate the potential viability losses of probiotics with very high inoculation levels may result in an inferior quality of the product (Olson & Aryana 2008); therefore choosing a technologically robust strain is a preferable way of achieving good quality probiotic yoghurt.

Yoghurt mild can be prepared by using *L. acidophilus* instead of *Lactobacillus bulgaricus* in combination with *Streptococcus thermophilus* as starter bacteria. Thus a probiotic *L. acidophilus* strain can be potentially used a starter provided that it is technologically suitable for the process (Heller 2001).

Viability and stability of probiotics in yoghurt has been improved by encapsulation in plain alginate beads (Kailasapathy & Sureeta 2004), in chitosan-coated alginate (Krasaekoopt *et al.* 2006; Capela *et al.* 2006), alginate-starch (Sultana *et al.* 2000; Kailasapathy 2006), alginate-prebiotic (Iyer & Kailasapathy 2005), alginate-pectin (Sandoval-Castilla *et al.* 2010), in whey protein-based matrix (Picot & Lacroix 2004) or by adding prebiotics or cysteine into yoghurt (Dave & Shah 1997a; Capela *et al.* 2006; Oliveira *et al.* 2009; Paseephol & Sherkat 2009). Encapsulation techniques of probiotics for yoghurt manufacture have been discussed in more detail in the review of Krasaekoopt *et al.* (2003).

The effect of packaging materials with different oxygen barrier functions on the survival of probiotic bacteria in yoghurt has been studied by Talwalkar *et al.* (2004). They did not detect any significant differences in the viability of *L. acidophilus* CSCC 2409 and *Bifidobacterium infantis* CSCC 1912 in yoghurts in different packages in the conditions tested, but nevertheless they concluded that in some conditions oxygen likely affects probiotic viability. Earlier, Dave and Shah had shown that the viability of *L. acidophilus* and *Bifidobacterium* spp. (strains specifics were not given) was improved when the dissolved oxygen concentration in yoghurt was lowered (Dave & Shah 1997a).

Cheese

The potential of various types of cheeses as a probiotic carrier has been widely explored. In these studies *Lactobacillus* and *Bifidobacterium* strains have been used as single probiotic cultures or in mixtures. Occasionally probiotics have been encapsulated before addition into cheese (Godward & Kailasapathy 2003; Özer *et al.* 2009) or prebiotics have been added together with probiotics into cheese (Buriti *et al.* 2007; Cardarelli *et al.* 2008). Lactobacilli have been added, for example, into fresh (cream) cheese (Buriti *et al.* 2007; Masuda *et al.* 2005), goat milk cheese (Gomes & Malcata 1998), Minas fresh cheese (Buriti *et al.* 2005a, 2005b), Turkish white cheese (Kasimoglu *et al.* 2004), semi-hard Argentinean cheese (Bergamini *et al.* 2005), Petit-Suisse cheese (Cardarelli *et al.* 2008) and Cheddar cheese (Gardiner *et al.* 1998, 2002; Ong & Shah 2009; Ong *et al.* 2006; Phillips *et al.* 2006). Bifidobacteria have been added e.g. into fresh cheese (Roy *et al.* 1997), goat milk cheese (Gomes *et al.* 1998), Canestrato Pugliese hard cheese (Corbo *et al.* 2001), Cheddar(-like) cheese (Daigle *et al.* 1999; Ong *et al.* 2006; Phillips *et al.* 2006; Ong & Shah 2009), Crescenza cheese (Corbo *et al.*

2001), Petit-Suisse cheese (Cardarelli *et al.* 2008) and cottage cheese (Blanchette *et al.* 1996). Although some species/strain-specific variation in the stability has been observed, typically the stability of the studied probiotic strains has either been satisfactory or quite good even after several weeks' storage at refrigerated temperatures. The effects of probiotic addition on the sensory properties of cheeses have typically been minor.

Since hard cheeses have a markedly higher pH than fermented milks such as yoghurt (4.8–5.6 vs. 3.7–4.3) they provide a better protection against low pH conditions. Furthermore, the structure (matrix) and the relatively high fat content of hard cheeses provides further protection against harmful conditions of the upper GI tract (Gardiner *et al.* 1999; Boylston *et al.* 2004; Roy 2005; Gomes da Cruz *et al.* 2009). On the other hand, the salting and ripening process, which changes the biochemical and microbiological parameters of cheese, has an impairing effect on probiotic viability. Furthermore, hard cheeses are seldom consumed in high enough amounts to allow obtaining the recommended daily dose of probiotics (typically about 10^9 CFUs). Fresh cheeses, like cottage cheeses, can be adjusted to low salt contents, and due to their shorter shelf life, refrigerated storage and higher consumption, they are probably better matrix candidates for probiotics than hard cheeses (Gomes da Cruz *et al.* 2009). Technological aspects related to probiotic cheeses are discussed in more detail in the review of Gomes da Cruz *et al.* (2009).

Other dairy-based products
Probiotics have also been added into quark, chocolate mousse, frozen fermented dairy desserts, ice cream, and spread. Information about probiotic stability in quark has not been published, only the nutritive characteristics of the product have been reported (Djuric *et al.* 2007). In chocolate mousse (made of milk cream, cocoa powder, chocolate powder, gelatine, emulsifiers, sucrose, skimmed milk powder, UHT skimmed milk, and optionally inulin) the viability of *L. paracasei* LBC 82 was retained during storage at 5°C up to four weeks. Frozen fermented dairy dessert is prepared similarly to ice cream but the starting material is yoghurt. Alginate encapsulation of probiotic *L. acidophilus* and *Bifidobacterium* spp. strains improved their survival in the dessert (Shah & Ravula 2000). During the frozen storage (at −20°C) of ice cream the stability has been variable between probiotic strains; either stable (Alamprese *et al.* 2002, 2005) or showing declining but still reasonable levels of living cells (Kailasapathy & Sultana 2003). Although ice-cream is a potential candidate carrier for probiotics, there are factors that can impair the viability and stability of probiotics. These include added, potentially antimicrobial flavourings (e.g. fruit/berry-based); incorporation of air in the structure during the beating step; and storage at frozen, but not very cold temperatures (Cruz *et al.* 2009).

A prototype of a reduced fat edible table spread (main ingredients being milk fats, soy oil and emulsifier) with probiotics (*L. casei, B. infantis*) has been described by Charteris *et al.* (2002). The stability of probiotics was studied in various modifications of the spread; in general the viability of bifidobacteria in the spread was poor compared to lactobacilli (which also declined in numbers) during the 12 weeks' storage in refrigerated conditions, and thus further improvement in the process and choice of other, more robust, probiotic strains is still needed.

There are several publications where probiotic-supplemented infant formulas have been studied for their health benefits. Probiotics incorporated into infant formulas include mainly *B. animalis* subsp. *lactis* Bb-12, but also *L. rhamnosus* LGG, *Bifidobacterium breve* C50, and *L. reuteri* ATCC 55730 (Isolauri *et al.* 2000; Thibault *et al.* 2004; Saavedra *et al.* 2004; Chouraqui *et al.* 2004; Bakker-Zierikzee *et al.* 2006). Sometimes extensively hydrolysed whey formula (Isolauri *et al.* 2000) or fermented formulas (Thibault *et al.* 2004; Chouraqui *et al.* 2004) were used. Infant formulas have to be exceptionally safe and of high quality. Thus in the development of infant formulas more emphasis has to be put on the selection of probiotic strain since the target consumer population is infants, and not adults who have stable and established gut microbiota.

18.4.2   Vegetable-based probiotic products

Vegetable and fruit juices are probably the most popular non-dairy probiotic food applications. Vegetable juices can be fermented or non-fermented whereas in fruit juices microbial fermentation is typically an unwanted phenomenon. Yoon and co-workers (Yoon *et al.* 2004, 2005, 2006) showed that probiotic lactobacilli (*L. acidophilus, L. casei* and *L. plantarum*) were able to grow and produce acid in non-supplemented tomato, beetroot and cabbage juice (final pH 3.4–5.0). The three strains showed variable stability in different juices. However, both *L. acidophilus* and *L. casei* were fairly stable in tomato juice. Since tomato juice had a low pH (approx. 3.5) acidity was not the only factor affecting probiotic stability in these studies. Also Champagne *et al.* (2009a) have successfully grown probiotic lactobacilli in cabbage juice. In the study of Savard *et al.* (2003) mixed vegetable juice (made of carrots, cabbage and onions; initial pH 6.3) was fermented with nine different probiotic *Lactobacillus* and *Bifidobacterium* strains. All strains grew in the medium but with variable final cell densities. When the fermented vegetable juice made of carrots, cabbage, beet and onions (pH 3.65 or 6.5) was stored at 4 °C for up to 90 days several of the probiotic strains showed fairly good stability at pH 3.65 for about one month, after which time the viability typically started to decline more rapidly. The stability was better in the juice with the higher pH. In the study of Ainsley Reid *et al.* (2007) the stability of the probiotic *L. rhamnosus* in a mixed vegetable juice (made of tomatoes, beets, carrots, spinach, celery, lettuce, parsley and watercress) with fairly high pH (4.35) was excellent over two weeks' storage at 4 °C.

Probiotic lactobacilli and bifidobacteria (together or without starter microbes) have been used to ferment soy, which is an important legume in the traditional Asian diet. Due to its bean flavour and the presence of raffinose and stachyose the applications of soybean are limited. Hence fermentation has been a popular means of modifying the properties of soy (Rivera-Espinoza & Gallardo-Navarro 2010). Both supplemented and non-supplemented soy beverages (or soy milks) have proved to be suitable carriers for probiotics (Garro *et al.* 1999; Chumchuere & Robinson 1999; Garro *et al.* 2004; Otieno *et al.* 2005; Wang *et al.* 2006; Tang *et al.* 2007; Farnworth *et al.* 2007; Champagne *et al.* 2009b). Furthermore, soy-based frozen desserts and soy cheese (sufu) have been used as a carrier for probiotic organisms (Heenan *et al.* 2004; Liu *et al.* 2006). Similarly to other food applications the stability of probiotics in soy-based products has been strain-specific.

Compared to vegetable juices there is much less information about the survival of probiotic on the actual vegetables. Valerio *et al.* (2006) and Lavermicocca *et al.* (2005) have shown that artichokes (with added *L. plantarum* and *L. paracasei* strains) and olives (with added *L. rhamnosus* (including LGG), *L. paracasei, B. bifidum,* and *Bifidobacterium longum* strains) preserved in brine, can be used as carrier foods for probiotics.

18.4.3   Fruit-based probiotic products

Fruit juices typically contain prohibitory levels of organic acids (Vinderola *et al.* 2002a) and have a low pH. Thus natural fruit juices are not good growth media or carriers for probiotic bacteria. The juice's pH is an important determinant of probiotic viability: pH values below 4 are typically detrimental to most probiotic strains (Savard *et al.* 2003; Ainsley Reid *et al.* 2007; Sheehan *et al.* 2007). Probiotic bacteria vary in their tolerance to organic acids and low pH. Lactobacilli (especially *L. acidophilus* and *L. casei* groups) are generally considered to be more resistant to acidic environments than bifidobacteria (Champagne *et al.* 2005). Bifidobacteria are reported to be sensitive to pH values below 4.6 (Boylston *et al.* 2004), and thus fruit juices (with typical pH values between 3 and 4) are poor supporters of their viability and stability. However, the acid resistance of bifidobacteria, like lactobacilli, varies and *B. animalis* strains are clearly more acid resistant than the strains of other *Bifidobacterium* species (Mättö *et al.* 2004).

In addition to pH the raw materials of the juice and the nature of organic acids they contain affect the viability of probiotic bacteria. It has been shown, for example, that at the same pH cranberry juice is more inhibitory to probiotics than pineapple juice, probably due to high levels of benzoic acids it contains (Sheehan *et al.* 2007). In addition to acids, fruits, especially berries, also contain various phenolic compounds which are inhibitory to bacteria (Puupponen-Pimiä *et al.* 2005; Howell 2007). However, depending on the juice, the probiotic strain and the formulation conditions the stability in juice can still be acceptable (at least 10^6–10^7 CFU/ml) after a couple of weeks' cold storage.

In the study of Sheehan *et al.* (2007) *Lactobacillus salivarius, B. animalis* subsp. *lactis, L. casei, L. rhamnosus* and *L. paracasei* were added into orange juice (pH 3.65) and pineapple juice (pH 3.4) and stored at 4°C for up to 12 weeks. *L. casei* and *L. rhamnosus* were the most robust strains in the orange juice, whereas *L. paracasei* was the most robust strain in the pineapple juice. In general, strains survived better in the orange juice than in the pineapple juice. One important factor for the survival in the orange juice was its higher pH compared to pineapple juice.

In the study of Saarela *et al.* (2006a) *B. animalis* subsp. *lactis* cells were freeze-dried with either reconstituted skim milk or sucrose as a carrier and freeze-dried cells were then formulated into three fruits' juice (made of orange, grape and passion fruit; pH 3.7) and stored at 4°C for six weeks. The storage stability of the sucrose-formulated cells proved to be better than that of the skim milk formulated cells. When the similarly formulated juices were stored at 20°C the decline in viability was more rapid. In another study by Saarela *et al.* (2006b) the stability of *L. rhamnosus* fresh cells formulated with different carriers (sucrose, oat flour, wheat dextrin and polydextrin) was studied in apple juice (pH 3.5) for 12 weeks at 4°C and 20°C. Oat fibre-formulated cells showed the best stability at both temperatures. Surprisingly the two studied *L. rhamnosus* strains (VTT E-97800 and LGG) formulated with oat flour were more stable at 20°C compared to 4°C. Champagne *et al.* (2008) added *L. rhamnosus* R0011 cells into sorbate-containing commercial apple-pear-raspberry juice (pH 3.6–3.9) and studied the effect of storage and handling conditions on the probiotic stability. Although the *L. rhamnosus* numbers dropped during storage and handling (temperature, time and gas atmosphere were the main variables) the authors concluded that the consumers can expect good viability over a few weeks of storage in a refrigerator, even if the juice bottles have been opened. In another study Champagne and Gardner (2008) added various probiotic *Lactobacillus* strains into commercial mixed fruit drink (containing pineapple, apple, orange, pear and/or grape, passion fruit and lemon juices; peach, strawberry, mango and kiwi purees; yoghurt powder and many other ingredients, pH 4.2) for stability studies. Several of the strains (including *L. rhamnosus, L. brevis, L. acidophilus, L. fermentum, L. reuteri*, and *L. plantarum*) had very good stability in the product (at 4°C) even after 80 days, whereas two *L. acidophilus* strains showed poor stability. The fairly high pH of the drink and the presence of milk components may have contributed to the general good survival of the probiotic strains. Ding and Shah (2008) compared the stability of free and alginate-encapsulated lactobacilli and bifidobacteria in orange and apple juices (pH 2.8–3.0). Encapsulated probiotics had better survival during storage at 4°C in both juices; the difference was much larger in apple juice where free probiotic cells showed poor survival (regardless of the strain applied).

Rößle *et al.* (2010) introduced a new fruit-based application for probiotics. They dipped fresh apple wedges into *L. rhamnosus* LGG solution, drained the wedges and then dipped them into anti-browning agent, drained the wedges again, and packed them into modified atmosphere packages. After the storage of wedges at 2–4°C for 10 days LGG levels were about 10^8 CFU/g, thus showing a reasonable stability.

18.4.4   Cereal-based probiotic products

Cereal-based probiotic products enable combining two health-promoting aspects, health-benefiting microbes and fibres (which can potentially be prebiotic). Largely water insoluble fibres of cereals could also function as probiotic protectants during processing, in foods, and in the GI tract (Charalampopoulos *et al.* 2002b;

Saarela *et al.* 2006b; Michida *et al.* 2006). The growth of probiotics in various cereal-based media has been reported by several authors (Jaskari *et al.* 1998; Kontula *et al.* 1998; Charalampopoulos *et al.* 2002a; Laine *et al.* 2003; Helland *et al.* 2004; Kedia *et al.* 2007). The stability of probiotic strains in cereal-based products can be quite good, but typically strain dependent (Mårtensson *et al.* 2002). Commercial oat-based drinks/gruels that contain probiotic bifidobacteria (Pitkala *et al.* 2007) or *L. plantarum* (Sen *et al.* 2002; Angelov *et al.* 2006) have been developed, and the oat-based drink with different fruit/berry flavours (ProViva) has proved quite popular among consumers.

In the study of Saarela *et al.* (2006b) probiotic *L. rhamnosus* strains (LGG and VTT E-97800), freeze-dried with sucrose or different fibre carriers were added in chocolate into breakfast oat cereals. The stability of the strains formulated either with sucrose or polydextrin was quite good during seven months storage at 20 °C, whereas oat fibre formulated cells did not perform well in this application.

18.4.5   Meat-based probiotic foods

Some meat-based foods can also be used as carrier matrices for probiotics. Meat matrix as such is a suitable carrier for many probiotics, but meat processing steps often involve heating which excludes the possibility of using probiotics. Thus probiotic applications are restricted to fermented meats (typically dry sausages), which are processed without heating (Rivera-Espinoza & Gallardo-Navarro 2010). Typically only *Lactobacillus* genus bacteria, which can also naturally be found in meat products, have been used in probiotic meat manufacture. Some *L. rhamnosus, L. paracasei, L. plantarum*, and *L. reuteri* strains have proved suitable for sausage fermentation (Erkkilä *et al.* 2001; Jahreis *et al.* 2002; Klingberg & Budde 2006; Muthukumarasamy & Holley 2006). In addition to functioning as a carrier matrix for probiotics sausage matrix has also been shown to protect the viability *L. plantarum* in the GI tract (Klingberg & Budde 2006). Alginate encapsulation has been applied to improve the viability of *L. reuteri* in sausages after drying (Muthukumarasamy & Holley 2006).

18.5   Future trends

Probiotics are today found in a wide range of food products. Since probiotics are today consumed globally and their markets are rapidly increasing in many countries outside Europe and the United States, we will likely see an increase in the variety and volume of probiotic plant-based foods. For example in Asia, fermented plant-based foods are commonly consumed and adding probiotics into these seems like a natural way of widening the range of probiotic food applications. Also probiotic foods targeted to specific consumer groups (infants, children, elderly, athletes, etc.) will likely become more important in the future.

All food applications have some kind of limitations regarding the viability and stability of probiotics. These limitations typically involve factors such as the acidity of the food matrix and storage time and temperature of the product. The presence of organic acids is perhaps the biggest individual challenge to probiotic viability in the food matrix. A lot of effort has been put on the acid protection by various means, including encapsulation. For the short term, (some) protection has been achieved, but since organic acids are small molecules and they tend to diffuse easily through various barriers, the long-term protection (e.g. during several weeks storage) has proved a very challenging task. Therefore new technological innovations are needed in this area. Currently the best way to ensure probiotic stability in the products is still to individually select a suitable probiotic strain for a specific food application. Selecting a strain with good technological properties will also be a key factor when novel food applications for probiotics are developed in the future. This goes together with tailoring the processing conditions to enable the incorporation of viable probiotic cells. However, there are limits to modifying food processing parameters and thus many food applications (e.g. those involving extensive heating steps) will remain outside probiotic applications. Since the health benefits of dead bacterial cells have raised some interest in the research field (Wagner et al. 2000; Mottet & Michetti 2005; Zhang et al. 2005), it may be possible that in the future we can incorporate probiotics practically to any food and do not need worry whether they are alive or not. However, this remains a big 'if', since the health effects of dead bacterial cells have been very little studied so far.

Another development in the area is the rapid accumulation of information about lactic acid bacterial and bifidobacterial genome sequences (see, e.g., http://wishart.biology.ualberta.ca/BacMap/index.html). Emerging knowledge of the genes important for the technological functionality can be used to monitor the presence/activity of single individual genes in potential probiotic strains, or alternatively it can be used to genetically modify probiotic strains (which so far has been avoided, mainly due the negative consumer attitudes towards 'gene manipulation'). Yet another option is to utilise this information to select strains with desired properties, for example from traditionally home-made fermented products or from plant material in nature.

Fermentation is an ancient way to store food and improve its safety and nutritional value. Home-made fermented foods are still nowadays commonly produced in the developing countries, especially in the rural areas, although their consumption is declining (Watson et al. 1996; Johns & Sthapit 2004). Non-commercial fermented products contain vast and largely unknown diversity of lactic acid bacteria (and also other microbes), among which novel probiotic strains could potentially be identified. However this rich source of microbes should be tapped quickly before these products are replaced with commercial products.

18.6   Sources of further information and advice

More information about the potential probiotic health effects is available in the following recently published meta-analysis studies and systematic reviews.

Chmielewska, A. and Szajewska, H. 2010, 'Systematic review of randomised controlled trials: Probiotics for functional constipation', *World Journal of Gastroenterology*, **16**, 69–75.

Deshpande, G., Rao, S. and Patole S. 2007, 'Probiotics for prevention of necrotising enterocolitis in preterm neonates with very low birthweight: a systematic review of randomised controlled trials', *Lancet*, **369**(9573), 1614–20.

Elahi, B., Nikfar, S., Derakhshani, S., Vafaie, M., and Abdollahi, M. 2008, 'On the benefit of probiotics in the management of pouchitis in patients underwent ileal pouch anal anastomosis: A meta-analysis of controlled clinical trials', *Digestive Diseases and Sciences*, **53**(5), 1278–84.

Hoveyda, N., Heneghan, C., Mahtani, K.R., Perera, R., Roberts, N., and Glasziou, P. 2009, 'A systematic review and meta-analysis: probiotics in the treatment of irritable bowel syndrome', *BMC Gastroenterology*, **9**, 15–25.

McFarland, L.V. 2009, 'Evidence-based review of probiotics for antibiotic-associated diarrhea and *Clostridium difficile* infections', *Anaerobe*, **5**, 274–80.

McFarland, L.V. 2007, 'Meta-analysis of probiotics for the prevention of traveler's diarrhea', *Travel Medicine and Infectious Disease*, **5**(2), 97–105.

Osborn, D.A. and Sinn, J.K. 2007, 'Probiotics in infants for prevention of allergic disease and food hypersensitivity', *Cochrane Databaseof Systematic Reviews*, Oct 17 (4): CD006475.

Rolfe, V.E., Fortun, P.J., Hawkey, C.J. and Bath-Hextall, F. 2006, 'Probiotics for maintenance of remission in Crohn's disease', *Cochrane Database of Systematic Reviews*, Oct 18 (4): CD004826.

Takahashi, O., Noguchi, Y., Omata, F., Tokuda, Y. and Fukui, T. 2007, 'Probiotics in the prevention of traveler's diarrhea: meta-analysis', *Journal of Clinical Gastroenterology*, **41**(3), 336–7.

Tong, J.L., Ran, Z.H., Shen, J., Zhang, C.X. and Xiao S.D. 2007, 'Meta-analysis: the effect of supplementation with probiotics on eradication rates and adverse events during *Helicobacter pylori* eradication therapy', *Alimentary Pharmacology & Therapeutics*, **25**(2), 155–68.

Introduction of a Qualified Presumption of Safety (QPS) approach for assessment of selected microorganisms referred to EFSA – Opinion of the scientific committee can be found at http://www.efsa.europa.eu/EFSA/efsa_locale-1178620753812_1178667590178.htm

18.7   References

Ainsley Reid, A., Champagne, C.P., Gardner, N., Fustier, P. and Vuillemard, J.C. 2007, 'Survival in food systems of *Lactobacillus rhamnosus* R011 microentrapped in whey protein gel particles', *Journal of Food Science*, vol. 72, no. 1, pp. 31–37.

Alamprese, C., Foschino, R., Rossi, M., Pompei, C. and Corti, S. 2005, 'Effects of *Lactobacillus rhamnosus* GG addition in ice cream', *International Journal of Dairy Technology*, vol. 58, no. 4, pp. 200–206.

Alamprese, C., Foschino, R., Rossi, M., Pompei, C. and Savani, L. 2002, 'Survival of *Lactobacillus johnsonii* La1 and influence of its addition in retail-manufactured ice cream produced with different sugar and fat concentrations', *International Dairy Journal*, vol. 12, no. 2–3, pp. 201–208.

Angelov, A., Gotcheva, V., Kuncheva, R. and Hristozova, T. 2006, 'Development of a new oat-based probiotic drink', *International Journal of Food Microbiology*, vol. 112, no. 1, pp. 75–80.

Anonymous 2002, *Guidelines for the evaluation of probiotics in food*. Joint FAO/WHO working group report on drafting guidelines for the evaluation of probiotics in food.

Anonymous 2009a, *EU digestive health ingredients market*. Frost & Sullivan, M426–88.

Anonymous 2009b, *U.S. digestive health ingredients markets*. Frost & Sullivan, N4F7–88.

Antunes, A.E.C., Grael, E.T., Moreno, I., Rodrigues, L.G., Dourado, F.M., *et al.* 2007, 'Selective enumeration and viability of *Bifidobacterium animalis* subsp. *lactis* in a new fermented milk product', *Brazilian Journal of Microbiology*, vol. 38, pp. 173–177.

Antunes, A.E.C., Silva, É.R.A., van Dender, A.G.F., Marasca, E.T.G., Moreno, I., *et al.* 2009, 'Probiotic buttermilk-like fermented milk product development in a semiindustrial scale: Physicochemical, microbiological and sensory acceptability', *International Journal of Dairy Technology*, vol. 62, no. 4, pp. 556–563.

Bakker-Zierikzee, A.M., Tol, E.A.F., Kroes, H., Alles, M.S., Kok, F.J. and Bindels, J.G. 2006, 'Faecal SIgA secretion in infants fed on pre-or probiotic infant formula', *Pediatric Allergy and Immunology*, vol. 17, no. 2, pp. 134–140.

Bergamini, C.V., Hynes, E.R., Quiberoni, A., Suárez, V.B. and Zalazar, C.A. 2005, 'Probiotic bacteria as adjunct starters: Influence of the addition methodology on their survival in a semi-hard Argentinean cheese', *Food Research International*, vol. 38, no. 5, pp. 597–604.

Blanchette, L., Roy, D., Bélanger, G. and Gauthier, S.F. 1996, 'Production of cottage cheese using dressing fermented by bifidobacteria', *Journal of Dairy Science*, vol. 79, no. 1, pp. 8–15.

Bolduc, M.-P., Raymond, Y., Fustier, P., Champagne, C.P. and Vuillemard, J.-C. 2006, 'Sensitivity of bifidobacteria to oxygen and redox potential in non-fermented pasteurized milk', *International Dairy Journal*, vol. 16, no. 9, pp. 1038–1048.

Boylston, T.D., Vinderola, C.G., Ghoddusi, H.B. and Reinheimer, J.A. 2004, 'Incorporation of bifidobacteria into cheeses: Challenges and rewards', *International Dairy Journal*, vol. 14, no. 5, pp. 375–387.

Buriti, F.C.A., Cardarelli, H.R., Filisetti, T.M.C.C. and Saad, S.M.I. 2007, 'Synbiotic potential of fresh cream cheese supplemented with inulin and *Lactobacillus paracasei* in co-culture with *Streptococcus thermophilus*', *Food Chemistry*, vol. 104, no. 4, pp. 1605–1610.

Buriti, F.C.A., da Rocha, J.S., Assis, E.G. and Saad, S.M.I. 2005a, 'Probiotic potential of Minas fresh cheese prepared with the addition of *Lactobacillus paracasei*', *Lebensmittel-Wissenschaft und-Technologie*, vol. 38, no. 2, pp. 173–180.

Buriti, F.C.A., da Rocha, J.S. and Saad, S.M.I. 2005b, 'Incorporation of *Lactobacillus acidophilus* in Minas fresh cheese and its implications for textural and sensorial properties during storage', *International Dairy Journal*, vol. 15, no. 12, pp. 1279–1288.

Capela, P., Hay, T.K.C. and Shah, N.P. 2006, 'Effect of cryoprotectants, prebiotics and microencapsulation on survival of probiotic organisms in yoghurt and freeze-dried yoghurt', *Food Research International*, vol. 39, no. 2, pp. 203–211.

Cardarelli, H.R., Buriti, F.C.A., Castro, I.A. and Saad, S.M.I. 2008, 'Inulin and oligofructose improve sensory quality and increase the probiotic viable count in potentially synbiotic Petit-Suisse cheese', *LWT – Food Science and Technology*, vol. 41, no. 6, pp. 1037–1046.

Carr, J.P. and Ibrahim, S.A. 2005, 'Viability of bifidobacteria in commercial yogurt products in North Carolina', *Milchwissenschaft*, vol. 60, no. 4, pp. 414–416.

Champagne, C.P., Savard, T. and Barrette, J. 2009a, 'Production of lactic acid bacteria on spent cabbage juice', *International Journal of Food, Agriculture and Environment*, vol. 7, no. 2, pp. 82–87.

Champagne, C.P. and Gardner, N.J. 2008, 'Effect of storage in a fruit drink on subsequent survival of probiotic lactobacilli to gastro-intestinal stresses', *Food Research International*, vol. 41, no. 5, pp. 539–543.

Champagne, C.P., Gardner, N.J. and Roy, D. 2005, 'Challenges in the addition of probiotic cultures to foods', *Critical Reviews in Food Science and Nutrition*, vol. 45, no. 1, pp. 61–84.

Champagne, C.P., Green-Johnson, J., Raymond, Y., Barrette, J. and Buckley, N. 2009b, 'Selection of probiotic bacteria for the fermentation of a soy beverage in combination with *Streptococcus thermophilus*', *Food Research International*, vol. 42, no. 5–6, pp. 612–621.

Champagne, C.P., Raymond, Y. and Gagnon, R. 2008, 'Viability of *Lactobacillus rhamnosus* R0011 in an apple-based fruit juice under simulated storage conditions at the consumer level', *Journal of Food Science*, vol. 73, no. 5, pp. 221–226.

Charalampopoulos, D., Pandiella, S.S. and Webb, C. 2002a, 'Growth studies of potentially probiotic lactic acid bacteria in cereal-based substrates', *Journal of Applied Microbiology*, vol. 92, no. 5, pp. 851–859.

Charalampopoulos, D., Wang, R., Pandiella, S.S. and Webb, C. 2002b, 'Application of cereals and cereal components in functional foods: a review', *International Journal of Food Microbiology*, vol. 79, no. 1–2, pp. 131–141.

Charteris, W.P., Kelly, P.M., Morelli, L. and Collins, J.K. 2002, 'Edible table (bio)spread containing potentially probiotic *Lactobacillus* and *Bifidobacterium* species', *International Journal of Dairy Technology*, vol. 55, no. 1, pp. 44–56.

Charteris, W.P., Kelly, P.M., Morelli, L. and Collins, J.K. 1998, 'Ingredient selection criteria for probiotic microorganisms in functional dairy foods', *International Journal of Dairy Technology*, vol. 51, no. 4, pp. 123–136.

Chouraqui, J.P., Van Egroo, L.D. and Fichot, M.C. 2004, 'Acidified milk formula supplemented with *Bifidobacterium lactis*: impact on infant diarrhea in residential care settings', *Journal of Pediatric Gastroenterology and Nutrition*, vol. 38, no. 3, pp. 288–292.

Chumchuere, S. and Robinson, R.K. 1999, 'Selection of starter cultures for the fermentation of soya milk', *Food Microbiology*, vol. 16, no. 2, pp. 129–137.

Conway, P.L., Gorbach, S.L. and Goldin, B.R. 1987, 'Survival of lactic acid bacteria in the human stomach and adhesion to intestinal cells', *Journal of Dairy Science*, vol. 70, no. 1, pp. 1–12.

Corbo, M.R., Albenzio, M., De Angelis, M., Sevi, A. and Gobbetti, M. 2001, 'Microbiological and biochemical properties of Canestrato pugliese hard cheese supplemented with bifidobacteria', *Journal of Dairy Science*, vol. 84, no. 3, pp. 551–561.

Cruz, A.G., Antunes, A.E.C., Sousa, A.L.O.P., Faria, J.A.F. and Saad, S.M.I. 2009, 'Ice-cream as a probiotic food carrier', *Food Research International*, vol. 42, no. 9, pp. 1233–1239.

Culligan, E.P., Hill, C. and Sleator, R.D. 2009, 'Probiotics and gastrointestinal disease: successes, problems and future prospects', *Gut Pathogens*, vol. 1, 19–30.

Daigle, A., Roy, D., Bélanger, G. and Vuillemard, J.C. 1999, 'Production of probiotic cheese (Cheddar-like cheese) using enriched cream fermented by *Bifidobacterium infantis*', *Journal of Dairy Science*, vol. 82, no. 6, pp. 1081–1091.

Dave, R.I. and Shah, N.P. 1997a, 'Effect of cysteine on the viability of yoghurt and probiotic bacteria in yoghurts made with commercial starter cultures', *International Dairy Journal*, vol. 7, no. 8–9, pp. 537–545.

Dave, R.I. and Shah, N.P. 1997b, 'Viability of yoghurt and probiotic bacteria in yoghurts made from commercial starter cultures', *International Dairy Journal*, vol. 7, no. 1, pp. 31–41.

Ding, W.K. and Shah, N.P. 2008, 'Survival of free and microencapsulated probiotic bacteria in orange and apple juices', *International Food Research Journal*, vol. 15, no. 2, pp. 219–232.

Djuric, M.S., Ilicic, M.D., Milanovic, S.D., Caric, M. and Tekic, M.N. 2007, 'Nutritive characteristics of probiotic quarg as influenced by type of starter', *APTEFF*, vol. 38, pp. 1–19.

Donkor, O.N., Henriksson, A., Vasiljevic, T. and Shah, N.P. 2006, 'Effect of acidification on the activity of probiotics in yoghurt during cold storage', *International Dairy Journal*, vol. 16, no. 10, pp. 1181–1189.

Eckert, M. and Riker, P. 2007, 'Overcoming challenges in functional beverages', *Food Technology*, vol. 61, no. 3, pp. 20–26.

Erkkilä, S., Suihko, M.L., Eerola, S., Petäjä, E. and Mattila-Sandholm, T. 2001, 'Dry sausage fermented by *Lactobacillus rhamnosus* strains', *International Journal of Food Microbiology*, vol. 64, no. 1–2, pp. 205–210.

Farnworth, E.R., Mainville, I., Desjardins, M.P., Gardner, N., Fliss, I. and Champagne, C. 2007, 'Growth of probiotic bacteria and bifidobacteria in a soy yogurt formulation', *International Journal of Food Microbiology*, vol. 116, no. 1, pp. 174–181.

Fasoli, S., Marzotto, M., Rizzotti, L., Rossi, F., Dellaglio, F. and Torriani, S. 2003, 'Bacterial composition of commercial probiotic products as evaluated by PCR-DGGE analysis', *International Journal of Food Microbiology*, vol. 82, no. 1, pp. 59–70.

Fernández, M.F., Boris, S. and Barbés, C. 2003, 'Probiotic properties of human lactobacilli strains to be used in the gastrointestinal tract', *Journal of Applied Microbiology*, vol. 94, no. 3, pp. 449–455.

Gardiner, G., Ross, R.P., Collins, J.K., Fitzgerald, G. and Stanton, C. 1998, 'Development of a probiotic Cheddar cheese containing human-derived *Lactobacillus paracasei* strains', *Applied and Environmental Microbiology*, vol. 64, no. 6, pp. 2192–2199.

Gardiner, G., Stanton, C., Lynch, P.B., Collins, J.K., Fitzgerald, G. and Ross, R.P. 1999, 'Evaluation of Cheddar cheese as a food carrier for delivery of a probiotic strain to the gastrointestinal tract', *Journal of Dairy Science*, vol. 82, no. 7, pp. 1379–1387.

Gardiner, G.E., Bouchier, P., O'Sullivan, E., Kelly, J., Kevin Collins, J. *et al.* 2002, 'A spray-dried culture for probiotic Cheddar cheese manufacture', *International Dairy Journal*, vol. 12, no. 9, pp. 749–756.

Garro, M.S., de Valdez, G.F. and de Giori, G.S. 2004, 'Temperature effect on the biological activity of *Bifidobacterium longum* CRL 849 and *Lactobacillus fermentum* CRL 251 in pure and mixed cultures grown in soymilk', *Food Microbiology*, vol. 21, no. 5, pp. 511–518.

Garro, M.S., de Valdez, G.F., Oliver, G. and de Giori, G.S. 1999, 'Starter culture activity in refrigerated fermented soymilk', *Journal of Food Protection*, vol. 62, no. 7, pp. 808–810.

Gilliland, S.E., Reilly, S.S., Kim, G.B. and Kim, H.S. 2002, 'Viability during storage of selected probiotic lactobacilli and bifidobacteria in a yogurt-like product', *Journal of Food Science*, vol. 67, no. 8, pp. 3091–3095.

Godward, G. and Kailasapathy, K. 2003, 'Viability and survival of free and encapsulated probiotic bacteria in cheddar cheese', *Milchwissenschaft*, vol. 58, no. 11–12, pp. 624–627.

Gomes da Cruz, A., Alonso Buriti, F.C., Batista de Souza, C.H., Fonseca Faria, J.A. and Isay Saad, S.M. 2009, 'Probiotic cheese: Health benefits, technological and stability aspects', *Trends in Food Science and Technology*, vol. 20, no. 8, pp. 344–354.

Gomes, A.M.P. and Malcata, F.X. 1999, '*Bifidobacterium* spp. and *Lactobacillus acidophilus*: Biological, biochemical, technological and therapeutic properties relevant for use as probiotics', *Trends in Food Science and Technology*, vol. 10, no. 4–5, pp. 139–157.

Gomes, A.M.P. and Malcata, F.X. 1998, 'Development of probiotic cheese manufactured from goat milk: Response surface analysis via technological manipulation', *Journal of Dairy Science*, vol. 81, no. 6, pp. 1492–1507.

Gomes, A.M.P., Silva, M.L.P.C. and Malcata, F.X. 1998, 'Caprine cheese with probiotic strains: The effects of ripening temperature and relative humidity on proteolysis and lipolysis', *European Food Research and Technology*, vol. 207, no. 5, pp. 386–394.

Hansen, L.T., Allan-Wojtas, P.M., Jin, Y.L. and Paulson, A.T. 2002, 'Survival of Ca-alginate microencapsulated *Bifidobacterium* spp. in milk and simulated gastrointestinal conditions', *Food Microbiology*, vol. 19, no. 1, pp. 35–45.

Heenan, C.N., Adams, M.C., Hosken, R.W. and Fleet, G.H. 2004, 'Survival and sensory acceptability of probiotic microorganisms in a nonfermented frozen vegetarian dessert', *LWT-Food Science and Technology*, vol. 37, no. 4, pp. 461–466.

Helland, M.H., Wicklund, T. and Narvhus, J.A. 2004, 'Growth and metabolism of selected strains of probiotic bacteria in milk-and water-based cereal puddings', *International Dairy Journal*, vol. 14, no. 11, pp. 957–965.

Heller, K.J. 2001, 'Probiotic bacteria in fermented foods: Product characteristics and starter organisms', *American Journal of Clinical Nutrition*, vol. 73, no. 2 (SUPPL.), pp. 374S–379S.

Hernandez-Mendoza, A., Robles, V.J., Angulo, J.O., De La Cruz, J. and Garcia, H.S. 2007, 'Preparation of a whey-based probiotic product with *Lactobacillus reuteri* and *Bifidobacterium bifidum*', *Food Technology and Biotechnology*, vol. 45, no. 1, pp. 27–31.

Howell, A.B. 2007, 'Bioactive compounds in cranberries and their role in prevention of urinary tract infections', *Molecular Nutrition and Food Research*, vol. 51, no. 6, pp. 732–737.

Hughes, D.B. and Hoover, D.G. 1995, 'Viability and enzymatic activity of bifidobacteria in milk', *Journal of Dairy Science*, vol. 78, no. 2, pp. 268–276.

Isolauri, E., Arvola, T., Sutas, Y., Moilanen, E. and Salminen, S. 2000, 'Probiotics in the management of atopic eczema', *Clinical and Experimental Allergy*, vol. 30, no. 11, pp. 1605–1611.

Iyer, C. and Kailasapathy, K. 2005, 'Effect of co-encapsulation of probiotics with prebiotics on increasing the viability of encapsulated bacteria under in vitro acidic and bile salt conditions and in yogurt', *Journal of Food Science*, vol. 70, no. 1, pp. 18–23.

Jahreis, G., Vogelsang, H., Kiessling, G., Schubert, R., Bunte, C. and Hammes, W.P. 2002, 'Influence of probiotic sausage (*Lactobacillus paracasei*) on blood lipids and immunological parameters of healthy volunteers', *Food Research International*, vol. 35, no. 2–3, pp. 133–138.

Jaskari, J., Kontula, P., Siitonen, A., Jousimies-Somer, H., Mattila-Sandholm, T. and Poutanen, K. 1998, 'Oat β-glucan and xylan hydrolysates as selective substrates for *Bifidobacterium* and *Lactobacillus* strains', *Applied Microbiology and Biotechnology*, vol. 49, no. 2, pp. 175–181.

Jayamanne, V.S. and Adams, M.R. 2006, 'Determination of survival, identity and stress resistance of probiotic bifidobacteria in bio-yoghurts', *Letters in Applied Microbiology*, vol. 42, no. 3, pp. 189–194.

Johns, T. and Sthapit, B.R. 2004, 'Biocultural diversity in the sustainability of developing country food systems', *Food and Nutrition Bulletin*, vol. 25, no. 2, pp. 143–155.

Kailasapathy, K. and Rybka, S. 1997, '*L. acidophilus* and *Bifidobacterium* spp. – their therapeutic potential and survival in yogurt', *Australian Journal of Dairy Technology*, vol. 52, pp. 28–35.

Kailasapathy, K. 2006, 'Survival of free and encapsulated probiotic bacteria and their effect on the sensory properties of yoghurt', *LWT – Food Science and Technology*, vol. 39, no. 10, pp. 1221–1227.

Kailasapathy, K., Harmstorf, I. and Phillips, M. 2008, 'Survival of *Lactobacillus acidophilus* and *Bifidobacterium animalis* ssp. *lactis* in stirred fruit yogurts', *LWT – Food Science and Technology*, vol. 41, no. 7, pp. 1317–1322.

Kailasapathy, K. and Sultana, K. 2003, 'Survival and β-D-galactosidase activity of encapsulated and free *Lactobacillus acidophilus* and *Bifidobacterium lactis* in ice-cream', *Australian Journal of Dairy Technology*, vol. 58, no. 3, pp. 223–227.

Kailasapathy, K. and Sureeta, B.S. 2004, 'Effect of storage on shelf life and viability of freeze-dried and microencapsulated *Lactobacillus acidophilus* and *Bifidobacterium infantis* cultures', *Australian Journal of Dairy Technology*, vol. 59, no. 3, pp. 204–208.

Kasimoglu, A., Göncuöglu, M. and Akgu#t3, S. 2004, 'Probiotic white cheese with *Lactobacillus acidophilus*', *International Dairy Journal*, vol. 14, no. 12, pp. 1067–1073.

Kaur, I.P., Kuhad, A., Garg, A. and Chopra, K. 2009, 'Probiotics: Delineation of prophylactic and therapeutic benefits', *Journal of Medicinal Food*, vol. 12, no. 2, pp. 219–235.

Kedia, G., Wang, R., Patel, H. and Pandiella, S.S. 2007, 'Use of mixed cultures for the fermentation of cereal-based substrates with potential probiotic properties', *Process Biochemistry*, vol. 42, no. 1, pp. 65–70.

Klingberg, T.D. and Budde, B.B. 2006, 'The survival and persistence in the human gastrointestinal tract of five potential probiotic lactobacilli consumed as freeze-dried cultures or as probiotic sausage', *International Journal of Food Microbiology*, vol. 109, no. 1–2, pp. 157–159.

Kontula, P., von Wright, A. and Mattila-Sandholm, T. 1998, 'Oat bran β-gluco- and xylo-oligosaccharides as fermentative substrates for lactic acid bacteria', *International Journal of Food Microbiology*, vol. 45, no. 2, pp. 163–169.

Krasaekoopt, W., Bhandari, B. and Deeth, H. 2003, 'Evaluation of encapsulation techniques of probiotics for yoghurt', *International Dairy Journal*, vol. 13, no. 1, pp. 3–13.

Krasaekoopt, W., Bhandari, B. and Deeth, H.C. 2006, 'Survival of probiotics encapsulated in chitosan-coated alginate beads in yoghurt from UHT- and conventionally-treated milk during storage', *LWT – Food Science and Technology*, vol. 39, no. 2, pp. 177–183.

Laine, R., Salminen, S., Benno, Y. and Ouwehand, A.C. 2003, 'Performance of bifidobacteria in oat-based media', *International Journal of Food Microbiology*, vol. 83, no. 1, pp. 105–109.

Lavermicocca, P., Valerio, F., Lonigro, S.L., De Angelis, M., Morelli, L., *et al.* 2005, 'Study of adhesion and survival of lactobacilli and bifidobacteria on table olives with the aim of formulating a new probiotic food', *Applied and Environmental Microbiology*, vol. 71, no. 8, pp. 4233–4240.

Liu, D., Li, L., Yang, X., Liang, S. and Wang, J. 2006, 'Survivability of *Lactobacillus rhamnosus* during the preparation of soy cheese', *Food Technology and Biotechnology*, vol. 44, no. 3, pp. 417–422.

Lomax, A.R. and Calder, P.C. 2009, 'Probiotics, immune function, infection and inflammation: a review of the evidence from studies conducted in humans', *Current Pharmaceutical Design*, vol. 15, no. 13, pp. 1428–1518.

Lourens-Hattingh, A. and Viljoen, B.C. 2001, 'Yogurt as probiotic carrier food', *International Dairy Journal*, vol. 11, no. 1–2, pp. 1–17.

Mårtensson, O., Öste, R. and Holst, O. 2002, 'The effect of yoghurt culture on the survival of probiotic bacteria in oat-based, non-dairy products', *Food Research International*, vol. 35, no. 8, pp. 775–784.

Martín-Diana, A.B., Janer, C., Peláez, C. and Requena, T. 2003, 'Development of a fermented goat's milk containing probiotic bacteria', *International Dairy Journal*, vol. 13, no. 10, pp. 827–833.

Martínez-Villaluenga, C., Frías, J., Gómez, R. and Vidal-Valverde, C. 2006, 'Influence of addition of raffinose family oligosaccharides on probiotic survival in fermented milk during refrigerated storage', *International Dairy Journal*, vol. 16, no. 7, pp. 768–774.

Masco, L., Huys, G., De Brandt, E., Temmerman, R. and Swings, J. 2005, 'Culture-dependent and culture-independent qualitative analysis of probiotic products claimed to contain bifidobacteria', *International Journal of Food Microbiology*, vol. 102, no. 2, pp. 221–230.

Masuda, T., Yamanari, R. and Itoh, T. 2005, 'The trial for production of fresh cheese incorporated probiotic *Lactobacillus acidophilus* group lactic acid bacteria', *Milchwissenschaft*, vol. 60, no. 2, pp. 167–171.

Matsumoto, M., Ohishi, H. and Benno, Y. 2004, 'H-ATPase activity in *Bifidobacterium* with special reference to acid tolerance', *International Journal of Food Microbiology*, vol. 93, no. 1, pp. 109–113.

Mättö, J., Malinen, E., Suihko, M.-L., Alander, M., Palva, A. and Saarela, M. 2004, 'Genetic heterogeneity and functional properties of intestinal bifidobacteria', *Journal of Applied Microbiology*, vol. 97, no. 3, pp. 459–470.

Micanel, N., Haynes, I.N. and Playne, M.J. 1997, 'Viability of probiotic cultures in commercial Australian yogurts', *Australian Journal of Dairy Technology*, vol. 52, no. 1, pp. 24–27.

Michida, H., Tamalampudi, S., Pandiella, S.S., Webb, C., Fukuda, H. and Kondo, A. 2006, 'Effect of cereal extracts and cereal fiber on viability of *Lactobacillus plantarum* under gastrointestinal tract conditions', *Biochemical Engineering Journal*, vol. 28, no. 1, pp. 73–78.

Mottet, C. and Michetti, P. 2005, 'Probiotics: wanted dead or alive', *Digestive and Liver Disease*, vol. 37, no. 1, pp. 3–6.

Muthukumarasamy, P. and Holley, R.A. 2006, 'Microbiological and sensory quality of dry fermented sausages containing alginate-microencapsulated *Lactobacillus reuteri*', *International Journal of Food Microbiology*, vol. 111, no. 2, pp. 164–169.

Nighswonger, B.D., Brashears, M.M. and Gilliland, S.E. 1996, 'Viability of *Lactobacillus acidophilus* and *Lactobacillus casei* in fermented milk products during refrigerated storage', *Journal of Dairy Science*, vol. 79, no. 2, pp. 212–219.

Oliveira, R.P.S., Florence, A.C.R., Silva, R.C., Perego, P., Converti, A., *et al.* 2009, 'Effect of different prebiotics on the fermentation kinetics, probiotic survival and fatty acids profiles in nonfat symbiotic fermented milk', *International Journal of Food Microbiology*, vol. 128, no. 3, pp. 467–472.

Olson, D.W. and Aryana, K.J. 2008, 'An excessively high *Lactobacillus acidophilus* inoculation level in yogurt lowers product quality during storage', *LWT – Food Science and Technology*, vol. 41, no. 5, pp. 911–918.

Ong, L., Henriksson, A. and Shah, N.P. 2006, 'Development of probiotic Cheddar cheese containing *Lactobacillus acidophilus, Lb. casei, Lb. paracasei* and *Bifidobacterium* spp. and the influence of these bacteria on proteolytic patterns and production of organic acid', *International Dairy Journal*, vol. 16, no. 5, pp. 446–456.

Ong, L. and Shah, N.P. 2009, 'Probiotic cheddar cheese: Influence of ripening temperatures on proteolysis and sensory characteristics of cheddar cheeses', *Journal of Food Science*, vol. 74, no. 5, pp. S182–S191.

Østlie, H.M., Helland, M.H. and Narvhus, J.A. 2003, 'Growth and metabolism of selected strains of probiotic bacteria in milk', *International Journal of Food Microbiology*, vol. 87, no. 1–2, pp. 17–27.

Otieno, D.O., Ashton, J.F. and Shah, N.P. 2005, 'Stability of β-glucosidase activity produced by *Bifidobacterium* and *Lactobacillus* spp. in fermented soymilk during processing and storage', *Journal of Food Science*, vol. 70, no. 4, pp. M236–M241.

Özer, B., Kirmaci, H.A., Şenel, E., Atamer, M. and Hayalolu, A. 2009, 'Improving the viability of *Bifidobacterium bifidum* BB-12 and *Lactobacillus acidophilus* LA-5 in white-brined cheese by microencapsulation', *International Dairy Journal*, vol. 19, no. 1, pp. 22–29.

Paseephol, T. and Sherkat, F. 2009, 'Probiotic stability of yoghurts containing Jerusalem artichoke inulins during refrigerated storage', *Journal of Functional Foods*, vol. 1, no. 3, pp. 311–318.

Phillips, M., Kailasapathy, K. and Tran, L. 2006, 'Viability of commercial probiotic cultures (*L. acidophilus, Bifidobacterium* sp., *L. casei, L. paracasei* and *L. rhamnosus*) in cheddar cheese', *International Journal of Food Microbiology*, vol. 108, no. 2, pp. 276–280.

Picot, A. and Lacroix, C. 2004, 'Encapsulation of bifidobacteria in whey protein-based microcapsules and survival in simulated gastrointestinal conditions and in yoghurt', *International Dairy Journal*, vol. 14, no. 6, pp. 505–515.

Pitkala, K.H., Strandberg, T.E., Finne-Soveri, U.H., Ouwehand, A.C., Poussa, T. and Salminen, S. 2007, 'Fermented cereal with specific bifidobacteria normalizes bowel movements in elderly nursing home residents. A randomized, controlled trial', *Journal of Nutrition Health and Aging*, vol. 11, no. 4, pp. 305.

Puupponen-Pimiä, R., Nohynek, L., Alakomi, H.L. and Oksman-Caldentey, K.M. 2005, 'The action of berry phenolics against human intestinal pathogens', *Biofactors*, vol. 23, no. 4, pp. 243–251.

Reid, G., Jass, J., Sebulsky, M.T. and McCormick, J.K. 2003, 'Potential uses of probiotics in clinical practice', *Clinical Microbiology Reviews*, vol. 16, no. 4, pp. 658–672.

Rivera-Espinoza, Y. and Gallardo-Navarro, Y. 2010, 'Non-dairy probiotic products', *Food Microbiology*, vol. 27, no. 1, pp. 1–11.

Rodas, B.A., Angulo, J.O., De la Cruz, J. and Garcia, H.S. 2002, 'Preparation of probiotic buttermilk with *Lactobacillus reuteri*', *Milchwissenschaft*, vol. 57, no. 1, pp. 26–28.

Rößle, C., Auty, M.A.E., Brunton, N., Gormley, R.T. and Butler, F. 2010, 'Evaluation of fresh-cut apple slices enriched with probiotic bacteria', *Innovative Food Science and Emerging Technologies*, vol. 11, no. 1, pp. 203–209.

Roy, D. 2005, 'Technological aspects related to the use of bifidobacteria in dairy products', *Lait*, vol. 85, pp. 39–56.

Roy, D., Mainville, I. and Mondou, F. 1997, 'Selective enumeration and survival of bifidobacteria in fresh cheese', *International Dairy Journal*, vol. 7, no. 12, pp. 785–793.

Saarela, M., Hallamaa, K., Mattila-Sandholm, T. and Mättö, J. 2003, 'The effect of lactose derivatives lactulose, lactitol and lactobionic acid on the functional and technological properties of potentially probiotic *Lactobacillus* strains', *International Dairy Journal*, vol. 13, no. 4, pp. 291–302.

Saarela, M., Mogensen, G., Fondén, R., Mättö, J. and Mattila-Sandholm, T. 2000, 'Probiotic bacteria: Safety, functional and technological properties', *Journal of Biotechnology*, vol. 84, no. 3, pp. 197–215.

Saarela, M., Virkajärvi, I., Alakomi, H.-L., Sigvart-Mattila, P. and Mättö, J. 2006a, 'Stability and functionality of freeze-dried probiotic *Bifidobacterium* cells during storage in juice and milk', *International Dairy Journal*, vol. 16, no. 12, pp. 1477–1482.

Saarela, M., Virkajärvi, I., Nohynek, L., Vaari, A. and Mättö, J. 2006b, 'Fibres as carriers for *Lactobacillus rhamnosus* during freeze-drying and storage in apple juice and chocolate-coated breakfast cereals', *International Journal of Food Microbiology*, vol. 112, no. 2, pp. 171–178.

Saavedra, J.M., Abi-Hanna, A., Moore, N. and Yolken, R.H. 2004, 'Long-term consumption of infant formulas containing live probiotic bacteria: tolerance and safety', *American Journal of Clinical Nutrition*, vol. 79, no. 2, pp. 261–267.

Sanders, M.E., Walker, D.C., Walker, K.M., Aoyama, K. and Klaenhammer, T.R. 1996, 'Performance of commercial cultures in fluid milk applications', *Journal of Dairy Science*, vol. 79, no. 6, pp. 943–955.

Sandoval-Castilla, O., Lobato-Calleros, C., García-Galindo, H.S., Alvarez-Ramírez, J. and Vernon-Carter, E.J. 2010, 'Textural properties of alginate-pectin beads and survivability of entrapped *Lb. casei* in simulated gastrointestinal conditions and in yoghurt', *Food Research International*, vol. 43, no. 1, pp. 111–117.

Sarkar, S. 2008, 'Effect of probiotics on biotechnological characteristics of yoghurt: A review', *British Food Journal*, vol. 110, no. 7, pp. 717–740.

Savard, T., Gardner, N. and Champagne, C.-P. 2003, 'Growth of *Lactobacillus* and *Bifidobacterium* cultures in a vegetable juice medium, and their stability during storage in a fermented vegetable juice', *Sciences des Aliments*, vol. 23, no. 2, pp. 273–283.

Saxelin, M., Grenov, B., Svensson, U., Fonden, R., Reniero, R. and Mattila-Sandholm, T. 1999, 'The technology of probiotics', *Trends in Food Science & Technology*, vol. 10, no. 12, pp. 387–392.

Saxelin, M., Korpela, R. and Mäyrä-Mäkinen, A. 2003, 'Introduction: classifying functional dairy products', in *Functional Dairy Products*, eds. T. Mattila-Sandholm and M. Saarela, CRC Press, Woodhead Publishing Limited, England, pp. 244–262.

Schillinger, U. 1999, 'Isolation and identification of lactobacilli from novel-type probiotic and mild yoghurts and their stability during refrigerated storage', *International Journal of Food Microbiology*, vol. 47, no. 1–2, pp. 79–87.

Sen, S., Mullan, M.M., Parker, T.J., Woolner, J.T., Tarry, S.A. and Hunter, J.O. 2002, 'Effect of *Lactobacillus plantarum* 299 v on colonic fermentation and symptoms of irritable bowel syndrome', *Digestive Diseases and Sciences*, vol. 47, no. 11, pp. 2615–2620.

Shah, N.P. and Lankaputhra, W.E.V. 1997, 'Improving viability of *Lactobacillus acidophilus* and *Bifidobacterium* spp. in yogurt', *International Dairy Journal*, vol. 7, no. 5, pp. 349–356.

Shah, N.P., Lankaputhra, W.E.V., Britz, M.L. and Kyle, W.S.A. 1995, 'Survival of *Lactobacillus acidophilus* and *Bifidobacterium bifidum* in commercial yoghurt during refrigerated storage', *International Dairy Journal*, vol. 5, no. 5, pp. 515–521.

Shah, N.P. and Ravula, R.R. 2000, 'Microencapsulation of probiotic bacteria and their survival in frozen fermented dairy desserts', *Australian Journal of Dairy Technology*, vol. 55, no. 3, pp. 139–144.

Sheehan, V.M., Ross, P. and Fitzgerald, G.F. 2007, 'Assessing the acid tolerance and the technological robustness of probiotic cultures for fortification in fruit juices', *Innovative Food Science and Emerging Technologies*, vol. 8, no. 2, pp. 279–284.

Sultana, K., Godward, G., Reynolds, N., Arumugaswamy, R., Peiris, P. and Kailasapathy, K. 2000, 'Encapsulation of probiotic bacteria with alginate-starch and evaluation of survival in simulated gastrointestinal conditions and in yoghurt', *International Journal of Food Microbiology*, vol. 62, no. 1–2, pp. 47–55.

Talwalkar, A. and Kailasapathy, K. 2003, 'Metabolic and biochemical responses of probiotic bacteria to oxygen', *Journal of Dairy Science*, vol. 86, no. 8, pp. 2537–2546.

Talwalkar, A., Miller, C.W., Kailasapathy, K. and Nguyen, M.H. 2004, 'Effect of packaging materials and dissolved oxygen on the survival of probiotic bacteria in yoghurt', *International Journal of Food Science and Technology*, vol. 39, no. 6, pp. 605–611.

Tamime, A.Y., Saarela, M., Skriver, A., Mistry, V. and Shah, N.P. 2005, 'Production and maintaining viability of probiotic bacteria in dairy products', in *Probiotic Dairy Products*, ed. A.Y. Tamime, Blackwell Publishing Ltd, Oxford, UK, pp. 39–72.

Tang, A.L., Shah, N.P., Wilcox, G., Walker, K.Z. and Stojanovska, L. 2007, 'Fermentation of calcium-fortified soymilk with *Lactobacillus*: Effects on calcium solubility, isoflavone conversion, and production of organic acids', *Journal of Food Science*, vol. 72, no. 9, pp. M431–M436.

Temmerman, R., Scheirlinck, I., Huys, G. and Swings, J. 2003, 'Culture-independent analysis of probiotic products by denaturing gradient gel electrophoresis', *Applied and Environmental Microbiology*, vol. 69, no. 1, pp. 220–226.

Thibault, H., Aubert-Jacquin, C. and Goulet, O. 2004, 'Effects of long-term consumption of a fermented infant formula (with *Bifidobacterium breve* c50 and *Streptococcus thermophilus* 065) on acute diarrhea in healthy infants', *Journal of Pediatric Gastroenterology and Nutrition*, vol. 39, no. 2, pp. 147–152.

Valerio, F., De Bellis, P., Lonigro, S.L., Morelli, L., Visconti, A. and Lavermicocca, P. 2006, '*In vitro* and *in vivo* survival and transit tolerance of potentially probiotic strains carried by artichokes in the gastrointestinal tract', *Applied and Environmental Microbiology*, vol. 72, no. 4, pp. 3042–3045.

Vankerckhoven, V., Huys, G., Vancanneyt, M., Snauwaert, C., Swings, J., *et al.* 2008, 'Genotypic diversity, antimicrobial resistance and virulence factors of human isolates and probiotic cultures constituting two intraspecific groups in *Enterococcus faecium*', *Applied and Environmental Microbiology*, vol. 74, pp. 4247–4255.

Vinderola, C.G., Costa, G.A., Regenhardt, S. and Reinheimer, J.A. 2002a, 'Influence of compounds associated with fermented dairy products on the growth of lactic acid starter and probiotic bacteria', *International Dairy Journal*, vol. 12, no. 7, pp. 579–589.

Vinderola, C.G., Mocchiutti, P. and Reinheimer, J.A. 2002b, 'Interactions among lactic acid starter and probiotic bacteria used for fermented dairy products', *Journal of Dairy Science*, vol. 85, no. 4, pp. 721–729.

Wagner, R.D., Pierson, C., Warner, T., Dohnalek, M., Hilty, M. and Balish, E. 2000, 'Probiotic effects of feeding heat-killed *Lactobacillus acidophilus* and *Lactobacillus casei* to *Candida albicans*-colonized immunodeficient mice', *Journal of Food Protection*, vol. 63, no. 5, pp. 638–644.

Wang, Y.C., Yu, R.C. and Chou, C.C. 2006, 'Antioxidative activities of soymilk fermented with lactic acid bacteria and bifidobacteria', *Food Microbiology*, vol. 23, no. 2, pp. 128–135.

Watson, F.E., Ngesa, A., Onyang'o, J., Alnwick, D. and Tomkins, A.M. 1996, 'Fermentation – a traditional anti-diarrhoeal practice lost? The use of fermented foods in urban and rural Kenya', *International Journal of Food Sciences and Nutrition*, vol. 47, no. 2, pp. 171–179.

Wohlgemuth, S., Loh, G. and Blaut, M. 2009, 'Recent developments and perspectives in the investigation of probiotic effects', *International Journal of Medical Microbiology*, vol. 300, no. 1, pp. 3–10.

Yoon, K.Y., Woodams, E.E. and Hang, Y.D. 2004, 'Probiotication of tomato juice by lactic acid bacteria', *Journal of Microbiology and Biotechnology*, vol. 42, no. 4, pp. 315–318.

Yoon, K.Y., Woodams, E.E. and Hang, Y.D. 2005, 'Fermentation of beet juice by beneficial lactic acid bacteria', *LWT – Food Science and Technology*, vol. 38, no. 1, pp. 73–75.

Yoon, K.Y., Woodams, E.E. and Hang, Y.D. 2006, 'Production of probiotic cabbage juice by lactic acid bacteria', *Bioresource Technology*, vol. 97, no. 12, pp. 1427–1430.

Zhang, L., Li, N., Caicedo, R. and Neu, J. 2005, 'Alive and dead *Lactobacillus rhamnosus* GG decrease tumor necrosis factor-α-induced interleukin-8 production in Caco-2 cells', *Journal of Nutrition*, vol. 135, no. 7, pp. 1752–1756.

19

Functional foods for the gut: probiotics, prebiotics and synbiotics

A. Drakoularakou, R. Rastall and G. Gibson, University of Reading, UK

Abstract: The human large intestine is an intensively colonised area containing bacteria that are health positive, as well as pathogenic. Probiotics have a long history of use in humans as live microbial feed additions. In contrast, a prebiotic is a non digestible food ingredient that beneficially affects the host by targeting indigenous components thought to be positive. Main prebiotic targets at the moment are bifidobacteria and lactobacilli (although this may change as our knowledge of the flora diversity and functionality expands). Any dietary component that reaches the colon intact is a potential prebiotic, however much of the interest in the development of prebiotics is aimed at non-digestible oligosaccharides. For prebiotics (and probiotics) a determination of the health consequences that are associated with gut flora modulation (e.g. anti-pathogen activities, reduced inflammatory disorders, immunological effects, protective aspects for bowel cancer, neutralisation of certain toxins) is needed and research is ongoing.

Key words: human gut microbiology, dietary intervention, prebiotic oligosaccharides.

19.1 Introduction

In recent years views on the role of foods in human health have changed markedly. The emergence of health-conscious consumers with a proactive approach emphasising 'prevention over cure', the need to deal with an ageing population and the development of nutritional science have all helped to drive the growth of functional foods. These are foods which have properties beyond normal nutrition. Currently around 60% of functional foods in use in Europe are targeted at gastrointestinal health. To understand the basis of functional foods for the gut, it is important to understand first the composition of the gastrointestinal (GI) microbiota and its implications for human health.

19.2   The composition of gastrointestinal (GI) microbiota

The GI tract of healthy adults contains a very diverse population of microorganisms which increases in size and metabolic activity along the length of the GI tract (Gibson *et al.*, 2001). After ingestion of a meal, about 10^5 bacteria can be isolated from gastric contents. However, the bacterial count declines as the pH falls and few viable cells are recovered at pH 2–3, the normal pH of the stomach secretions (Press *et al.*, 1998). As such, the resident bacterial population of the stomach is estimated to be around 10^3/ml contents (Rathbone and Heatley, 1992).

Bacterial counts are higher in the small intestine and range from 10^4 to 10^7 per ml contents in the terminal ileum (Gibson and McCartney, 1998). One of the limiting factors is the relatively rapid transit time of luminal contents through the small intestine (usually 2–3 hours). Moving towards the colon, transit time is reduced and bacterial numbers begin to gradually increase. In the ileum water is absorbed, reducing the flow rate and thus allowing for bacterial multiplication. The upper small intestine is dominated by streptococci, staphylococci and lactobacilli, which show an increase in numbers along its length (Gibson *et al.*, 2001).

The large intestine, on the other hand, harbours an extremely complex microbial ecosystem. The colonic environment (particularly the distal colon) is more favourable to microbial colonisation, with a slow transit time (~70 hours) and pH of 5.5–6.8. Bacterial counts in colonic contents and faeces usually exceeds 10^{11}–10^{12}/g dry weight (Gibson, 1998). The adult human GI tract contains bacteria, archaea and eukarya. The main divisions (phyla) of bacteria that have been identified to date, and which appear to be the most dominant, are Bacteroidetes, Actinobacteria and Firmicutes (such as clostridia and eubacteria). Proteobacteria are also very common inhabitants but not as numerically dominant.

The main substrates available to the bacteria in the human colon are dietary carbohydrates that have escaped digestion in the small intestine. These include resistant starches, dietary fibre (cellulose, hemicellulose, pectin and inulin), and unabsorbed sugars and sugar alcohols (Roberfroid, 1999, 2000, 2002; Cummings *et al.*, 1989). Dietary carbohydrates are rapidly fermented by the saccharolytic bacteria such as *Bacteroides*, *Bifidobacterium*, *Ruminococcus*, *Eubacterium* and *Clostridium* (Salminen *et al.*, 1998). In the caecum and right colon, fermentation is very intense with high production of short-chain fatty acids, an acidic pH (5–6), and rapid bacterial growth. On the other hand, substrate in the left or distal colon is less available, the pH is close to neutral, putrefactive processes become quantitatively more important, and bacterial populations are stable.

The principal products of colonic bacterial fermentation are the short-chain fatty acids (SCFA) acetate, propionate and butyrate. Intermediate products of saccharolysis in the colon (such as lactate, ethanol and succinate) do not accumulate in the lumen as they are utilised by other bacterial species. A summary of different bacterial groups and the predominant products of carbohydrate breakdown are shown in Table 19.1. Approximately 300 mM SCFA are produced daily from bacterial fermentation in the human colon (Topping and Clifton, 2001). It has been suggested that over 95% of SCFA is absorbed through the colonic epithelium.

Table 19.1 Major metabolic end-products of the colonic microbiota and some of the bacterial groups implicated in their production

Metabolic products	Bacterial groups
Acetate	Bacteroides, bifidobacteria, butyrivibrio, clostridia, eubacteria, fusobacteria, lactobacilli, peptostreptococci, propionibacteria
Propionate	Bacteroides, propionibacteria, veillonella
Butyrate	Butyrivibrio, clostridia, eubacteria, fusobacteria, peptostreptococci
Ethanol	Bacteroides, bifidobacteria, clostridia, lactobacilli, peptostreptococci
Lactate	Actinomycetes, bacteroides, bifidobacteria, clostridia, enterococci, eubacteria, fusobacteria, lactobacilli, peptostreptococci, ruminococci
Succinate	Bacteroides, prevotella, ruminococci
Hydrogen	Clostridia, fusobacteria, ruminococci
Formate	Bacteroides, bifidobacteria, butyrivibrio, enterobacteria, eubacteria, ruminococci

Source: Gibson *et al.*, 1998.

The most abundant SCFA in the human colon is acetate. It crosses the colonic epithelium into the hepatic portal circulation and is eventually transferred to the liver. It is then distributed to peripheral tissues to be metabolised by muscle and brain cells (Salminen *et al.*, 1998). Propionate is mainly cleared by the liver. Its exact function is as yet unknown, but it is possible that it functions as a gluconeogenic precursor and could also be involved in the reduction of plasma lipid values (Gibson, 1998). The third physiologically important SCFA is butyrate, as it is the primary energy source for colonocytes accounting for 70% of their oxygen consumption. In epithelial cells, butyrate is metabolised via β-oxidation. This initially involves conversion to butyrl-CoA by the enzyme butyryl-CoAsynthetase and, in a series of reactions, a rapid conversion to acetyl-CoA. Butyrate serves as an energy yielding substrate in the colonocytes and can affect several cellular functions like proliferation and differentiation.

As well as playing a role in the production of SCFA, resident bacteria are a crucial line of resistance to colonisation by exogenous microbes and, therefore, are extremely important in prevention of invasion of tissues by pathogens. Several mechanisms have been implicated in the barrier effect. These include competiton for nutrients and colonisation sites, as well as direct inhibitory processes (e.g. the production of acids or peptides) (Guarner, 2006).

19.3 Probiotics

Cultured dairy products, together with other lactic acid fermented foods, have been part of the human diet for thousands of years and are considered to have therapeutic effects in many cultures. Elie Metchnikoff was the first to suggest a scientific basis for the consumption of fermented milk as beneficial to health (Metchnikoff, 1907). The apparent benefits of such products in improving digestive health provided a starting point for the development of the concept of probiotics.

The term probiotic, derived from the Greek meaning 'for life', was first used by Lilley and Stillwell (1965) to describe substances produced by one microorganism that stimulate the growth of another. Sperti (1971) later used the term 'probiotic' to describe tissue extracts that stimulate microbial growth. The terminology totally changed when Parker (1974) defined probiotics as 'organisms and substances which contribute to intestinal microbial balance'. This definition was further improved by Fuller (1989) who redefined probiotics as 'live microbial feed supplement which beneficially affects the host animal by improving its intestinal microbial balance'. A later definition was introduced by Salminen *et al.* (1999), who defined probiotics as 'preparations of microbial cells that have a beneficial effect on the health and well-being of the host'. The currently accepted FAO/WHO definition is 'live microorganisms which when administered in adequate amounts confer a health benefit on the host' (Anon., 2002)

Probiotic bacteria are generally (though not exclusively) lactic acid bacteria, notably species of *Lactobacillus* and *Bifidobacterium*. Some of these microorganisms originate from the intestinal tract of humans or other animals. Their wide use as starters in dairy products is based on the fact that not only do they provide fermented products with longer preservation time than the raw product, but they also have beneficial nutritional and health effects on consumers. In order to provide these effects the retailed product must contain a minimum probiotic content. The most recent proposals within the EU require that the minimum level of probiotic bacteria should be set at 10^7 CFU/g (EU/AGRI/38743/2003rev3).

A healthy microbiota has been considered to be one that is predominantly saccharolytic and comprises significant numbers of bifidobacteria and lactobacilli (Cummings *et al.*, 1989, 2001). The genera *Bifidobacterium* and *Lactobacillus* are generally pathogen free (though oral bifidobacteria (*B. dentium*) are considered pathogens). They are primarily carbohydrate-fermenting bacteria, unlike other groups, such as *Bacteroides* and *Clostridium* spp., members of which are also proteolytic and amino acid fermenting. The products of carbohydrate fermentation, principally short-chain fatty acids (SCFA) are beneficial to host health, while those of protein breakdown and amino acid fermentation, which include ammonia, phenols, indoles, thiols, amines and sulphides are not (Gibson *et al.*, 2001).

As well as contributing towards a healthy microbiota in the GI tract, lactic acid-producing bacteria, such as bifidobacteria and lactobacilli are also believed to play a significant role in the maintenance of colonisation resistance. There are several proposed mechanisms of antimicrobial action of probiotics against GI pathogens which cause infections. Probiotics are considered to produce inhibitory compounds such as organic acids which decrease luminal pH. Production of lactic and acetic acids by *Lactobacillus* and *Bifidobacterium* spp. appears to be the most likely mechanism of inhibition of pathogenic bacteria (Asahara *et al.*, 2001).

Probiotics also produce antimicrobial substances which can directly interfere with the growth of the pathogens (Ouwehand, 1999, 2004). Such compounds include peptides and proteins, which have been grouped into three classes: Class I which includes lantibiotics, Class II which includes small heat stable antimicrobial peptides and Class III which comprises large heat-stable antimicrobials. Adherence of probiotics to intestinal surfaces could also prevent pathogen adhesion through receptor competition or blocking of binding site of pathogens. The beneficial effects of probiotics may also be achieved through a variety of immunomodulation mechanisms including regulation of cytokine (such as IFN-γ, IFN-α and IL-12) production and enhancement of IgA secretion (Yan and Polk, 2004).

19.3.1 Effects of probiotics on GI disease states

GI infections such as diarrhoea can occur due to changes in the gut microbiota such as the establishment of an invading pathogen. Diarrhoeal diseases are still a major cause of morbidity and mortality in infants and children, causing many deaths each year. *Lactobacillus rhamnosus* GG and *Bifidobacterium animalis* subsp. *lactis* Bb12 have been associated with reduced incidence and duration of rotavirus diarrhoea in children (Guandalini *et al.*, 2000). Probiotics have also been linked to the prevention of traveller's diarrhoea (McFarland, 2007; Takahashi *et al.*, 2007).

Clostridium difficile is currently recognised as a very common cause of nosocomial infectious diarrhoea. The incidence of *C. difficile* has doubled in recent years and accounts for approximately 3 million cases of diarrhoea and colitis each year. Overall mortality associated with *C. difficile* infectious diarrhoea is estimated to be 17% but is even higher in the older adult population (Crogan and Evans, 2007). The majority of *C. difficile* infections are treated with antimicrobial agents such as antibiotics. However, such agents also have a non-specific impact on the normal gut microbiota. Probiotics have been suggested as an alternative treatment. McFarland (2000) described the effect of *S. boulardii* in a double-blind placebo-controlled human trial. *S. boulardii* was administered daily (at a dose of 3 g) together with vancomycin (for eradication) over a period of 28 days. Recurrence was significantly lower in the group consuming the probiotic. A proposed mechanism for the action of *S. boulardii* was the digestion of toxin A or B (produced by *C. difficile*) and the production of receptors for these toxins on intestinal mucoepithelium. The ability of *Lactobacillus plantarum* 299 V to prevent recurrence of *C. difficile*-associated diarrhoea (CDAD) has also been evaluated in a double-blind, placebo-controlled study (Wult *et al.*, 2003). Recurrent infections were observed in fewer of the patients receiving the probiotic strain than with patients treated with antibiotics.

Diarrhoea induced by antibiotics (AAD) can sometimes be attributed to the abnormal proliferation of *C. difficile* in the gut, because of the disturbed intestinal microbial balance induced by antibiotics. Many different probiotic strains have been studied for their effects on AAD. Asymptomatic *H. pylori* infected patients suffering from AAD were, for example, treated with *L. rhamnosus* GG, which significantly reduced diarrhoea, nausea and taste disturbance (Armuzzi *et al.*, 1999). In another study, *L. rhamnosus* GG was administered to children receiving antibiotics for respiratory infections, resulting in a reduced incidence of AAD (Arvola *et al.*, 1999). An overview of a range of studies on the use of probiotics for the treatment of AAD and *C. difficile* infections has been provided by McFarland (2009). Probiotic preparations such as *L. rhamnosus* GG, *L. acidophilus* and *B. animalis* subsp. *lactis* have also been evaluated for the prevention of side effects of *H. pylori* treatment (Cremonini *et al.*, 2002; Tong *et al.*, 2007).

Lactose intolerance is caused by a deficiency in the intestinal brush-border enzyme β-galactosidase (lactase), resulting in an inability to digest lactose. The common therapeutic approach tends to exclude milk and dairy products from the diet. However, this strategy may have serious nutritional disadvantages, chiefly for reduced intake of substances such as calcium, phosphorus and vitamins, and maybe associated with decreased bone mineral density. To overcome these limitations, several studies have been carried out to find alternative approaches, such as exogenous galactosidase, yogurt and probiotics for their bacterial lactase activity. These and other potential health benefits of probiotics are discussed in Reid *et al.* (2003), Culligan *et al.* (2009), Lomax and Calder (2009) and Wohlgemuth *et al.* (2009).

Inflammatory bowel disease (IBD) is a chronic inflammatory condition of the GI tract that can present either as ulcerative colitis (UC) or Crohn's disease (CD). The aetiology of this condition remains unknown but microbial influences are seen as a strong factor. Venturi *et al.* (1999) carried out a pilot study using the probiotic cocktail VSL#3, containing eight probiotic strains (*L. acidophilus, L.casei, L. bulgaricus, L. plantarum, B. longum, B. infantis, B. breve* and *Streptococcus salivarius* subsp. *thermophilus*), as maintenance treatment for patients with UC in remission to assess its impact on the faecal microbiota. 20 patients received 6 g/day of VSL#3 probiotic mixture for 12 months and were assessed clinically and endoscopically at baseline, at 6 and 12 months, and in the event of a relapse. 15 of the 20 patients (75%) remained in remission throughout the treatment period. In patients with pouchitis, treatment with a combined preparation of probiotics (VSL#3 probiotic cocktail and *Streptococcus salivarius*; containing 5×10^{11} bacteria per gram) dramatically reduced relapses (15% of patients with probiotics vs. 100% of the placebo group) (Gionchetti *et al.*, 2003). In addition, four months after the end of the feeding study, all patients with bacteriotherapy were in remission.

Irritable bowel syndrome (IBS) is a functional bowel disorder characterised by symptoms such as abdominal pain, diarrhoea and/or constipation (Drossman *et al.*, 2003). IBS is a poorly understood GI condition, which typically begins in early adult life and is believed to affect 3–15% of the general population in Western countries. Probiotics may have beneficial effects on altered colonic immune states (such as those be found in some IBS patients). In fact, promising evidence is provided by the study of O'Mahony *et al.* (2005), in which treatment of IBS with *Bifidobacterium infantis* normalised pro-inflammatory IL10/IL12-ratios towards an anti-inflammatory state. This was associated with significant improvement in IBS symptoms. Alteration of the colonic microbiota, using probiotics, may modify gut fermentation processes and hence gas production, colonic transit and fluid fluxes. In fact, abdominal bloating, distension and/or flatulence (which are dominant symptoms in many IBS patients) have been shown to improve significantly following probiotic treatment (Nobaek *et al.*, 2000; Bausserman and Michail, 2005; Kim *et al.*, 2005; O'Mahony *et al.*, 2005). A review of a number of studies on the use of probiotics in the treatment of IBS has been provided by Hoveyda *et al.* (2009).

19.4   Prebiotics and synbiotics

Prebiotics are a far more recent concept than probiotics, being first developed in the mid 1990s. Prebiotics have been defined as 'non-digestible food ingredients that beneficially affect the host by selectively stimulating the growth and/or activity of one, or a limited number of bacteria in the colon, and which may thus improve the health of the host' (Gibson and Roberfroid, 1995). A more recent and broader definition (ISAPP, 2008) is: 'A dietary prebiotic is a selectively fermented ingredient that results in specific changes in the composition and/or activity of the gastrointestinal microbiota, thus conferring benefit(s) upon host health.'

There are three very important criteria in order to classify a food ingredient as a prebiotic (Gibson and Roberfroid, 1999; Gibson *et al.*, 2004).

1 Resistance to gastric acidity, hydrolysis by mammalian enzymes and GI absorption.
2 Fermentation by intestinal microbiota.
3 Selective stimulation of the growth and/or activity of intestinal bacteria associated with health and well-being.

Prebiotics are distinct from most dietary fibres like pectin, celluloses or xylan which are not selectively metabolised in the gut. Dietary prebiotics are typically oligosaccharides that escape digestion in the upper gastrointestinal tract. Their common target is selective fermentation by *Bifidobacterium* and *Lactobacillus* species. For this reason they are sometimes referred to as bifidogenic factors. Prebiotics can affect human health indirectly, through the stimulation of bifidobacteria and lactobacilli, and directly through their physicochemical properties as dietary ingredients.

It is crucial that prebiotics are selectively fermented by their target bacterial groups, such as bifidobacteria. There are a number of *in vitro* studies which have suggested this selective stimulation of bifidobacteria and lactobacilli (Yazawa *et al.*, 1978; Yazawa and Tamura, 1982; Gibson, 1998; Hylla *et al.*, 1998). Several *in vivo* studies have shown similar results (Gibson *et al.*, 1995; Kleessen *et al.*, 1997, 2001; Kruse *et al.*, 1999; Rao, 2001; Boehm *et al.*, 2002). Other studies on selective fermentation of bifidobacteria specific to particular types of prebiotic are discussed later in this chapter.

Recently there has been a call to standardise methods for demonstrating a candidate prebiotic meets all three criteria required (Roberfroid, 2007), including the following:

- Resistance to gastric acidity, hydrolysis by mammalian enzymes and GI absorption: *in vitro* methods including determining resistance to acidic conditions and enzymatic hydrolysis; *in vivo* techniques such as the direct recovery of undigested molecules from the distal ileum and faeces.
- Fermentation by intestinal microbiota: *in vitro* methods such as anaerobic fermentation by mixed bacterial populations; *in vivo* methods such as analysis of faecal samples after oral feeding and measuring recovery of the tested prebiotic.
- Selective stimulation of the growth and/or activity of intestinal bacteria associated with health and well-being: *in vitro* techniques such as anaerobic sampling of faeces followed by reliable and quantitative microbiological analysis of the range of bacterial genera present.

On this basis, it has been suggested that only inulin and trans-galacto-oligosaccharides (TOS) have so far been fully validated as prebiotics, even though the evidence for other candidate prebiotics is promising (Roberfroid, 2007).

Mechanisms by which prebiotic oligosaccharides are selectively metabolised by beneficial members of the gut microbiota are not adequately understood at the present time. There are two general paradigms of prebiotic metabolism. The most documented of which is the possession by probiotic microorganisms of cell-associated exo-glycosidases. Such enzymes act by hydrolysis of monosaccharides from the non-reducing end of the oligosaccharide, which are then taken up by the cell. This mechanism has been shown to operate in *B. infantis*, which possesses cell-associated β-fructofuranosidase activity. An alternative mechanism is the uptake of intact oligosaccharides by probiotic organisms followed by intracellular metabolism, and there is some evidence that this mechanism may operate in some species (Kaplan and Hutkins, 2000). The extent to which these two mechanisms operate *in vivo* remains to be determined.

Prebiotics such as fructooligosaccharides (FOS) and galactooligosaccharides (GOS) are readily fermented in the proximal colon, suggesting any beneficial effects may not persist in the distal colon where colonic diseases such as ulcerative colitis and tumours originate (Roediger, 1980; Bufill, 1990; Macfarlane *et al.*, 1992; Lupton and Kurtz, 1993). One avenue of research has focused on developing prebiotics which persist to more distal regions of the colon, for example through enzymatic modification of polysaccharides (Olano-Martin *et al.*, 2000; Wichienchot *et al.*, 2006).

There are a number of studies associating prebiotics with the alleviation of conditions such as IBS and diarrhoea. A range of these studies are summarised in Table 19.2. A number of studies of the beneficial effects of prebiotics on human subjects have been reviewed by Saavendra and Tschemia (2002). There has been interest in effects of prebiotics on lipid metabolism, immunomodulation of the gut immune system, glycaemic control, gut hormones, weight loss and satiety (Parnell and Reimer, 2009). The books by Tannock (2002), Gibson and Rastall (2006), Gibson and Roberfroid (2008), Versalovic and Wilson (2008) and Charalampopoulos and Rastall (2009) all summarise a range of research on the selective stimulaton of bifidobacteria by prebiotics and the associated benefits for gut health.

Table 19.2   Examples of human intervention studies performed with prebiotics

Clinical condition	Prebiotic intervention and clinical outcome	Reference
Inflammatory bowel disease	24 g/day of inulin for 3 weeks reduced the endoscopic and histological pouchitis disease index score	Welters *et al.* (2002)
	Improved ulcerative colitis (UC) symptomology with a synbiotic (*B. longum*/Synergy 1 (FOS and inulin mixture)) approach that increased gut bifidobacteria	Furrie *et al.* (2005)
	Lactulose (20 g/d) showed beneficial effects in a study of IBD patients with a reduction in disease symptoms relative to controls	Szilagyi *et al.* (2002)
	FOS and inulin gave positive results in CD patients, with a significant reduction in disease severity in one small open label study	Lindsay *et al.* (2006)
	A mixture of FOS and inulin showed significant reductions in disease severity indices, reduction in pro-inflammatory immune markers and reduction in calprotectin, a validated marker of intestinal inflammation	Konikoff and Denson (2006)
Antibiotic-associated diarrhoea	Daily ingestion of 12 g of FOS reduced episodes of diarrhoea in 142 patients with *C. difficile* induced diarrhoea	Lewis *et al.* (2005)
Traveller's diarrhoea	244 healthy subjects travelling to high or medium risk destinations for traveller's diarrhoea received either 10 g of FOS or placebo for 2 weeks before travelling and then for the 2 weeks they were away. The prevalence of diarrhoea was lower in the prebiotic group and less severe attacks of diarrhoea were recorded.	Cummings *et al.* (2001)

Continued

Table 19.2   Continued

Clinical condition	Prebiotic intervention and clinical outcome	Reference
	The positive effects of GOS in reducing diarrhoea were confirmed	Drakoularakou *et al.* (2010)
Bowel cancer	sc-FOS (short chain FOS) was investigated in a study on adenoma and adenoma-free patients. Feeding 10 g/day sc-FOS resulted in positive effects in biomarkers in the adenoma-free patients	Boutron-Ruault *et al.* (2005)
	Synbiotic: a FOS and inulin mixture (Synergy 1) together with *L. rhamnosus* GG and *B. animalis* subsp. *lactis* Bb-12. The study was a 12-week double-blind, placebo-controlled trial in cancer patients and polypectomised individuals. Colorectal cell proliferation and genotoxicity were significantly reduced and the intestinal barrier function increased	Rafter *et al.* (2007)
Calcium absorption and bone health	Inulin type-fructans enhanced calcium absorption primarily via the colonic mucosa in humans	Abrams *et al.* (2005)
	When 100 young adolescents received 8 g/day of short and long chain inulin fructans for a year, a significant increase in calcium absorption was seen and moreover led to greater bone mineral density	Abrams *et al.* (2005)
Childhood diarrhoea	A significant decrease in diarrhoea, vomiting and fever in a study of young children in a day-care centre. Infants were fed 2 g/day FOS or placebo for 21 days in a double-blind trial	Waligora-Dupriet *et al.* (2007)
Irritable bowel syndrome	Feeding of GOS caused improvements in IBS following prebiotic-based modulation of gut bifidobacteria. This included statistically significant effects on gut function and typical IBS symptoms (FOS).	Silk *et al.* (2009)

FOS = fructooligosaccharide; GOS = galactooligosaccharide.

19.4.1   Fructooligosaccharides

Fructooligosaccharides (FOS) are one of the major classes of bifidogenic oligosaccharides as far as production volume and use are concerned. They are polymers of D-fructose joined by β-(2–1) bonds. Molecules with a degree of polymerisation (DP) between 3 and 5 are referred to as oligofructose. Those with a DP between 2 and 60 are referred to as inulin. This section discusses FOS in general followed by a more detailed discussion of inulin given its particularly widespread use.

FOS occur naturally in a range of plants such as chicory, onion, garlic, tomato and banana. Commercially available inulin and oligofructose are mainly produced from chicory and beet sugar, with very small scale production also from dahlia tubers and agave. FOS can be manufactured by the transglycosylation of sucrose by the enzyme β-fructofuranosidase. High concentrations of starting material are required. Glucose, small amounts of fructose and unreacted sucrose are all by-products of the reaction, but these can be removed using chromatographic procedures to obtain FOS of higher purity (Nakakuki, 2003). FOS can also be produced via the enzymatic hydrolysis of inulin. An overview of the production steps of FOS is shown in Fig. 19.1.

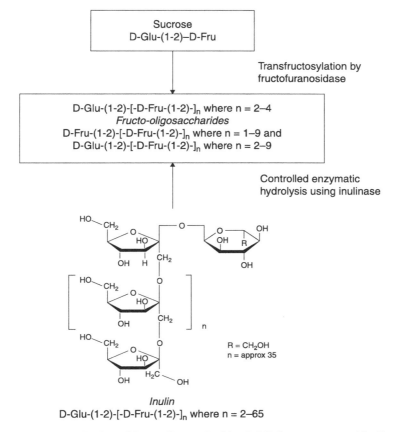

Fig. 19.1   Production of fructooligosaccharides (FOS) from sucrose and inulin.

A number of studies have shown that FOS are resistant to hydrolysis by human digestive enzymes, that they reach the colon and are then fermented by the colonic microbiota, making them potential prebiotics (Molis *et al.*, 1996; Ellegard *et al.*, 1997; Andersson *et al.*, 1999; Roberfroid, 1999). Other studies have focused on their selective stimulation of target bacteria. A study by Wang and Gibson (1993) showed preferential fermentation of FOS by bifidobacteria, while populations of *Escherichia coli* and *Clostridium perfringens* remained at relatively low levels. A later study by Gibson and Wang (1994) determined the bifidogenic effect of oligofructose in single stage continuous culture systems inoculated with human faecal bacteria, while Kaplan and Hutkins (2000) found that 12 of the 16 *Lactobacillus* strains and 7 of 8 *Bifidobacterium* strains they studied were able to ferment FOS on MRS agar.

A number of *in vivo* studies have also shown that ingestion of FOS has selectively stimulated the growth of bifidobacteria and inhibited the growth of clostridia (Gibson *et al.* 1995; Kleessen *et al.*, 1997; Kruse *et al.*, 1999). Subsequent studies have similarly demonstrated a major shift in the intestinal bacterial composition after ingestion of FOS, with bifidobacteria increasing significantly (Bouhnik *et al.*, 1997; Marx *et al.*, 2000; Tuohy *et al.*, 2001a, b; Harmsen *et al.*, 2002; Flickinger and Fahey, 2002; Kolida *et al.*, 2002; Biedrzycka and Bielecka, 2004; Sangeetha *et al.*, 2005).

19.4.2   Inulin

Perhaps the most widely used FOS is inulin. As has been noted, inulin has a chain length of between 2 and 60+ fructose units with β-(2–1) links and with a glucose terminal end linked by an α-(2–1) bond. Many plants contain inulin, notably plants of the Compositae family (Davidson and Maki, 1999; Lopez-Molina *et al.*, 2005). Inulin is extracted mainly from the artichoke via enzymatic hydrolysis, though it can also be derived from chicory and dahlias. Standard methods of extraction, purification and isolation of inulin from plants significantly reduce the degree of polymerisation (DP) of the product (Moerman *et al.*, 2004). This change in DP affects inulin sweetness, water-binding capacity and digestibility, reducing both its value as an ingredient in further processing and its prebiotic activity. Techniques to increase the DP of inulin include ultrafiltration and the use of transgenic plants designed specifically to synthesise high chain-length inulin (Hellwege *et al.*, 2000 and Moerman *et al.*, 2004).

Inulin's prebiotic efficacy has been documented in a number of studies (Yazawa *et al.*, 1978; Yazawa and Tamura, 1982; Gibson *et al.*, 1995; Campbell *et al.*, 1997; Roberfroid *et al.*, 1998; Menne *et al.*, 2000; Cherbut, 2002; Roberfroid, 2002). Its bifodogenic effect has been linked to immune system stimulation and anti-mutagenic effects on colonocytes (Jenkins *et al.*, 1999; Roberfroid, 1999; Guigoz *et al.*, 2002), as well as inhibition of the growth of clostridia (Gibson *et al.*, 1995; Hopkins and Macfarlane, 2003) and other pathogens (Shiba *et al.*, 2003; van Nuenen *et al.*, 2003; Servin, 2004). It has also been linked to vitamin B production (Deguchi *et al.*, 1985) and reduction of the hypercholesterolaemic effects of some foods (Davidson and Maki, 1999). Because inulin resists digestion in the stomach and small intestine, it has also been considered as a protective envelope for drugs targeting the diseases associated with the distal colon such as Crohn's disease and ulcerative colitis (Fuchs, 1993; Chourasia and Jain, 2002). A review of human trials using inulin to improve immune function has been provided by Roberfroid (2007).

19.4.3   Galactooligosaccharides

Galactooligosaccharides (GOS) consist of a number of β-(1–6) linked and β-(1–4) galactopyranosyl units linked to a terminal glucopyranosyl residue through an α-(1–4) glycosidic bond. They have been reported in fermented milk as a result of β-galactosidase activity of starter bacterial cultures (Sako et al., 1999). These oligosaccharides are synthesised from lactose by a β-galactosidase transfer reaction, resulting in the formation of a family of di- to hexasaccharides, with the end products depending on the source of the enzyme. The enzyme transfers the galactose moiety of a β-galactosidase to an acceptor containing a hydroxyl group. Galactose is formed when the acceptor is water, whereas trisaccharides are formed when the acceptor is lactose. Trisaccharides can, in turn, act as acceptors, resulting in the formation of tetrasaccharides, pentasaccharides and hexasaccharides (Crittenden and Playne, 1996). An overview of the production process for GOS is shown in Fig. 19.2.

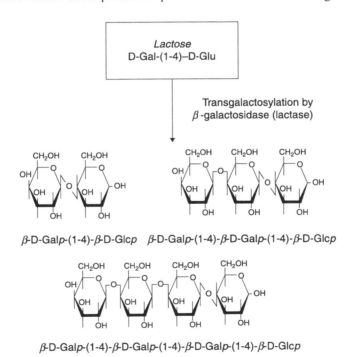

Fig. 19.2   Production of galactooligosaccharides (GOS) from lactose. Gal, galactose; Glc, glucose (Tungland and Meyer, 2002).

A number of *in vivo* studies have shown that faecal bifidobacterial levels are stimulated by consumption of GOS (Ito *et al.*, 1993; Bouhnik *et al.*, 1997). More recent studies by Boehm *et al.* (2002) and Chung and Day (2002) showed GOS were readily fermented by *Bifidobacterium* and *Lactobacillus* spp., but not by *Salmonella* sp. or *E. coli*.

19.4.4   Trans-galactooligosaccharides

Trans-galactooligosaccharides (TOS) are a mixture of oligosaccharides produced from lactose by transgalactosylation. They are linear oligomers consisting of varying proportions of D-glucose and D-galactose, primarily in 1–4 and 1–6 linkages (Alles *et al.*, 1999). They resist digestion by β-galactosidases in the small intestine and enter the colon where, like other dietary fibres, they are fermented by the colonic micobiota. β-galactosidases have been extracted from different probiotic strains of bifidobacteria and used to synthesise TOS in the presence of lactose (Rabiu *et al.*, 2001).

It has been demonstrated that fermentation of TOS is selective for bifidobacteria (Tanaka *et al.*, 1983; Ito *et al.*, 1993; Rowland and Tanaka, 1993; Bouhnik *et al.*, 1997; Alles *et al.*, 1999; Moro *et al.*, 2005). Such studies have also suggested potential health benefits such as a reduction in faecal nitroreductase activity and decreased levels of indole and isovaleric acid. It has also been suggested that TOS inhibits pathogens such as *E. coli* (EPEC) from binding to human colonic cells where they can cause infection (Shoaf *et al.*, 2006).

19.4.5   New candidate prebiotics and synbiotics

As our knowledge of gut microbial diversity expands, along with our understanding of the implications of this diversity for health, new candidate prebiotics are being identified. Among the current candidates are polydextrose, soybean oligosaccharides, lactosucrose, isomalto-oligosaccharides, gluco-oligosaccharide, xylo-oligosaccharide, palatinos, gluconic acid, gentio-oligosaccharides, mannan oligosaccharide, lactose, hemicellulose, resistant starch and its derivatives, oat bran, oligosaccharides from melibiose, β-glucans, N-acetylchitooligosaccharides, sugar alcohols such as lactitol, sorbitol and maltitol. An example of this kind of development is BiMuno, a synthetic lactose based oligosaccharide synthesised from enzymes in *B. bifidum* 41171. BiMuno has been tested *in vitro* in pigs and in humans for its prebiotic effect (Depeint *et al.*, 2008; Vulevic *et al.*, 2008). It has also been linked to improvements in conditions such as irritable bowel syndrome (Silk *et al.*, 2009) and diarrhoea (Drakoularakou *et al.*, 2010).

Synbiotics are defined as 'a mixture of probiotics and prebiotics that beneficially affects the host by improving the survival and implantation of live microbial dietary supplements in the GI tract' (Gibson and Roberfroid, 1995). Synbiotics are designed to beneficially affect the host by:

- improving survival and implantation of probiotics in the colon;
- selectively stimulating the growth or activating the metabolism of health promoting bacteria (including probiotics) in the colon;
- improving the GI tract microbial composition.

A number of studies have suggested a synergistic effect in combining probiotics and prebiotics (Roberfroid, 1998; Rowland *et al.*, 1998; Schaafsma *et al.* 1998). Though less developed than research into prebiotics, this remains a promising area for future research.

19.5   Conclusions

Major advances have been made in the application of pharmaceutical-based interventions for improving human health. Nevertheless, the incidence of both acute and chronic disorders remains high. Drug based therapies are often inefficient, expensive and may have unwarranted side effects. Moreover, the indiscriminate use of antibiotics has led to a reduction in potency and efficiency. As the population continues to age, there is increasing susceptibility among consumers to morbidity and mortality. In later years, there is more emphasis on long-term care rather than treatment. This necessitates a more prophylactic approach. Attention has therefore turned towards dietary ingredients that help to improve health and treat disease.

The realisation of the importance of gut microbiology in human health and nutrition has led to a major increase in research into probiotic and prebiotic products. There is significant evidence to suggest that prebiotics, for example, have great potential as agents to improve or maintain a balanced intestinal microbiota to enhance health and well-being. However, the evidence in some cases, whilst promising, is neither complete nor conclusive, and there is a need both for further research and agreement on standard methods which will provide definitive and comparable data. With a new generation of molecular microbiological techniques emerging, and the possibility of developing detailed profiles of target bacteria, it will be easier both to test candidate prebiotics and tailor them to achieve specific health outcomes.

19.6   References

Abrams, S.A., Griffin, I.J., Hawthorne, K.M., Liang, L., Gunn, S.K., *et al.* (2005). A combination of prebiotic short- and long-chain inulin-type fructans enhances calcium absorption and bone mineralization in young adolescents. *American Journal of Clinical Nutrition*, **82**, 471–476.

Alles, M.S., Hartemink, R., Meyboom, S., Harryvan, J.L., Van Laere, K., *et al.* (1999). Effect of transgalactooligosaccharides on the composition of the human intestinal microflora and on putative risk markers for colon cancer. *American Journal of Clinical Nutrition*, **69**, 980–991.

Andersson, H.B., Elegard, L.H. and Bosaeus, I.G. (1999). Nondigestibility characteristics of inulin and oligofructose in humans. *Journal of Nutrition*, **129**, 1428S–1429S.

Anon. (2002). *Guidelines for the evaluation of probiotics in food.* Joint FAO/WHO working group report on drafting guidelines for the evaluation of probiotics in food.

Armuzzi, A., Gasbarrini, A., Franceschi, F., Ojetti, V., Candelli, M., *et al.* (1999). Efficacy of *Lactobacillus* GG in decreasing antibiotic-associated gastrointestinal morbidity during *H. pylori* eradication regimen. *Gut,* **45** (Suppl. 3), 121–125.

Arvola, T., Laiho, K. and Torkkeli, S. (1999). Prophylactic *Lactobacillus* GG reduces antibiotic-associated diarrhea in children with respiratory infections: a randomized study. *Pediatrics,* **104**, 64–78.

Asahara, T., Nomoto, K., Shimizu, K., Watanuki, M. and Tanaka, R. (2001). Increased resistance of mice to *Salmonella enterica serovar Typhymurium* infection by synbiotic administration of bifidobacteria and transgalactosylated oligosaccharides. *Journal of Applied Microbiology,* **91**, 985–996.

Bausserman, M. and Michail, S. (2005). The use of *Lactobacillus* GG in irritable bowel syndrome in children: a double-blind randomized control trial. *Journal of Pediatrics,* **147**, 197–201.

Biedrzycka, E. and Bielecka, M. (2004). Prebiotic effectiveness of fructans of different degrees of polymerisation, *Trends Food Sci Technol,* **15**, 255–267.

Boehm, G., Lidestri, M., Casetta, P., Jelinek, J., Negretti, F., *et al.* (2002). Supplementation of a bovine milk formula with an oligosaccharide mixture increases counts of faecal bifidobacteria in preterm infants. *Archives of Disease in Childhood: Fetal and Neonatal,* **86**, 178–181.

Bouhnik, Y., Flourie, B., D'Agay-Abensour, L., Pochart, P., Gramet, G., *et al.* (1997). Administration of *trans*galacto-oligosaccharides increases fecal bifidobacteria and modifies colonic fermentation metabolism in healthy humans. *Journal of Nutrition,* **127**, 444–448.

Boutron-Ruault, M.C., Marteau, P., Lavergne-Slove, A., Myara, A. and Gerhardt, M.F. (2005). Effects of a 3-mo consumption of short-chain fructo-oligosaccharides on parameters of colorectal carcinogenesis in patients with or without small or large colorectal adenomas. *Nutrition and Cancer,* **53**, 160–168.

Bufill, J. (1990). Colorectal cancer: evidence for distinct genetic categories based on proximal or distal tumor location. *Annals of Internal Medicine,* **113**, 779–788.

Campbell, J.H., Fahey, G.C. and Wolf, B.W. (1997). Selected indigestible oligosaccharides affect large bowel mass, cecal and fecal short-chain fatty acids, pH and microflora in rats. *Journal of Nutrition,* **127**, 130–6.

Charalampopoulos, D. and Rastall, R.A. [editors] (2009), *Prebiotics and Probiotics Science and Technology.* Springer, New York.

Cherbut, C. (2002). Inulin and oligofructose in the dietary fibre concept. *British Journal of Nutrition,* **87** (Supplement 2), S159–S162.

Cherbut, C., Michel, C. and Lecannu, G. (2003). The prebiotic characteristics of fructooligosaccharides are necessary for reduction of TNBS-induced colitis in rats. *Journal of Nutrition,* **133**, 21–27.

Chourasia, M. and Jain, S. (2002). Pharmaceutical approaches to colon targeted drug delivery systems. *Journal of Pharmacy and Pharmacology,* **6**, 33–66.

Chung, C.H. and Day, D.F. (2002). Glucooligosaccharides from *Leuconostoc mesenteroides* B-742 (ATCC 13146): a potential prebiotic. *Journal of Industrial Microbiology and Biotechnology,* **29**, 186–199.

Cremonini, F., Di Caro, S. and Nista, E.C. (2002). Meta-analysis: The effect of probiotic administration on antibiotic associated diarrhea. *Alimentary Pharmacology Therapies,* **16**, 1461–1467.

Crogan, N.L. and Evans, B.C. (2007). *Clostridium difficile*: an emerging epidemic in nursing homes. *Geriatric Nursing,* **28**, 161–164.

Crittenden, R.G and Playne, M.J. (1996). Production, properties and applications of food-grade oligosaccharides. *Trends in Food Science and Technology,* 7, 353–361.

Culligan, E.P., Hill, C. and Sleator, R.D. (2009). Probiotics and gastrointestinal disease: successes, problems and future prospects. *Gut Pathogens,* **1**, 19–30.

Cummings, J.H., Christie, S. and Cole, T.J. (2001). A study of fructo oligosaccharides in the prevention of travellers' diarrhoea. *Alimentary Pharmacology Therapy*, **15**, 1139–1145.

Cummings, J.H., Macfarlane, G.T. and Drasar, B.D. (1989). 'The gut microflora and its significance', in Whitehead, R. (ed), *Gastrointestinal Pathology*, Edinburgh: Churchill-Livingstone.

Cummings, J.H., Macfarlane, G.T. and Enlglyst, H.N. (2001). Prebiotic digestion and fermentation. *American Journal of Clinical Nutrition*, **73**, 415S–420S.

Davidson, M.H. and Maki, K.C. (1999). Effects of dietary inulin on serum lipids. *Journal of Nutrition*, **129**, 1474S–1477S.

Deguchi, Y., Morishita, T. and Mutai, M. (1985). Comparative studies on synthesis of water-soluble vitamins among human species of bifidobacteria. *Agricultural and Biological Chemistry*, **49**, 13–19.

Depeint, F., Tzortzis, G., Vulevic, J., I'anson, K. and Gibson GR. (2008). Prebiotic evaluation of a novel galactooligosaccharide mixture produced by the enzymatic activity of *Bifidobacterium bifidum* NCIMB 41171, in healthy humans: a randomized, double-blind, crossover, placebo-controlled intervention study. *American Journal of Clinical Nutrition*, **87**, 785–791.

Drakoularakou, A., Tzortzis, G., Rastall, R.A. and Gibson, G.R. 2010. A double-blind, placebo-controlled, randomized human study assessing the capacity of a novel galacto-oligosaccharide mixture in reducing travellers' diarrhoea. *European Journal of Clinical Nutrition*, **64**, 146–152.

Drossman, D.A., Camilleri, M., Mayer, E.A. and Whitehead, W.E. (2003). AGA technical review on irritable bowel syndrome. *Gastroenterology*, **123**, 2108–2131.

Ellegard, L., Andersson, H. and Bosaeus, I. (1997). Inulin and oligofructose do not influence the absorption of cholesterol, or the excretion of cholesterol, Ca, Mg, Zn, Fe or bile acids but increases energy excretion in ileostomy subjects. *European Journal of Clinical Nutrition*, **51**, 1–5.

Flickinger, E.A. and Fahey, G.C. (2002). Pet food and feed applications of inulin, oligofructose and other oligosaccharides. *British Journal of Nutrition*, **87**, S297–S300.

Fuchs, A. (1993). 'Production and utilization of inulin', in Suzuki, M. and Chatterton, N. (eds), *Science and Technology of Fructans*, CRC Press, Boca Raton, FL, 319–352.

Fuller, R. (1989). Probiotics in man and animals. *Journal of Applied Bacteriology*, **66**, 356–378.

Furrie, E., Macfarlane, S., Kennedy, A., Cummings, J.H., Walsh, S.V., *et al.* (2005). Synbiotic therapy (*Bifidobacterium longum*/Synergy 1) initiates resolution of inflammation in patients with active ulcerative colitis: a randomised controlled pilot trial. *Gut*, **54**, 242–249.

Gibson, G.R. (1998). Dietary modulation of the human gut microbiota using prebiotics. *British Journal of Nutrition*, **80**(4), S209–S210.

Gibson, G.R. and McCartney, A.L. (1998). Modifications of the gut flora by dietary means. *Biochemical Society Transactions*, **26**, 222–228.

Gibson G.R. and Rastall R.A. [editors] (2006) *Prebiotics: Development and Application*. Chichester: John Wiley and Sons Ltd.

Gibson G.R. and Roberfroid MB [editors] (2008) *A Handbook of Prebiotics*. Taylor and Francis, Boca Raton.

Gibson, G.R. and Roberfroid, M.B. (1995). Dietary modulation of the human colonic microbiota: introducing the concept of prebiotics. *Journal of Nutrition*, **125**, 1401–1412.

Gibson, G.R. and Roberfroid, M.B. (eds) (1999). *Colonic Microbiota, Nutrition and Health*. Kluwer Academic Publishers, Dordrecht, the Netherlands.

Gibson, G.R. and Wang, X. (1994). Enrichment of bifidobacteria from human gut contents by oligofructose using continuous culture. *FEMS Microbiology Letters*, **118**, 121–128.

Gibson, G.R., Beatty, E.R., Wang, X. and Cummings, J.H. (1995). Selective stimulation of bifidobacteria in the human colon by oligofructose and inulin. *Gastroenterology*, **108**(4), 975–982.

Gibson, G.R., Ottaway, P.B. and Rastall, R.A. (2001). *Prebiotics: New Developments in Functional Foods*. Chadwick House Group Ltd, UK.

Gibson, G.R., Probert, H.M., Van Loo, J., Rastall, R.A. and Roberfroid, M.B. (2004). Dietary modulation of the human colonic microbiota: updating the concept of prebiotics. *Nutrition Research Reviews*, **17**, 259–275.

Gionchetti, P., Rizzello, F., Helwig, U., Venturi, A., Lammers, K.M., *et al.* (2003). Prophylaxis of pouchitis onset with probiotic therapy: a double-blind, placebo-controlled trial. *Gastroenterology*, **124**(5), 1535–1538.

Guandalini, S., Pensabene, L. and Zikri, M.A. (2000). *Lactobacillus GG* administered in oral rehydration solution to children with acute diarrhea: a multicenter European trial. *Journal of Pediatric Gastroenterology and Nutrition*, **30**, 54–60.

Guarner, F. (2006). Enteric flora in health and disease. *Digestion*, **73** (suppl. 1), 5–12.

Guigoz, Y., Rochat., F., Perruisseau-Carrier, G., Rochat, I. and Schriffen, E. (2002). Effects of oligosaccharides on the faecal flora and non-specfic immune system in elderly people. *Nutrition Research*, **22**, 13–25.

Harmsen, H.M.J, Raangs G.C., He T., Degener, J.E, and Welling, G.W. (2002). Extensive set of 16S rRNA probes for detection of bacteria in human faeces. *Applied and Environmental Microbiology*, **68** (2), 2982–2990.

Hellwege, E.M., Czapla, S., Jahnke, A., Willmitzer, L. and Heyer, A.G. (2000). Transgenic potato (*Solanum tuberosum*) tubers synthesize the full spectrum of inulin molecules naturally occurring in globe artichoke (*Cynara scolymus*) roots. *Proceedings of the National Academy of Sciences of the United States of America*, **97**, 8699–8704.

Hopkins, M.J. and Macfarlane, G.T. (2003). Nondigestible oligosaccharides enhance bacterial colonisation resistance against *Clostridium difficile in vitro*. *Applied and Environmental Biology*, **69**, 1920–1927.

Hoveyda, N., Heneghan, C., Mahtani, K. R., Perera, R., Roberts, N. and Gasziou, P. (2009). A systematic review and meta-analysis: probiotics in the treatment of irritable bowel syndrome, *BMC Gastroenterology*, **9**, 15–25.

Hylla, S., Gostner, A., Dusel, G., Anger, H., Bartram, H., *et al.* (1998). Effects of resistant starch on the colon in healthy volunteers: possible implications for cancer prevention. *American Journal of Clinical Nutrition*, **67**, 136–142.

International Scientific Association for Probiotics and Prebiotics (ISAPP) (2008). 6th Meeting of the International Scientific Association of Probiotics and Prebiotics. London, Ontario.

Ito, M., Deguchi, Y., Matsumoto, K., Kimura, M., Onodera, N. and Yajima, T. (1993). Influence of galactooligosaccharides on the human fecal microflora. *Journal of Nutritional Science and Vitaminology*, **39**, 635–640.

Jenkins, D.J., Kendall., C. and Vuksan, V. (1999). Inulin, oligofructose and intestinal function. *Journal of Nutrition*, **129**, 1431S–1433S.

Kaplan, H. and Hutkins, R.W. (2000). Fermentation of fructooligosaccharides by lactic acid bacteria and bifidobacteria. *Applied and Environmental Microbiology*, **66**(6), 2682–2684.

Kim, H.J., Vazquez Roque, M.I., Camilleri, M., Stephens, D., Burton, D.D., *et al.* (2005). A randomized controlled trial of a probiotic combination VSL# 3 and placebo in irritable bowel syndrome with bloating. *Neurogastroenterology Motility*, **17**, 687–696.

Kleessen, B., Hartman, L. and Blaut, M. (2001). Oligofructose and long chain inulin influence the gut microbial ecology of rats associated with human faecal flora. *British Journal of Nutrition*, **86**, 291–300.

Kleessen, B., Sykura, B., Zunft, H.J. and Blaut, M. (1997). Effects of inulin and lactose on faecal microflora, microbial activity, and bowel habit in elderly constipated persons. *American Journal of Clinical Nutrition*, **65**, 1397–1402.

Kolida, S., Tuohy, K. and Gibson, G. R. (2002). Prebiotic effects of inulin and oligofructose. *British Journal of Nutrition*, **87**, S193–S197.

Konikoff, M.R. and Denson, L.A. (2006). Role of fecal calprotectin as a biomarker of intestinal inflammation in inflammatory bowel disease. *Inflammatory Bowel Disease*, **12**, 524–534.

Kruse, H.P., Kleessen, B. and Blaut, M. (1999). Effects of inulin on faecal bifidobacteria in human subjects. *British Journal of Nutrition*, **82** (5), 375–382.

Lewis, S., Burmeister, S. and Brazier, J. (2005). Effect of the prebiotic oligofructose on relapse of *Clostridium difficile*-associated diarrhea: a randomized, controlled study. *Clinical Gastroenterology Hepatology*, **3**, 442–448.

Lilly, D.M. and Stillwell, R.H. (1965). Probiotics: growth promoting factors produced by microorganisms. *Science*, **147**, 747–748.

Lindsay, J.O., Whelan, K., Stagg, A.J., Gobin, P. and Al-Hassi, H.O. (2006). Clinical, microbiological, and immunological effects of fructo-oligosaccharide in patients with Crohn's disease. *Gut*, **55**, 348–355.

Lomax, A.R. and Calder, P.C. (2009). Probiotics, immune function, infection and inflammation: a review of the evidence from studies conducted in humans. *Current Pharmaceutical Design*, **15**(13), 128–151.

Lopez-Molina, D., Navarro-Martinez, M.D., Rojas-Melgarejo, F., Hiner, A., Chazarra, S. and Rodriguez-Lopez, J.N. (2005). Molecular properties and prebiotic effects of inulin obtained from artichoke. *Phytochemistry*, **66**, 1476–1484.

Lupton, J.R. and Kurtz, P.P. (1993). Relationship of colonic luminal short-chain fatty acids and pH to *in vivo* cell proliferation in rats. *Journal of Nutrition*, **123**, 1522–1530.

Macfarlane, G.T., Gibson, G.R. and Cummings, J.H. (1992). Comparison of fermentation reactions in different regions of the human colon. *J. Applied Bacteriology*, **72**, 57–64.

Marx, S.P., Winkler, S. and Hartmeier, W. (2000). Metabolisation of β-(2,6)-linked fructose-oligosaccharides by different bacteria, *FEMS Microbiol Lett*, **192**, 163–169.

McFarland, L.V. (2000). A review of the evidence of health claims for biotherapeutic agents. *Microbial Ecology in Health and Disease*, **12**, 65–76.

McFarland, L.V. (2007). Meta-analysis of probiotics for the prevention of traveller's diarrhea. *Travel Medicine and Infectious Disease*, **5** (2), 97–105.

McFarland, L.V. (2009). Evidence-based review of probiotics for antibiotic-associated diarrhea and *Clostridium difficile* infections. *Anaerobe*, **5**, 274–280.

Menne, E., Guggenbuhl, N. and Roberfroid, M. (2000). Fn-type chicory inulin hydrolyzate has a prebiotic effect in humans. *Journal of Nutrition*, **130**, 197–9.

Metchnikoff, E. (1907) *The Prolongation of Life*. London: William Heinemann.

Moerman, F.T., Van Leeuwen, M.B. and Delcour, J.A. (2004). Enrichment of higher molecular weight fractions in inulin. *Journal of Agricultural and Food Chemistry*, **52**, 3780–3783.

Molis, C., Flourie, B., Ouarne, F., Gailing, MF., Lartigue, S., Guibert, A., Bornet, F. and Galmiche, J.P. (1996). Digestion, excretion, and energy value of fructooligosaccharides in healthy humans. *American Journal of Clinical Nutrition*, **64** (3), 324–328.

Moro, G., Stahl, B., Fanaro, S., Jelinek, J., Boehm, G. and Coppa, G. (2005). Dietary prebiotic oligosaccharides are detectable in the faeces of formula-fed infants. *Acta Paediactrica*, **94**, 27–30.

Nakakuki, T. (2003). Development of functional oligosaccharides in Japan. *Advanced Dietary Fibre Technology*, **15** (82), 57–64.

Nobaek, S., Johansson, M.L., Molin, G., Ahrné, S. and Jeppsson, B. (2000). Alteration of intestinal microflora is associated with reduction in abdominal bloating and pain in patients with irritable bowel syndrome. *American Journal of Gastroenterology*, **95**, 1231–1238.

Olano-Martin, E., Mountzouris, K., Gibson, G. R. and Rastall, R. (2000). In vitro fermentability of dextran, oligodextran and maltodextran by human gut bacteria. *British Journal of Nutrition*, **83**, 247–255.

O'Mahony, L., McCarthy, J., Kelly, P., Hurley, G., Luo, F. *et al.* (2005). *Lactobacillus* and *Bifidobacterium* in irritable bowel syndrome: symptom responses and relationship to cytokine profiles. *Gastroenterology*, **128**, 541–551.

Ouwehand, A., Kurvinen, T. and Päivi Rissanen, P. (2004). Use of a probiotic *Bifidobacterium* in a dry food matrix, an *in vivo* study. *International Journal of Food Microbiology*, **95**, 103–106.

Ouwehand, A.C., Kirjavainen, P.V., Shortt, C. and Salminen, S. (1999). Probiotics: mechanisms and established effects. *International Dairy Journal*, **9**, 43–52.

Parker, R.B. (1974). Probiotics: the other half of the antibiotic story. *Animal Nutrition and Health*, **29**, 4–8.

Parnell, J.A. and Reimer, R.A. (2009). Weight loss during oligofructose supplementation is associated with decreased ghrelin and increased peptide YY in overweight and obese adults. *American Journal of Clinical Nutrition*, **89**, 1751–1759.

Press, A.G., Hauptmann, I.A., Hauptmann, L., Fuchs, B. and Ramadori, G. (1998). Gastrointestinal pH profiles in patients with inflammatory bowel disease. *Alimentary Pharmacology and Therapeutics*, **12**, 673–678.

Rabiu, B., Jay, A., Gibson, G.R. and Rastall, R.A. (2001). Synthesis and fermentation properties of novel galacto-oligosaccharides by [beta]-galactosidases from *Bifidobacterium* species. *Applied and Environmental Microbiology*, **67**, 2526–2530.

Rafter, J., Bennett, M., Caderni, G., Clune, Y. and Hughes, R. (2007). Dietary synbiotics reduce cancer risk factors in polypectomized and colon cancer patients. *American Journal of Clinical Nutrition*, **85**, 488–496.

Rao, V. (2001). The prebiotic properties of oligofructose at low intake levels. *Nutrition Research*, **21**, 843–848.

Rathbone, B.J. and Heatley, R.V. (1992). *Helicobacter pylori* and Gastroduodenal Disease, 2nd edn, Blackwell Scientific Publications, Oxford.

Reid, G., Jass, J., Sebulsky, M.T. and McCormick, J.K. (2003). Potential uses of probiotics in clinical practice. *Clinical Microbiology Reviews*, **16**(4), 658–672.

Roberfroid, M.B. (1998). Prebiotics and synbiotics: concepts and nutritional properties. *Br. J. Nutr.*, **130**, S396–S402.

Roberfroid, M.B. (1999). Caloric value of inulin and oligofructose. *Journal of Nutrition*, **129**, 1436S–1437S.

Roberfroid, M.B. (2000). Probiotics and prebiotics: are they functional foods? *American Journal of Clinical Nutrition*, **71**, S1682–S1687.

Roberfroid, M.B. (2002). Functional foods: concepts and application to inulin and oligofructose. *British Journal of Nutrition*, **87** (Suppl. 2), S139–S143.

Roberfroid, M.B. (2007). Prebiotics: the concept revisited. *Journal of Nutrition*, **137**, 830S–837S.

Roberfroid, M.B., Van Loo, F. and Gibson, G.R. (1998). The bifidogenic nature of chicory inulin and oligofructose. *Journal of Nutrition*, **128**, 11–19.

Roediger, W.E. (1980). The colonic epithelium in ulcerative colitis: an energy-deficiency disease? *Lancet*, **2**, 712–715.

Rowland, I.R., Rumney, C.J., Coutts, J.T. and Lievense, L.C. (1998). Effect of *Bifidobacterium longum* and inulin on gut bacterial metabolism and carcinogen-induced aberrant crypt foci in rats. *Carcinogenesis*, **19**, 281–285.

Rowland, I.R. and Tanaka, R. (1993). The effects of transgalactosylated oligosaccharides on gut flora metabolism in rats associated with a human faecal microflora. *Journal of Applied Bacteriology*, **74**, 667–674.

Saavendra, J. M and Tschemia, A. (2002). Human studies with probiotics and prebiotics: clinical implications. *British J. Nutr.*, **87**: S241–S246.

Sako, T., Matsumoto, K. and Tanaka, R. (1999). Recent progress on research and applications of non-digestible galacto-oligosaccharides. *International Dairy Journal*, **9**, 69–80.

Salminen, A.C, Bouley, C., Boutron-Ruault, M.C., Cummings, J.H, Frank, A., *et al.* (1998). Functional food science and gastrointestinal physiology and function. *British Journal of Nutrition*, **80** (Suppl. 1), S147–S171.

Salminen, E., Ouwehand, A., Benno, Y. and Lee, Y.K. (1999). Probiotics: how they should be defined? *Trends in Food Science and Technology*, **10**, 107–110.

Sangeetha, P.T., Ramesh, M.N. and Prapulla, S.G. (2005). Recent trends in the microbial production, analysis and application of fructooligosaccharides. *Trends Food Sci. Technol.*, **16**, 442–457.

Schaafsma, G., Meuling, W., van Dokkum, W. and Bouley, C. (1998). Effects of a milk product, fermented with *Lactobacillus acidophilus* and with fructo-oligosaccharides added, on blood lipids in male volunteers. *European Journal of Clinical Nutrition*, **52**, 436–440.

Servin, A. L. (2004). Antagonistic activities of lactobacilli and bifidobacteria against microbial pathogens. *FEMS Microbiology Reviews*, **28**, 405–440.

Shiba, T., Aiba, Y., Ishikawa, H., Ushiyama, A., Takagi, A., *et al.* (2003). The suppressive effect of bifidobacteria on *Bacteroides vulgaris*, a putative pathogenic microbe in inflammatory bowel disease. *Microbiology and Immunology*, **47**, 371–378.

Shoaf, K., Mulvey, G., Armstrong, G. and Hutkins, R. (2006). Prebiotic galactooligosaccharides reduce adherence of enteropathogenic *Escherichia coli* to tissue culture cells. *Infection and Immunity*, IAI.01030–06.

Silk, D.B., Davis, A., Vulevic, J., Tzortzis, G. and Gibson, G.R. (2009). Clinical trial: the effects of a trans-galactooligosaccharide prebiotic on faecal microbiota and symptoms in irritable bowel syndrome. *Alimentary Pharmacology and Therapy* **29**, 508–518.

Sperti, G.S. (1971). *Probiotics*. Avi Publishing Co., West Point, CT.

Szilagyi, A., Rivard, J. and Shrier, I. (2002). Diminished efficacy of colonic adaptation to lactulose occurs in patients with Inflammatory Bowel Disease in remission. *Digestive Diseases and Sciences*, **47**, 2811–2822.

Takahashi, O., Noguchi, Y., Omata, F., Tokuda Y. and Fakui, Y. (2007). Probiotics in the prevention of traveler's diarrhea: meta-analysis. *Journal of Clinical Gastroenterology*, **41** (3), 336–7.

Tanaka, R., Takayama, H., Morotomi, M., Kuroshima, T., Ueyama, S., *et al.* (1983). Effects of administration of TOS and *Bifidobacterium breve* 4006 on the human fecal microflora. *Bifidobacteria Microflora*, **2**, 17–24.

Tannock, G. [editor] (2002). *Probiotics and Prebiotics*. Norfolk: Caister Academic Press.

Tong, J.L., Ran, Z.H., Shen, J., Zhang, C.X. and Xiao, S.D. (2007). Meta-analysis: the effect of supplementation with prebiotics on eradication rates and adverse events during *Helicobacter pylori* eradication therapy. *Alimentary Pharmocology and Therapeutics*, **25**(2), 155–168.

Topping, D.L. and Clifton, P.M. (2001). Short chain fatty acids and human colonic function: roles of resistant starch and non-starch polysaccharides. *Physiological Reviews*, **81** (3), 1031–1063.

Tungland, B.C. and Meyer, D. (2002). Nondigestible oligo-and polysaccharides (dietary fiber): their physiology and role in human health and food. *Comprehensive Reviews in Food Science and Food Safety*, **1**, 73–92.

Tuohy, K.M., Finlay, R.K., Wynne, A.G. and Gibson, G.R. (2001a). A human volunteer study on the effects of HP-inulin-gut bacteria enumerated using FISH. *Anaerobe*, **7**, 113–118.

Tuohy, K.M., Kolida, S., Lustenberger, A. and Gibson, G.R. (2001b). The prebiotic effects of biscuits containing partially hydrolysed guar gum and fructooligosaccharides-a human volunteer study. *British Journal of Nutrition*, **86**, 341–348.

van Nuenen, M., Meyer, P. and Venema, K. (2003). The effect of various inulins and *Clostridium difficile* on the metabolic activity of the human colonic microbiota *in vitro*. *Microbial Ecology in Health and Disease*, **15**, 137–144.

Venturi, A., Gionchetti, P., Rizzello, F., Johansson, R., Zucconi, E., *et al.* (1999). Impact on the composition of the faecal flora by a new probiotic preparation: preliminary data on maintenance treatment of patients with ulcerative colitis. *Alimentary Pharmacology Therapy*, **13**, 1103–1108.

Versalovic, J. and Wilson, M. [editors] (2008) *Therapeutic Microbiology*. Washington: ASM Press.

Vulevic, J., Drakoularakou, A., Yaqoob, P., Tzortzis, G. and Gibson, G.R. (2008). Modulation of the fecal microflora profile and immune function by a novel trans-galactooligosaccharide mixture (B-GOS) in healthy elderly volunteers. *American Journal of Clinical Nutrition*, **88**, 1438–1446.

Waligora-Dupriet AJ, Campeotto F., Nicolis I, Bonet A, Soulaines, P. *et al.* (2007) Effect of oligofructose supplementation on gut microflora and well-being in young children attending a day care centre. International Journal of Food Microbiology **113**, 108–113.

Wang, X. and Gibson, G.R. (1993). Effects of the *in vivo* fermentation of oligofructose and inulin by bacteria growing in the human large intestine. *Journal of Applied Bacteriology*, **75** (4), 373–380.

Welters, C.F., Heineman, E., Thunnissen, F.B., van den Bogaard, A.E., Soeters, P.B. and Baeten, C.G. (2002) Effect of dietary inulin supplementation on inflammation of pouch mucosa in patients with an ileal pouch-anal anastomosis. *Diseases of the Colon and Rectum*, **45**, 621–627.

Wichienchot, S., Prasertsan, P., Hongpattarakere, T., Gibson, G.R. and Rastall, R. (2006). In vitro fermentation of mixed linkage glucooligosaccharides produced by gluconobacter oxydans NCIMB 4943 by the human colonic micoflora. *Current Issues in Intestinal Microbiology*, **7**, 7–12.

Wohlgemuth, S., Loh, G. and Blaut, M. (2009). Recent developments and perspectives in the investigation of probiotic effects. *International Journal of Medical Microbiology*, **300** (1), 3–10.

Wult, M., Hagslatt, M.L. and Odenholt, I. (2003). *Lactobacillus plantarum* for the treatment of recurrent *Clostridium difficile* diarrhoea: a double-blind, placebo-controlled trial. *Scandinavian Journal of Infections Diseases*, **35**, 365–367.

Yan, F. and Polk, D.B. (2004). Commensal bacteria in the gut: learning who our friends are. *Current Opinion in Gastroenterology*, **20**, 565–567.

Yazawa, K., Imai, K. and Tamura, Z. (1978). Oligosaccharides and polysaccharides specifically utilizable by bifidobacteria. *Chemical and Pharmaceutical Bulletin*, **26**, 3306–3311.

Yazawa, K. and Tamura, Z. (1982). Search for sugar sources for selective increase of bifidobacteria. *Bifidobacteria Microflora*, **1**, 39–44.

20

Bioactive milk proteins, peptides and lipids and other functional components derived from milk and bovine colostrum

H. J. Korhonen, MTT Agrifood Research Finland, Finland

Abstract: Research-based evidence on the health-promoting effects of milk components is accumulating rapidly. This development has laid the basis for use of bioactive milk components as ingredients for functional dairy products. Also, fractionation and marketing of bioactive milk components is emerging as a new lucrative sector for the dairy industries and specialized bio-industries. This chapter focuses on the health-promoting properties and applications of a range of bioactive proteins, peptides, lipids and other minor components derived from bovine colostrum and milk.

Key words: milk, colostrum, bioactive components, health-promoting properties, commercial applications.

20.1 Introduction

The importance of colostrum to the newborn in protection against pathogens and in securing healthy growth and development is well documented. Colostrum contains plenty of immunologically and physiologically active components which are found also in the mature milk but usually in much lower concentrations. These bioactive components comprise specific proteins, polypeptides, growth factors, lipids and carbohydrates.

Over the last two decades major advances have taken place with regard to the science, technology and commercial applications of many of these bioactive components. In particular, the advent of health-promoting functional foods has increased scientific and commercial interest in exploitation of these beneficial components for human health (Pihlanto and Korhonen, 2003; Playne *et al.*, 2003; Rowan *et al.*, 2005; Recio *et al.*, 2009; Ko and Kwak, 2009; Korhonen, 2009a). To this end, chromatographic and membrane separation techniques have been developed to fractionate and purify many of these components on an industrial scale from colostrum, milk and cheese whey (Korhonen, 2002; Kitts and Weiler, 2003; Pouliot and Gauthier, 2006; Korhonen and Pihlanto, 2007; Kulozik, 2009; Sichien *et al.*, 2009; Vercruysse *et al.*, 2009).

Manufacture of bioactive milk ingredients has emerged as a lucrative sector for dairy industries and specialized bio-industries. Colostrum and whey-derived bioactive ingredients have already been commercialized for example in products that strenghten the immune system, reduce elevated blood pressure, combat gastrointestinal infections, help in weight management and prevent osteoporosis (Miller *et al.*, 2000; Krissansen, 2007; Luhovyy *et al.*, 2007; Heaney, 2009; Kris-Etherton *et al.*, 2009; Parodi, 2009). There is also increasing evidence that consumption of low-fat milk and milk whey proteins in particular reduces the risk of metabolic syndrome, which is manifested by various chronic diseases such as obesity, hypertension and diabetes type 2 (Ha and Zemel, 2003; Choi *et al.*, 2005; Mensink, 2006; Pfeuffer and Schrezenmeir, 2006a; Elwood *et al.*, 2008; Lamarche, 2008; Möller *et al.*, 2008; Akhavan *et al.*, 2009; Engberink *et al.*, 2009; Schaafsma, 2009; Veldhorst *et al.*, 2009).

A growing body of evidence from observational studies suggests an inverse relationship between calcium and vitamin D status and dairy food intake and the development of the insulin resistance syndrome and diabetes type 2 (Tremblay and Gilbert, 2009). Also, intake of milk and some of its components have been associated with a lower risk of certain cancer types, e.g. breast, prostate and colon cancer (Parodi, 1998, 2005, 2009; Bounous, 2000; Zimecki and Kruzel, 2007; Lamarche, 2008). Beyond nutritional properties, colostrum and milk seem capable of delivering many health benefits to humans by provision of specific bioactive components. Figure 20.1 illustrates such major bioactive components found in colostrum and milk and suggests their potential health effects and interactions in the matrix. This chapter gives an overview of these components focusing on bioactive proteins, peptides and lipids which have been the subject of intensive research in recent years.

20.2   Bioactive proteins

20.2.1   Caseins and whey proteins

Among the bioactive milk components, proteins have proven particularly interesting because of the many different bioactivities they exert, in addition to their well documented nutritional and functional properties (Kanwar *et al.*, 2009). Furthermore, milk proteins possess additional physiological functions due to the numerous bioactive peptides that are encrypted within intact proteins (Korhonen, 2009b).

One litre of cow's milk contains about 35 grams of protein, of which casein constitutes about 80% and whey proteins 20% (7 grams per litre). Whole casein is known to have a good nutritive value owing to its valuable amino acid composition and calcium, phosphate and several trace elements linked chemically with the

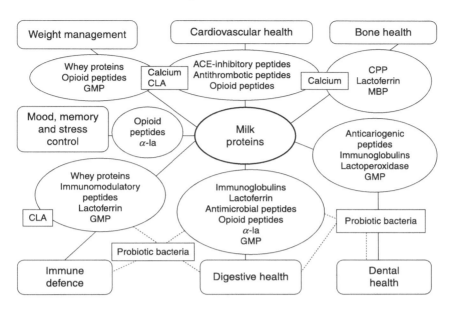

Fig. 20.1 Potential health targets of major milk proteins and bioactive peptides derived from milk proteins, including potential interactions with other milk components and probiotic bacteria. Abbreviations: ACE = angiotensin-converting enzyme, α-la = alpha-lactalbumin, CLA = conjugated linoleic acid, GMP = glycomacropeptide, MBP = milk basic protein.

casein molecule. Moreover, individual casein fractions αs1-, αs2-, β- and κ-casein fractions and caseinates have proven biologically active and also a good source of different bioactive peptides (Akuzawa *et al.*, 2009). These bioactivities include e.g. immunomodulatory (Bennett *et al.*, 2005; Silva and Malcata, 2005; Gauthier *et al.*, 2006b), antihypertensive (López-Expósito *et al.*, 2007; Phelan *et al.*, 2009; Saito, 2008; del Mar Contreras *et al.*, 2009), antimicrobial (López-Expósito and Recio, 2006; Pan *et al.*, 2007), antioxidative (Pihlanto, 2006) and opioid-like (Hartman and Meisel, 2007).

Much research has been carried out on casein-derived bioactive peptides that are encrypted within the primary structures of intact casein. Casein peptides are not active within the parent protein but can be released and activated during enzymatic hydrolysis, microbial fermentation and during gastrointestinal digestion. Once absorbed, casein peptides have potential to exert numerous biological effects in the body. Important tasks for the production of functional foods containing bioactive peptides are to either enhance their bioavailability from their natural source or create novel foods via the addition and/or fortification of isolated or enriched fractions of bioactive peptides. Selected biological effects of casein-derived bioactive peptides and their applications in the food industry will be discussed later on in this review.

Recent findings suggest that casein hydrolysates provide a potential source of highly functional ingredients for different food applications. Examples of such ingredients are the hypotensive tripeptides Val-Pro-Pro and Ile-Pro-Pro which are derived from both β-casein and κ-casein and are already commercially exploited in many countries (Saito, 2008). Otherwise, industrial manufacture of casein fractions for dietary purposes has not progressed to any significant extent, so far.

On the other hand, the whey proteins have attained increasing commercial interest, because the whey protein complex and several individual proteins have been implicated in a number of physiologically beneficial effects (Schaafsma, 2006a, b; Madureira *et al.*, 2007; Smithers, 2008; Kekkonen and Peuhkuri, 2009; Ko and Kwa, 2009). The whey protein complex contains a great variety of proteins which differ from each other in their chemical structure, functional properties and biological functions. The best-characterized whey proteins are alpha-lactalbumin (α-la), beta-lactoglobulin (β-lg), immunoglobulins (Ig), lactoferrin (LF) and glycomacropeptide (GMP) (Table 20.1). The specific characteristics have been used in isolation of individual proteins from whey, but the purity has proven a critical factor in assessing the biological activity of a purified component. The major whey proteins can nowadays be isolated using industrial or semi-industrial scale processing techniques (Chatterton *et al.*, 2006; Korhonen and Pihlanto, 2007; Gokawi, 2009; Vercruysse *et al.*, 2009).

The total whey protein complex and several individual proteins have been implicated in a number of physiologically beneficial effects, as listed in Table 20.2. Of particular interest at present are the potential beneficial effects of whey proteins and biologically active peptides on many chronic diseases, e.g. obesity, type 2 diabetes and hypertension.

Table 20.1   Major bioactive whey proteins of bovine colostrum and milk: concentrations and molecular weights

Protein	Concentration (g/l)		Molecular weight (Daltons)
	Colostrum	Milk	
β-Lactoglobulin	8.0	3.3	18 400
α-Lactalbumin	3.0	1.2	14 200
Immunoglobulins (IgG, IgM, IgA)	20–150	0.5–1.0	150 000–900 000
Glycomacropeptide	2.5	1.2	8000
Lactoferrin	1.5	0.1	80 000
Lactoperoxidase	0.02	0.03	78 000
Lysozyme	0.0004	0.0004	14 000
Milk basic protein	N.A.	N.A	10 000–17 000
Growth factors	50 μg–40 mg/l	<1 μg–2 mg/l	6400–30 000

Compiled from Pihlanto and Korhonen (2003) and Korhonen and Pihlanto (2007); N.A. = not announced.

Table 20.2 Potential health benefits delivered by whey proteins

Health benefit	Whey proteins involved	Reference
Improved physical performance, prevention of muscular atrophy, faster recovery after exercise	Total whey protein hydrolysates, immunoglobulins, growth factors	Crittenden *et al.*, 2009 Ha and Zemel, 2003 Krissansen, 2007
Satiety and weight management	Total whey protein concentrates, glycomacropeptide, lactoferrin	Luhovyy *et al.*, 2007 Pilvi *et al.*, 2009 Schaafsma, 2006a,b Veldhorst *et al.*, 2009
Reduction of blood pressure and cholesterol	α-Lactalbumin and β-lactoglobulin hydrolysates (peptides), glycomacropeptide	Lòpez-Fandino *et al.*, 2006 Murray and FitzGerald, 2007 Saito, 2008
Stimulation of insulin production and reduction of postprandial glycemia	Total whey protein concentrates	Blouet *et al.*, 2007 Frid *et al.*, 2005
Prevention of microbial infections	Immunoglobulins, lactoferrin, lactoperoxidase system	Korhonen and Marnila, 2006, 2009 Ochoe, 2009 Seifu *et al.*, 2005
Prevention of mucosal inflammation	Whey protein concentrates, α-lactalbumin, lactoferrin	Chatterton *et al.*, 2006 Mezzaroba *et al.*, 2006
Wound care and repair	Growth factors	Pouliot *et al.*, 2006 Smithers, 2008
Anti-cancer effects	Total whey proteins and hydrolysates, lactoferrin	Bounous, 2000 Parodi, 1998, 2005 Zimecki and Kruzel, 2007
Improved cognitive functions, anti-stress effects	α-Lactalbumin	Markus *et al.*, 2002
Hypoallergenic effects	Whey protein hydrolysates	Crittenden and Bennett, 2005

20.2.2 Immunoglobulins

Immunoglobulins (Ig) are present in colostrum of all lactating species and provide primary passive protection to the newborn offspring against invading pathogenic microorganisms (Bostwick *et al.*, 2000; Zhao *et al.*, 2006; Stelwagen *et al.*, 2009). In bovine colostrum Ig account for up to 70–80% of the total protein content, whereas in milk they account for only 1–2% of total protein (Marnila and Korhonen, 2002). Ig preparations concentrated from bovine colostrum or cheese whey are commercially available in many countries. These products are targeted to farm animals as colostrum supplements and to humans as dietary supplements to boost or support various body functions, such as protection against microbial infections and general well-being without any specific microbial target (Scammell, 2001; Tripathi and Vashishtha, 2006; Struff and Sprotte, 2007). The scientific clinical evidence related to colostral supplements remains, however, disputed. At present, the proven benefits seem mainly to be associated with a faster recovery from long endurance physical training among athletes (Crittenden *et al.*, 2009). The Ig carry the biological function of specific antibodies as they are formed in the body as a response to an immunogenic stimulus. The concentration of specific antibodies, against pathogenic microorganisms can be raised in colostrum and milk by immunizing cows with vaccines made of pathogens or their antigens (Korhonen *et al.*, 2000). Advances in bioseparation techniques have made it possible to fractionate and enrich such antibodies and formulate so-called immune milk preparations (Korhonen, 2004; Mehra *et al.*, 2006). Oral administration of these preparations has proven successful in connection of many microbial infections in humans. The concept of 'immune milk' origins from the studies of Petersen and Campbell who in the 1950s first suggested that orally administered colostrum from hyperimmunized cows could provide passive immune protection for humans (Campbell and Petersen, 1963; Wheeler *et al.*, 2007). Over the last 30 years, a great number of clinical studies have demonstrated that immune milk preparations can be effective in prevention of human and animal diseases caused by different pathogenic microbes, e.g. rotavirus, *Escherichia coli, Candida albicans, Clostridium difficile, Shigella flexneri, Streptococcus mutans, Cryptosporidium parvum* and *Helicobacter pylori*. The therapeutic efficacy of these preparations has, however, proven quite limited (Korhonen *et al.*, 2000; Korhonen and Marnila, 2006, 2009; Hammarström and Weiner, 2008). A few immune milk products are on the market in some countries but the unclear regulatory status of these products has emerged as a constraint for global commercialization (Hoerr and Bostwick, 2002; Mehra *et al.*, 2006). The globally increasing problem of antibiotic-resistant strains which have led to serious endemic hospital infections may in future offer an interesting approach for development of suitably designed immune milk products. The safety of hyperimmune milk products has been established by the US Food and Drug Administration (FDA), based on animal and human studies which have not shown any adverse effects from these products (Gingerich and McPhillips, 2005; Krissansen, 2007; Young *et al.*, 2007).

20.2.3 Lactoferrin

LF is an iron-binding glycoprotein found in colostrum, milk and other body secretions and cells of most mammalian species (Conesa *et al.*, 2008). In comparison to bovine colostrum (1.5 g/l) human colostrum is a very rich source (up to 5 g/l) of this multifunctional compound. LF confers many biological activities, such as antimicrobial, antioxidative, anti-inflammatory, anticancer and immune regulatory properties (Lönnerdal, 2003; Valentini and Antonini, 2005; Wakabayashi *et al.*, 2006; Pan *et al.*, 2007; Zimecki and Kruzel, 2007; Legrand *et al.*, 2008; Marnila and Korhonen, 2009). In addition, several antimicrobial peptides, such as lactoferricin B f(18–36) and lactoferrampin f(268–284) can be cleaved from LF by the action of pepsin (Wakabayashi *et al.*, 2003). The biological properties of LF have been subject of scientific research since the discovery of this 'red protein' in the early 1960s (Groves, 1960). Initially, the role was confined largely to antimicrobial activity alone but now the multi-functionality of LF is well recognized. Ingested LF has been suggested to exert antibacterial and antiviral activities in the intestine, in part through a direct effect on pathogens, but possibly also affecting mucosal immune function. The latter function is most likely mediated by LF being taken up by cells via a unique receptor-mediated pathway and affecting gene transcription (Lönnerdal, 2009). The bactericidal effect of LF can be augmented by the action of lysozyme or antibodies (Pan *et al.*, 2007). Also, a synergistic antibacterial effect has been demonstrated between LF and lactoferricin against *E. coli* and *Staphylococcus epidermidis* (López-Expósito *et al.*, 2008). Interestingly, LF can augment susceptibility of bacteria to certain antibiotics, such as vancomycin, penicillin and cephalosporins.

The *in vitro* antimicrobial activity of LF and its peptide derivatives has been demonstrated against a wide range of pathogenic microbes, including enteropathogenic *E. coli, Clostridium perfringens, C. albicans, Haemophilus influenzae, H. pylori* and *Listeria monocytogenes* and viruses, including hepatitis C, HIV-1, cytomegalovirus, poliovirus, rotavirus and herpes simplex virus (Fernaud and Evans, 2003; Jenssen and Hancock, 2009; Ochoa and Cleary, 2009). Also, LF and lactoferricin have proven antimicrobial against microorganisms causing mastitis suggesting their potential prophylactic or therapeutic role in combating udder diseases in cows (Lacasse *et al.*, 2008).

At present, LF is considered to play an important role in the body's innate defence system against microbial infections and degenerative processes induced, for example by free oxygen radicals. Furthermore, the antitumor activity of LF has been studied intensively and several mechanisms have been suggested, e.g. iron-chelation related antioxidative property, immunoregulatory and anti-inflammatory functions (Wakabayashi *et al.*, 2006; Legrand *et al.*, 2008). In lacteal secretions, the major known or speculated *in vivo* activities of LF are:

- Defence against infections of the mammary gland and the gastrointestinal tract (antimicrobial activity, regulation of the immune system).
- Nutritional effects (bioavailability of iron, source of amino acids).
- Mitogenic and trophic activities on the intestinal mucosa and gastrointestinal tract associated lymphoid tissue and on bone tissue.
- Antineoplastic activity in gastrointestinal tract.

A great number of animal and human studies performed during the last three decades have shown that oral administration of LF can exert several beneficial effects on the health of humans and animals (Weinberg, 2003; Legrand *et al.*, 2008; Lönnerdal, 2009). Animal studies have demonstrated that LF can suppress the overgrowth and translocation of certain intestinal bacteria, but does not affect intestinal bifidobacteria. Also, oral administration of LF and lactoferricin reduce the infection rate of *H. pylori, Toxoplasma gondii*, candidiasis and prevent clinical symptoms of influenza virus infection in humans (Costantino and Guaraldi,

2008; Koikawa *et al.*, 2008; Ochoa *et al.*, 2008). Further human studies have demonstrated that orally ingested LF and related compounds improve nutritional status by reducing iron-deficient anemia and drug induced intestinal inflammation, colitis, arthritis and decrease mortality caused by endotoxin shock. Also, LF stimulates weight gain in pre-weaning calves (Teraguchi *et al.*, 2004). Cornish *et al.* (2006) have shown that oral LF administration to mice regulates the bone cell activity and increases bone formation. If confirmed in human studies, this result could open possibilities of using LF as a therapeutic agent in osteoporosis. Based on animal studies, Zimecki and Kruzel (2007) have suggested that bovine LF administration could be beneficial also in stress-related neurodegenerative disorders and treatment of certain cancer types. The anticarcinogenic properties of LF and lactoferricin have been demonstrated in many animal models and cell line studies (Kim *et al.*, 2009; Lizzi *et al.*, 2009; Marnila and Korhonen, 2009). Clinical studies are, however, required to confirm these results in humans. Encouraging results have been obtained in an intervention trial by Hayes *et al.* (2006) where patients with progressive advanced tumours were given orally recombinant human lactoferrin (talactoferrin) in doses varying from 1.5 g to 9 g daily, using a two weeks on–two weeks off therapy. Among eight patients who could be evaluated radiologically, the tumour growth rate had decreased in seven cases.

In human studies reviewed by Wakabayashi *et al.* (2006) bovine LF has been shown to increase eradication rate of *H. pylori* gastritis when administered in connection of triple therapy. Also, LF ingestion has decreased the incidence of bacteremia and severity of infection in neutropenic patients. In further human studies LF has been shown to alleviate symptoms of hepatitis C virus infection, and to reduce small intestine permeability in drug induced intestinal injury. Also, LF ingestion and topical application have proven beneficial in the cure of tinea pedis. An earlier study on infants has demonstrated that oral administration of bovine LF preparations increased the number of bifidobacteria in fecal flora and the serum ferritin level while the numbers of *Enterobacteriaceae, Streptococcus* and *Clostridium* decreased (Roberts *et al.*, 1992). Recently, King *et al.* (2007) have shown that supplementation of bovine LF to healthy infants for 12 months was associated with fewer lower respiratory tract illnesses and higher hematocrits as compared to the control group which received regular infant formula.

In another human study on pregnant women Paesano *et al.* (2006) reported that oral intake of 100 mg of bovine LF twice a day for 30 days increased significantly the haemoglobin and total iron concentration in blood serum as compared to the control group which received ferrous sulphate 520 mg per day, respectively. In a recent study on healthy human males Mulder *et al.* (2008) demonstrated that a daily oral intake of 100 mg of lactoferrin for 7 days, followed by 200 mg of lactoferrin for another 7 days resulted in statistically significant increases of many immunological parameters. These results suggest that oral supplements of bovine LF may be a useful adjunct in boosting natural defence mechanisms, in particular T-cell activation and antioxidant status. In a recent study Manzoni *et al.* (2009) demonstrated that supplementation of 100 mg/d of bovine LF alone or in combination with a probiotic strain *Lactobacillus rhamnosus* LGG (6×10^9 colony-forming units/d) from birth until day 30 of life reduced significantly the incidence of a first episode of late-onset sepsis in very low-birth-weight neonates. No adverse effects or intolerances to treatments occurred.

Increasing evidence about the potential health benefits of LF has created growing interest in producing LF industrially from cheese whey or by means of recombination technique (Tomita *et al.*, 2008). Purified LF for ingredient use is now manufactured by many companies and commercial products containing added LF have been launched on the market in Asian countries, in particular. Such commercial applications of LF include e.g. yoghurt, baby foods and infant formulas. In addition, LF has been applied in different dietary supplements as such or in combination with bovine colostrum and/or probiotic bacteria. Due to potential synergistic actions LF has been incorporated together with lysozyme and lactoperoxidase into human oral health care products, such as toothpastes, mouth-rinses, moisturising gels and chewing gums (Wakabayashi *et al.*, 2006; Weinberg, 2007). Food and Drug Administration (FDA) of United States have granted bovine LF a 'Generally Recognized As Safe' (GRAS, GRN 67) status and approved the use of bovine LF (at not more than 2% by weight) as a spray to reduce microbial contamination on the surface of raw beef carcasses. It can be envisaged that the usage of LF as an ingredient in functional foods and pharmaceutical preparations will increase considerably in the coming years. Also, accumulating evidence about the clinical efficacy of LF may in future make this natural compound an alternative or adjunct means to prevent or even cure certain pathologic conditions in humans.

20.2.4   α-Lactalbumin

α-Lactalbumin is the predominant whey protein in human milk and accounts about 20% of the proteins in bovine whey. The health benefits of α-la have long been obscured but recent research suggests that this protein can provide beneficial effects in many molecular forms, such as the intact whole protein molecule, peptides of the partly hydrolysed protein and amino acids of the fully digested protein (Chatterton *et al.*, 2006). α-Lactalbumin is a good source of the essential amino acids tryptophan and cysteine which are precursors of serotonin and glutathione, respectively. As these biomolecules are important for the cognitive functions, it has been speculated that the oral administration of α-la could improve the ability to cope with stress. This hypothesis has been supported by a study of Markus *et al.* (2002) who observed that α-la improved cognitive functions in stress-vulnerable subjects by increased brain tryptophan and serotonin activity. In another clinical study Scrutton *et al.* (2007) demonstrated that daily administration of 40 g of α-la to healthy women increased plasma tryptophan levels and its ratio to neutral amino acids but no changes in emotional processing was observed. Furthermore, there is significant evidence from animal model studies that α-la can provide protective effect against induced gastric mucosal injury caused by intake of ethanol or non-steroid anti-inflammatory drugs (NSAID) (Mezzaroba *et al.*,

2005). α-Lactalbumin is rich in cysteine and it has been demonstrated that an intake of cysteine-rich whey protein diet improves glycaemic control and alleviates sucrose-induced oxidative stress and also development of insulin resistance in rats fed a high sucrose diet (Blouet *et al.*, 2007). Moreover, intake of whey proteins, and α-la in particular, has been suggested to be associated with body composition and satiety affecting food intake (Schaafsma, 2006a, b; Luhovyy *et al.*, 2007). These effects may be related at least partially to the branched-chain amino acids leucine, isoleucine and valine which are high in α-la. In recent animal model and human studies leucine has been shown to be important for, e.g. synthesis of muscle protein, regulation of insulin production and deposition of body fat (Belobrajdic *et al.*, 2004; Frid *et al.*, 2005; Donato *et al.*, 2006; Nilsson *et al.*, 2007). Interesting results were obtained in a recent mouse model study by Pilvi *et al.* (2009) who studied the effect of different whey protein-containing high-Ca diets on the weight loss and weight regain in a model of diet-induced obesity. Weight loss by energy restriction was performed on four different high-Ca diets (1.8% CaCO3) containing different whey proteins (18% of energy): α-la, β-lg, LF and whey protein isolate (WPI). After seven weeks of energy restriction some of the mice were killed and the rest were fed with the same diets *ad libitum* for seven weeks. The results showed that the mice on the LF diet lost significantly more weight than mice on the WPI diet. The body fat content in the α-la and LF groups was significantly lower than in the WPI group (P < 0.05) and the LF group differed significantly even from the β-lg group (P < 0.05). *Ad libitum* feeding after weight loss resulted in weight regain in all groups and only the α-la diet significantly reduced fat accumulation during weight regain. The authors concluded that a high-Ca diet with α-la significantly improved the outcome of weight loss and subsequent weight regain during the feeding of a high-fat diet in mice, in comparison with WPI. These animal studies are encouraging in view of the potential use of α-la in dietary regimes targeting at reducing the risk of development of diabetes type two and obesity. Intervention trials in humans are required to confirm these results. Another suitable field of application for bovine α-la and its hydrolysates are infant formulas owing to the high degree of amino acid homology to human α-la. Based on its high degree of amino acid homology to human α-la, bovine α-la and its hydrolysates are well suited as an ingredient for infant formulas. A few α-la enriched formulas have been commercialized.

20.2.5 β-Lactoglobulin

β-Lactoglobulin is the major whey protein in bovine milk accounting for about 50% of the proteins in whey but is not found in human milk. β-Lactoglobulin poses a variety of functional and nutritional characteristics that have made this protein a versatile ingredient material for many food and biochemical applications. β-Lactoglobulin has excellent heat-set gelation properties and has found a wide range of applications in products where water-binding and texturization are required. β-Lactoglobulin exhibits a number of biological activities, including antiviral, prevention of pathogen adhesion, anticarcinogenic and hypocholesterolemic effects (Chatterton *et al.*, 2006). Furthermore, β-lg has the ability to bind hydrophobic components, for example retinol and long-chain fatty acids. It also may play a role in the absorption and subsequent metabolism of fatty acids. Like α-la, β-lg has proven an excellent source of peptides with a wide range of bioactivities, such as antihypertensive, antimicrobial, antioxidative, anticarcinogenic, immunomodulatory, opioid, hypocholesterolemic and other metabolic effects (Hernandez-Ledesma *et al.*, 2008). In view of the abundance of β-lg in bovine whey and its postulated biological properties, this protein fraction would warrant more basic research.

20.2.6   Lactoperoxidase

Lactoperoxidase (LP) is a glycoprotein-based enzyme which occurs naturally in colostrum, milk and many other human and animal secretions. LP represents the most abundant enzyme in milk (about 30 mg/l) and can be recovered in substantial quantities from whey using chromatographic techniques (Chiu and Etzel, 1997; Kussendrager and Hooijdonk, 2000). LP catalyses an antimicrobial system consisting of the thiocyanate anion (SCN-) and hydrogen peroxide to generate short-lived oxidation products, primarily hypothiocyanate (OSCN-), which kill or inhibit the growth of a wide range of microorganisms, including bacteria, viruses, fungi, molds and protozoa (Seifu *et al.*, 2005). The LP system is known to be bactericidal against many Gram-negative pathogenic and spoilage bacteria and bacteriostatic against many Gram-positive bacteria. Also, it is inhibitory *in vitro* to *Candida albicans* and the malaria causing protozoan *Plasmodium falciparium* as well as inactivates *in vitro* the HIV type 1 and polio virus. Since the discovery of the antimicrobial mechanism of the LP system in the early 1960s (Reiter and Oram, 1967) considerable amount of research has been conducted to establish its biological importance. Nowadays the LP system is considered to be an important part of the natural host defence system in mammals, the protective function being mediated by several mechanisms (Boots and Floris, 2006). One of these functions is to extend the freshness of raw milk as bovine milk contains naturally all necessary components to make the system functional. The natural concentrations of thiocyanate and hydrogen peroxide ($H^2 O^2$) can, however, be critical in milk and the activation of the system usually requires addition of a source of these two components. The effectiveness of the activated LP system has been demonstrated in many field trials worldwide (Anon., 2005; Seifu *et al.*, 2005). Since 1991, the LP system has been approved by the Codex Alimentarius Committee of FAO/ WHO for preservation of raw milk under conditions where facilities for milk cooling are insufficient. The method is now being employed for raw milk preservation in many developing countries but in some countries the safety of this system is still under consideration. The LP system has found also other applications, for example in dental health care products and animal feeds. Other potential applications for this natural antimicrobial system could be found in preservation of different products, for example meat, fish, vegetables, fruits and even live flowers (Boots and Floris, 2006).

20.2.7   Glycomacropeptide

GMP is a C-terminal glycopeptide f (106–169) released from the κ-casein molecule by the action of chymosin. GMP is hydrophilic and remains in the whey fraction in the cheese manufacturing process. GMP contains a significant (50–60% of total GMP) carbohydrate fraction which is composed of galactose, N-acetyl-galactosamine and N-neuraminic acid. The non-glycosylated form of GMP is often termed caseinomacropeptide or CMP. Pure GMP can be recovered in large quantities from cheese whey (up to 20% of proteins) by chromatographic or ultrafiltration techniques (Thomä-Worringer et al., 2006; Kulozik, 2009). The potential biological activities of GMP have received much attention in recent years. It has been shown in many studies that GMP inactivates in vitro microbial toxins of E. coli and V. cholerae, inhibits in vitro adhesion of cariogenic bacteria and influenza virus, modulates immune system responses, promotes growth of bifidobacteria, suppresses gastric hormone activities and regulates blood circulation through antihypertensive and antithrombotic activity (Manso and López-Fandino, 2004). Rhoades et al. (2005) have demonstrated that GMP inhibits effectively in vitro adhesion of pathogenic (VTEC and EPEC) E. coli strains to human HT29 colon carcinoma cells whereas probiotic Lactobacillus strains were inhibited to a lesser extent.

Owing to its glycoprotein nature GMP has interesting nutritional and physico-chemical properties. GMP is rich in branched-chain amino acids and low in methionine, which makes it a useful ingredient in diets for patients suffering from hepatic diseases. GMP contains no phenylalanin making it suitable for patients suffering from phenylketonuria. Results from animal model studies have suggested that the high sialic acid content of GMP may deliver beneficial effects for brain development and improvement of learning ability (Wang et al., 2001). A number of experimental studies have further suggested that GMP may have a role in regulation of intestinal functions (Manso and Lopéz-Fandino, 2004). This argument is based on the findings that GMP has been found to inhibit gastric secretions and slow down stomach motility by means of stimulating the release of cholecystokinin (CKK), the satiety hormone involved in controlling food intake and digestion in the duodenum of animals and humans (Yvon et al., 1994). In this context, an interesting finding is that intact GMP and fragments of this macropeptide have been detected in human blood plasma after milk or yoghurt ingestion (Chabance et al., 1998). This would suggest that GMP may be produced in the gut before being absorbed into the circulation. In recent years, commercial GMP or CMP containing products have been launched on the market being targeted for appetite control and weight management. The clinical efficacy of such products remains, however, to be established. A short-term intervention trial failed to show any effect on satiety when 2.0 grams of CMP was administered daily to healthy human subjects (Gustafson et al., 2001).

In a recent animal model study Royle et al. (2008) demonstrated that both GMP and a whey protein isolate (WPI) decreased weight gain and altered body composition of male Wistar rats. Burton-Freeman (2008) found that GMP had no effect or on satiety on food intake 75 minutes after ingestion but did reduce daily food intake. In a recent randomized double blind acute satiety study by Clifton *et al.* (2009) 20 overweight or obese males consumed four 50 g preloads of GMP (two GMP preparations, GPM depleted whey and glucose) with a three-day interval between treatments. There was no significant difference in CCK levels, subjective measures of satiety or food intake between treatments at the given preload level. In another intervention trial (Keogh and Clifton, 2009) for six months on overweight subjects, milk protein-based meal replacements achieved a meaningful weight loss with benefits on markers of cardiovascular disease risk but GMP had no additional effect. Zemel (2004) has suggested that whey proteins and dairy calcium contribute to limiting body fat accumulation and offer thus advantages in maintaining optimal body composition. Another interesting finding is that GMP may have an active, beneficial role in modulation of gut microbiota, as this macropeptide has been shown to promote the growth of bifidobacteria (Manso and López-Fandino, 2004). There is some recent indication from mouse model studies that bifidobacteria may affect the weight gain. Further research in human subjects is needed to elucidate the influence of GMP on weight management.

20.2.8   Growth factors

It is now well documented that colostrum and milk contain several factors which promote or inhibit the growth of different cell types (Gauthier *et al.*, 2006a; Pouliot and Gauthier, 2006). The best characterized growth factors are BTC (beta cellulin), EGF (epidermal growth factor), FGF1 and FGF2 (fibroblast growth factor), IGF-I and IGF-II (insulin-like growth factor), TGF-β1 and TGF-β2 (transforming growth factor) and PDGF (platelet-derived growth factor). The concentration of growth factors is highest in colostrum during the first hours after calving and decreases substantially thereafter (Elfstrand *et al.*, 2002; Montoni *et al.*, 2009). Chemically the growth factors are polypeptides and their molecular masses range between 6000 and 30 000 Daltons. It is noteworthy that the growth factors present in milk seem to withstand relatively well pasteurization and even UHT (ultra high temperature) heat treatment of milk (Gauthier *et al.*, 2006a). In recent years, several pilot or semi-industrial methods have been developed for extraction of different growth factors from bovine colostrum and cheese whey (Piot *et al.*, 2004; Akbache *et al.*, 2009).

The growth factors have been associated with many physiological functions affecting, for example, skin, intestinal tract and bone health (Tripathi and Vashishtha, 2006). Contradictory results have been reported on the stability of growth factors in the gastrointestinal tract. Many animal model studies have shown that EGF, IGF-I, and both TGF forms can provoke various local effects on the gut mucosa and can be absorbed intact or partially from intestine into blood circulation (Gauthier *et al.*, 2006a). Accordingly, the growth factors may stimulate in the body a variety of local and systemic functions. Several health-related applications have been proposed for growth factors extracted from bovine colostral or cheese whey. Playford *et al.* (2000) have suggested that colostrum-based products containing active growth factors could be applied to prevent the side-effects of non-steroid anti-inflammatory drugs (NSAIDs) and symptoms of arthritis. An acid casein extract rich in TGF-$\beta2$ has been tested successfully in children suffering from Crohn's disease. Another growth factor extract from cheese whey has shown promising results in animal models and humans in treatment of oral mucositis and wound healing, for example leg ulcers (Smithers, 2008). Other potential applications could be treatment of psoriasis, induction of oral tolerance in the newborn children against allergies and cytoprotection against intestinal damages caused by chemotherapy.

Another interesting protein complex isolated from whey is milk basic protein (MBP) which consists of several low-molecular compounds, such as kininogen and cystatin and HMG-like protein. In cell culture and animal model studies BMP has been shown to stimulate bone formation and simultaneously suppress bone resorption (Kawakami, 2005). The bone-strenghtening effects of BMP have been confirmed in human trials and the product has been evaluated for safety and commercialized in Japan.

20.3   Bioactive peptides

Bioactive peptides have been defined as specific protein fragments that have a positive impact on body functions or conditions and may ultimately influence health (Kitts and Weiler, 2003). The activity of peptides is based on their inherent amino acid composition and sequence. The size of active sequences may vary from two to twenty amino acid residues, and many peptides are known to reveal multi-functional properties. Milk proteins have been studied for presence of bioactive amino acid sequences since late 1970s and are now considered the most important source of bioactive peptides. The best characterized ones include antihypertensive, antithrombotic, antimicrobial, antioxidative, immunomodulatory and opioid peptides. At present, totally more than two hundred bioactive peptide sequences have been identified from caseins and whey proteins. Their production, functionality and potential applications have been reviewed in many articles and book chapters over the last ten years (Clare and Swaisgood, 2000; Pihlanto and Korhonen, 2003; Korhonen and Pihlanto, 2003, 2006, 2007; Baldi *et al.*, 2005; Silva and Malcata, 2005; Meisel, 2005, 2009; López-Fandino *et al.*, 2006; Gobbetti *et al.*, 2007; Jauhiainen and Korpela, 2007; López-Expósito *et al.*, 2007; Murray and FitzGerald, 2007; Saito, 2008; Korhonen, 2009b, c; Phelan *et al.*, 2009).

20.3.1   Occurrence in dairy products

It is now well documented that bioactive peptides are formed in the manufacturing and maturation processes of various fermented dairy products as a result of proteolytic action by added microbial cultures. In screening studies a great variety of bioactive peptides has been found in fermented dairy products, such as yoghurt, sour milk, dahi, kefir, quark and different types of cheese, eg. Cheddar, Edam, Emmental, Gouda and many Italian varieties (Singh *et al.*, 1997; FitzGerald and Murray, 2006; Gobbetti *et al.*, 2007). The occurrence, specific activity and amount of bioactive peptides in fermented dairy products depend on many factors, such as type of starters used, type of product, time of fermentation and storage conditions (Saito *et al.*, 2000; Ardö *et al.*, 2007; Ong *et al.*, 2007; Bütikofer *et al.*, 2008; Paul and Somkuti, 2009). Ong and Shah (2008) demonstrated that Cheddar cheeses made with the addition of probiotic *Lactobacillus casei 279*, *L. casei* LAFTI® L26 or *L. acidophilus* LAFTI® L10 had significantly higher angiotensin-converting enzyme (ACE) inhibitory activity than those without any probiotic adjunct. These probiotic adjuncts are known to improve proteolysis and enhance flavour during Cheddar cheese ripening. It is noteworthy that in fermented dairy products peptides with different bioactivities (e.g. calcium binding, antihypertensive, antioxidative, immunomodulatory and antimicrobial), can be found at the same time.

The formation of peptides can be regulated to some extent by starter and adjunct cultures used but the stability of desired peptides during storage seems difficult to control. For example, the ACE-inhibitory activity increases during cheese maturation, but decreases when the proteolysis exceeds a certain level (Ryhänen *et al.*, 2001; Bütikofer *et al.*, 2007, 2008). Apart from generation during the ripening process, more bioactive peptides are likely to be formed in the gastrointestinal tract upon ingestion of a fermented dairy product. This was demonstrated under *in vitro* conditions by Parrot *et al.* (2003) who showed that consecutive digestion of the water-soluble extract (WSE) of Emmental cheese with pepsin and trypsin, respectively, induced an increase in ACE inhibition as compared with undigested WSE. Similar results were obtained by Ardö *et al.* (2009) who evaluated the impact of heat-treated *Lactobacillus helveticus* CNRZ 303 culture on the formation, accumulation and hydrolysis of bioactive peptides during ripening of semi-hard cheese. During ripening, the formation of antioxidative and phosphopeptides peptides were observed and they were further hydrolysed by *Lb. helveticus* enzymes. Also, ACE-inhibitory peptides accumulated during the ripening period of nine months but no hydrolysis by *Lb. helveticus* enzymes was noted. Further increased ACE inhibition was observed when the cheese samples were digested *in vitro* by Corolase PP (Röhm, Germany) enzyme preparation simulating gastrointestinal enzymes.

Hernández-Ledesma *et al.* (2004) evaluated the ACE-inhibitory activity of several commercial fermented milks and fresh cheeses and found that most of these products showed moderate ACE-inhibitory activity. The ACE-inhibitory activity of these commercial products remained stable or increased after simulated gastrointestinal digestion with pepsin and Corolase PP. Also, ACE-inhibitory peptides have been detected in yoghurt made from ovine milk (Chobert *et al.*, 2005) and in kefir made from caprine milk (Quiros *et al.*, 2005). The potential *in vivo* effect of fermented cheese or fermented milk products containing naturally formed antihypertensive peptides on blood pressure of hypertensive subjects remain to be studied. On the other hand, many clinical studies have shown that fermented liquid milk products supplemented or enriched with specific antihypertensive peptides are effective in reduction of blood pressure in moderately hypertensive subjects (Murray and FitzGerald, 2007; Saito, 2008; Kekkonen and Peuhkuri, 2009).

Calcium-binding casein phosphopeptides (CPPs) have been identified in casein hydrolysates, milk-based infant formulae, and fermented dairy products, such as cheese and yoghurt (Gagnaire *et al.*, 2001; Kawahara *et al.*, 2005; Miquel *et al.*, 2005; Dupas *et al.*, 2009). CPPs may also arise from αs_1-, αs_2-, and β-casein digestion in the gut (FitzGerald, 1998).

20.3.2   Production systems

Bioactive peptides are inactive within the sequence of their parent protein molecule and can be released in the following ways: (a) hydrolysis by digestive enzymes, (b) fermentation of milk with proteolytic starter cultures, and (c) proteolysis by microbial or plant-derived enzymes (Korhonen and Pihlanto, 2007; Korhonen, 2009c; Vercruysse *et al.*, 2009). In many studies, the above methods have been combined successfully to generate novel functional peptides. In the following, examples of biopeptides produced by the above techniques will be described.

Gastrointestinal enzymes pepsin, trypsin and chymotrypsin have been shown to release a great number of antihypertensive peptides, CPPs, antibacterial, immunomodulatory and opioid peptides both from casein (α-, β- and κ-casein) and whey protein (α-la, β-lg and GMP) fractions (López-Fandino *et al.*, 2006; Ferreira *et al.*, 2007; del Mar Contreras *et al.*, 2009). Also, commercial proteolytic enzymes, such as Alcalase, Flavourzyme, Thermolysin and Subtilisin have been employed to release various bioactive peptides both from caseins and whey proteins (Pihlanto-Leppälä *et al.*, 2000; Otte *et al.*, 2007). Ortiz-Chao *et al.* (2009) obtained novel, potent ACE-inhibitory peptide mixtures from the hydrolysis of β-lg using Protease N Amano, a food-grade commercial proteolytic preparation (Amano Enzyme Inc., Nagoya, Japan). The heptapeptide SAPLRVY was isolated and characterized corresponding to b-lg f(36–42). It expressed an IC50 value of 8 mM, which was considerably lower than the most potent ACE inhibitory peptides derived from bovine β-lg reported, so far. The IC50 value was defined as the concentration of peptide in mg protein/ml required to inhibit 50% of the original ACE activity. Antihypertensive peptides and antimicrobial peptides are the most studied ones and at present more than 150 hypotensive peptides have been identified from different milk proteins (Korhonen, 2009b; Phelan *et al.*, 2009).

Many lactic acid bacteria (LAB) and probiotic strains are highly proteolytic and formation of bioactive peptides can, therefore, be anticipated in milk fermentation processes. Indeed, the release of bioactive peptides from milk proteins by means of microbial fermentation is now well documented (Hernandez-Ledesma *et al.*, 2004; Hayes *et al.*, 2007a, b; Murray and FitzGerald, 2007; Mills *et al.*, 2009). A great number of dairy cultures and probiotic strains have been associated with the release of bioactive peptides but *Lactobacillus helveticus* strains, in particular, have proven highly prominent in releasing antihypertensive peptides. The best studied peptides are the ACE-inhibitory tripeptides Val-Pro-Pro (VPP) and Ile-Pro-Pro (IPP) (Yamamoto *et al.*, 2003; Lopez-Fandino *et al.*, 2006;

Saito, 2008). These amino acid sequences are present in β- and κ-casein fractions and GMP and can be released by both microbial and pepsin treatments. Also yoghurt bacteria, cheese starter bacteria and commercial probiotic bacteria have been shown to produce different bioactive peptides in milk during fermentation (Gomez-Ruiz *et al.*, 2002; Fuglsang *et al.*, 2003; Gobbetti *et al.*, 2004; Chen *et al.*, 2007). Virtanen *et al.* (2006) studied the production of antioxidant activity during fermentation of milk with 25 LAB strains. It was demonstrated that the development of antioxidant activity was strain-specific with *Leuconostoc mesenteroides* ssp. *cemoris* strains, *Lactobacillus jensenii* (ATCC 25258) and *Lb. acidophilus* (ATCC 4356) showing the highest activity. The activity correlated positively with the degree of proteolysis suggesting that peptides were responsible for the antioxidative property. Donkor *et al.* (2007) studied the proteolytic activity of several dairy cultures and probiotic strains (*Lb. acidophilus, Bifidobacterium animalis subsp. lactis* and *Lactobacillus casei*) as determinant of growth and *in vitro* ACE-inhibitory activity in milk fermented with these single cultures. All the cultures released ACE-inhibitory peptides during growth with a *Bifidobacterium. longum* strain, the probiotic *Lb. acidophilus* strain showing the strongest ACE-inhibitory activity. Chen *et al.* (2007) observed that fermentation of milk with a commercial starter culture mixture of five LAB strains followed by hydrolysis with a microbial protease increased ACE inhibitory activity of the hydrolysate. Two strong ACE-inhibitory tripeptides (Gly-Thr-Trp) and (Gly-Val-Trp) were identified and an antihypertensive effect of the hydrolysate containing these peptides was demonstrated in an animal model study using spontaneously hypertensive rats (SHR). In a similar study Tsai *et al.* (2008) fermented milk with yoghurt bacteria (*Streptococcus thermophilus, Lactobacillus bulgaricus*) and a protease Flavourzyme was added at the beginning of fermentation. An ACE-inhibitory peptide Tyr-Pro-Tyr-Tyr was identified in the whey fraction and oral administration for 8 weeks of this whey reduced systolic and diastolic blood pressure 15.9 and 15.6 mm Hg, respectively, in SHR. Pihlanto-Leppälä *et al.* (1998) have demonstrated that fermentation of milk with starter cultures alone was not enough to generate ACE inhibitory activity, but a further digestion with pepsin and trypsin was necessary. It can be expected that similar events may happen also under *in vivo* conditions in the gastrointestinal tract when ingesting fermented dairy products. In a recent study, Paul and Somkuti (2009) demonstrated that antimicrobial and hypotensive polypeptides released from LF by pepsin remain mostly intact at pH 4.5 when added into yoghurt at the end of the fermentation process. Thus, the health-promoting qualities of fermented liquid or semi-solid dairy foods may be increased by supplementation with bioactive peptides.

Various technologies have been applied for the enrichment and isolation of bioactive peptides from the hydrolysates of milk proteins (Korhonen and Pihlanto, 2007; Vercruysse *et al.*, 2009). For this purpose, membrane filtration systems, chromatographic methods and selective precipitation have been developed up to semi-industrial or industrial scale and many companies manufacture now specific peptide concentrates.

20.3.3   Functionality

A great number of *in vitro* and experimental studies conducted since the 1980s have demonstrated the wide functionality of bioactive peptides released from bovine milk proteins. These studies suggest that such peptides may exert physiological effects, for example on the gastrointestinal, cardiovascular, endocrine, immune, nervous and other body systems. A majority of animal model and human studies have concerned antihypertensive, mineral-binding and anticariogenic peptides. The antihypertensive capacity of many milk peptides has been indicated in many *in vitro* and rat model studies (Murray and FitzGerald, 2007; Haque and Chand, 2008; Saito, 2008). In these studies, the tripeptides VPP and IPP have proven the most effective ones (Nakamura *et al.*, 1995; Sipola *et al.*, 2002; Jauhiainen *et al.*, 2005; De Leeuw *et al.*, 2009). In human studies moderate or significant reduction of blood pressure has been observed in mildly hypertensive subjects after consumption of fermented dairy products or tablets containing these peptides (Seppo *et al.*, 2003; Hirota *et al.*, 2007; Boelsma and Kloek, 2009). Reductions of 1.5 to 14.0 mm Hg for systolic blood pressure (SBP) and 0.5 to 6.8 mm Hg for diastolic blood pressure (DBP), compared with placebo have been recorded. Effective dosages of lactotripeptides (VPP and IPP) range from 3.07 to 52.5 mg/d (Korhonen, 2009c). Blood pressure-lowering effects of lactotripeptides are typically measured after 4–6 weeks of treatment. Maximum blood pressure reductions approximate 13 mmHg of SBP and 8 mmHg of DBP, respectively, after active treatment compared with placebo, are likely reached after 8–12 weeks of treatment.

The absorption from the gastrointestinal tract into circulation and dose-dependent antihypertensive effect *in vivo* of VPP and IPP has been established in rat model and human studies (Hata *et al.*, 1996; Masuda *et al.*, 1996; Aihara *et al.*, 2005; Jauhiainen *et al.*, 2007b). Foltz *et al.* (2007) showed in a placebo-controlled, full crossover intervention study that IPP was absorbed intact from a fermented milk drink into circulation of healthy human subjects. On the other hand, several recent studies have not established any significant effect of drinks containing ACE-inhibitory peptides (Lee *et al.*, 2007) or VPP and IPP peptides on blood pressure in human subjects with mild hypertension (Engberink *et al.*, 2008; van der Zander *et al.*, 2008; van Mierlo *et al.*, 2009). Also, the three recent meta-analyses have resulted in non-conclusive results about the efficacy of milk derived biopeptides in reduction of hypertension (Pripp, 2008; Xu *et al.*, 2008; Usinger *et al.*, 2009).

A recent study by Turpeinen *et al.* (2009) has suggested that the beneficial effects of tripeptides on cardiovascular functions can be combined with other dietary components, for example with cholesterol-lowering plant sterols. The effects of a spread containing IPP, VPP and plant sterols were studied in subjects with mild hypertension and elevated LDL cholesterol. 62 subjects consumed 20 g/day spread containing 4.2 mg milk peptides and 2 g plant sterol esters or placebo for 10 weeks. A significant decrease was seen in SBP ($p = 0.026$), but not in DBP ($p = 0.53$). Also, total cholesterol and LDL cholesterol decreased significantly, whereas HDL cholesterol, and triacylglycerols remained unchanged. The results suggest that a spread containing bioactive milk peptides and plant sterols has a beneficial effect on two major cardiovascular risk factors, blood pressure and plasma lipids, in hypertensive, dyslipidemic subjects.

Apart from ACE-inhibitory activity, the lactotripeptides VPP and IPP have been shown to exert a beneficial effect on arterial stiffness of hypertensive rats (Jäkälä *et al.*, 2009) and mildly hypertensive human subjects (Jauhiainen *et al.*, 2007a). Another possible mechanism for antihypertensive action of milk protein derived peptides is stimulation of nitric oxide production by endothelial cells. A novel whey derived peptide (NOP-47) has been shown *in vitro* to increase endothelial nitric oxide synthesis. In a recent randomized, placebo-controlled, crossover study on healthy human subjects, a two week of supplementation with a single dose of 5 g/day of NOP-47 peptide improved vascular function as compared with placebo (Ballard *et al.*, 2009). In view of the great public health importance of hypertension, the potential beneficial impact of antihypertensive effects of milk derived peptides deserves further research.

Calcium-binding phosphopeptides (CCPs) have been studied for the potential health effects, for example enhancement of calcium bioavailability, but the results obtained in animal and human studies have been inconclusive (Meisel and Fitzgerald, 2003). Instead, the anticariogenic effect of some CPPs is well documented in animal and human studies (Reynolds, 2003; Aimutis, 2004; Morgan *et al.*, 2008) and such specific peptides have been commercialized.

20.3.4 Applications

Commercially marketed products which contain milk protein-derived bioactive peptides are now available in many countries. These products are, for example, dairy and fruit based drinks, confectionery, chewing gum, pastilles and capsules. They are claimed to possess antihypertensive, anticariogenic, mineral-binding or stress-relieving properties (Hartman and Meisel, 2007; Korhonen, 2009b). Examples of these commercial ingredients and their applications are listed in Table 20.3. So far, the best studied peptide products are the fermented milk products Calpis® and Evolus® which are targeted to subjects having a mild hypertension. The blood pressure reducing effects of both products have been established in many human studies (Hata *et al.*, 1996; Seppo *et al.*, 2003; Aihara *et al.*, 2005; Jauhiainen *et al.*, 2005). These products contain the two ACE-inhibitory tripeptides VPP and IPP. The Japanese product Calpis® is fermented with a culture containing *Lb. helveticus* and *S. cerevisiae* (Saito, 2008) and the Finnish product Evolus® is produced using a *Lb. helveticus* LBK-16 H strain in milk fermentation (Seppo *et al.*, 2003).

CPPs have been studied for the potential health effects, for example enhancement of calcium bioavailability, but the results obtained in animal and human studies have been inconclusive (Hartman and Meisel, 2007). A casein hydrolysate (CE90CPP) containing enriched CPPs has, however, been commercialized with a health claim. Various dental care products, e.g. Recaldent®, containing CPPs have been launched on the market in some countries (Reynolds, 2003). Other interesting applications of bioactive peptides are Lactium®, Vivinal Alpha® and Cysteine peptide® products which claim to deliver stress-relieving effects. PeptoPro® is

Table 20.3 Commercial dairy products and ingredients based on bioactive peptides

Brand name	Type of product	Functional bioactive peptides	Health/function claims	Manufacturer
Calpis	Sour milk	Val-Pro-Pro, Ile-Pro-Pro, derived from β-casein and κ-casein	Reduction of blood pressure	Calpis Co., Japan
Evolus	Fermented milk	Val-Pro-Pro, Ile-Pro-Pro, derived from β-casein and κ-casein	Reduction of blood pressure	Valio Oy, Finland
BioZate	Hydrolysed whey protein isolate	β-Lactoglobulin fragments	Reduction of blood pressure	Davisco, USA
BioPURE-GMP	Whey protein isolate	κ-Casein f(106–169) (glycomacropeptide)	Anticariogenic, antimicrobial, antithrombotic	Davisco, USA
ProDiet F200/Lactium	Flavoured milk drink, confectionery, capsules	α_{s1}-casein f(91–100) (Tyr-Leu-Gly-Tyr-Leu-Glu-Gln-Leu-Leu-Arg)	Relief of stress symptoms	Ingredia, France
Recaldent	Chewing gum	Calcium casein peptone-calcium phosphate	Anticariogenic	Cadbury Adams, USA
Festivo	Fermented low-fat hard cheese	α_{s1}-Casein f(1–9) α_{s1}-Casein f(1–6) α_{s1}-Casein f(1–7)	Contains bioactive peptides which are shown to reduce blood pressure *in vitro*	MTT Agrifood Research, Finland
Cysteine Peptide	Ingredient	Milk protein derived peptide	Aids sleep	DMV International, the Netherlands
C12 Peption	Ingredient	Casein derived dodeca-peptide FFVAPFPEVFGK*	Reduction of blood pressure	DMV International, the Netherlands
Capolac	Ingredient	Caseinophosphopeptide	Helps mineral absorption	Arla Foods Ingredients, Sweden

PeptoPro	Flavoured drink	Casein derived di- and tripeptides	Improves athletic performance and muscle recovery after exercise	DSM Food Specialties, the Netherlands
Vivinal Alpha	Ingredient	α-Lactalbumin rich whey protein hydrolysate	Aids relaxation and sleep	Borculo Domo Ingredients (BDI), the Netherlands
Praventin	Capsule	Lactoferrin enriched whey protein hydrolysate	Helps reduce acne	DMV International, the Netherlands

Source: modified from Korhonen and Pihlanto (2006).

* One-letter amino acid code.

targeted to improve athletic performance and recovery from physical exercise (Korhonen, 2009b).

20.3.5   Conclusions

The current global interest in developing health-promoting functional foods provides a timely opportunity to tap the myriad of innate bioactive milk components for inclusion in such formulations. Moving from science to commercial applications seems now appropriate as the fundamental biological properties and mechanism of action of milk proteins, bioactive peptides and growth factors are reasonably well established. Also, industrial or semi-industrial scale processing techniques are available for fractionation and isolation of such components from colostrum and milk. These components present an excellent source for different applications in health-promoting foods. In fact, fractionation and marketing of bioactive milk ingredients is emerging as a new lucrative sector for the dairy industries and specialized bio-industries. Much as a result of this development the dairy industry has achieved a leading role in the development of functional foods and has already commercialized many milk protein and peptide-based products which can be consumed as part of a regular healthy diet. It can be envisaged that in the near future more similar products will be launched on worldwide markets. They could be targeted to infants, elderly and immune-compromised people as well as to maintain good health status and prevent diet-related chronic diseases. In view of the current global trend of increasing prevalence of obesity and related diseases, type two diabetes, in particular, more experimental research should be focused on bioactive milk peptides which can regulate appetite and manage blood glucose balance. Other new areas where more research with bioactive milk proteins and peptides is warranted are impairment of cognitive functions, memory-related diseases and mood control. In this context, antioxidative and opioid properties of many milk peptides may be worth further investigations. Also, potential to reduce oxidative stress in the body via oral administration of antioxidative peptides may be of considerable interest in view of the inflammatory events caused by radical oxygen species (ROS) in the living cells.

In conclusion, beyond being an excellent source of essential nutrients milk promises to deliver many health benefits to humans of all ages by provision of specific bioactive factors. Thus, they can be part of a healthy diet and lifestyle to prevent or reduce high blood pressure.

20.4   Bioactive lipids

Bovine milk fat is composed of more than 400 different fatty acids which are primarily found as triglycerides esterified to the glycerol molecule backbone (Walstra et al., 2006). Most of milk fat is used for human consumption in different forms of traditional dairy products, such as liquid milk, cream, butter, ghee, cheese and ice cream. In most industrialized countries consumption of butter and other high-fat dairy products has been on the decline due to a negative nutritional image of milk fat. According to the current conception the intake of milk fat is associated with an increased risk to develop coronary heart disease (CHD) or metabolic syndrome (MacRae, *et al.*, 2005; Mensink, 2006). This property is claimed to be correlated primarily to certain saturated long-chain fatty acids, notably lauric (C12:0), myristic (C14:0) and palmitic (C16:0) acids, which are considered atherogenic by increasing plasma cholesterol and LDL-levels (Kris-Etherton and Yu, 1997). These fatty acids comprise about 35% of total milk fat. Other long-chain fatty acids in milk fat, such as stearic acid (C18:0) and short-chain acids (C4:0–C10:0) are considered neutral, whereas linoleic (C18:1) or linolenic (C18:2) acids may reduce cholesterol level (Jensen, 2002). On the other hand, some minor components of milk fat, especially conjugated linoleic acid (CLA), sphingomyelin, butyric acid, and ether lipids may have beneficial effects on health (Parodi, 2004, 2009; German and Dillard, 2006; Shingfield *et al.*, 2008; Churruca *et al.*, 2009).

20.4.1 Conjugated linoleic acid

CLA refers to a collection of positional and geometrical isomers of *cis*-9, *cis*-12-octadecadienoic acid (C18:2) with a conjugated double bond system. The major CLA isomer in milk fat is 9-cis, 11-*trans*, also called rumenic acid (Collomb *et al.*, 2006). CLA is formed partially by bioconversion of polyunsaturated fatty acids in the rumen by anaerobic bacteria, e.g. *Butyrovibrio fibrisolvens* and primarily endogenously by Δ9-desaturation of vaccenic acid in the mammary gland of lactating cows (Griinari *et al.*, 2000; Churruca *et al.*, 2009). Milk fat is the richest natural source of CLA and contents ranging from 2 to 53.7 mg/g fat have been recorded in different studies (Collomb *et al.*, 2006). The wide range of CLA values can be attributed to various factors such as feeding regime, forage preservation, geographical regions and breed of cows. A number of studies have confirmed that pasture feeding can increase significantly CLA concentrations as compared to indoor winter feeding. Also, the grass composition of pasture seems to affect the CLA level of milk. Cows grazed in the alpine region were found to produce milk with almost 2–3 times higher concentration of CLA as compared to the milk of cows grazed in the lowlands (Collomb *et al.*, 2001). Several experimental studies have demonstrated that feeding cows with meals containing plant oils and/or marine oils can effectively increase the CLA content of milk. The majority of these studies suggest that concentrates rich in linoleic acid (rapeseed, soybean, sunflower) have a better impact than other polyunsaturated plant oils (peanut, linseed) whereas the dietary fish oils and their combination with plant oils appear even more effective than plant oils alone (Shingfield *et al.*, 2005).

The effects of manufacturing conditions on the content of CLA in milk and dairy products have been studied extensively (Collomb *et al.*, 2006) and CLA enriched milk has been shown to produce softer butter than butter from ordinary milk. In cheese manufacture, processing seems to have only minor effects on the CLA content of final products but the properties of cheeses manufactured from CLA-enriched milk differ from control cheeses (Chamba *et al.*, 2006; Bisig *et al.*,

2007). In Cheddar and Edam types the texture of cheese made of CLA enriched milk was softer than in control cheese but no major differences were observed in the organoleptic properties (Ryhänen *et al.*, 2001; Avramis *et al.*, 2003). In organic milk and organic dairy products the CLA content has been shown to be higher in comparison to conventionally produced milk and products (Bisig *et al.*, 2007).

Possibilities to increase the CLA content of dairy products with microbial cultures have been investigated in many studies (Sieber *et al.*, 2004; Bisig *et al.*, 2007). Many dairy starter cultures, such as propionibacteria, lactobacilli and bifidobacteria have been found to be able to convert linoleic acid into CLA in culture media; however, inconsistent results have been obtained about CLA production by these cultures in yoghurt and cheese (Xu *et al.*, 2005). Bisig *et al.* (2007) have suggested that dairy products could be enriched with CLA produced in a special culture medium. Recently, Florence *et al.* (2009) demonstrated that organic milks fermented with several strains of bifidobacteria and yoghurt cultures contained significantly higher amounts of CLA than the same milk before fermentation, whereas CLA amounts did not change during fermentation of conventional milk. Supplementation of milk with different prebiotic compounds has been shown to further stimulate production of CLA by probiotic bacteria (Oliveira *et al.*, 2009).

During the past twenty years a large number of animal model studies have demonstrated multiple health benefits for dietary CLA. Such positive effects include anticarcinogenic, antiatherogenic, antidiabetic, antiobesity and enhancement of immune system (Pariza *et al.*, 2001; Belury, 2002; Pfeuffer and Schrezenmeir, 2006b; Field *et al.*, 2009). The effects seem to be mediated primarily by two CLA isomers: *cis*-9, *trans*-11 and *trans*-10, *cis*-12 but the impact may differ depending on the isomer. In milk fat the *cis*-9, *trans*-11 isomer amounts to 75–90% of total CLA. The average total daily dietary intake of CLA is estimated to range between 95 and 440 mg and differs from country to country. Optimal dietary intake remains to be established but it has been proposed that a daily intake of 3.0 to 3.5 grams of CLA is required to provide anticarcinogenic response in humans (Collomb *et al.*, 2006). Strong evidence from animal trials supports an influence of CLA intake on lowering of body weight and fat mass and increase in lean body mass. Human studies carried out do not support, however, any weight loss-inducing effect of CLA but suggest a lowering effect on body fat associated with an increase in lean body mass (Larsen *et al.*, 2003; Schoeller *et al.*, 2009).

Contradictory results have been reported in animal and human studies regarding the antidiabetic effect of CLA. The antiatherogenic effect of CLA also has been a controversial issue. In rodents and humans, dietary CLA supplementation has produced inconsistent results, as far as the reduction of serum cholesterol and triglyceride levels are concerned (Terpstra, 2004). A great number of *in vitro* experiments and animal trials have been conducted with regard to anticarcinogenic effects of synthetic CLA and rumenic acid enriched milk fat (Ip *et al.*, 2003; Parodi, 2004; Lee and Lee, 2005). A majority of these studies support the role for dietary CLA in protection against various types of cancer (e.g. breast, prostate and colon cancer), but the underlying mechanisms remain obscure. Further studies are warranted, as at present relevant human experimental data are scarce. An epidemiological study (Aro *et al.*, 2000) has suggested an inverse association between dietary and serum CLA and risk of breast cancer in postmenopausal women. Another cohort study has suggested that the high intake of CLA containing dairy foods may reduce the risk of colorectal cancer (Larsson *et al.*, 2005). Recently Churruca *et al.* (2009) reviewed the potential biological effects of CLA isomers and concluded as follows:

> Although the cis-9,trans-11 isomer is mainly responsible for the anticarcinogenic effect, the trans-10,cis-12 isomer reduces body fat and it is referred as the most effective isomer affecting blood lipids. As far as insulin function is concerned, both isomers seem to be responsible for insulin resistance in humans. Finally, with regard to the immune system it is not clear whether individual isomers of CLA could act similarly or differently.

20.4.2   Other bioactive lipids

Another biologically interesting lipid group in milk fat is the polar lipids, which are mainly located in the milk fat globule membrane (MFGM). It is a highly complex biological structure that surrounds the fat globule stabilizing it in the continuous aqueous phase of milk and preventing from enzymatic degradation by lipases (Mather, 2000; Spitsberg, 2005; Dewettinck *et al.*, 2008; Mezouari and Pouliot, 2009). The membrane consists about 60% of proteins and 40% of lipids that are mainly composed of triglycerides, cholesterol, phospholipids and sphingolipids (Rombaut and Dewettinck, 2006; Jimenez-Flores and Brisson, 2008). The polar lipid content of raw milk is reported to range between 9.4 and 35.5 mg per 100 g of milk. The major phospholipid fractions are phosphatidylethanolamine and phosphatidylcholine followed by smaller amounts of phosphatidylserine and phosphatidylinositol. The major sphingolipid fraction is sphingomyelin with smaller portions of ceramides and gangliosides (Jensen, 2002). In processing of milk into different dairy products, the polar lipids are preferentially enriched in the aqueous phases like skimmed milk, butter milk and butter serum (Sichien *et al.*, 2009).

The polar lipids in milk are gaining increasing interest due to their nutritional and technolocical properties. These compounds are secondary messengers involved in transmembrane signal transduction and regulation, growth, proliferation, differentiation and apoptosis of cells. Further they play a role in neuronal signaling, are linked to age-related diseases, blood coagulation, immunity and inflammatory responses (Pettus *et al.*, 2004). In particular, sphingolipids and their derivatives are considered highly bioactive components possessing anticancer, cholesterol-lowering and antibacterial activities (Rombaut and Dewettinck, 2006). Furthermore, butyric acid and butyrate have been shown to inhibit development of colon and mammary tumours (Parodi, 2003). These promising results from cell culture and animal model studies require further confirmation and human clinical studies but suggest that sphingolipid-rich foods or supplements could be beneficial in the prevention of certain cancer types and bowel-related diseases.

20.5   Other bioactive components

In addition to major bioactive components described above, bovine mammary secretions are known to contain a great number of other indigenous minor bioactive components with distinct characteristics. These include hormones, cytokines, oligosaccharides, nucleotides and specific proteins. A few of the best characterized of these factors will be described briefly below.

A large number of hormones of either steroidic or peptidic origin are found in bovine colostrum and milk (Grosvenor *et al.*, 1993; Jouan *et al.*, 2006). These molecules belong to the following main categories: gonadal hormones (estrogens, progesterone, androgens), adrenal (glucocorticoids) pituitary (prolactin, growth hormone) and hypothalamic hormones (gonadotropin-releasing hormone, luteinising-hormone-releasing hormone, thyrotropin-releasing hormone and somatostatin). Other hormones of interest are bombesin, calcitonin, insulin, melatonin and parathyroid hormone. These hormones occur in very small concentrations (picograms or nanograms per millilitre) and the highest quantities are usually found in colostrum, declining thereafter drastically at the onset of the main lactation period. For example the concentration of prolactin found in colostrum varies between 500 and 800 ng/ml compared to 6–8 ng/ml in mature milk (Jouan *et al.*, 2006). The biological significance of hormones occurring in mammary secretions is not fully elucidated but in general they are considered important both in the regulation of specific functions of the mammary gland and in the growth of the newborn, including development and maturation of its gastrointestinal and immune systems. Hormones in colostrum could also temporarily regulate the activity of some endocrine glands until the newborn's hormonal system reaches maturity (Bernt and Walker, 1999). There is some evidence from animal model and human studies that oral ingestion of melatonin-enriched milk improves sleep and diurnal activity (Valtonen *et al.*, 2005). Naturally melatonin-rich milk (milk obtained during the night or in the dark), has been commercialized in some countries.

Nucleotides, nucleosides and nucleobases belong to the non-protein-nitrogen fraction of milk. These components are suggested to be acting as pleiotrophic factors in the development of brain functions (Schlimme *et al.*, 2000). Because of the important role of nucleotides in infant nutrition, some infant and follow-on formulas have been supplemented with specific ribonucleotide salts. Also nucleotides could have significance as exogenous anticarcinogens in the control of intestinal tumour development (Michaelidou and Steijns, 2006).

Bovine colostrum contains relatively high concentrations of cytokines (such as IL-1 (interleukin), IL-6, TNF-α (tumor necrosis factor), IF-γ (interferon), and IL-1 receptor antagonist), but their levels decline markedly in mature milk (Kelly, 2003). The biological role of these components and their potential applications have been reviewed recently (Struff and Sprotte, 2007; Wheeler *et al.*, 2007). Using proteomic techniques, Fong *et al.* (2008) identified 120 novel protein fractions from bovine whey. Among the minor whey proteins many biologically active specific molecules and complexes, such as proteose-peptones, serum albumin, osteopontin and the enzymes lysozyme and xanthine oxidase have been characterized (Mather, 2000; Fox and Kelly, 2006; Recio *et al.*, 2009).

As described earlier, the milk fat globule membrane contains several lipid and protein fractions (e.g. butyrophilin, CD36, mucin and fatty acid binding protein) that have shown specific biological functions and these components have been reviewed recently (Spitsberg, 2005; Fong *et al.*, 2007; Jimenez-Flores and Brisson, 2008; Recio *et al.*, 2009). Colostrinin™ (CLN) is a proline-rich polypeptide complex which was originally isolated from ovine colostrum. Colostrinin has been identified and isolated also from bovine colostrum in the form of a peptide complex with a molecular mass around 14 000 Daltons (Sokolowska *et al.*, 2008). In *in vitro* and animal studies, ovine colostrinin has been shown to exert immunomodulatory properties. A recent clinical study (Billikiewicz and Gaus, 2004) suggested that colostrinin is beneficial in the treatment of mild or moderate Alzheimer's disease. The mechanism of action remains, however, to be elucidated and the efficacy confirmed in further clinical studies.

Human milk contains significant concentrations (5–10 g/l) of complex oligosaccharides which are considered to exert different health benefits to the newborn (Kunz *et al.*, 2000; Kunz and Rudloff, 2006). They may contribute to the growth of beneficial flora in the intestine, stimulation of the immune system and defence against microbial infections. Similar oligosaccharides and glycoconjugates are present in bovine milk and colostrum but in much smaller concentrations (Gopal and Gill, 2000; Martin *et al.*, 2001; Schaafsma, 2008; Hickey, 2009). The low concentration and complex nature of these compounds have hindered their characterization and utilization in healthcare and food industries. Recent advances in analytical techniques have, however, enabled a more detailed structural and functional analysis of bovine milk derived oligosaccharides. Also membrane separation based processes have been developed for the recovery of sialyloligosaccharides from cheese whey. Such ingredients could find applications as a prebiotic component in functional foods and infant formulas (Mehra and Kelly, 2006).

20.6 Conclusions

Over the last 20 years, bovine colostrum and milk have proven a valuable natural source for biologically active components, beyond their well-known nutritional attributes. The bioactive properties have been demonstrated in *in vitro* and *in vivo* experiments and the mechanisms of action have been identified for many native milk components. In particular, this is true for a few individual protein fractions, such as immunoglobulins, lactoferrin, lactoperoxidase system and more recently for whey proteins alpha-lactalbumin and beta-lactoglobulin. These components are found in abundance in cheese whey which earlier has been considered as an invaluable waste-product of cheese manufacture. The recent advent of bioactive peptides derived from milk proteins has vastly expanded our understanding about the physiological role of milk proteins, not only as a good source of amino acids but also as nutrients which actively can regulate and promote human health.

In recent years, considerable progress has also been recorded in research concerning properties of specific milk fat fractions, notably CLA, as well as oligosaccharides and derivatives of lactose. These components and bioactive peptides warrant more research in view of their potential beneficial health benefits. Industrial or semi-industrial scale processing techniques are now available for fractionation and isolation of major proteins from colostrum and milk. Such purified or enriched components can be used as active ingredients for functional foods targeted to certain consumer groups. A few colostral or cheese whey derived proteins, peptides, growth factors and lipid fractions are already manufactured commercially and have found focused fields of applications, thus adding commercial value to colostrum and cheese whey. On the other hand, there is a need to further substantiate in clinical human trials the claimed health benefits of above-mentioned individual milk components. Many of these components have posed health-promoting effects when investigated under laboratory conditions or in animal model studies, while human studies with the same components have failed to produce positive results. Such failures could be attributed to many factors, for example study design, dose, target population or metabolic/physiological differences between test animals and human subjects.

Another point to consider in human studies is the potential synergistic or antagonistic action by other nutrients in the regular diet. To avoid such interference targeted delivery technologies or protective food matrices could perhaps provide a practical solution. Further research is needed to elucidate this issue when pursuing to maximize the health-promoting effects of various milk bioactives.

20.7   Future trends

The current global interest in developing health-promoting functional foods provides a timely opportunity to tap the myriad of innate bioactive milk components for inclusion in such formulations. Milk bioactives present an excellent source of well-characterized natural ingredients for different applications in functional foods. In fact, manufacture and marketing of milk bioactives appear as a lucrative new field of business, also for the traditional dairy industry. It can be envisaged that in the near future several breakthrough products based on these ingredients will be launched on worldwide markets. They could be targeted to infants, elderly and immune-compromised people as well as to improve performance and prevent diet-related chronic diseases related to the metabolic syndrome, in particular. It is obvious that in this respect a special emphasis will be put on exploitation of bioactive peptides. New emerging technologies, such as micro- or nanoencapsulation may offer feasible solutions for improving stability and bioavailability of such peptides in various food products and during digestion. Furthermore, molecular studies are needed to assess the mechanisms by which bioactive components exert their activities. For this approach, it is necessary to employ new nutrigenomic techniques, for example proteomics and metabolomics (Smilowitz et al., 2005; German, 2009). By developing such novel facilities it will be possible to study the impact of milk bioactives on the expression of genes, and hence optimize the nutritional and health effects of these compounds. This research area is currently considered highly challenging and will revolutionize the nutrient research in the near future. Moreover, there is a need to study and exploit the health potential of other minor components occurring naturally in colostrum and milk. In future studies more emphasis should also be given to the health-promoting potential hidden in the vast range of traditional dairy products consumed worldwide.

20.8   References

Aihara K, Kajimoto O, Hirata H, Takahashi R, Nakamura Y (2005), 'Effect of powdered fermented milk with *Lactobacillus helveticus* on subjects with high-normal blood pressure or mild hypertension', *J Am Coll Nutr*, **24**, 257–265.

Aimutis, W R (2004), 'Bioactive properties of milk proteins with particular focus on anticariogenesis', *J Nutr*, **134**, 989–95.

Akbache A, Lamiot E, Moroni O, Turgeon S, Gauthier S F, Pouliot Y (2009), 'Use of membrane processing to concentrate TGF-β2 and IGF-I from bovine milk and whey', *J Membrane Sci*, **20**, 435–40.

Akhavan T, Panahi S, Anderson G H, Luhovyy B L (2009), 'Application of dairy-derived ingredients in food intake and metabolic regulation', in Corredig M, *Dairy-derived Ingredients – Food and Nutraceutical Uses*, Cambridge, Woodhead, pp. 212–37.

Akuzawa R, Miura T, Kawakami H (2009), 'Bioactive components in caseins, caseinates and cheeses', in Park Y, *Bioactive Components in Milk and Dairy Products*, Iowa, Wiley-Blackwell, pp. 217–33.

Anon. (2005), 'Benefits and potential risks of the lactoperoxidase system of raw milk preservation', Report of an FAO/WHO technical meeting. FAO Headquarters, Rome.

Ardö Y, Lilbaek H, Kristiansen K R, Zakora M, Otte J (2007), 'Identification of large phosphopeptides from β-casein that characteristically accumulate during ripening of the semi-hard cheese Herrgård', *Int Dairy J*, **17**, 513–24.

Ardö; Y, Pripp A H, Lillevang S K (2009), 'Impact of heat-treated *Lactobacillus helveticus* on bioactive peptides in low-fat, semi-hard cheese', *Aust J Dairy Technol*, **64**, 58–62.

Aro A, Männistö; S, Salminen I, Ovaskainen M-L, Kataja V, Uusitupa M (2000), 'Inverse association between dietary and serum conjugated linoleic acid and risk of breast cancer in postmenopausal women', *Nutr Cancer*, **38**, 151–57.

Avramis C A, Wang H, McBride B W, Wright T C, Hill A R (2003), 'Physical and processing properties of milk, butter, and Cheddar cheese from cows fed supplemental fish meal', *J Dairy Sci*, **86**, 2568–76.

Baldi A, Politis I, Pecorini C, Fusi E, Chronopoulou R, Dell'Orto V (2005), 'Biological effects of milk proteins and their peptides with emphasis on those related to the gastrointestinal ecosystem', *J Dairy Res*, **72** (Special Issue), 66–72.

Ballard K D, Bruno R S, Seip R L, Quann E E, Volk B M, *et al.* (2009), 'Acute ingestion of a novel whey-derived peptide improves vascular endothelial responses in healthy individuals: a randomized, placebo controlled trial', *Nutr J*, **8**(1), 34.

Belobrajdic D P, McIntosh G H, Owens J A (2004), 'A high-whey protein diet reduces body weight gain: a longitudinal study of adolescents,' *J Nutr*, **134**, 1454–58.

Belury M A (2002), 'Dietary conjugated linoleic acid in health: Physiological effects and mechanisms of action', *Ann Rev Nutr*, **22**, 505–31.

Bennett L E, Crittenden R, Khoo E, Forsyth S (2005), 'Evaluation of immune-modulatory dairy peptide fractions', *Austr J Dairy Technol*, **60**, 106–09.

Bernt K M, Walker W A (1999), 'Human milk as carrier of biochemical messages', *Acta Pediatr*, **430**(Suppl), 27–41.

Billikiewicz A, Gaus W (2004), 'Colostrinin (a naturally occurring proline-rich, polypeptide mixture) in the treatment of Alzheimer's disease', *J Alzheimer's Dis*, **6**, 17–26.

Bisig W, Eberhard P, Collomb M, Rehberger B (2007), 'Influence of processing on the fatty acid composition and the content of conjugated linoleic acid in organic and conventional dairy products – a review', *Lait*, **87**, 1–19.

Blouet C, Mariotti F, Mikogami T, Tome D, Huneau J (2007), 'Meal cysteine improves postprandial glucose control in rats fed a high-sucrose meal', *J Nutr Biochem*, **18**(8), 519–24.

Boelsma E, Kloek J (2009), 'Lactotripeptides and antihypertensive effects: a critical review', *Br J Nutr*, **101**(6), 776–86.

Boots J-W, Floris R (2006), 'Lactoperoxidase: From catalytic mechanism to proactical applications', *Int Dairy J*, **16**, 1272–76.

Bostwick E F, Steijns J, Braun S (2000), 'Lactoglobulins', in Naidu A S, *Natural Food Antimicrobial Systems*, Florida, CRC Press, pp. 133–58.

Bounous G (2000), 'Whey protein concentrate (WPC) and glutathione modulation in cancer treatment', *Anticancer Res*, **20**, 4785–92.

Burton-Freeman B M (2008), 'Glycomacropeptide (GMP) is not critical to whey-induced satiety, but may have a unique role in energy intake regulation through cholecystokinin (CCK)', *Physiol Behav*, **93**, 379–87.

Bütikofer U, Meyer J, Sieber R, Walther B, Wechsler D (2008), 'Occurrence of the angiotensin-converting enzyme-inhibiting tripeptides Val-Pro-Pro and Ile-Pro-Pro in different cheese varieties of Swiss origin', *J Dairy Sci*, **91**, 29–38.

Bütikofer U, Meyer J, Sieber R, Wechsler D (2007), 'Quantification of the angiotensin-converting enzyme-inhibiting tripeptides Val-Pro-Pro and Ile-Pro-Pro in hard, semi-hard and soft cheeses', *Int Dairy J*, **17**, 968–75.

Campbell B, Petersen W E (1963), 'Immune milk – a historical survey', *Dairy Sci Abstr*, **25**, 345–58.

Chabance B, Marteau P, Rambaud J C, Migliore-Samour D, Boynard M, *et al.* (1998), 'Casein peptide release and passage to the blood in humans during digestion of milk or yogurt', *Biochimie*, **80**, 155–65.

Chamba J-F, Chardigny J-M, Gnädig S, Perreard E, Chappaz S, *et al.* (2006), 'Conjugated linoleic acid (CLA) content of French Emmental cheese: Effect of the season, region of production, processing and culinary preparation', *Lait*, **86**, 407–80.

Chatterton D E W, Smithers G, Roupas P, Brodkorb A (2006), 'Bioactivity of β-lactoglobulin and α-lactalbumin- technological implications for processing', *Int Dairy J*, **16**, 1229–40.

Chen G-W, Tsai J-S, Sun Pan B (2007), 'Purification of angiotensin I-converting enzyme inhibitory peptides and antihypertensive effect of milk produced by protease-facilitated lactic fermentation', *Int Dairy J*, **17**, 641–47.

Chiu C K, Etzel M R (1997), 'Fractionation of lactoperoxidase and lactoferrin from bovine whey using a cation exchange membrane', *J Food Sci*, **62**, 996–1000.

Chobert J-M, El-Zahar K, Sitohy M, Dalgalarrondo M, Métro F, *et al.* (2005), 'Angiotensin I-converting-enzyme (ACE)- inhibitory activity of tryptic peptides of ovine β-lactoglobulin and of milk yoghurts obtained by using different starters', *Lait*, **85**, 141–52.

Choi H K, Willet W C, Stampfer M J, Rimm E, Hu F B (2005), 'Dairy consumption and risk of type 2 diabetes mellitus in men: a prospective study', *Arch Intern Med*, **165**, 997–1003.

Churruca I, Fernández-Quintela A, Portillo M P (2009), 'Conjugated linoleic acid isomers: Differences in metabolism and biological effects', *Biofactors*, **35**(1), 105–11.

Clare D A, Swaisgood H E (2000), 'Bioactive milk peptides: A prospectus', *J Dairy Sci*, **83**, 1187–95.

Clifton P M, Keogh J B, Woonton B W, Taylor C M, Janakiewski F, De Silva K (2009), 'Effect of glycomacropeptides (GMP) on satiety hormones and food intake', *Aust J Dairy Technol*, **64**, 29–31.

Collomb M, Bütikofer U, Sieber R, Bosset J O, Jeangros B (2001), 'Conjugated linoleic acid and *trans* fatty acid compositionof cow's milk fat produced in lowlands and highlands', *J Dairy Res*, **68**, 519–23.

Collomb M, Schmid A, Sieber R, Wechsler D, Ryhänen E-L (2006), 'Conjugated linoleic acids in milk fat: Variation and physiological effects', *Int Dairy J*, **16**, 1347–61.

Conesa C, Sánchez L, Rota C, Pérez M-D, Calvo M, *et al.* (2008), 'Isolation of lactoferrin from milk of different species: Calorimetric and antimicrobial studies', *Comp. Biochem Physiol. B*, 150, 131-9. doi: 10.1016/j.cbpb.2008.02.005

Cornish J, Palmano K, Callon K E, Watson M, Lin J M, *et al.* (2006), 'Lactoferrin and bone; structure-activity relationships', *Biochem Cell Biol*, **84**(3), 297–302.

Costantino D, Guaraldi C (2008), 'Preliminary evaluation of a vaginal cream containing lactoferrin in the treatment of vulvovaginal candidosis', *Minerva Ginecol*, **60**(2), 121–25.

Crittenden R G, Bennett L E (2005), 'Cow's milk allergy: A complex disorder', *J Am Coll Nutr*, **24** (Suppl 6), S582–91.

Crittenden R, Buckley J, Cameron-Smith D, Brown A, Thomas K, Dawey S (2009), 'Functional dairy protein supplements for elite athletes', *Aust J Dairy Technol*, **64**(1), 133–37.

Crittenden R, Buckley J, Cameron-Smith D, Brown A, Thomas K, Dawey S (2009), 'Functional dairy protein supplements for elite athletes', *Aust J Dairy Technol*, **64**(1), 133–137.

De Leeuw P W, Van der Zander K, Kroon A A, Rennenberg R M, Koning M M (2009), 'Dose-dependent lowering of blood pressure by dairy peptides in mildly hypertensive subjects', *Blood Press*, **18**(1–2), 44–50.

del Mar Contreras M, Carron R, Montero M J, Ramos M, Recio I (2009), 'Novel casein-derived peptides with antihypertensive activity', *Int Dairy J*, **19**(10), 566–73.

Dewettinck K, Rombaut R, Thienpont N, Trung Le T, Messens K, Van Camp J (2008), 'Nutritional and technological aspects of milk fat globule membrane material', *Int Dairy J*, **18**, 436–57.

Donato J Jr, Pedrosa R G, Cruzat V F, Pires I S, Tirapegui J (2006), Effects of leucine supplementation on the body composition and protein status of rats submitted to food restriction, *Nutrition*, **22**, 520–27.

Donkor O, Henriksson A, Vasiljevic T, Shah N P (2007), 'Proteolytic activity of dairy lactic acid bacteria and probiotics as determinant of growth and in vitro angiotensin-converting enzyme inhibitory activity in fermented milk, *Lait*, **86**, 21–38.

Dupas C, Adt I, Cottaz A, Boutrou R, Molle D, Jardin J, Jouvet T, Degraeve P (2009), 'A chromatographic procedure for semi-quantitative evaluation of caseinophosphopeptides in cheese', *Dairy Sci Technol*, **89**, 519–29.

Elfstrand L, Lindmark-Månsson H, Paulsson M, Nyberg L, Åkesson B (2002), 'Immunoglobulins, growth factors and growth hormone in bovine colostrums and the effects of processing,' *Int Dairy J*, **12**, 879–87.

Elwood P C, Givens D I, Beswick A D, Fehily A M, Pickering J E, Gallacher J (2008), 'The survival advantage of milk and dairy consumption: an overview of evidence from cohort studies of vascular diseases, diabetes and cancer', *J Am Coll Nutr*, **27**(6), S723–34.

Engberink M F, Hendriksen M A, Schouten E G, van Rooij F J, Hofman A, *et al.* (2009), 'Inverse association between dairy intake and hypertension: the Rotterdam Study', *Am J Clin Nutr*, **89**(6), 1877–83.

Engberink M F, Schouten E G, Kok F J, van Mierlo L A, Brouwer I A, Geleijnse J M (2008), 'Lactotripeptides show no effect on human blood pressure: results from a double-blind randomized controlled trial', *Hypertens*, **51**, 399–405.

Fernaud S, Evans RW (2003), 'Lactoferrin – a multifunctional protein with antimicrobial properties', *Molec Immunol*, **40**, 395–405.

Ferreira I M P L V O, Pinho O, Mota M V, Tavares P, Pereira A, *et al.* (2007), 'Preparation of ingredients containing an ACE-inhibitory peptide by tryptic hydrolysis of whey protein concentrates', *Int Dairy J*, **17**, 481–87.

Field C J, Blewett H H, Proctor S, Vine D (2009), 'Human health benefits of vaccenic acid', *Appl Physiol Nutr Metab*, **34**(5), 979–91.

FitzGerald R J (1998), 'Potential uses of caseinophosphopeptides', *Int Dairy J*, **8**, 451–57.

FitzGerald R J, Murray B A (2006), 'Bioactive peptides and lactic fermentations,' *Int J Dairy Technol*, **59**, 118–25.

Florence A C R, Da Silva R C, Do Espirito Santo A P, Gioielli L A, Tamime A Y, De Oliveira M N (2009), 'Increased CLA content in organic milk fermented by bifidobacteria or yoghurt cultures', *Dairy Sci Technol*, **89**, 541–53.

Foltz M, Meynen E E, Bianco V, van Platerink C, Koning T M, Klock J (2007), 'Angiotensin converting enzyme inhibitoy peptides from a lactotripeptide-enriched milk beverage are absorbed intact into the circulation', *J Nutr*, **137**, 953–58.

Fong B Y, Norris C S, MacGibbon A K H (2007), 'Protein and lipid composition of bovine milk-fat-globule-membrane', *Int Dairy J*, **17**, 275–88.

Fong B Y, Norris C S, Palmano K M (2008), 'Fractionation of bovine whey proteins and characterization by proteomic characteristics', *Int Dairy J*, **18**, 23–46.

Fox P F, Kelly A L (2006), 'Indigenous enzymes in milk: Overview and historical aspects – Part 1', *Int Dairy J*, **16**, 500–16.

Frid A H, Nilsson M, Holst J J, Bjorck I M (2005), 'Effect of whey on blood glucose and insulin responses to composite breakfast and lunch meals in type 2 diabetic subjects', *Am J Clin Nutr*, **82**, 69–75.

Fuglsang A, Rattray F P, Nilsson D, Nyborg N C B (2003), 'Lactic acid bacteria: inhibition of angiotensin converting enzyme *in vitro* and *in vivo*', *Ant van Leeuw*, **83**, 27–34.

Gagnaire V, Molle D, Herrouin M, Leonil J (2001), 'Peptides identified during Emmental cheese ripening: origin and proteolytic systems involved', *J Agric Food Chem*, **49**, 4402–13.

Gauthier S F, Pouliot Y, Maubois J-L (2006a), 'Growth factors from bovine milk and colostrum: composition, extraction and biological activities', *Lait*, **86**, 99–126.

Gauthier S F, Pouliot Y, Saint-Sauveur D (2006b), 'Immunomodulatory peptides obtained by the enzymatic hydrolysis of whey proteins', *Int Dairy J*, **16**, 1315–23.

German B (2009), 'Genomics and milk', *Aust J Dairy Technol*, **64**(1), 94–101.

German J B, Dillard C J (2006), 'Composition, structure and absorption of milk lipids: a source of energy, fat-soluble nutrients and bioactive molecules', *Crit Rev Food Sci Nutr*, **46**, 57–92.

Gingerich D A, McPhillips C A (2005), 'Analytical approach to determination of safety of milk ingredients from hyperimmunized cows', *Regulat Toxicol Pharmacol*, **41**(2), 102–12.

Gobbetti M, Minervini F, Rizzello C G (2004), 'Angiotensin I-converting-enzyme-inhibitory and antimicrobial bioactive peptides', *Int J Dairy Technol*, **57**, 172–88.

Gobbetti M, Minervini F, Rizzello C G (2007), 'Bioactive peptides in dairy products', in Hui Y H, *Handbook of Food Products Manufacturing: Health, Meat, Milk, Poultry, Seafood, and Vegetables*, John Wiley & Sons, Inc., Hoboken, NJ, pp. 489–517.

Gokawi S (2009), 'New technologies for isolation and analysis of bioactive compounds', in Park Y, *Bioactive Components in Milk and Dairy Products*, Iowa, Wiley-Blackwell, pp. 329–45.

Gomez-Ruiz J A, Ramos M, Recio I (2002), 'Angiotensin-converting enzyme-inhibitory peptides in Manchego cheeses manufactured with different starter cultures', *Int Dairy J*, **12**, 697–706.

Gopal P, Gill H S (2000), 'Oligosaccharides and glycoconjugates in bovine milk and colostrum', *Br J Nutr*, **84** (Suppl 1), S69–74.

Griinari J M, Corl B A, Lacy S H, Choinard P Y, Nurmela K V, Bauman D E (2000), 'Conjugated linoleic acid is synthesized endogenously in lactating dairy cows by Δ9-desaturase', *J Nutr*, **130**, 2285–91.

Grosvenor C E, Picciano M F, Baumrucker C R (1993), 'Hormones and growth factors in milk', *Endocrine Rev*, **14**, 710–28.

Groves M L (1960), 'The isolation of a red protein from milk', *J Am Chem Soc*, **82**, 3345–50.

Gustafson D R, McMahon D J, Morrey J, Nan R (2001), 'Appetite is not influenced by a unique milk peptide: caseinomacropeptide (CMP)', *Appetite*, **36**, 157–63.

Ha E, Zemel M B (2003), 'Functional properties of whey, whey components, and essential amino acids: mechanisms underlying health benefits for active people', *J Nutr Biochem*, **14**, 251–58.

Hammarström L, Krüger Weiner C (2008), 'Targeted antibodies in dairy-based products', *Adv Exp Med Biol*, **606**, 321–44.

Haque E, Chand R (2008), 'Antihypertensive and antimicrobial bioactive peptides from milk proteins', *Eur Food Res Technol*, **227**, 7–15.

Hartmann R, Meisel H (2007), 'Food-derived peptides with biological activity: from research to food applications', *Curr Opin Biotechnol*, **18**, 1–7.

Hata Y, Yamamoto M, Ohni H, Nakajima K, Nakamura Y, Takano T (1996), 'A placebo-controlled study of the effect of sour milk on blood pressure in hypertensive subjects', *Am J Clin Nutr*, **64**, 67–71.

Hayes M, Ross P, Fitzgerald G F, Stanton C (2007a), 'Putting microbes to work: dairy fermentation, cell factories, and bioactive peptides, Part 1: Overview', *Biotechnol J*, **2**, 426–34.

Hayes M, Stanton C, Fitzgerald G F, Ross P (2007b), 'Putting microbes to work: dairy fermentation, cell factories, and bioactive peptides, Part 2: Bioactive peptide functions', *Biotechnol J*, **2**, 435–49.

Hayes T G, Falchook G F, Varadhachary G R, Smith D P, Davis L D, *et al.* (2006), 'Phase I trial of oral talactoferrin alfa in refractory solid tumors', *Invest New Drugs*, **24**(3), 233–40.

Heaney R P (2009) 'Dairy and bone health', *J Am Coll Nutr*, **28** (Suppl 1), S82–90.

Hernández-Ledesma B, Amigo L, Ramos M, Recio I (2004), 'Angiotensin converting enzyme inhibitory activity in commercial fermented products. Formation of peptides under simulated gastrointestinal digestion', *J Agric Food Chem*, **52**, 1504–10.

Hernández-Ledesma B, Recio I, Amigo L (2008), 'beta-Lactoglobulin as source of bioactive peptides', *Amino Acids*, **35**, 257–65.

Hickey R (2009), 'Harnessing milk oligosaccharides for nutraceuticcal applications', in Corredig M, *Dairy-derived Ingredients–Food and Nutraceutical Uses*, Cambridge, Woodhead, pp. 308–43.

Hirota T, Ohki K, Kawagishi R, Kajimoto Y, Mizuno S, Nakamura Y (2007), 'Casein hydrolysate containing the antihypertensive tripeptides Val-Pro-Pro and Ile-Pro-Pro improves vascular endothelial function independent of blood pressure–lowering effects: Contribution of the inhibitory action of angiotensin-converting enzyme', *Hypertens Res*, **30**, 489–96.

Hoerr R A, Bostwick E F (2002), 'Commercializing colostrum based products: a case study of Galagen Inc.', *Int Dairy Fed Bull*, **375**, 33–46.

Ip M M, Masso-Welch P A, Ip C (2003), 'Prevention of mammary cancer with conjugated linoleic acid: Role of the stroma and the epithelium', *J Mammary Gland Neoplasia*, **8**, 103–18.

Jäkälä P, Jauhiainen T, Korpela R, Vapaatalo H (2009), 'Milk protein-derived bioactive tripeptides Ile-Pro-Pro and Val-Pro-Pro protect endothelial function in vitro in hypertensive rats', *J Func Foods*, **1**(3), 266–73.

Jauhiainen T, Korpela R (2007), 'Milk peptides and blood pressure', *J Nutr*, **137**, S825–29.

Jauhiainen T, Rönnback M, Vapaatalo H, Wuolle K, Kautiainen H, Korpela R. (2007a), '*Lactobacillus helveticus* fermented milk reduces arterial stiffness in hypertensive subjects', *Int Dairy J*, **17**, 1209–11.

Jauhiainen T, Vapaatalo H, Poussa T, Kyrönpalo S, Rasmussen M, Korpela R (2005), '*Lactobacillus helveticus* fermented milk reduces blood pressure in 24-h ambulatory blood pressure measurement', *Am J Hypertens*, **18**, 1600–05.

Jauhiainen T, Wuolle K, Vapaatalo H, Kerojoki O, Nurmela K, *et al.* (2007b), 'Oral absorption, tissue distribution and excretion of a radiolabelled analog of a milk-derived antihypertensive peptide, Ile-Pro-Pro, in rats', *Int Dairy J*, **17**, 1216–23.

Jensen R G (2002), 'Invited review: The composition of bovine milk lipids: January 1995 to December 2000', *J Dairy Sci*, **85**, 295–350.

Jenssen H, Hancock R E W (2009), 'Antimicrobial properties of lactoferrin', *Biochimie*, **91**, 19–29.

Jimenez-Flores R, Brisson G (2008), 'The milk fat globule membrane as an ingredient: why, how, when?', *Dairy Sci Technol*, **88**, 5–18.

Jouan P-N, Pouliot Y, Gauthier S F, Laforest J-P (2006) 'Hormones in milk and milk products: A survey', *Int Dairy J*, **16**, 1408–14.

Kanwar J R, Kanwar R K, Sun X, Punj V, Matta H, *et al.* (2009), 'Molecular and biotechnological advances in milk proteins in relation to human health', *Curr Protein Pept Sci*, **10**(4), 308–38.

Kawahara T, Aruga K, Otani H (2005), 'Characterization of caseinophosphopeptides from fermented milk products', *J Nutr Sci Vitaminol*, **51**, 377–81.

Kawakami H (2005), 'Biological significance of milk basic protein (MBP) for bone health', *Food Sci Technol Res*, **11**, 1–8.

Kekkonen R, Peuhkuri K (2009), 'Bioactive milk protein and peptide functionality', in Corredig M, *Dairy-derived Ingredients-Food and Nutraceutical Uses*, Cambridge, Woodhead, pp. 238–68.

Kelly G S (2003), 'Bovine colostrums: A review of clinical uses', *Altern Med Rev*, **8**, 378–94.

Keogh J B, Clifton P M (2009), 'Weight loss using meal replacements high in glycomacropeptide-enriched whey powder', *Aust J Dairy Technol*, **64**, 32–33.

Kim Y, Kim M J, Han K S, Imm J Y, Oh S, Kim S H (2009), 'Anticancer activity of lactoferrin isolated from caprine colostrum on human cancer cell lines', *Int J Dairy Technol*, **62**, 277–81.

King Jr, J C, Cummings G E, Guo N, Trivedi L, Readmond B X, *et al.* (2007), 'A double-blind, placebo-controlled, pilot study of bovine lactoferrin supplementation in bottle-fed infants', *J Pediatr Gastroenterol Nutr*, **44**, 245–51.

Kitts D D, Weiler K (2003), 'Bioactive proteins and peptides from food sources. Applications of bioprocesses used in isolation and recovery', *Curr Pharm Des*, **9**, 1309–23.

Ko S, Kwak H-S (2009). 'Bioactive components in whey products', in Park Y, *Bioactive Components in Milk and Dairy Products*, Iowa, Wiley-Blackwell, pp. 263–285.

Koikawa N, Nagaoka I, Yamaguchi M, Hamano H, Yamauchi K, Sawaki K (2008), 'Preventive effect of lactoferrin intake on anemia in female long distance runners', *Biosci Biotechnol Biochem*, **72**(4), 931–35.

Korhonen H (2002), 'Technology options for new nutritional concepts', *Int J Dairy Technol*, **55**, 79–88.

Korhonen H (2004), 'Isolation of immunoglobulins from colostrum', *Int Dairy Fed Bull*, **389**, 78–81.

Korhonen H (2009a), 'Bioactive components in bovine milk', in Park Y, *Bioactive Components in Milk and Dairy Products*, Iowa, Wiley-Blackwell, pp. 15–42.

Korhonen H (2009b), 'Bioactive milk proteins and peptides: from science to functional applications', *Aust J Dairy Technol* **64**, 16–25.

Korhonen H (2009c), 'Bioactive milk peptides: from science to applications', *J Funct Foods*, **1**(2), 177–87.

Korhonen H, Marnila P (2006), 'Bovine milk antibodies for protection against microbial human diseases', in Mine Y, Shahidi F, *Nutraceutical Proteins and Peptides in Health and Disease*, Boca Raton, CRC Press, Taylor & Francis Group, pp. 137–59.

Korhonen H, Marnila P (2009), 'Bovine milk immunoglobulins against microbial human diseases', in Corredig M, *Dairy-derived Ingredients – Food and Nutraceutical Uses*, Cambridge, Woodhead, pp. 269–89.

Korhonen H, Marnila P, Gill H (2000), 'Bovine milk antibodies for health: a review', *Br J Nutr*, **84** (Suppl 1), S1–7.

Korhonen H, Pihlanto A (2003), 'Food-derived bioactive peptides – opportunities for designing future foods', *Curr Pharm Des*, **9**, 1297–1308.

Korhonen H, Pihlanto A (2006), 'Technological options for the production of health-promoting proteins and peptides derived from milk and colostrum', *Curr Pharm Des*, **13**(8), 829–43.

Korhonen H, Pihlanto A (2007), 'Bioactive peptides from food proteins', in Hui Y H, *Handbook of Food Products Manufacturing: Health, Meat, Milk, Poultry, Seafood, and Vegetables*, John Wiley & Sons, Inc., Hoboken, NJ, pp. 5–38.

Kris-Etherton P M, Grieger J A, Hilpert K F, West S G (2009), 'Milk products, dietary patterns and blood pressure management', *J Am Coll Nutr*, **28** (Suppl 1), S103–19.

Kris-Etherton P M, Yu S (1997), 'Individual fatty acid effects on plasma lipids and lipoproteins: human studies', *Am J Clin Nutr*, **65**, S1628–44.

Krissansen G W (2007), 'Emerging health properties of whey proteins and their clinical implications', *J Am Coll Nutr*, **26**(6), S713–23.

Kulozik U (2009), 'Novel approaches for the separation of dairy components and manufacture of dairy ingredients', in Corredig M, *Dairy-derived Ingredients – Food and Nutraceutical Uses*, Cambridge, Woodhead, pp. 3–23.

Kunz C, Rudloff S (2006), 'Health promoting aspects of milk oligosaccharides', *Int Dairy J*, **16**, 1341–46.

Kunz C, Rudloff S, Baier W, Klein N, Strobel S (2000), 'Oligosaccharides in human milk: Structural, functional, and metabolic aspects', *Ann Rev Nutr*, **20**, 699–722.

Kussendrager K D, van Hooijdonk A C M (2000), 'Lactoperoxidase: physico-chemical properties, occurrence, mechanism of action and applications', *Br J Nutr*, **84** (Suppl 1), 19–25.

Lacasse P, Lauzon K, Diarra M S, Petitclerc D (2008), 'Utilization of lactoferrin to fight antibiotic-resistant mammary gland pathogens', *J Anim Sci*, **86** (Suppl 13), 66–71.

Lamarche B (2008), 'Review of the effect of dairy products on non-lipid risk factors for cardiovascular disease', *J Am Coll Nutr*, **27**(6), S741–46.

Larsen TM, Tourbro S, Astrup A (2003), 'Efficacy and safety of dietary supplements containing CLA for the treatment of obesity: Evidence from animal and human studies', *J Lipid Res*, **44**, 2234–41.

Larsson S C, Bergkvist L, Wolk A (2005), 'High-fat dairy food and conjugated linoleic acid intakes in relation to colorectal cancer incidence in the Swedish mammography cohort', *Am J Clin Nutr*, **82**, 894–900.

Lee K W, Lee H, J (2005), 'Role of the conjugated linoleic acid in the prevention cancer', *Crit Rev Food Sci Nutr*, **45**, 135–44.

Lee Y-M, Skurk T, Hennig M, Hauner H (2007), 'Effect of a milk drink supplemented with whey peptides on blood pressure in patients with mild hypertension', *Eur J Nutr*, **46**, 21–27.

Legrand D, Pierce A, Elass E, Carpenter M, Mariller C, Mazurier J (2008), 'Lactoferrin structure and functions', in Bösze Z, *Bioactive Components of Milk*, Springer, New York, pp. 163–94.

Lizzi A R, Carnicelli V, Clarkson M M, Di Giulio A, Oratore A, (2009), 'Lactoferrin derived peptides: mechanisms of action and their perspectives as antimicrobial and antitumoral agents', *Mini Rev Med Chem*, **9**, 687–95.

Lönnerdal B (2003), 'Nutritional and physiologic significance of human milk proteins', *Am J Clin Nutr*, **77**, S1537–43.

Lönnerdal B (2009), 'Nutritional roles of lactoferrin', *Curr Opin Clin Nutr Metab Care*, **12**(3), 293–97.

López-Expósito I, Pellegrini A, Amigo L, Recio I (2008), 'Synergistic effect between different milk-derived peptides and proteins', *J Dairy Sci*, **91**, 2184–89.

López-Expósito I, Quiros A, Amigo L, Recio I (2007), 'Casein hydrolysates as a source of antimicrobial, antioxydant and antihypertensive peptides', *Lait*, **87**, 241–49.

López-Expósito I, Recio I (2006), 'Antibacterial activity of peptides and folding variants from milk proteins', *Int Dairy J*, **16**, 1294–1305.

López-Fandino R, Otte J, van Camp J (2006), 'Physiological, chemical and technological aspects of milk-protein-derived peptides with antihypertensive and ACE-inhibitory activity', *Int Dairy J*, **16**, 1277–93.

Luhovyy B L, Akhavan T, Anderson G H (2007), 'Whey proteins in the regulation of food intake and satiety', *J Am Coll Nutr*, **26**, S704–12.

MacRae J, O'Reilly L, Morgan P (2005), 'Desirable characteristics of animal products from a human health perspective', *Livestock Prod Sci*, **94**, 95–103.

Madureira A R, Pereira C I, Gomes A M P, Pintado M E, Malcata F X (2007), 'Bovine whey proteins – Overview on their main biological properties', *Food Res Int*, **40**, 1197–1211.

Manso M A, López-Fandino R (2004), '*K*-Casein macropeptides from cheese whey: Physicochemical, biological, nutritional, and technological features for possible uses', *Food Rev Int*, **20**, 329–55.

Manzoni P, Rinaldi M, Cattani S, Pugni L, Romeo M G, *et al.* (2009), 'Bovine lactoferrin supplementation for prevention of late-onset sepsis in very low-birth-weight neonates: A randomized trial', *J Am Med Assoc*, **302**(13), 1421–28.

Markus C R, Olivier B, de Haan E H (2002), 'Whey protein rich in α-lactalbumin increases the ratio of plasma tryptophan to the sum of the large neutral amino acids and improves cognitive performance in stress-vulnerable subjects', *Am J Clin Nutr*, **75**, 1051–56.

Marnila P, Korhonen H (2002), 'Immunoglobulins,', in Roginski H, Fuquay J W, Fox P F, *Encyclopedia of Dairy Sciences*, London, Academic Press, pp. 1950–56.

Marnila P, Korhonen H (2009), 'Lactoferrin for human health', in Corredig M, *Dairy-derived Ingredients – Food and Nutraceutical Uses*, Cambridge, Woodhead, pp. 290–307.

Martin M J, Martin-Sosa S, Garcia-Pardo I A, Hueso P (2001), 'Distribution of bovine sialoglycoconjugates during lactation', *J Dairy Sci*, **84**, 995–1000.

Masuda O, Nakamura Y, Takano T (1996), 'Antihypertensive peptides are present in aorta after oral administration of sour milk containing these peptides to spontaneously hypertensive rats', *J Nutr* **126**, 3063–68.

Mather I H (2000), 'A review and proposed nomenclature for major proteins of the milk-fat globule membrane', *J Dairy Sci*, **83**, 203–47.

Mehra R, Kelly P (2006), 'Milk oligosaccharides: Structural and technological aspects', *Int Dairy J*, **16**, 1334–40.

Mehra R, Marnila P, Korhonen H (2006), 'Milk immunoglobulins for health promotion: A review', *Int Dairy J*, **16**(11), 1262–71.

Meisel H (2005), 'Biochemical properties of peptides encrypted in bovine milk proteins', *Curr Med Chem*, **12**, 1905–19.

Meisel H (2009), 'Functional milk-protein-derived peptides,' *Eur Dairy Mag*, **21**(3), 12–18.

Meisel H, FitzGerald R J (2003), 'Biofunctional peptides from milk proteins: mineral binding and cytomodulatory effects', *Curr Pharm Des*, **9**, 1289–95.

Mensink R P (2006), 'Dairy products and the risk to develop type 2 diabetes or cardiovascular disease', *Int Dairy J*, **16**, 1001–04.

Mezouari S, Pouliot Y (2009), 'Lipids from the milk fat globule membrane as a health ingredient: Composition, properties and technological aspects,' in Corredig M, *Dairy-derived Ingredients – Food and Nutraceutical Uses*, Cambridge, Woodhead, pp. 344–67.

Mezzaroba L F H, Carvalho J E, Ponezi A N, Antônio M A, Monteiro K M, *et al.* (2005), 'Antiulcerative properties of bovine α-lactalbumin', *Int Dairy J*, **16**(9), 943–1118.

Michaelidou A, Steijns J (2006), 'Nutritional and technological aspects of minor bioactive components in milk and whey: Growth factors, vitamins and nucleotides', *Int Dairy J*, **16**, 1421–26.

Miller G D, DiRienzo D D, Reusser M E, McCarron D A (2000), 'Benefits of dairy product consumption on blood pressure in humans: A summary of the biomedical literature', *J Am Coll Nutr*, **19** (No. 90002), S147–64.

Mills S, Stanton C, Ross R P (2009), 'Microbial production of bioactives: from fermented functional foods to probiotic mechanisms', *Aust J Dairy Technol*, **64**, 41–49.

Miquel E, Gomez J A, Alegra A, Barber R, Farr R, Recio I (2005), 'Identification of casein phosphopeptides released after simulated digestion of milk-based infant formulas', *J Agric Food Chem*, **53**, 3426–33.

Möller N P, Scholz-Ahrens K E, Roos N, Schrezenmeir J (2008), 'Bioactive peptides and proteins from foods: Indication for health effects', *Eur J Nutr*, **47**, 171–82.

Montoni A, Gauthier S F, Richard C, Poubelle P E, Chouinard Y, Pouliot Y (2009), 'Bovine colostrum as substrate for the preparation of growth factor-enriched protein extracts: Identifying the optimal collection period during lactation', *Dairy Sci Technol*, **89**, 511–18.

Morgan M V, Adams G G, Bailey D L, Tsao C E, Fischman S L, Reynolds E C (2008), 'The anticariogenic effect of sugar-free chewing gum containing CPP-ACP nanocomplexes on approximal caries determined using digital bitewing radiography', *Caries Res*, **42**, 171–84.

Mulder A M, Connellan P A, Oliver C J Morris C A, Stevenson (2008), 'Bovine lactoferrin supplementation supports immune and antioxidant status in healthy human males', *Nutr Res*, **28**(9), 583–89.

Murray B A, FitzGerald R J (2007), 'Angiotensin converting enzyme inhibitory peptides derived from food proteins: Biochemistry, bioactivity and production', *Curr Pharm Des*, **13**, 773–91.

Nakamura Y, Yamamoto M, Sakai K, Okubo A, Yamazaki S, Takano T (1995), 'Purification and characterization of angiotensin I-converting enzyme inhibitors from sour milk', *J Dairy Sc*, **78**, 777–83.

Nilsson M, Holst J J, Bjorck I M (2007), 'Metabolic effects of amino acid mixtures and whey protein in healthy subjects: studies using glucose-equivalent drinks', *Am J Clin Nutr*, **85**, 996–1004.

Ochoa T J, Chea-Woo E, Campos M, Pecho I, Prada A, *et al.* (2008), 'Impact of lactoferrin supplementation on growth and prevalence of *Giardia* colonization in children', *Clin Infect Dis*, **46**(12), 1881–83.

Ochoa T J, Cleary T G (2009), 'Effect of lactoferrin on enteric pathogens', *Biochimie*, **91**, 30–34.

Oliveira R P S, Florence A C R, Silva R C, Perego P, Converti A, *et al.* (2009), 'Effect of different prebiotics on the production of nonfat symbiotic fermented milk', *Int J Food Microbiol*, **128**, 467–72.

Ong L, Henriksson A, Shah N P (2007), 'Angiotensin converting enzyme-inhibitory activity in Cheddar cheeses made with the addition of probiotic *Lactobacillus casei* sp', *Lait*, **87**, 149–65.

Ong L, Shah N P (2008), 'Release and identification of angiotensin-converting enzyme inhibitory peptides as influenced by ripening temperatures and probiotic adjuncts in Cheddar cheeses', *LWT-Food Sci Technol*, **41**, 1555–66.

Ortiz-Chao P, Go'mez-Ruiz J A, Rastall R A, Mills D, Cramer R, *et al.* (2009), 'Production of novel ACE inhibitory peptides from b-lactoglobulin using Protease N Amano', *Int Dairy J*, **19**, 69–76.

Otte J, Shalaby S M, Zakora M, Pripp A H, El-Shabrawy S A (2007), 'Angiotensin-converting enzyme inhibitory activity of milk protein hydrolysates: Effect of substrate, enzyme and time of hydrolysis', *Int Dairy J*, **17**, 488–503.

Paesano R, Torcia F, Berlutti F, Pacifici E, Ebano V, *et al.* (2006), 'Oral administration of lactoferrin increases hemoglobin and total serum iron in pregnant women', *Biochem Cell Biol*, **84**(3), 377–80.

Pan Y, Lee A, Wan J, Coventry M J, Michalski W P, *et al.* (2006), 'Antiviral properties of milk proteins and peptides', *Int Dairy J*, **16**(11), 1252–61.

Pan Y, Rowney M, Guo P, Hobman P (2007), 'Biological properties of lactoferrin: an overview', *Aust J Dairy Technol*, **62**, 31–42.

Pariza M W, Park Y, Cook M E (2001), 'The biological active isomers of conjugated linoleic acid', *Progr Lipid Res*, **40**, 283–98.

Parodi P (2005), 'Dairy product consumption and the risk of breast cancer', *J Am Coll Nutr*, **24**, S556–68.

Parodi P W (1998), 'A role for milk proteins in cancer prevention', *Aust J Dairy Technol*, **53**, 37–47.

Parodi P W (2003), 'Anti-cancer agents in milkfat', *Aust J Dairy Technol*, **58**, 114–18.

Parodi P W (2004), 'Milk fat in human nutrition', *Aust J Dairy Technol*, **59**, 3–59.

Parodi P W (2009), 'Has the association between saturated fatty acids, serum cholesterol and coronary heart disease been over emphasized?', *Int Dairy J*, **19**(7), 345–61.

Parrot S, Degraeve P, Curia C, Martial-Gros A (2003), '*In vitro* study on digestion of peptides in Emmental cheese: analytical evaluation and influence on angiotensin I converting enzyme inhibitory peptides', *Nahrung*, **47**, 87–94.

Paul M, Somkuti G A (2009), 'Degradation of milk-based bioactive peptides by yogurt fermentation bacteria', *Lett Appl Microbiol*, **49**, 345–50.

Pettus B J, Chalfant C E, Hannun Y A (2004), 'Shingolipids in inflammation: Roles and implications', *Curr Molec Med*, **4**, 405–18.

Pfeuffer M, Schrezenmeir J (2006a), 'Milk and the metabolic syndrome', *Obes Revs* **8**, 109–18.

Pfeuffer M, Schrezenmeir J (2006b), 'Impact of *trans* fatty acids of ruminant origin compared with those from partially hydrogenated vegetable oils on CHD risk', *Int Dairy J*, **16**, 1383–88.

Phelan M, Aherne A, Fitzgerald R J, O'Brien N M (2009), 'Casein-derived bioactive peptides: Biological effects, industrial uses, safety aspects and regulatory status', *Int Dairy J*, **19**(11), 643–54.

Pihlanto A (2006), 'Antioxidative peptides derived from milk proteins', *Int. Dairy J.* 2006, 16, 1306–1314.

Pihlanto A, Korhonen H (2003), 'Bioactive peptides and proteins', in Taylor S L, *Advances in Food and Nutrition Research*, Elsevier Inc., San Diego, pp. 175–276.

Pihlanto-Leppälä A, Koskinen P, Piilola K, Tupasela T, Korhonen H (2000), 'Angiotensin I-converting enzyme inhibitory properties of whey protein digests: concentration and characterization of active peptides', *J Dairy Res*, **67**, 53–64.

Pihlanto-Leppälä A, Rokka T, Korhonen H (1998), 'Angiotensin I-converting enzyme inhibitory peptides derived from bovine milk proteins', *Int Dairy J*, **8**, 325–31.

Pilvi T K, Harala S, Korpela R, Mervaala E M (2009), 'Effects of high-calcium diets with different whey proteins on weight loss and weight regain in high-fat-fed C57BL/6J mice', *Br J Nutr*, **102**(3), 337–41.

Piot M, Fauquant J, Madec M-N, Maubois J-L (2004), 'Preparation of serocolostrum by membrane microfiltration', *Lait*, **84**, 333–41.

Playford R J, MacDonald C E, Johnson W S (2000), 'Colostrum and milk-derived peptide growth factors for the treatment of gastrointestinal disorders', *Am J Clin Nutr*, **72**, 5–14.

Playne M J, Bennett L E, Smithers G W (2003), 'Functional dairy foods and ingredients', *Aust J Dairy Technol*, **58**, 242–64.

Pouliot Y, Gauthier S F (2006), 'Milk growth factors as health products: Some technological aspects', *Int Dairy J*, **16**, 1415–20.

Pripp A H (2008), 'Effect of peptides derived from food proteins on blood pressure: a meta-analysis of randomized controlled trials', *Food Nutr Res*, **52**, 1–9.

Quiros A, Hernandez-Ledesma B, Ramos M, Amigo L, Recio I (2005), 'Angiotensin-converting enzyme inhibitory activity of peptides derived from caprine kefir', *J Dairy Sci*, **88**, 3480–87.

Recio I, Moreno E J, López-Fandino R (2009), 'Glycosylated dairy components: Their roles in nature and ways to make use of their functionality in dairy products', in Corredig M, *Dairy-derived Ingredients – Food and Nutraceutical Uses*, Cambridge, Woodhead, pp. 170–211.

Reiter B, Oram J D (1967), 'Bacterial inhibitors in milk and other biological fluids', *Nature*, **216**, 328–30.

Reynolds E C (2003), 'Dairy components in oral health', *Aust J Dairy Technol*, **58**, 79–81.

Rhoades J R, Gibson G R, Formentin K, Beer M, Greenberg N, Rastall R A (2005), 'Caseinoglycomacropeptide inhibits adhesion of pathogenic *Escherichia coli* strains to human cells in culture', *J Dairy Sci*, **88**, 3455–59.

Roberts A K, Chierici R, Sawatzki G, Hill M J, Volpato S, Vigi V (1992), 'Supplementation of an adapted formula with bovine lactoferrin: 1. Effect on the infant faecal flora', *Acta Paediatr*, **81**(2), 119–24.

Rombaut R, Dewettinck K (2006), 'Properties, analysis and purification of milk polar lipids', *Int Dairy J*, **16**, 1362–73.

Rowan A M, Haggarty N W, Ram S (2005), 'Milk bioactives: discovery and proof of concept', *Aust J Dairy Technol*, **60**, 114–20.

Royle P J, McIntosh G H, Clifton P M (2008), 'Whey protein isolate and glycomacropeptide decreases weight gain and alters body composition in male Wistar rats', *Br J Nutr*, **100**, 88–93.

Ryhänen E-L, Pihlanto-Leppälä A, Pahkala E (2001), 'A new type of ripened; low-fat cheese with bioactive properties', *Int Dairy J*, **11**, 441–47.

Saito T (2008), 'Antihypertensive peptides derived from bovine casein and whey proteins', *Adv Exp Med Biol*, **606**, 295–317.

Saito T, Nakamura T, Kitazawa H, Kawai Y, Itoh T (2000), 'Isolation and structural analysis of antihypertensive peptides that exist naturally in Gouda cheese', *J Dairy Sci*, **83**, 1434–40.

Scammell A W (2001), 'Production and uses of colostrum', *Aust J Dairy Technol*, **56**(2), 74–82.

Schaafsma G (2006a), 'Health issues of whey proteins: 1. Protection of lean body mass', *Curr Topics Nutrac Res*, **4**, 113–22.

Schaafsma G (2006b), 'Health issues of whey proteins: 2. Weight management', *Curr Topics Nutrac Res*, **4**, 123–26.

Schaafsma G (2008), 'Lactose and lactose derivatives as bioactive ingredients in human nutrition', *Int Dairy J*, **18**(5), 458–65.

Schaafsma G (2009), 'Health benefits of milk beyond traditional nutrition', *Aust J Dairy Technol*, **64**(1), 113–16.

Schlimme E, Martin D, Meisel H (2000), 'Nucleosides and nucleotides: natural bioactive substances in milk and colostrum', *Br J Nutr*, **84** (Suppl 1), S59–68.

Schoeller D A, Watras A C, Whigham L D (2009), 'A meta-analysis of the effects of conjugated linoleic acid on fat-free mass in humans', *Appl Physiol Nutr Metab*, **34**(5), 975–78.

Scrutton H, Carbonnier A, Cowen P J, Harmer C (2007), 'Effects of (alpha)-lactalbumin on emotional processing in healthy women', *J Psychopharmacol*, **21**(5), 519–24.

Seifu E, Buys E M, Donkin E F (2005), 'Significance of the lactoperoxidase system in the dairy industry and its potential applications: A review', *Trends Food Sci Technol*, **16**, 137–54.

Seppo L, Jauhiainen T, Poussa T, Korpela R (2003), 'A fermented milk high in bioactive peptides has a blood pressure-lowering effect in hypertensive subjects', *Am J Clin Nutr*, **77**, 326–30.

Shingfield K J, Chilliard Y, Toivonen V, Kairenius P, Givens DI (2008), 'Trans fatty acids and bioactive lipids in ruminant milk', *Adv Exp Med Biol*, **606**, 3–65.

Shingfield K J, Reynolds C K, Lupoli B, Toivonen V, Yurawecz M P, *et al.* (2005), 'Effect of forage type and proportion of concentrate in the diet on milk fatty acid composition in cows given sunflower oil and fish oil', *Animal Sci*, **80**, 225–38.

Sichien M, Thienpont N, Fredrick, E, Trung Le T, Van Camp J, Dewettinck K (2009), 'Processing means for milk fat fractionation and production functional compounds', in Corredig M, *Dairy-derived Ingredients – Food and Nutraceutical Uses*, Cambridge, Woodhead, pp. 68–102.

Sieber R, Collomb M, Aeschlimann A, Jelen P, Eyer H (2004), 'Impact of microbial cultures on conjugated linoleic acid in dairy products-a review', *Int Dairy J*, **14**, 1–15.

Silva S V, Malcata F X (2005), 'Caseins as source of bioactive peptides', *Int Dairy J* **15**, 1–15.

Singh T K, Fox P F, Healy A (1997), 'Isolation and identification of further peptides in the diafiltration retentate of the water-soluble fraction of Cheddar cheese', *J Dairy Res*, **64**, 433–43.

Sipola M, Finckenberg P, Korpela R, Vapaatalo H, Nurminen M-L (2002), 'Effect of long-term intake of milk products on blood pressure in hypertensive rats', *J Dairy Res*, **69**, 103–11.

Smilowitz J T, Dillard C J, German J B (2005), 'Milk beyond essential nutrients: the metabolic food', *Aust J Dairy Technol*, **60**, 77–83.

Smithers G W (2008), 'Whey and whey proteins – from 'gutter-to-gold'', *Int Dairy J*, **18**, 695–704.

Sokolowska A, Bednarz R, Pacewicz M, Georgiades J A, Wilusz T, Polanowski A (2008), 'Colostrum from different mammalian species- A rich source of colostrinin', *Int Dairy J*, **18**, 204–09.

Spitsberg V L (2005), 'Bovine milk fat globule membrane as a potential nutraceutical', *J Dairy Sci*, **88**, 2289–94.

Stelwagen K, Carpenter E, Haigh B, Hodgkinson A, Wheeler T T (2009), 'Immune components of bovine colostrum and milk', *J Anim Sci*, **87**, 3–9.

Struff W G, Sprotte G (2007), 'Bovine colostrum as a biologic in clinical medicine: a review', *Int J Clin Pharmacol Therap*, **45**, 193–202.

Teraguchi S, Wakabayashi H, Kuwata H, Yamauchi K, Tamura Y (2004), 'Protection against infections by oral lactoferrin: evaluation in animal models', *Biometals*, **17**, 231–34.

Terpstra A H M (2004), 'Effect of conjugated linoleic acid on body composition and plasma lipids in human: An overview of the literature', *Am J Clin Nutr*, **79**, 352–61.

Thomä-Worringer C, Sörensen J, López-Fandino R (2006), 'Health effects and technological features of caseinomacropeptide', *Int Dairy J*, **16**, 1324–33.

Tomita M, Wakabayashi H, Shin K, Yamauchi K, Yaeshima T, Iwatsuki K (2008), 'Twenty-five years of research on bovine lactoferrin appications', *Biochimie*, Epub ahead. doi: 10.1016/j.biochi.2008.05.021

Tremblay A, Gilbert J-A (2009), 'Milk products, insulin resistance syndrome and type 2 diabetes', *J Am Coll Nutr*, **28** (Suppl 1), S91–102.

Tripathi V, Vashishtha B (2006), 'Bioactive compounds of colostrum and its application', *Food Rev Int*, **22**, 225–44.

Tsai J-S, Chen T-J, Sun Pan B, Gong S-D, Chung M-Y (2008), 'Antihypertensive effect of bioactive peptides produced by protease-facilitated lactic acid fermentation of milk', *Food Chem*, **106**, 552–58.

Turpeinen A, Kumpu M, Rönnback M, Seppo L, Kautiainen H, *et al.* (2009), 'Antihypertensive and cholesterol-lowering effects of a spread containing bioactive peptides IPP and VPP and plant sterols', *J Func Foods*, **1**(3), 260–65.

Usinger L, Ibsen H, Jensen L (2009), 'Does fermented milk possess antihypertensive effect in humans?', *J Hypertens*, **27**(6), 1115–20.

Valenti P, Antonini G (2005), 'Lactoferrin: an important host defence against microbial and viral attack', *Cell Mol Life Sci*, **62**(22), 2576–87.

Valtonen M, Niskanen L, Kangas A P, Koskinen T (2005), 'Effect of melatonin-rich night-time milk on sleep and activity in elderly institutionalized subjects', *Nordic J Psyc*, **59**, 217–21.

van der Zander K, Bots ML, Bak A A A, Koning M M G, de Leeuw P W (2008), 'Enzymatically hydrolyzed lactotripeptides do not lower blood pressure in mildly hypertensive subjects', *Am J Clin Nutr*, **88**, 1697–1702.

van Mierlo L A J, Koning M M G, van der Zander K, Draijer R (2009), 'Lactotripeptides do not lower blood pressure in untreated whites: Results from 2 controlled multicenter crossover studies', *Am J Clin Nutr*, **89**, 617–623.

Veldhorst M A, Nieuwenhuizen A G, Hochstenbach-Waelen A, van Vught A J, Westerterp K R, *et al.* (2009), 'Dose-dependent satiating effect of whey relative to casein or soy', *Physiol Behav*, **96**(4–5), 675–82.

Vercruysse L, Van Camp J, Dewettinck K, Smagghe G (2009), 'Production and enrichment of bioactive peptides derived from milk proteins', in Corredig M, *Dairy-derived Ingredients – Food and Nutraceutical Uses*, Cambridge, Woodhead, pp. 51–67.

Virtanen T, Pihlanto A, Akkanen S, Korhonen H (2006), 'Development of antioxidant activity in milk whey during fermentation with lactic acid bacteria', *J Appl Microbiol*, **102**, 106–15.

Wakabayashi H, Takase M, Tomita M (2003), 'Lactoferricin derived from milk protein lactoferrin', *Curr Pharm Des*, **9**(16), 1277–87.

Wakabayashi H, Yamauchi K, Takase M (2006), 'Lactoferrin research, technology and applications', *Int Dairy J*, **16**, 1241–51.

Walstra P, Wouters J, Geurts T J (2006), *Dairy Technology: Principles of Milk properties and Processes*, 2nd edition. Chapter 2: Milk Components, CRC Press, New York, pp. 27–105.

Wang B, Brand-Miller J, McVeagh P, Petocz P (2001), 'Concentration and distribution of sialic acid in human milk and infant formulas', *Am J Clin Nutr*, **74**, 510–15.

Weinberg E D (2003), 'The therapeutic potential of lactoferrin', *Exp Opin Investig Drugs*, **12**(5), 841–51.

Weinberg E D (2007), 'Antibiotic properties and applications of lactoferrin', *Curr Pharm Des*, **13**(8), 801–11.

Wheeler T T, Hodgkinson A J, Prosser CG and Davis S R (2007), 'Immunen components of colostrum and milk – a historical perspective', *J. Mamm Gland Biol. Neoplasia*, **12**, 237–47.

Xu J-Y, Qin L-Q, Wang P-Y, Li W, Chang C (2008), 'Effect of milk tripeptides on blood pressure: A meta-analysis of randomized controlled trials', *Nutr*, **24**, 933–40.

Xu S, Boylston T D, Glatz B A (2005), 'Conjugated linoleic acid content and organoleptic attributes of fermented milk products produced with probiotic bacteria', *J Agric Food Chem*, **53**, 9064–72.

Yamamoto N, Ejiri M, Mizuno S (2003), 'Biogenic peptides and their potential use', *Curr Pharm Des*, **9**, 1345–55.

Young K W, Munro I C, Taylor S L, Veldkamp P, van Dissel J T (2007), 'The safety of whey protein concentrate derived from the milk of cows immunized against *Clostridium difficile*', *Regul Toxicol Pharmacol*, **47**(3), 317–26.

Yvon M, Beucher S, Guilloteau P, Le Huerou-Luron I, Corring T (1994), 'Effects of caseinomacropeptide (CMP) on digestion regulation', *Reprod Nutrit Dev*, **34**, 527–37.

Zemel M B (2004), 'Role of calcium and dairy products in energy partitioning and weight management', *Am J Clin Nutr*, **79** (Suppl), S907–12.

Zhao Y, Jackson S M, Aitken R (2006), 'The bovine antibody repertoire', *Dev & Comp Immunol*, **30**, 175–86.

Zimecki M, Kruzel M L (2007), 'Milk-derived proteins and peptides of potential therapeutic and nutritive value', *J Exp Ther Oncol*, **6**(2), 89–106.

21

Functional meat products

K. Arihara and M. Ohata, Kitasato University, Japan

Abstract: Although studies of functional meat products have been limited until recently, it should be possible to develop novel meat products with potential health benefits by increasing or introducing bioactive properties. This chapter initially describes meat consumption and human health, looking at the potential benefits of representative meat-derived bioactive components, such as conjugated linoleic acid, histidyl dipeptides, and L-carnitine. The chapter then goes on to look at the development of functional meat products. It focuses on the possibility of novel functional meat products utilizing meat protein-derived bioactive peptides, probiotics and prebiotics. Along with the scientific basis for peptides and probiotics, the application of these concepts to meat products is emphasized.

Key words: meat, functional meat products, bioactive peptides, probiotics, prebiotics.

21.1   Introduction

Meat is an excellent source of proteins with high biological value (Lawrie and Ledward, 2006). Meat proteins contain well balanced essential amino acids, particularly sulphated amino acids. Meat also plays an important role in supplying our diet with minerals and vitamins (Mulvihill, 2004). The bioavailability of minerals found in meat is superior to those found in vegetables. Consumers, however, often associate meat and meat products with a negative health image viewing meat as a source of high fat, saturated fatty acids and cholesterol (Chan, 2004; Fernández-Ginés *et al.*, 2005; Ovesen, 2004a, 2004b; Valsta *et al.*, 2005). Many consumers associate meat consumption with chronic illnesses, such as cardiovascular diseases, some types of cancer and obesity. Additionally, a high intake of sodium chloride, which is a basic ingredient for most meat products (e.g. sausages), has been linked to hypertension (Ruusunen and Puolanne, 2005).

During the past few decades, much attention has been paid to the tertiary functions of foods (Sloan, 2008). Tertiary functions are the roles of food components in preventing diseases by modulating physiological systems. Due to increasing concerns for health, efforts have been made by food industries in many countries to develop new foods with tertiary functions. These foods are known as functional foods. Although studies of functional meat products have been limited until recently, it should be possible to develop new meat products with potential health benefits by increasing or introducing bioactive properties (Arihara, 2004, 2006a, 2006b; Arihara and Ohata, 2008; Fernández-Ginés *et al.*, 2005; Jiménez-Colmenero, 2007a, 2007b; Jiménez-Colmenero *et al.*, 2001, 2006).

There are diverse possible strategies for developing healthier meat and meat products, including functional foods (Fernández-Ginés *et al.*, 2005; Jiménez-Colmenero, 2007a; Jiménez-Colmenero *et al.*, 2001, 2006). Although all aspects, from animal production to product processing, should be considered for designing healthier meat products, this chapter focuses on functional meat products mainly from the viewpoint of food processing. Along with meat consumption and human health, the potential benefits of representative meat components on health are described. An overview of meat-based functional products is presented and the development of novel functional meat products which utilize bioactive peptides, probiotics and prebiotics is particularly focused on.

21.2   Meat consumption and human health

Undoubtedly, meat is an excellent source of the nutrients required for human health. However, the fat content of meat has been associated with the incidence of some diseases, such as atherosclerosis and obesity (Biesalski, 2005). Consumption of red meat proteins has also been associated with colon cancer in some epidemiological studies (MacIntosh and Le Leu, 2001). In this section the consumption of major meat components and human nutrition are described briefly.

21.2.1   Proteins
Along with poultry, fish and eggs, meat is categorized in the protein food group in the food guide pyramid (Lachance and Fisher, 2005). Meat is a fundamental source of essential amino acids, since it contains an abundance of proteins with high biological value. The nine amino acids which are indispensable for human nutrition are tryptophan, threonine, leucine, isoleucine, lysine, methionine, phenylalanine, valine and histidine. Tyrosine and cystine also perform critical roles in human nutrition and should be included in a nutritional assessment of food proteins. Most meat and meat products contain high levels of these essential amino acids and of tyrosine and cystine.

The consumption of red meat has been associated with colorectal cancer in many, although not all, epidemiological studies. There is some evidence that the risk of colorectal cancer increases if a red meat derived protein is consumed twice a day or more (MacIntosh and Le Leu, 2001). There is a potential value to examining long-term meat consumption, assessing its link to the risk of cancer and reviewing the evidence that prolonged high consumption of red meat may increase the risk of colorectal cancer (Chao *et al.*, 2005). However, since few studies have examined the risk in relation to long-term meat intake or the association of meat with rectal cancer, the idea that the concentration of meat protein in a diet determines the cancer risk is still controversial.

21.2.2   Minerals and vitamins

Meat is a good source of iron, zinc, selenium, and B vitamins in the diet (Biesalski, 2005; Higgs, 2000; Mulvihill, 2004). The percentages of micronutrients contributed to the diet by meat and meat products are as follows: 14% iron, 30% zinc, 14% vitamin B2, 21% vitamin B6, 22% vitamin B12, 19% vitamin D, and 37% niacin (Mulvihill, 2004). Red meat especially contains an abundance of iron (e.g. 2.1 mg of iron per 100 g of fillet steak). Most of the iron in meat exists as a part of haem in myoglobin. Haem is a highly absorbable form of iron. Meat proteins enhance the absorption of iron. Zinc in meat is also highly bioavailable. Some muscle organ meats, such as heart and gizzard, are also good sources of riboflavin, niacin, pantothenic acid, and vitamin B6.

21.2.3   Fat and fatty acids

Consumers often associate meat and meat products with a negative health image. This unfortunate image of meat is mainly because of the fat, saturated fatty acids and cholesterol it contains and its association with chronic illnesses, such as cardiovascular diseases, some types of cancer and obesity (Chan, 2004; Fernández-Ginés *et al.*, 2005; Ovensen, 2004a, 2004b; Valsta *et al.*, 2005). It is recommended that dietary fat provides between 15 and 30% of the total energy in the diet, that less than 10% of calorie intake should be from saturated fatty acids (SFA) and that 6–10% and 10–15% of that should be from polyunsaturated fatty acids (PUFA) and from monounsaturated fatty acids (MUFA) respectively. Furthermore, less than 1% of that should be from trans fatty acids and cholesterol intake should be limited to less than 300 mg per day.

Meat fat contains less than 50% SFA and up to 65–70% unsaturated fatty acids (Jiménez-Colmenero, 2007a). Various modifications, including reduced fatty acid levels, raised MUFA and PUFA levels, improved n-6:n-3 PUFA balances, and limited cholesterol contents, can be achieved by animal breeding and feeding, material formulation and technical processing (Jiménez-Colmenero *et al.*, 2006). Many studies have demonstrated the possibility of changing the image of meat and meat products by the addition, elimination and reduction of fat and fatty acids (Jiménez-Colmenero, 2007a). Since meat and meat products contain high percentages of SFA and less fatty acids from the n-6 family (e.g. linoleic acid), replacement of such fatty acids in meat with vegetable oils would mean a great improvement in their nutritional value. Olive oil contains the highest level of MUFA of the vegetable oils. If meat fat were replaced with olive oil, a notable improvement in nutritional quality could be expected (Barberá, 2008).

21.3   Meat-based bioactive compounds

As previously discussed, meat is an excellent source of proteins with a high biological value and valuable minerals and vitamins. In addition to these basic nutrients, attention has also been paid to meat-based bioactive compounds. Utilizing or emphasizing the physiological activities of such bioactive compounds originating from meat is one possible approach for developing functional meat products. Meat-based bioactive compounds, such as conjugated linoleic acid (CLA), histidyl dipeptides (carnosine and anserine), L-carnitine, glutathione, taurine, coenzyme Q10, creatine, choline, balenine, creatinine, lipoic acid, putrescine, spermidine, and spermine have been studied for their physiological properties (Arihara and Ohata, 2008; Williams, 2007). Since the feeding conditions of animals affect the contents of CLA and L-carnitine in meat (Krajcovicova-Kudlackova et al., 2000; Mir et al., 2004), healthier meats would be produced through modification of the animal feed. As representative meat-based bioactive compounds, CLA, histidyl dipeptides and L-carnitine (Fig. 21.1) are described here.

21.3.1   Conjugated linoleic acid

Conjugated linoleic acids (CLAs) have attracted considerable attention as representative nutraceutical compounds found in beef and milk. They were

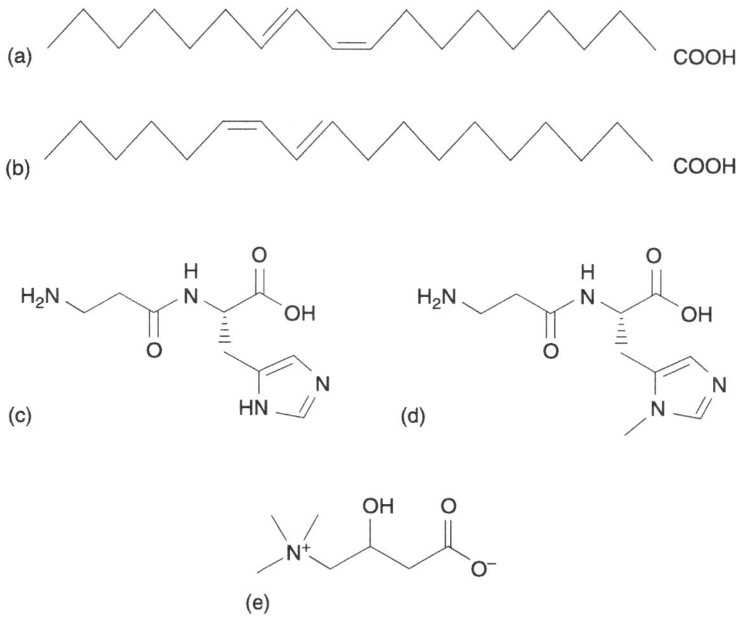

Fig. 21.1   Representative meat-based bioactive compounds: (a) conjugated linoleic acid (c9,t11-isomer); (b) conjugated linoleic acid (t10,c12-isomer); (c) carnosine; (d) anserine; (e) L-carnitine.

initially found in cooked ground beef (Pariza *et al.*, 1983). Later, they were found in meat and milk of ruminants (Gnadig *et al.*, 2000; Nagao and Yanagita, 2005; Watkins and Yong, 2001).

Since rumen bacteria convert linoleic acid to CLA by their isomerases, CLA is rich in the fat of ruminant animals and beef fat contains 3.1–8.5 mg CLA per g of fat (Hasler, 1988). CLA is composed of a group of positional and geometric isomers of octadecadienoic acid. The most common CLA isomer found in beef is octadeca-*c*9, *t11*-dienoic acid (Fig. 21.1a). Much attention has been paid to this CLA isomer due to its bioactive activity (anticarcinogenicity). Commercially available supplements utilized for many studies usually contains several CLA isomers (e.g. *c*9, *t*11: 41%; *t*10, *c*12: 44%; *t*9, *t*11/*t*10, *t*12: 7%). Although some studies demonstrated that the *t*10, *c*12 isomer (Fig. 21.1b) has stronger physiological activities than those of the *c*9, *t*11 isomer, most animal products such as beef and cow's milk contain only trace amounts of the *t*10, *c*12 CLA isomer.

The CLA content of milk and beef is affected by several factors, such as breed, age and feed composition (Dhiman *et al.*, 2005). CLA content in products sourced from grass-fed animals is more than three times greater than that in products from animals fed a diet of 50% hay and silage with 50% grain. The CLA content was also reported to be higher in beef from cattle fed a diet containing soy oil (Lorenzen *et al.*, 2007). The CLA content of foods can be increased by heat treatments, such as cooking and processing (Herzallah *et al.*, 2005). Lactic acid bacteria also promote the formation of CLA. The effect of lactic acid bacteria on the formation of CLA in media and fermented dairy products has been studied (Alonso *et al.*, 2003; Coakley *et al.*, 2003; Sieber *et al.*, 2004; Xu *et al.*, 2005). Such bacterial conversion would be expected in fermented meat products. Epidemiological studies have suggested that high intakes of high-fat dairy foods and CLA may reduce the risk of colorectal cancer (Larsson *et al.*, 2005). Besides anti-carcinogenic properties, CLA also has anti-atherosclerotic, antioxidative and immunomodulative properties (Azain, 2003).

21.3.2   Histidyl dipeptides

Various endogenous antioxidants including tocopherols, ubiquinone, cartenoids, ascorbic acid, glutathione, lipoic acid, uric acid, spermine, carnosine and anserine, have been found in skeletal muscle (Decker *et al.*, 2000). Both carnosine (β-alanyl-L-histidine, Fig. 21.1c) and anserine (N-β-alanyl-1-methyl-L-histidine, Fig. 21.1d) are antioxidative histidyl dipeptides and are the most abundant antioxidatives in meats. The consumption of antioxidant-rich foods prevents oxidative damage in our body (Lindsay, 2000). This is attributed to the neutralization and reduced release of free radicals by antioxidants (Langseth, 2000). The antioxidative properties of carnosine and anserine may result from their ability to chelate transition metals such as copper (Brown, 1981).

The concentrations of carnosine and anserine in meat vary depending on the animal species and cut of meat. The concentration of carnosine in meat ranges from 500 mg/kg in a chicken thigh to 2700 mg/kg in a pork shoulder. Anserine is especially abundant in chicken muscle (e.g., 980 mg/kg in skeletal muscle). These peptides have been reported to assist in wound healing, recovery from fatigue and prevention of diseases related to oxidative stress. Since anserine is more resistant to digestion than carnosine, the physiological function of anserine would be more effective than carnosine in the human body. For this reason, functional food ingredients with high concentrations of anserine (approx. 98%) purified from fish extracts have been developed in Japan.

Park *et al.* (2005) demonstrated the bioavailability of carnosine by determining its concentration in human plasma after ingestion of beef. Increasing attention to meat-based bioactive compounds has resulted in the development of a new sensitive procedure for determining these compounds (Mora *et al.*, 2007).

21.3.3 L-carnitine

L-carnitine (β-hydroxy-γ-trimethyl amino butyric acid, Fig. 21.1e) is found in the skeletal muscle of various animals (Shimada *et al.*, 2005) and is especially abundant in beef (e.g. 1300 mg per kg of the thigh). It transports long-chain fatty acids across the inner mitochondrial membranes, where they are processed by β-oxidation to produce biological energy. L-carnitine can also help energy production in muscle, when we are doing hard exercise and assists the human body in lowering the levels of cholesterol and in absorbing calcium. A study demonstrated that L-carnitine blocked apotosis and prevented skeletal muscle myopathy in heart failure (Vescovo *et al.*, 2002). Many products containing L-carnitine have been marketed in the United States and Japan. Some products are advertised as having several beneficial effects, such as greater endurance and fast recovery from fatigue.

21.4   Development of functional meat products

There are various possible strategies for developing healthier meat and functional meat products (Jiménez-Colmenero, 2007b; Jiménez-Colmenero *et al.*, 2001). All stages, from animal production to product processing, have to be considered. As previously discussed, by modifying animal feed, the composition (e.g., conjugated linoleic acid) of animal products can be improved. Additionally, the functional characteristics of meat products can be changed by introducing food ingredients considered to be beneficial for health or by eliminating components that are considered harmful. Approaches for the modification and improvement of meat products suggested by Fernández-Ginés *et al.* (2005), Jiménez-Colmenero (2007a) and Jiménez-Colmenero *et al.* (2006) are summarized in Table 21.1.

21.4.1   Functional meat products

Low-fat or fat-free meat products have been developed prolifically in many countries with the United States at the head of the list (Jiménez-Colmenero *et al.*,

Table 21.1   Representative approaches for developing functional meat products

Reduction
Sodium chloride
Fat and/or cholesterol
Allergens (vegetable and egg proteins)
Biogenic amines

Modification
Fatty acid (selection of breeds)
n-6:n-3 PUFA (linseed feed)

Addition
Vegetable oils (olive oil)
Fish oils
Conjugated linoleic acid
Plant-based proteins (soy protein)
Natural extracts
Nuts (walnuts)
Vitamins C and E
Minerals (Ca, Se, Fe, Mg, Mn)
Plant sterols
Phytate
Probiotic lactic acid bacteria
Dietary fibers (apple, pear, citrus)
Oligosaccharides
L-carnitine

2006). Sugar-free meat products such as roast ham, sausages and bacon have also been developed in Japan (Fig. 21.2). In addition to these 'free' and 'low' types of products, meat products in which additional physiologically functional properties have been added are also being produced. Functional ingredients for meat products such as vegetable proteins, fibers (e.g. oats, sugar beet, soy beans, apples, peas), antioxidants and probiotics (intestinal *Lactobacillus* and *Bifidobacterium*), can now be listed (Fernández-Ginés *et al.*, 2005; Jiménez-Colmenero, 2007a; Jiménez-Colmenero *et al.*, 2006) and studies for meat products with functional ingredients were reviewed by Fernández-Ginés *et al.* (2005).

Japan is the first country to have formulated a specific regulatory approval process for functional foods. In 1991, the concept of foods for specified health use (FOSHU) was established by the Japanese Ministry of Health and Welfare. FOSHU are foods that, based on the knowledge of the relationship between foods or food components and health, are expected to have certain health benefits and have been licensed to bear the label claiming that the person using them may expect to obtain that health benefit through the consumption of these foods. Most FOSHU products utilize physiologically functional ingredients. As of April 2010, 936 FOSHU products have been approved in Japan. Dietary fibers and soy proteins have been utilized for developing FOSHU meat products (Arihara, 2004). There are now pork sausage products containing indigestible dextrin, a water-soluble dietary fiber prepared from potato, which claim to have beneficial effects

(a)

(b)

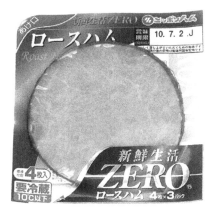
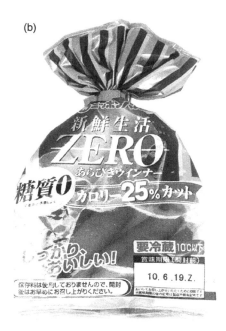

Fig. 21.2   Sugar-free meat products 'Zero' (Nippon Meat Packers, Inc., Japan). (a) Sliced roast ham; (b) pork Vienna-type sausage.

on intestinal disorders. Another product available is a sausage containing soy proteins which claims to help maintain acceptable blood cholesterol levels.

In addition to the FOSHU products, meat products with additional functional food ingredients, such as fibers, vegetable proteins and minerals (e.g. calcium), have been developed in Japan. Soy proteins are popular vegetable proteins for their various health-enhancing activities (e.g. prevention of cardiovascular diseases, cancer and osteoporosis). A sausage with additional potato starch was also developed in the United States (Pszczola *et al.*, 2002). Dietary fibers like these improve intestinal microflora such as prebiotics, as described in a later section, and contribute to the reduction of fat intake. Healthier lipid formulation is also a critical approach to develop meat-based functional foods. Technological options for the replacement of meat fats with various non-meat fats (i.e. plant and fish fats) were reviewed extensively by Jiménez-Colmenero (2007b)

People who suffer from allergies are often affected by allergens in foods. Meat is less allergenic than common allergy-inducing foods, such as milk, eggs and soy (Tanabe and Nishimura, 2005), but meat products (e.g. sausages) often utilize vegetable, egg and/or milk proteins as ingredients. There is, however, a series of meat products named 'Apilight' including sausages, hamburgers steaks and meat balls, (Fig. 21.3) which are beneficial for people suffering from food allergies. These products are made with a formulation that eliminates ingredients causing

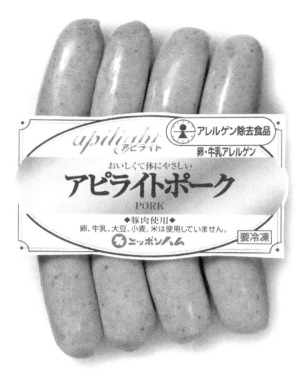

Fig. 21.3   Allergen-free pork frankfurter 'Apilight pork' (Nippon Meat Packers, Inc., Japan).

allergic symptoms. Apilight meat products have been approved as allergen-free products by the Japanese Ministry of Health and Welfare. Gluten-free and/or lactose-free meat products have also been developed in some countries (Jiménez-Colmenero *et al.*, 2006). There is increasing evidence that even meat can cause allergic symptoms in very sensitive patients. Chicken allergy was the most prevalent (4.5%) among various meat allergies in Japanese children (Iikura *et al.*, 1999). Studies also show that beef allergy occurs with an incidence of 3.3–6.5% in children with atopic dermatitis (Fiocchi *et al.*, 2000). Heat and enzymatic treatments are effective methods for reducing the allergenicity of meat allergens (Tanabe and Nishimura, 2005). High-pressure treatment also can change the antigenicity of some food proteins (Han *et al.*, 2002).

21.4.2   Utilization of meat protein-derived peptides
Meat protein-derived peptides are a group of bioactive components of meat (Arihara, 2006a; Arihara and Ohata, 2008). Studies show that numerous bioactive peptides are generated from food proteins, such as milk, soy, fish and meat proteins

(Gobbetti, *et al.*, 2007; Korhonen and Pihlanto, 2003, 2007; Mine and Shahidi, 2005; Pihlanto and Korhonen, 2003). As representative bioactivities of such peptides, antihypertensive, antioxidative, antithrombotic, hypocholesterolemic, antimicrobial, mineral binding, prebiotic, immunomodulatory and opioid activities have been studied. Angiotensin I-converting enzyme (ACE) inhibitory peptides are the most extensively studied of these bioactive peptides (Meisel *et al.*, 2005; Vermeirssen *et al.*, 2004). Since some of these peptides have antihypertensive effects by oral administration, they have been utilized for functional foods (Arihara, 2004, 2006a). However, functional meat products with bioactive peptides, including ACE-inhibitory peptides, have not been developed.

21.4.3   Generation of peptides from meat proteins

Although most food proteins contain bioactive sequences, those sequences are inactive within the parent proteins. Peptides with respective bioactivities are generated from native proteins by proteolytic digestion. Processes of protein digestion for the generation of peptides from meat proteins include digestion, aging, fermentation and protease treatment (Fig. 21.4). Meat proteins are attacked by proteolytic enzymes (e.g. pepsin, trypsin, chymotripsin, elastase and carboxypeptidase) during gastrointestinal digestion (Pihlanto and Korhonen, 2003). Although there has been no clear evidence that bioactive peptides are generated from meat proteins in human intestinal tracts, their generation has been shown in several *in vitro* studies. Some gastrointestinal digestive enzymes generated ACE-inhibitory activity from pork proteins (Arihara *et al.*, 2001). ACE-inhibitory activity was also generated from some meat proteins (myosin, actin, tropomyosin and troponin) by pancreatic protease treatment (Katayama *et al.*, 2003a).

Meat contains various muscle endogenous proteases and meat proteins are hydrolyzed by these enzymes during aging (Etherington, 1984; Koohmaraie, 1994; Toldrá, 2007). Thus, the content of amino acids and peptides increases in aged meat (Mikami *et al.*, 1995; Nishimura *et al.*, 1988). Although enzymatic hydrolysis of meat proteins during aging results in an improvement in sensory properties, there have been no reports of bioactive peptides being generated in meat during aging or storage. Studies, however, would be expected to show that meat aging improves bioactivity. Meat proteins are hydrolyzed during the fermentation and ripening of dry sausages. Both muscle endogenous and microbial proteolytic enzymes are involved in the fermentation of meat products and contribute to the development of sensory properties of fermented meat products

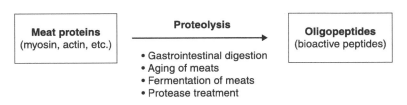

Fig. 21.4   Generation of bioactive peptides from meat proteins.

(Hammes *et al.*, 2003; Hierro *et al.*, 1999; Toldrá, 2004). ACE-inhibitory and antihypertensive activities were generated from porcine skeletal muscle proteins by lactic acid bacteria (Arihara *et al.*, 2004). Since small peptides have been identified in dry-cured ham (Sentandreu *et al.*, 2003), some such peptides generated from meat proteins could have bioactivities. Also, Sentandreu and Toldrá (2007a, 2007b) suggested that the proteolytic action of porcine muscle dipeptidyl peptidases during the ripening period of dry-cured ham could contribute to the generation of ACE-inhibitory peptides.

The most effective procedure for producing bioactive peptides on an industrial scale is enzymatic treatment. Various commercially available proteases have been utilized for the production of peptides from food proteins (Pihlanto and Korhonen, 2003). Many bioactive peptides have been experimentally prepared using commercial proteases (Korhonen and Pihlanto, 2003, 2007) and proteolytic enzymes have been used for meat tenderization in the meat industry (Dransfield and Etherington, 1981). Although bioactive peptides might be generated in meat treated with enzymatic tenderization, efforts have not been directed towards such studies. Since the effects of commercial proteases on the breakdown of meat protein and the sensory properties of fermented sausages have been demonstrated (Bruna *et al.*, 2000), such treatments could be used for developing functional meat products containing bioactive peptides.

21.4.4   Meat protein-derived bioactive peptides

ACE-inhibitory peptides have been studied most extensively among the bioactive peptides derived from meat proteins (Arihara, 2006a; Arihara and Ohata, 2008; Vercruysse *et al.*, 2005). A summary of bioactive peptides, including ACE-inhibitory peptides, generated from meat proteins is shown in Table 21.2. Some ACE-inhibitory peptides generated from meat proteins have demonstrated antihypertensive properties when administered orally to spontaneously hypertensive rats (Arihara *et al.*, 2005a; Fujita *et al.*, 2000; Nakashima *et al.*, 2002). Two ACE-inhibitory peptides, Met-Asn-Pro-Pro and Ile-Thr-Thr-Asn-Pro, which are found in the myosin-heavy chain sequence, showed antihypertensive properties (Nakashima *et al.*, 2002).

Meat protein-derived bioactive peptides, other than the ACE-inhibitory peptides, are still limited. Some antioxidative peptides have been identified in the enzymatic hydrolyzates of meat proteins (Arihara *et al.*, 2005b; Saiga *et al.*, 2003b). Hydrolyzates from porcine myofibrillar proteins generated by papain or actinase E exhibited high levels of antioxidative activity (Saiga *et al.*, 2003b). Asp-Ala-Gln-Glu-Lys-Leu-Glu, which is found in the actin sequence, showed the highest level of activity among five identified peptides. In another study, three antioxidative peptides (Asp-Leu-Tyr-Ala, Ser-Leu-Tyr-Ala, and Val-Trp) were isolated from the enzymatic hydrolyzates of porcine skeletal muscle (Arihara *et al.*, 2005b). In addition to the bioactive peptides described above, prebiotic (Arihara *et al.*, 2006) and hypocholesterolemic (Morimatsu *et al.*, 1996) peptides have been studied. Apart from bioactivities, meat protein-derived peptides also

Table 21.2 Bioactive peptides derived from meat proteins

Bioactivity	Sequence*	Muscle protein source	References
Antihypertensive	IKW	Chicken muscle protein	Fujita et al., 2000
(ACE inhibitory)	LKA	Chicken muscle creatine kinase	Fujita et al., 2000
	LKP	Chicken muscle aldolase	Fujita et al., 2000
	LAP	Chicken muscle protein	Fujita et al., 2000
	VWI	Porcine muscle actin	Arihara et al., 2005b
	ITTNP	Porcine myosin	Nakashima et al., 2002
	MNPPK	Porcine myosin	Nakashima et al., 2002
	FQKPKR	Chicken muscle myosin	Fujita et al., 2000
	VLAQYK	Bovine muscle protein	Jang and Lee, 2005
	FKGRYYP	Chicken muscle creatine kinase	Fujita et al., 2000
	VFPMNPPK	Fermented pork myosin	Arihara et al., 2004
	IVGRPRHQG	Chicken muscle actin	Fujita et al., 2000
	RMLGQTPTK	Porcine muscle troponin C	Katayama et al., 2003b, 2004
	GFXGTXGLXGF	Chicken muscle collagen	Saiga et al., 2003a
Antioxidative	VW	Porcine muscle	Arihara et al., 2005b
	DLYA	Porcine muscle	Arihara et al., 2005b
	SLYA	Porcine muscle	Arihara et al., 2005b
	DLQEKLE	Porcine muscle actin	Saiga et al., 2003a
Prebiotic	ELM	Porcine muscle	Arihara et al., 2006

* The one-letter amino acid codes were used.

contribute to the organo-leptic properties of meat (Nishimura and Kato, 1988; Nishimura et al., 1988).

Bioactive peptides generated from food proteins, such as milk and soy proteins, have been used as functional ingredients. For example, several food products containing ACE-inhibitory peptides have been marketed for hypertensives (Arihara, 2006b). Although bioactive peptides have not yet been made use of in the meat industry, such peptides are promising candidates for ingredients of functional meat products. Also, bioactive peptides (hydrolyzates) generated from meat proteins could be developed as novel functional food ingredients.

21.4.5 Probiotic and prebiotic meat products

Utilization of probiotics and prebiotics is one of main trends in developing functional foods. In the dairy industry, traditional fermented dairy products have been rediscovered and reborn as functional foods (Farnworth, 2008). The rediscovery of traditional fermented meat products as functional foods is therefore an appropriate and interesting next step in this direction. Although the preservation of meat by fermentation has been carried out for thousands of years and lactic acid starter cultures have been used for dry sausages since the 1950s (Työppönen et al., 2003), probiotics and prebiotics are both relatively new concepts in the meat industry. Ansorena and Astiasarán (2007) described the possibility of the development of novel, healthier, dry-fermented sausages that could minimize the negative features of meat. The following instructions and changes were listed for producing these dry-fermented sausages: (1) modification of mineral content, (2) fat modifications, (3) incorporation of fiber into formulation, and (4) utilization of probiotic bacteria. This section includes a discussion of the potential benefits of probiotics and prebiotics for meat products.

21.4.6   Probiotics and meat fermentation

Probiotics are defined as 'live microorganisms which when administered in adequate amounts confer a health benefit on the host' (Anonymous, 2002). Probiotic bacteria, mainly intestinal *Lactobacillus* and *Bifidobacterium*, show various physiological functions, such as modulation of intestinal flora, prevention of diarrhea, improvement of constipation, lowering faucal enzyme activities, lowering blood cholesterol level, modulation of immune responses, prevention of food allergies, prevention of cancer and act as an adjuvant in *Helicobacter pylori* treatment (Agrawal, 2005; Stanton *et al.*, 2003). Further desirable properties of probiotic strains include their human origin, resistance to acid and bile toxicity, adherence to human intestinal cells, colonization of the human gut, antagonism against pathogenic bacteria, production of antimicrobial substances, immune modulation properties and history of safe use in humans (Brassart and Schiffrin, 2000).

The research and development of meat products with probiotic bacteria has been discussed in recent years (Ammor and Mayo, 2007; Ansorena and Astiasarán, 2007; Arihara, 2004, 2006a, 2006b; Cocconcelli and Fontana, 2008; Hammes *et al.*, 2003; Kröckel, 2006; Leroy *et al.*, 2008; Työppönen *et al.*, 2003; De Vuyst *et al.*, 2008). Promising target meat products with probiotics and prebiotics include fermented sausages (i.e. dry sausages, Fig. 21.5), since such products are processed without heat treatment and probiotic bacteria can survive in the final meat products. Although the market for probiotic meat products is still very limited, some probiotic meat products have already been marketed in Germany and Japan (Arihara, 2006b). A German producer developed a salami product containing intestinal bacterial strains (*Lactobacillus casei, Bifidobacterium* spp.) in 1998. In the same year, a Japanese producer began to market a new type of meat spread product fermented with intestinal lactobacilli (*L. rhamnosus* FERM P-15120). Strain FERM P-15120 has been screened from the collection of human intestinal lactobacilli (Sameshima *et al.*, 1998). Since this strain was resistant to sodium nitrite and sodium chloride and grew at $20\,^{\circ}$C, it was a suitable starting point for the development of further probiotic meat products. This strain also proved resistant to gastric acid and bile while passing through the gastrointestinal tracts.

L. gasseri is one of the predominant lactic acid bacteria in human intestinal tracts, and has been utilized for use in probiotics. *L. gasseri* JCM1131 was shown to be applicable for meat fermentation as a potentially probiotic strain (Arihara *et al.*, 1998). *L. rhamnosus* is also representative of human intestinal lactic acid bacteria and it too has been widely utilized for use in probiotics. For example,

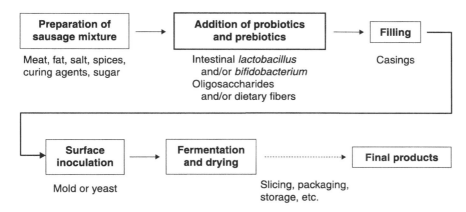

Fig. 21.5   Example of processing scheme for probiotic and prebiotic dry sausages.

products containing *L. rhamnosus* GG strain have been marketed in more than 30 countries. Erkkilä *et al.* (2000, 2001a, 2001b) tested the applicability of probiotic strains *L. rhamnosus* GG, LC-705 and VTT-97800 on dry sausage fermentation with the result that strains GG and E-97800 were found to be suitable for use as probiotic starter cultures in fermenting dry sausage.

Furthermore, several studies have demonstrated the possibility of utilizing probiotic strains of lactic acid bacteria and bifidobacteria for meat products (Klingberg *et al.*, 2005; Klingberg and Budde, 2006; Leroy *et al.*, 2006; Pennacchia, *et al.*, 2004, 2006; Rebucci *et al.*, 2007; Ruiz-Moyano, 2008). Muthukumarasamy and Holly (2006, 2007) studied the effectiveness of a microencapsulation technique for protecting probiotic bacteria during sausage processing. Most studies on the utilization of probiotic strains for meat fermentation have focused on the growth of bacteria in meat and their influence on the sensory properties and inactivation of pathogenic bacteria. Bunte *et al.* (2000) and Jahreis *et al.* (2002) carried out remarkable studies on the utilization of probiotic lactobacilli for fermented sausages. They used healthy volunteers and demonstrated that the ingestion of meat products with probiotic strains of *L. paracasei* LTH2579 had some beneficial physiological effects. The levels of CD4 T helper cells were elevated and the phagocytosis index increased after ingestion of the product.

21.4.7   Prebiotics for meat products

Prebiotic ingredients are added in foods for their nutritional and physiological advantages (Roberfroid, 2008; Tanaka and Sako, 2003). Prebiotics were initially defined as 'non-digestible food ingredients that beneficially affect the host by selectively stimulating the growth and/or activity of one or a limited number of bacteria in the colon and thus improve the health of the host' (Gibson and

Roberfroid, 1995). Later, this definition was updated to 'a selectively fermented ingredient that allows specific changes, both in the composition and/or activity in the gastrointestinal microflora that confers benefits' (Gibson *et al.*, 2004). This change came about after representative prebiotic substances, oligosaccharides and dietary fibers were used to enhance the growth of probiotic bacteria (Holzapfel and Schillinger, 2002; Roberfroid, 2008; Tanaka and Sako, 2003).

In the meat industry, prebiotic ingredients have been used for fat replacement, texture and stability improvement and fiber functionality. The addition of fibers to meat products has been widely practiced (Jiménez-Colmenero *et al.*, 2006) and has been shown to improve the water binding properties, texture and emulsion stability of meat products. Antioxidant dietary fibers (e.g. grape fiber) would also be effective inhibitors of lipid oxidation for meat products (Sáyago-Ayerdi *et al.*, 2009). As described above, most FOSHU products utilize functional ingredients to help in the maintenance of a healthy human body. As an example of FOSHU meat products, a pork Vienna-type sausage product containing indigestible dextrin and a water-soluble dietary fiber made from potato starch, which claims to have beneficial effects on intestinal disorders (prebiotic effect), has now been approved.

In addition to oligosaccharides and dietary fibers, the presence of prebiotic peptides has also been studied (Arihara, 2006a; Liepke *et al.*, 2002). Many studies have shown that hydrolyzates of milk proteins stimulate the growth of lactic acid bacteria (Brody, 2000). However, most of these activities have been estimated to be carbohydrate parts of glycosylated peptides (Idota *et al.*, 1994). Liepke *et al.* (2002) first reported nonglycosylated peptides that selectively stimulate the growth of *Bifidobacterium*. Apart from protein-derived peptides, Etoh *et al.* (2000) discovered a growth-stimulating peptide for *Bifidobacterium bifidum* from natural rubber serum. Arihara *et al.* (2006) found that the hydrolyzate of porcine skeletal muscle proteins enhanced the growth of *Bifidobacterium* strains. One of the corresponding prebiotic peptides was identified as Glu-Leu-Met. Although Glu-Leu-Met showed the growth-promoting activity of *B. bifidum*, neither the dipeptides (Glu-Leu, Leu-Met) or amino acids (Glu, Leu, Met), which are parts of the tripeptide, showed growth-promoting activity.

21.5   Future trends of functional meat products

In recent years, increasing attention has been paid to functional meat products (Arihara, 2004, 2006a, 2006b; Arihara and Ohata, 2008; Fernández-Ginés *et al.*, 2005; Jiménez-Colmenero, 2007a, 2007b; Jiménez-Colmenero *et al.*, 2001, 2006). Since meat and meat products are an important part of the diet in most developed countries, healthier meat and meat products would significantly contribute to human health. Technically, it has already become possible to develop and produce various functional meat products. However, there are still some hurdles in developing and marketing novel functional meat products. For example, many consumers regard meat and meat products as unhealthy, unlike milk and dairy products (Biesalski,

2005). Functional meat products are unconventional for most consumers and further efforts are required to demonstrate the benefits of meat and meat products for human health. Along with the accumulation of scientific evidence, it is important to inform consumers of the exact functional value of meat products.

The utilization of meat-based bioactive compounds, including bioactive peptides generated from meat proteins, is a possible approach for the development of functional meat products. The generation of peptides from meat proteins by proteolytic digestion is also expected for the improvement of their sensory characteristics (Bruna *et al.*, 2000; Toldrá, 2004). An accumulation of bioactive peptides in meat products by fermentation is a good strategy for developing functional meat products. A combination of fermentation by probiotic bacteria and the generation of bioactive peptides would also assist in this.

Gibson and Roberfroid (1995) first proposed the concept of synbiotics, which is a mixture of probiotics and prebiotics. Synbiotics are foods containing both probiotic bacteria and prebiotic substances to provide a diet in which the growth of the probiotic bacteria is enhanced by the prebiotics, thus promoting the chance of the probiotic bacteria becoming established in the gut and conferring a health benefit (Ziemer and Gibson, 1998). Along with probiotics, the uses of prebiotics and synbiotics for the development of novel fermented functional meat products are expected to be explored. Such efforts for developing novel meat products would open up a new market.

21.6   Sources of further information and advice

Further information regarding functional meat products can be obtained from the following articles.

Ansorena D and Astiasarán I (2007), 'Functional meat products', in Toldrá F, *Handbook of Fermented Meat and Poultry*, Hoboken, Wiley-Blackwell, 257–266.

Arihara K (2006), 'Functional properties of bioactive peptides derived from meat proteins', in Nollet L M L and Toldrá F, *Advanced Technologies for Meat Processing*, Boca Raton, CRC Press, 245–274.

Arihara K (2006), 'Strategies for designing novel functional meat products', *Meat Sci*, **74**, 219–229.

Arihara K and Ohata M (2008), 'Bioactive compounds in meat', in Toldrá F, *Meat Biotechnology*, New York, Springer, 231–249.

De Vuyst L, Falony G, and Leroy F (2008), 'Probiotics in fermented sausages', *Meat Sci*, **80**, 75–78.

Fernández-Ginés J M, Fernández-López J, Sayas-Barberá E, and Pérez-Alvarez J A (2005), 'Meat products as functional foods: a review', *J Food Sci*, **70**, R37–43.

Jiménez-Colmenero F (2007a), 'Functional foods based on meat products', in Hui Y H, *Handbook of Food Products Manufacturing – Principles, bakery, beverages, cereals, cheese, confectionary, fats, fruits, and functional foods*, Hoboken, John Wiley & Sons, 989–1015.

Jiménez-Colmenero F (2007b), 'Healthier lipid formulation approaches in meat-based functional foods. Technological options for replacement of meat fats by non-meat fats', *Trends Food Sci Technol*, **18**, 567–578.

Jiménez-Colmenero F, Reig M, and Toldrá F (2006), 'New approaches for the development of functional meat products', in Nollet L M L and Toldrá F, *Advanced Technologies for Meat Processing*, Boca Raton, CRC Press, 275–308.

21.7 References

Agrawal R (2005), 'Probiotics: an emerging food supplement with health benefits', *Food Biotechnol*, **19**, 227–246.

Alonso L, Cuesta E P, and Gilliland S E (2003), 'Production of free linoleic acid by *Lactobacillus acidophilus* and *Lactobacillus casei* of human intestinal origin', *J Dairy Sci*, **86**, 1941–1946.

Ammor M S and Mayo B (2007), 'Selection criteria for lactic acid bacteria to be used as functional starter cultures in dry sausage production: an update', *Meat Sci*, **76**, 138–146.

Anonymous (2002), 'Guidelines for the evaluation of probiotics in food', Report of a joint FAO/WHO working group on drafting guidelines for the evaluation of probiotics in food, London and Ontario, 30 April and 1 May 2002.

Ansorena D and Astiasarán I (2007), 'Functional meat products', in Toldrá F, *Handbook of Fermented Meat and Poultry*, Hoboken, Wiley-Blackwell, 257–266.

Arihara K (2004), 'Functional Foods', in Jensen W K, Devine C, and Dikeman M, *Encyclopedia of Meat Sciences*, Oxford, Elsevier, 492–499.

Arihara K (2006a), 'Functional properties of bioactive peptides derived from meat proteins', in Nollet L M L and Toldrá F, *Advanced Technologies for Meat Processing*, Boca Raton, CRC Press, 245–274.

Arihara K (2006b), 'Strategies for designing novel functional meat products', *Meat Sci*, **74**, 219–229.

Arihara K and Ohata M (2008), 'Bioactive compounds in meat', in Toldrá F, *Meat Biotechnology*, New York, Springer, 231–249.

Arihara K, Ota H, Itoh M, Kondo Y, Sameshima T, *et al.* (1998), '*Lactobacillus acidophilus* group lactic acid bacteria applied to meat fermentation', *J Food Sci*, **63**, 544–547.

Arihara K, Nakashima Y, Mukai T, Ishikawa S, and Itoh M (2001), 'Peptide inhibitors for angiotensin I-converting enzyme from enzymatic hydrolysates of porcine skeletal muscle proteins', *Meat Sci*, **57**, 319–324.

Arihara K, Nakashima Y, Ishikawa S, and Itoh M (2004), 'Antihypertensive activities generated from porcine skeletal muscle proteins by lactic acid bacteria', in *Abstracts of 50th International Congress of Meat Science and Technology*, August 2004, Helsinki, Finland, p. 236.

Arihara K, Ishikawa S, Itoh M, Akimoto M, Nakashima Y, and Kanai S (2005a), 'Antihypertensive peptides derived from meat proteins', *Japan patent* (No. 2005-175085).

Arihara K, Tomita K, Ishikawa S, Itoh M, Akimoto M, and Sameshima T (2005b), 'Anti-fatigue peptides derived from meat proteins', *Japan patent* (No. 2005-234407).

Arihara K, Ishikawa S, and Itoh M (2006), '*Bifidobacterium* growth promoting peptides derived from meat proteins', *Japan patent* (No. 2006-8738).

Azain M J (2003), 'Conjugated linoleic acid and its effects on animal products and health in single-stomached animals', *Proceed Nutr Soc*, **62**, 319–328.

Barberá E S (2008), 'The use of olive oil in processing meat products', in Fernández-López J, *Technological Strategies for Functional Meat Products Development*, Kerala, India, Transworld Research Network, 139–162.

Biesalski H-K (2005), 'Meat as a component of a healthy diet – are there any risks or benefits if meat is avoided in the diet?', *Meat Sci*, **70**, 509–524.

Brassart D and Schiffrin E J (2000), 'Pre- and probiotics', in Schmidl M K and Labuza T P, *Essentials of Functional Foods*, Gaithersburg, Aspen Publication, 205–216.

Brody E P (2000), 'Biological activities of bovine glycomacropeptide', *Br J Nutr*, **84**, S39–46.

Brown C E (1981), 'Interactions among carnosine, anserine, ophidine and copper in biochemical adaptation', *J Theor Biol*, **88**, 245–256.

Bruna J M, Fernandez M, Hierro E M, Ordonez J A, and de la Hoz L (2000), 'Combined use of pronase E and a fungal extract (*Penicillium aurantiogriseum*) to potentiate the sensory characteristics of dry fermented sausages', *Meat Sci*, **54**, 135–145.

Bunte C, Hertel C, and Hammes W P (2000), 'Monitoring and survival of *Lactobacillus paracasei* LTH2579 in food and the human intestinal tract', *Syst Appl Microbiol*, **23**, 260–266.

Chan W (2004), 'Macronutrients in meat', in Jensen W K, Devine C, and Dikeman M, *Encyclopedia of Meat Sciences*, Oxford, Elsevier, 614–618.

Chao A, Thun M J, Connell C J, McCullough M L, Jacobs E J, *et al.* (2005), 'Meat consumption and risk of colorectal cancer', *J Am Med Assoc*, **293**, 172–182.

Coakley M, Ross R P, Nordgren M, Fitzerald G, Devery R, and Stanton C (2003), 'Conjugated linoleic acid biosynthesis by human-derived *Bifidobacterium* species', *J Appl Microbiol*, **94**, 138–145.

Cocconcelli P S and Fontana C (2008), 'Characteristics and applications of microbial starters in meat fermentation', in Toldrá F, *Meat Biotechnology*, New York, Springer, 129–148.

Decker E A, Livisay S A, and Zhou S (2000), 'Mechanisms of endogenous skeletal muscle antioxidants: chemical and physical aspects', in Decker E A, Faustman C, and Lopez-Bote C J, *Antioxidants in Muscle Foods*, New York, Wiley-Interscience, 25–60.

De Vuyst L, Falony G, and Leroy F (2008), 'Probiotics in fermented sausages', *Meat Sci*, **80**, 75–78.

Dhiman T R, Nam S H, and Ure A L (2005), 'Factors affecting conjugated linoleic acid content in milk and meat', *Crit Rev Food Sci Nutr*, **45**, 463–482.

Dransfield E and Etherington D (1981), 'Enzymes in the tenderization of meat', in Nagodawithana T and Reed G, *Enzymes and Food Processing*, London, Applied Science Publishers, 177–194.

Erkkilä S, Venäläinen M, Hielm S, Petäjä E, Puolanne E, and Mattila-Sandholm T (2000), 'Survival of *Escherichia coli* O157:H7 in dry sausage fermented by probiotic lactic acid bacteria', *J Sci Food Agric*, **80**, 2101–2104.

Erkkilä S, Suihko M-L, Eerola S, Petäjä E, and Mattila-Sandholm T (2001a), 'Dry sausages fermented by *Lactobacillus rhamnosus* strains', *Int J Food Microbiol*, **64**, 205–210.

Erkkilä S, Petäjä E, Eerola S, Lilleberg L, Mattila-Sandholm T, and Suihko M-L (2001b), 'Flavour profiles of dry sausages fermented by selected novel meat starter cultures', *Meat Sci*, **58**, 111–116.

Etherington D J (1984), 'The contribution of proteolytic enzymes to postmortem changes in muscle', *J Anim Sci*, **59**, 1644–1650.

Etoh S, Asamura K, Obu A, Sonomoto K, and Ishizaki A (2000), 'Purification and identification of a growth-stimulating peptide for Bifidobacterium bifidum from natural rubber serum powder', *Biosci Biotechnol Biochem*, **64**, 2083–2088.

Farnworth E R (2008), *Handbook of Fermented Functional Foods* (2nd edition). Boca Raton, CRC Press.

Fernández-Ginés J M, Fernández-López J, Sayas-Barberá E, and Pérez-Alvarez J A (2005), 'Meat products as functional foods: a review', *J Food Sci*, **70**, R37–43.

Fiocchi A, Restani P, and Riva E (2000), 'Beef allergy in children', *Nutrition*, **16**, 454–457.

Fujita H, Yokoyama K, and Yoshikawa M (2000), 'Classification and antihypertensive activity of angiotensin I-converting enzyme inhibitory peptides derived from food proteins', *J Food Sci*, **65**, 564–569.

Gibson G R and Roberfroid M B (1995), 'Dietary modulation of the human colonic microbiota: introducing the concept of prebiotics', *J Nutr*, **125**, 1401–1412.

Gibson G R, Probert H M, Van Loo J A E, Rastall R A, and Roberfroid M B (2004), 'Dietary modulation of the human colonic microflora: Updating the concept of prebiotics', *Nutr Res Rev*, **17**, 259–275.

Gnadig S, Xue Y, Berdeaux O, Chardigny J M, and Sebedio J-L (2000), 'Conjugated linoleic acid (CLA) as a functional ingredient', in Mattila-Sandholm T and Saarela M, *Functional Dairy Products*, Boca Raton, CRC Press, 263–298.

Gobbetti M, Minervini F, and Rizzello C G (2007), 'Bioactive peptides in dairy products', in Hui Y H, *Handbook of Food Products Manufacturing – Health, meat, milk, poultry, seafood, and vegetables*, Hoboken, John Wiley & Sons, 489–517.

Hammes W P, Haller D, and Gänzle M G (2003), 'Fermented meat', in Farnworth E R, *Handbook of Fermented Functional Foods*, Boca Raton, CRC Press, 251–275.

Han G D, Matsuo M, Ikeuchi Y, and Suzuki A (2002), 'Effects of heat and high-pressure treatments on high-pressure treatments on antigenicity of beef extract', *Biosci Biotechnol Biochem*, **66**, 202–205.

Hasler C M (1988), 'Functional foods: their role in disease prevention and health promotion', *Food Technol*, **52**(10), 63–70.

Herzallah S M, Humeid M A, and Al-Ismail K M (2005), 'Effects of heating and processing methods of milk and dairy products on conjugated linoleic acid and trans fatty acid isomer content', *J Dairy Sci*, **88**, 1301–1310.

Hierro E, de la Hoz L, and Ordonez J A (1999), 'Contribution of the microbial and meat endogenous enzymes to the free amino acid and amine contents of dry fermented sausages', *J Agric Food Chem*, **47**, 1156–1161.

Higgs J D (2000), 'The changing nature of red meat: 20 years of improving nutritional quality', *Trend Food Sci Technol*, **11**, 85–95.

Holzapfel W H and Schillinger U (2002), 'Introduction to pre- and probiotics', *Food Res Int*, **35**, 109–116.

Idota T, Kawakami H, Nakajima I (1994), 'Growth-promoting effects of N-acetyl-neuraminic acid containing substances on bifidobacteria', *Biosci Biotechnol Biochem*, **58**, 1720–1722.

Iikura Y, Imai Y, Akasawa A, Fujita K, Hoshiyama K, *et al.* (1999), 'Frequency of immediate-type food allergy in children in Japan', *Int Arch Aller Immun*, **16**, 454–457.

Jahreis G, Vogelsang H, Kiessling G, Schubert R, Bunte C, and Hammes W P (2002), 'Influence of probiotic sausage (*Lactobacillus paracasei*) on blood lipids and immunological parameters of healthy volunteers', *Food Res Int*, **35**, 133–138.

Jang A and Lee M (2005), 'Purification and identification of angiotensin converting enzyme inhibitory peptides from beef hydrolysates', *Meat Sci*, **69**, 653–661.

Jiménez-Colmenero F (2007a), 'Functional foods based on meat products', in Hui Y H, *Handbook of Food Products Manufacturing – Principles, bakery, beverages, cereals, cheese, confectionary, fats, fruits, and functional foods*, Hoboken, John Wiley & Sons, 989–1015.

Jiménez-Colmenero F (2007b), 'Healthier lipid formulation approaches in meat-based functional foods. Technological options for replacement of meat fats by non-meat fats', *Trends Food Sci Technol*, **18**, 567–578.

Jiménez-Colmenero F, Carballo J, and Cofrades S (2001), 'Healthier meat and meat products: their role as functional foods', *Meat Sci*, **59**, 5–13.

Jiménez-Colmenero F, Reig M, and Toldrá F (2006), 'New approaches for the development of functional meat products', in Nollet L M L and Toldrá F, *Advanced Technologies for Meat Processing*, Boca Raton, CRC Press, 275–308.

Katayama K, Fuchu H, Sakata A, Kawahara S, Yamauchi K, *et al.* (2003a), 'Angiotensin I-converting enzyme inhibitory activities of porcine skeletal muscle proteins following enzyme digestion', *Asian-Aust J Anim Sci*, **16**, 417–424.

Katayama K, Tomatsu M, Fuchu H, Sugiyama M, Kawahara S, *et al.* (2003b), 'Purification and characterization of an angiotensin I-converting enzyme inhibitory peptide derived from porcine troponin C', *Anim Sci J*, **74**, 53–58.

Katayama K, Tomatsu M, Kawahara S, Yamauchi K, Fuchu H, *et al.* (2004), 'Inhibitory profile of nonapeptide derived from porcine troponin C against angiotensin I-converting enzyme', *J Agric Food Chem*, **52**, 771–775.

Klingberg T D and Budde B B (2006), 'The survival and persistence in the human gastrointestinal tract of five potential probiotic lactobacilli consumed as freeze-dried cultures or as probiotic sausage', *Int J Food Microbiol*, **109**, 157–159.

Klingberg T D, Axelsson L, Naterstad K, Elsser D, and Budde B B (2005), 'Identification of potential probiotic starter cultures for Scandinavian-type fermented sausages', *Int J Food Microbiol*, **105**, 419–431.

Koohmaraie M (1994), 'Muscle proteinases and meat aging', *Meat Sci*, **36**, 93–104.

Korhonen H and Pihlanto A (2003), 'Food-derived bioactive peptides: opportunities for designing future foods', *Cur Pharm Des*, **9**, 1297–1308.

Korhonen H and Pihlanto A (2007), 'Bioactive peptides from food proteins', in Hui Y H, *Handbook of Food Products Manufacturing – Health, meat, milk, poultry, seafood, and vegetables*, Hoboken, John Wiley & Sons, 5–37.

Krajcovicova-Kudlackova M, Simoncic R, Bederova A, Babinska K, and Beder I (2000), 'Correlation of carnitine levels to methionine and lysine intake', *Phys Res*, **49**, 399–402.

Kröckel L (2006), 'Use of probiotic bacteria in meat products', *Fleischwirtschaft*, **86**, 109–113.

Lachance P A and Fisher M C (2005), 'Reinvention of the food guide pyramid to promote health', *Adv Food Nutr Res*, **49**, 1–39.

Langseth L (2000), 'Antioxidants and their effect on health', in Schmidl M K and Labuza T P, *Essentials of Functional Foods*, Gaithersburg, Aspen Publication, 303–317.

Larsson S C, Bergkvist L, and Wolk A (2005), 'High-fat dairy food and conjugated linoleic acid intakes in relation to colorectal cancer incidence in the Swedish Mammography Cohort', *Am J Clin Nutr*, **82**, 894–900.

Lawrie R A and Ledward D A (2006), 'Meat and human nutrition', in Lawrie R A and Ledward D A, *Lawrie's Meat Science*, Boca Raton, CRC Press, 342–357.

Leroy F, Verluyten L, and De Vuyst L (2006), 'Functional meat starter cultures for improved sausage fermentation', *Int J Food Microbiol*, **106**, 270–285.

Leroy F, Falony G, and De Vuyst L (2008), 'Latest developments in probiotics', in Toldrá F, *Meat Biotechnology*, New York, Springer, 217–229.

Liepke C, Adermann K, Raida M, Magert H-J, Forssman W-G, and Zucht H-D (2002), 'Human milk provides peptides highly stimulating the growth of bifidobacteria', *Eur J Biochem*, **269**, 712–718.

Lindsay D G (2000), 'Maximizing the functional benefits of plants foods', in Gibson G R and Williams C M, *Functional Foods*, Boca Raton, CRC Press, 183–208.

Lorenzen C L, Golden J W, Martz F A, Grün I U, Ellersieck M R, *et al.* (2007), 'Conjugated linoleic acid content of beef differs by feeding regime and muscle', *Meat Sci*, **75**, 159–167.

MacIntosh M and Le Leu R K (2001), 'The influence of dietary proteins on colon cancer risks', *Nutr Res*, **21**, 1053–1066.

Meisel H, Walsh D J, Murry B, and FitzGerald R J (2005), 'ACE inhibitory peptides', in Mine Y and Shahidi F, *Nutraceutical Proteins and Peptides in Health and Disease*, Boca Raton, CRC Press, 269–315.

Mikami M, Nagao M, Sekikawa M, and Miura H (1995), 'Changes in peptide and free amino acid contents of different bovine muscle homogenate during storage', *Anim Sci Technol (Japan)*, **66**, 630–638.

Mine Y and Shahidi F (2005), *Nutraceutical Proteins and Peptides in Health and Disease*, Boca Raton, CRC Press.

Mir P S, McAllister T A, Scott S, Aalhus J, Baron V, *et al.* (2004), 'Conjugated linoleic acid-enriched beef production', *Am J Clin Nutr*, **79**, S1207–1211.

Mora L, Sentandreu M A and Toldrá F (2007), 'Hydrophilic chromatographic determination of carnosine, anserine, balenine, creatine, and creatinine', *J Agric Food Chem*, **55**, 4664–4669.

Morimatsu F, Ito M, Budijanto S, Watanabe I, Furukawa Y, and Kimura S (1996), 'Plasma cholesterol-suppressing effect of papain-hydrolyzed pork meat in rats fed hypercholesterolemic diet', *J Nutr Sci Vitaminol*, **42**, 145–153.

Mulvihill B (2004), 'Micronutrients in meat', in Jensen W K, Devine C, and Dikeman M, *Encyclopedia of Meat Sciences*, Oxford, Elsevier, 618–623.

Muthukumarasamy P and Holley R A (2006), 'Microbiological and sensory quality of dry fermented sausages containing alginate-microencapsulated *Lactobacillus reuteri*', *Int J Food Microbiol*, **111**, 164–169.

Muthukumarasamy P and Holley R A (2007), 'Survival of *Escherichia coli* O157:H7 in dry fermented sausages containing micro-encapsulated probiotic lactic acid bacteria', *Food Microbiol*, **24**, 82–88.

Nagao K and Yanagita T (2005), 'Conjugated fatty acids in food and their health benefits', *J Biosci Bioeng*, **100**, 152–157.

Nakashima Y, Arihara K, Sasaki A, Ishikawa S, and Itoh M (2002), 'Antihypertensive activities of peptides derived from porcine skeletal muscle myosin in spontaneously hypertensive rats', *J Food Sci*, **67**, 434–437.

Nishimura T and Kato H (1988), 'Mechanisms involved in the improvement of meat taste during postmortem aging', *Food Sci Technol Int Tokyo*, **4**, 241–249.

Nishimura T, Rhue M R, Okitani A, and Kato H (1988), 'Components contributing to the improvement of meat taste during storage', *Agric Biol Chem*, **52**, 2323–2330.

Ovesen L (2004a), 'Cardiovascular and obesity health concerns', in Jensen W K, Devine C, and Dikeman M, *Encyclopedia of Meat Sciences*, Oxford, Elsevier, 623–628.

Ovesen L (2004b), 'Cancer health concerns', in Jensen W K, Devine C, and Dikeman M, *Encyclopedia of Meat Sciences*, Oxford, Elsevier, 628–633.

Pariza M W, Loretz L J, Storkson J M, and Holland N C (1983), 'Mutagens and modulator of mutagenesis in fried ground beef', *Cancer Res*, **43** (Suppl.), S2444–2446.

Park Y J, Volpe S L, and Decker E A (2005), 'Quantitation of carnosine in humans plasma after dietary consumption of beef', *J Agric Food Chem*, **53**, 736–739.

Pennacchia C, Ercolini D, Blaiotta G, Pepe O, Mauriello G, and Villani F (2004), 'Selection of *Lactobacillus* strains from fermented sausages for their potential use as probiotics', *Meat Sci*, **67**, 309–317.

Pennacchia C, Vaughan E E, and Villani F (2006), 'Potential probiotic *Lactobacillus* strains from fermented sausages: further investigations on their probiotic properties', *Meat Sci*, **73**, 90–101.

Pihlanto A and Korhonen H (2003), 'Bioactive peptides and proteins', *Adv Food Nutr Res*, **47**, 175–276.

Pszczola D E, Katz F, and Giese J (2002), 'Research trends in healthful foods', *Food Technol*, **54**(10), 45–52.

Rebucci R, Sangalli L, Fava M, Bersani C, Cantoni C, and Baldi A (2007), 'Evaluation of functional aspects in *Lactobacillus* strains isolated from dry fermented sausages', *J Food Qual*, **30**, 187–201.

Roberfroid M B (2008), 'Prebiotics: concept, definition, criteria, methodologies, and products', in Gibson G R and Roberfroid M B, *Handbook of Prebiotics*, Boca Raton, CRC Press, 39–68.

Ruiz-Moyano S, Martin A, Benito M J, Nevado F P, and De Guia Coordo B A M (2008), 'Screening of lactic acid bacteria and bifidobacteria for potential probiotic use in Iberian dry fermented sausages', *Meat Sci*, **80**, 715–721.

Ruusunen M and Puolanne E (2005), 'Reducing sodium intake from meat products', *Meat Sci*, **70**, 531–541.

Saiga A, Okumura T, Makihara T, Katsuta S, Shimizu T, *et al.* (2003a), 'Angiotensin I-converting enzyme inhibitory peptides in a hydrolyzed chicken breast muscle extract', *J Agric Food Chem*, **51**, 1741–1745.

Saiga A, Tanabe S, and Nishimura T (2003b), 'Antioxidant activity of peptides obtained from porcine myofibrillar proteins by protease treatment', *J Agric Food Chem*, **51**, 3661–3667.

Sameshima T, Magome C, Takeshita K, Arihara K, Itoh M, and Kondo Y (1998), 'Effect of intestinal *Lactobacillus* starter cultures on the behaviour of *Staphylococcus aureus* in fermented sausage', *Int J Food Microbiol*, **41**, 1–7.

Sayago-Ayerdi S G, Brenes A, and Goni I (2009), 'Effect of grape antioxidant dietary fiber on the lipid oxidation of raw and cooked chicken hamburgers', LWT-Food Sci Technol, **42**, 971–976.

Sentandreu M A and Toldrá F (2007a) 'Oligopeptides hydrolysed by muscle dipeptidyl peptidases can generate angiotensin-I converting enzyme inhibitory dipeptides', *Eur Food Res Technol*, **224**, 785–790.

Sentandreu M A and Toldrá F (2007b) 'Evaluation of ACE inhibitory activity of dipeptides generated by the action of porcine muscle dipeptidyl peptidases', *Food Chem*, **102**, 511–515.

Sentandreu M A, Stoeva S, Aristoy M C, Laib K, Voelter W, and Toldrá F (2003), 'Identification of small peptides generated in Spanish dry-cured ham', *J Food Sci*, **68**, 64–69.

Shimada K, Sakura Y, Fukushima M, Sekikawa M, Kuchida K, and Mikami M (2005), 'Species and muscle differences in L-carnitine levels in skeletal muscles based on a new simple assay', *Meat Sci*, **68**, 357–362.

Sieber R, Collomb M, Aeschlimann A, Jelen P, and Eyer H. (2004), 'Impact of microbial cultures on conjugated linoleic acid in dairy products – a review', *Int Dairy J*, **14**, 1–15.

Sloan A E (2008), 'The top 10 functional food trends', *Food Technol*, **62**(4), 25–44.

Stanton C, Desmond C, Coakley M, Collins J K, Fitzgerald G, and Ross P, (2003), 'Challenges facing development of probiotic-containing functional foods', in Farnworth E R, *Handbook of Fermented Functional Foods*, Boca Raton, CRC Press, 27–58.

Tanabe S and Nishimura T (2005), 'Meat allergy', in Mine Y and Shahidi F, *Nutraceutical Proteins and Peptides in Health and Disease*, Boca Raton, CRC Press, 482–491.

Tanaka R and Sako T (2003), 'Prebiotics', in Roginski H, Fuquay J W and Fox P F, *Encyclopedia of Dairy Sciences*, London, Academic Press, 2256–2276.

Toldrá F (2004), 'Dry', in Jensen W K, Devine C, and Dikeman M, *Encyclopedia of Meat Sciences*, Oxford, Elsevier, 360–365.

Toldrá F (2007), 'Biochemistry of meat and fat', in Toldrá F, *Handbook of Fermented Meat and Poultry*, Hoboken, Wiley-Blackwell, 51–58.

Työppönen S, Petäjä E, and Mattila-Sandholm T (2003), 'Bioprotectives and probiotics for dry sausages (review)', *Int J Food Microbiol*, **83**, 233–244.

Valsta L M, Tapanainen H, and Mannisto S (2005), 'Meat fats in nutrition', *Meat Sci*, **70**, 525–530.

Vercruysse L, Van Camp J, and Smagghe G (2005), 'ACE inhibitory peptides derived from enzymatic hydrolysates of animal protein: a review', *J Agric Food Chem*, **53**, 8106–8115.

Vermeirssen V, Camp J V, and Verstraete W (2004), 'Bioavailability of angiotensin I converting enzyme inhibitory peptide (review article)', *Br J Nutr*, **92**, 357–366.

Vescovo G, Ravara B, Gobbo V, Sandri M, Angelini A, Dalla Libera L (2002), 'L-Carnitine: A potential treatment for blocking apotosis and preventing skeletal muscle myopathy in heart failure', *Am J Physiol*, **283**, C802–810.

Watkins B A and Yong L (2001), 'Conjugated linoleic acid: the present state of knowledge', in Wildman R E C, *Handbook of Nutraceuticals and Functional Foods*, Boca Raton, CRC Press, 445–476.

Williams P G (2007), 'Nutritional composition of red meat', *Nutr Diet*, **64** (Suppl 4), S113–119.

Xu S, Boylston T D, and Glatz B A (2005), 'Conjugated linoleic acid content and organoleptic attributes of fermented milk products produced with probiotic bacteria', *J Agric Food Chem*, **53**, 9064–9072.

Ziemer C J and Gibson G R (1998), 'An overview of probiotics, prebiotics and synbiotics in the functional food concept: perspectives and future strategies', *Int Dairy J*, **8**, 473–479.

22

Functional soy products

C. W. Xiao, Health Canada and University of Ottawa, Canada

Abstract: Consumption of soy foods has a long history and is becoming increasingly popular. This chapter has summarized the current status of soy consumption worldwide, soybean composition, and potential bioactive components. The major functional soy foods including fermented soybeans natto, γ-aminobutyric acid-enriched tempeh-like (GABA-tempeh), aglycone-rich functional soy beverages, soy yogurt, glyceollins-enriched soy yogurt, monascus-fermented soybean extract, okara-based soy foods, functional soy peptides, and their potential health benefits have been reviewed. The safety concerns such as estrogenic, anti-estrogenic effects and anti-thyroid actions of soy as well as future trends in research and development of functional soy foods have also been discussed.

Key words: soy food, phytoestrogen, health effects, chronic disease, safety.

22.1 Introduction

Soy foods have been consumed for more than 1000 years in Asian countries. Soybean is one of the most predominant legumes cultivated worldwide. Because of their potential health benefits, consumption of soy foods/products is steadily rising in last two decades, especially in Western countries. In particular, a dramatic increase occurred after the approval of a food labeling health claim for soy proteins in the reduction of heart disease risk by the US Food and Drug administration in 1999 (US Food and Drug Administration, 1999). Similar health claims have also been approved by other countries including Japan, the United Kingdom, South Africa, the Philippines, Brazil, Indonesia, Korea and Malaysia to date (Xiao, 2008).

Traditional soy foods can be divided into fermented and nonfermented groups by their preparation. Nonfermented soy foods include fresh green soybeans, whole dry soybeans, soy nuts, soy sprouts, whole-fat soy flour, soy milk, tofu, soy-based infant formulas, okara and yuba. Fermented soy foods include tempeh, miso, soy sauces, natto and fermented tofu and soy milk products (Golbitz, 1995).

To satisfy the taste of Western consumers, many 'Western-style' soy foods have been developed, such as tofu hot dogs, tofu ice cream, veggie burgers, tempeh burgers, soy yogurt, soy cheeses, and soy pancake mix.

Soy proteins and their associated isoflavones as well as soy oil are the most studied components in soybeans and their products for the potential effects on human health. According to epidemiological investigations and clinical trials, a variety of health benefits have been linked to consumption of soy foods, and are particularly attributable to the proteins and isoflavones. Additionally, fermented soy foods have additive beneficial effects than nonfermented ones because of the novel bioactive components produced during bacterial fermentations. This chapter will mainly focus on the soy foods containing known component(s) with bioactive functions and having potentials to be used in the prevention and treatment of human diseases.

22.2   Major compositions of soybeans

Dry soybean contains about 35–40% protein, 19% oil, 28% carbohydrate including 17% dietary fibre, 5% minerals and vitamins. Soy proteins are mainly comprised of two storage globulins, 11S glycinin and 7S β-conglycinin (Torres et al., 2006). Glycinin has 5 subunits, G1, G2, G3, G4, and G5, and each subunit contains two polypeptide chains – A (acidic) and B (basic) – while β-conglycinin has α, α' and β subunits. These proteins contain all amino acids essential to human nutrition, which makes soy products almost equivalent to animal sources in protein quality but with less saturated fat, no cholesterol and lactose (Young, 1991).

Isoflavones (ISF) are one of the most studied bioactive compounds and are closely associated with the proteins in soybeans. ISF are major soy phytoestrogens present in soy foods (Anthony et al., 1996). Soy foods and soy-based infant formulas are rich sources of ISF and contain about 1–4.2 mg ISF/g, while soy ISF supplements contain up to 500 mg ISF/g. Genistin, daidzin and glycitein are the main soy ISF. Both genistin and daidzin are present as glycosides in soybeans and in most soy foods consumed in the Western countries. Glycoside ISF are difficult to absorb unless hydrolysed and converted to the bioactive aglycones, genistein and daidzein, by intestinal microbiota or in vitro fermentation (Miniello et al., 2003).

22.3   Soy consumption in different populations

Soy consumptions are quite variable among different populations. The average daily intakes of soy are around 30 g in Japan, 20 g in Korea, 10 g in Hong Kong, 8 g in China, and <1 g in the United States. The average ISF consumptions are 50–100 mg/day in Asian countries, 1–2 mg/day in the US and Canada, <1 mg/day in UK and 28–47 mg/day in four-month-old infants fed soy formulas.

Average plasma concentrations of ISF are: 1640 nmol/L for genistein, 1160 nmol/L for daidzein in infants fed soy formulas (Setchell et al., 1997);

492.7 nmol/L for genistein, 282.5 nmol/L for daidzein in Japanese men; and 33.2 nmol/L for genistein, 17.9 nmol/L for daidzein in British men (Morton *et al.*, 2002). These data indicate that soy formula-fed infants are a group exposed to the highest amount of soy ISF.

22.4   Functional soy foods

Many traditional soy foods were made by fermentation with different bacteria. During fermentations, enzymes produced by bacteria can hydrolyse soy proteins or ISF glycosides into peptides or ISF aglycones. Many of these peptides and ISF aglycones can be absorbed into blood stream and function as hormones, growth factors or cytokines through receptor-dependent or independent mechanisms. Moreover, these bacteria can also synthesize and release bioactive components such as menaquinone-7, nattokinase, dipicolinic acid and γ-aminobutyric acid into the fermented products, which play important roles in modulating human physiological functions. This section will describe the major functional soy foods including fermented soybeans natto, tempeh, aglycone-rich functional soy beverages and pasta, Monascus-fermented soybean extract (MFSE), functional soy yogurts, okara-based soy foods and functional soy-derived bioactive peptides.

22.4.1   Natto

Natto is a traditional Japanese soy food made from boiled or steamed soybeans through salt-free fermentation with *Bacillus subtilis* (natto). A variety of substances with different biological effects can be produced during fermentation, which makes the fermented soybeans very different from original beans in many aspects.

Menaquinone-7 and bone health
In the process of natto fermentation, *Bacillus subtilis* (natto), a Gram-positive endospore-forming bacterium, can synthesize menaquinone-7 (MK-7) that is a type of vitamin K2. Vitamin K2 is a cofactor of γ-glutamyl carboxylase, a key enzyme responsible for the conversion of undercarboxylated osteocalcin to carboxylated osteocalcin by transforming the glutamyl residues of osteocalcin into carboxyglutamic acid residues; carboxylated osteocalcin has a high affinity for calcium ions in hydroxyapatite and regulates the growth of these crystals. Therefore, vitamin K plays an important role in the regulation of bone metabolism and prevention of osteoporosis. The content of MK-7 in natto is over 100 times more than in various kinds of cheese (Table 22.1) (Kamao *et al.*, 2007).

The beneficial effects of MK-7 from natto or supplementation on bone metabolism and prevention of bone loss have been demonstrated in both humans and animal studies. For instance, feeding ovariectomized (OVX) rats the diets containing MK-7 remarkably increased serum and femoral MK-7 levels and prevented OVX-induced decrease in the femoral dry weight and calcium content. Intake of natto without or with added MK-7 also significantly elevated serum

Table 22.1 Menaquinone-7 contents in several food items

Food item	MK-7 (μg/100 g)
Pulses	
Cotton tofu (hard type)	N.D.
Silken tofu (soft type)	N.D.
Deep-fried bean curd	N.D.
Natto (fermented soybeans)	939 ± 753
Hikiwari natto (chopped natto)	827 ± 194
Black bean natto	796 ± 93
Milk and dairy products	
Whole milk	N.D.
Cream	N.D.
Yogurt, plain (whole-milk type)	0.1 ± 0.2
Processed cheese	0.3 ± 0.1

N.D., not detectable.
Adapted from Kamao *et al.* (2007).

MK-7 concentrations, prevented the OVX-induced decreases in the femoral dry weight and calcium content (Yamaguchi *et al.*, 1999) and significantly prevented the decrease in serum γ-carboxylated osteocalcin concentration and mineral density induced by OVX (Tsukamoto 2004; Yamaguchi *et al.*, 2000).

In addition, intake of natto or MK-7 may also play a role in preventing the bone deterioration caused by aging. It has been shown that presence of MK-7 significantly prevented the reduction of bone formation biomarkers including calcium content, alkaline phosphatase activity and deoxyribonucleic acid (DNA) in the cultured femoral-diaphyseal and -metaphyseal tissues obtained from elderly female rats (50-week-old) (Yamaguchi *et al.*, 2002). On the other hand, MK-7 completely inhibited the decrease in calcium content and suppressed the formation of the osteoclast-like multinucleated cells (Yamaguchi and Ma, 2001) in the bone tissues induced by the bone-resorbing factor, parathyroid hormone (PTH) and prostaglandin E(2) (PGE2) (Tsukamoto, 2004). These findings suggest that MK-7 may have a dual role in the regulation of bone metabolism: stimulating bone formation and suppressing bone degeneration.

In the postmenopausal women, the total hip bone mineral density (BMD) and the rates of changes in BMD at the femoral neck and at the distal third of the radius were positively associated with natto intake. However, the other soybean products did not have the same effects. Therefore, natto intake may help prevent postmenopausal bone loss through the effects of MK-7 or bioavailable isoflavones, which are more abundant in natto than in other soybean products (Ikeda *et al.*, 2006). Interestingly, the serum vitamin K2 (menaquinone-7; MK-7) levels in postmenopausal women show a large geographic difference in Japan and are associated with the amount of natto consumption. Moreover, the incidence of hip fractures in women and natto consumption in each prefecture throughout Japan are strongly negatively correlated. These findings suggest the possibility that higher MK-7 level resulting from natto consumption may contribute to the relatively lower fracture risk (Kaneki *et al.*, 2001). In healthy premenopausal women, intake of natto for one year significantly increased bone specific alkaline phosphatase (BAP), an indicator of bone formation, and decreased undercarboxylated osteocalcin (Katsuyama *et al.*, 2004). In the normal males, dietary intake of MK-7 or occasional or frequent intake of natto significantly increased serum MK-7 and γ-carboxylated osteocalcin concentrations (Tsukamoto *et al.*, 2000).

Nattokinase and fibrinolytic activity

Nattokinase (NK) is a potent fibrinolytic (clot dissolving) enzyme discovered in natto by Dr. Hiroyuki Sumi in the 1980s. It is an extracellular enzyme secreted by *B. subtilis* natto (Sumi *et al.*, 1987). The fibrinolytic activity of NK is four times greater than that of plasmin, a major enzyme responsible for lysis of blood clot (Fujita *et al.*, 1995). This novel enzyme can be easily extracted with saline, and consists of 275 amino acid residues. Its molecular weight is 27.7 kDa and pI = 8.6. NK is a subtilisin-like serine protease and exhibits 99.5% homology with subtilisin E in their DNA sequences (Nakamura *et al.*, 1992). NK not only digested fibrin but also the plasmin substrate H-D-Val-Leu-Lys-pNA (S-2251) (Sumi *et al.*, 1987).

Oral administration of NK (or natto) enhanced the fibrinolytic activity in the plasma and increased the production of tissue plasminogen activator (t-PA), a protein involved in catalyzing the conversion of plasminogen to plasmin, and resulted in the lysis of the thrombi in the dogs with experimentally induced thrombosis (Sumi *et al.*, 1990). Natto extracts containing NK inactivate plasminogen activator inhibitor type 1 and then potentiate fibrinolytic activity. Further, dietary supplementation with natto extracts containing NK suppresses neointima formation induced by endothelial injury at femoral artery and enhances thrombolysis at the site of endothelial injury in rats (Suzuki *et al.*, 2003a, 2003b). NK administered intraduodenally can be absorbed from rat intestinal tract and detected in the plasma 3 and 5 h after administration. The cleavage of fibrinogen in the plasma could even be detectable within 0.5 h after administration (Fujita *et al.*, 1995).

Intake of NK (2000 Fibrinolysis Units/capsule) for eight weeks reduced both systolic and diastolic blood pressures (−5.55 mmHg and −2.84 mmHg, respectively) in the subjects with prehypertension or stage 1 hypertension (Kim *et al.*, 2008). Ingestion of NK (2 capsules/day of 2000 FU/capsule) for two months significantly reduced the plasma levels of coagulation factors – fibrinogen, factor VII and factor VIII in all groups of subjects including healthy volunteers, or patients with cardiovascular risk factors, or patients undergoing dialysis. Fibrinogen, factor VII, and factor VIII levels were decreased by 7–10%, 7–14%, 17–19%, respectively (Hsia *et al.*, 2009). Fibrinogen is a strong and independent risk factor for cardiovascular diseases (CVD) (Eidelman *et al.*, 2003; Kannel, 2005; Koenig, 2003; Lefevre *et al.*, 2004). Factor VII and factor VIII are highly related to increased risk of CVD (Cushman *et al.*, 1996; Kannel, 2005). This result suggests that consumption of natto may have beneficial effects on blood clotting-related CVD such as stroke and atherosclerosis.

Formation of amyloid fibrils is linked to various diseases such as Alzheimer's disease, prion disease and systematic amyloidosis. Degradation or clearance of amyloid is one of the strategies utilized in the prevention or treatment of amyloid-related diseases. Results from *in vitro* studies have demonstrated that NK extracted from *Bacillus subtilis* (natto) dose-dependently degraded Aβ40 amyloid fibrils, insulin amyloid fibrils, and huPrP amyloid fibrils formed from synthetic human prion peptide (Hsu *et al.*, 2009). In addition, NK has been shown to dose-dependently reduce aggregation of red blood cells and lower blood viscosity *in vitro* at physiological concentrations achieved in animal studies (Pais *et al.*, 2006).

Antioxidative functions

Natto was fractioned into a water-soluble high-molecular-weight viscous substance (HMWVS, MW > 100 K), a low-molecular-weight viscous substance (LMWVS, MW < 100 K) and soybean water extract (SWE). LMWVS had the strongest radical scavenging activity for hydroxyl and superoxide anion radicals. Presence of LMWVS and SWE attenuated the oxidation of rat plasma low-density lipoprotein (LDL) *in vitro*. These results indicate that natto fractions have inhibitory effects on LDL oxidation as a result of their radical scavenging activity (Iwai *et al.*, 2002a). Feeding rats the diets containing LMWVS and SWE lowered plasma triglyceride and total cholesterol levels, inhibited copper-oxidation of plasma and LDL *ex vivo* and reduced lipid peroxidation in liver and aorta *in vivo*. However, the antioxidant enzymes were unchanged by dietary natto extracts, indicating that these natto fractions may have direct antioxidant functions. These findings suggest that consumption of natto may be useful in the prevention of arteriosclerosis through reduction of lipid peroxidation and improvement of lipid profile (Iwai *et al.*, 2002b).

Antibacterial function

Natto has been known to have potent antibacterial function, and was used for the treatment of bacterial infectious diseases (Senbon *et al.*, 1940). The main effective component identified in natto is dipicolinic acid (DPA, 2,6-pyridinedicarboxylic acid) produced by natto bacteria during fermentation (Udo, 1936). Its average content in various kinds of natto is 17.60 ± 17.40 mg/100 g, while the content in natto bacteria is much higher, at 1772 to 3644 mg/100 g of dry weight of bacteria. Dipicolinic acid is effective against a variety of microorganisms such as *Aspergillus oryzae, Penicillium spp.*, pathogenic colon *bacillus, Escherichia O-157*, and yeasts (Sumi *et al.*, 1999).

22.4.2   Tempeh

Tempeh is a traditional fermented Indonesian soy food, and prepared from soaked and cooked soybeans by salt-free aerobic fermentation using the mold *Rhizopus*. During the fermentation, dense cottony mycelium produced binds the soybeans together to form a compact cake. Enzymes synthesized by the mold can hydrolyse soybean constituents to release bioactive peptides, and inactivate or eliminate antinutritional components. Enzymatic hydrolysis also plays a role in the development of a desirable texture, flavour and aroma of the product (Hachmeister *et al.*, 1993).

Tempeh is one of the most widely accepted and studied mold-fermented products, and contains high levels of γ-aminobutyric acid (GABA), other free amino acids and peptides. GABA is a ubiquitous nonprotein amino acid and is produced primarily by the α-decarboxylation of glutamic acid catalyzed by the enzyme glutamate decarboxylase (Brown and Shelp, 1997). Glutamic acid is one of the most abundant amino acids present in soybeans.

Contents of GABA in tempeh are quite variable and affected by the strains of *Rhizopus* species and the fermentation conditions. For example, GABA content was about 30 mg/100 g dry fermented soybeans in the aerobically fermented soybeans using *Rhizopus microsporus* var. *oligosporus* IFO 8631, while the anaerobically cultivation was about 370 mg/100 g dry weight. Among different strains of *Rhizopus* species, *R. microsporus* var. *oligosporus* IFO 32002 and IFO 32003 produced the highest amounts of GABA, 1740 mg and 1500 mg/100 g dry fermented soybeans, respectively (Table 22.2) (Aoki *et al.*, 2003b).

Tempeh is shown to have antioxygenic effects. The antioxidant activities in the water-soluble fraction of GABA-tempeh are higher than in both soybean and conventional tempeh. It is believed that ISF aglycones, free amino acids and peptides, which increased during aerobic and anaerobic fermentations, might be the effective components responsible for the antioxidant activity (Watanabe *et al.*, 2007). Consumption of GABA-enriched soy foods reduces the elevation of systolic blood pressure in spontaneously hypertensive rats (SHR) at a concentration of as low as 0.3 mg GABA/rat/day (Aoki *et al.*, 2003a). The hypotensive effect of GABA appears to be mediated through renal sympathetic nerves since GABA inhibited the development of hypertension in sham-operated SHR but not in renal-denervated SHR (Hayakawa *et al.*, 2005). GABA is also a depressive neurotransmitter in the sympathetic nervous system (Kuriyama *et al.*, 1993),

Table 22.2   GABA content in soybeans fermented by several strains of *Rhizopus*

Strains	GABA content (mg/100 g dry fermented soybeans)
Rhizopus microsporus var. *oligosporus* IFO 8631	720
Rhizopus microsporus var. *oligosporus* IFO 31987	810
Rhizopus microsporus var. *oligosporus* IFO 32002	1740
Rhizopus microsporus var. *oligosporus* IFO 32003	1500
Rhizopus oryzae IFO 4705	770
Rhizopus oryzae IFO 4770	510
Rhizopus oryzae IFO 5438	770
Rhizopus oryzae IFO 5780	420
Rhizopus oryzae IFO 9364	620

Source: Aoki *et al.* (2003b) (with permission).

improves discrimination learning in rats (Ishikawa and Saito, 1978) and relieve the discomfort symptoms that appear during the menopausal or presenile period such as sleeplessness, depression and autonomic disorder (Okada *et al.*, 2000). Highly purified GABA is used as medication for amelioration of the brain bloodstream in Japan (Aoki *et al.*, 2003a).

22.4.3 Aglycone-rich soy beverages

The major soy ISF, genistin and daidzin, are present in the form of glycosides in soybeans and most nonfermented soy foods (Anthony *et al.*, 1996; Miniello *et al.*, 2003). After ingestion, glycoside ISF are hydrolysed and converted to the aglycones, genistein and daidzein, by both intestinal mucosal and bacterial β-glucosidase (Miniello *et al.*, 2003; Setchell, 1998). Many traditional Asian soy foods are fermented and contain high levels of aglycone ISF that are more bioavailable and active than the glycoside ISF (Table 22.3).

Many of the lactic acid bacteria (LAB) have β-glucosidase activity, and are able to convert ISF glucosides to aglycones during soymilk fermentation (Chien *et al.*, 2006; Chun *et al.*, 2007; Donkor and Shah, 2008; Marazza *et al.*, 2009). Marazza *et al.* examined 63 strains of different *Lactobacillus* species, and found that *Lactobacillus rhamnosus* CRL981 contains the highest levels of β-glucosidase and can proliferate in soymilk. After 12 hours of fermentation with *Lactobacillus rhamnosus* CRL981, glucoside ISF can be completely hydrolysed to aglycones (Table 22.4) (Marazza *et al.*, 2009). Chun *et al.* tested four LAB, *Lactobacillus paraplantarum* KM, *Enterococcus durans* KH, *Streptococcus salivarius* HM and *Weissella confusa* JY, isolated from humans, for their capabilities of converting ISF glucosides to aglycones in soymilk. The glucoside concentrations were significantly decreased in soymilks fermented with either *L. paraplantarum* KM, *S. salivarius* HM, or *W. confusa* JY with fermentation time. Among them, *L. paraplantarum* KM was the best, resulting in 100%, 90%, and 61% hydrolysis of genistin, daidzin and glycitin, respectively, in six hours. The aglycone concentrations in soymilk fermented with *L. paraplantarum* KM were six and seven-fold higher than the initial levels of daidzein and genistein, respectively,

Table 22.3   Isoflavone glycosides and aglycones in soy foods (mg/kg dry wt)

Soy foods	Glycosides		Aglycones	
	Genistin	Daidzin	Genistein	Daidzein
Soy milk	1680	1337	98	141
Tofu	2087	1513	116	113
Tempeh	296	103	434	298
Miso	64	54	745	516
Soybean paste	160	90	514	404

Adapted from Coward *et al.* (1993) *J. Agric. Food Chem.*, **41**: 1961–7.

Table 22.4 Changes of isoflavones in soymilk after fermentation for 12 hours

Bacterial strains	Fermentation time (h)	Glucosides			Aglycones		
		Daidzin	Genistin	Glycitin	Daidzein	Genistein	Glycitein
					(mg/L)		
L. rhamnosus CR981*	0	4.80 ± 0.12	20.1 ± 0.15		3.30 ± 0.20	8.40 ± 0.22	
	12	0	0		14.50 ± 0.17	33.0 ± 0.30	
				(µmol/g dry soymilk)			
L. paraplantarum KM**	0	3.50 ± 0.09	4.2 ± 0.27	0.73 ± 0.02	0.87 ± 0.02	1.00 ± 0.06	0.25 ± 0.01
	12	0.32 ± 0.03	0	0.12 ± 0.02	5.17 ± 0.07	7.85 ± 0.24	1.35 ± 0.12
E. durans KH**	0	3.54 ± 0.09	4.20 ± 0.27	0.73 ± 0.02	0.87 ± 0.02	1.00 ± 0.06	0.25 ± 0.01
	12	3.25 ± 0.08	3.77 ± 0.06	0.77 ± 0.01	1.06 ± 0.07	1.68 ± 0.02	0.33 ± 0.00
S. salivarius HM**	0	3.54 ± 0.09	4.21 ± 0.27	0.73 ± 0.02	0.87 ± 0.02	1.00 ± 0.06	0.25 ± 0.01
	12	0.58 ± 0.04	1.01 ± 0.03	0.70 ± 0.07	4.57 ± 0.24	6.10 ± 0.11	0.44 ± 0.03
W. confusa JY**	0	3.54 ± 0.09	4.21 ± 0.27	0.73 ± 0.02	0.87 ± 0.02	1.00 ± 0.06	0.25 ± 0.01
	12	0.47 ± 0.03	1.30 ± 0.05	0.59 ± 0.01	4.87 ± 0.09	5.86 ± 0.14	0.59 ± 0.05

Adapted from: *Marazza *et al.* (2009), ** Chun *et al.* (2007).

after six hours of fermentation. However, changes in the daidzin and genistin levels were not significant in soymilk fermented with *E. durans* KH (Table 22.4) (Chun *et al.*, 2007).

Hypolipidemic effects
Treatment of preadipocyte 3T3-L1 cells with Soypro, a soymilk fermented with LAB isolated from Kimchi, significantly reduced the content of cellular triglyceride and inhibited cell differentiation. Expression of genes for peroxisome proliferator-activated receptor-γ2 and CCAAT/enhancer binding protein-α, transcription factors of adipocyte differentiation had also been down-regulated. Moreover, feeding of the high-fat diet-induced obese Sprague Dawley rats with Soypro for six weeks lowered LDL cholesterol levels (Kim *et al.*, 2008). In five-month-old ovariectomized Syrian hamsters, feeding *bifidobacterium*-fermented soy milk for four weeks significantly lowered the atherogenic index value, plasma triglyceride level and hepatic total cholesterol contents (Kikuchi-Hayakawa *et al.*, 2000).

Anticarcinogenesis effects
Ingestion of *Bifidobacterium*-fermented soy milk reduced 2-amino-1-methyl-6-phenylimidazo [4, 5-b] pyridine-induced mammary carcinogenesis in rats. The incidences (percentage of rats with tumors) of mammary gland tumors were significantly lower in the fermented soy milk (FSM)-fed rats than in the control rats (51% vs 71%). Mammary tumor multiplicities (number of tumors per rat) were also smaller in the rats fed 10% FSM than in the control group (1.2 ± 0.2 vs 2.6 ± 0.5). Furthermore, feeding of FSM reduced the sizes of mammary tumors. It is believed that the chemopreventive components in FSM might be ISF aglycones, genistein and daidzein, produced during fermentation because similar effects have also been observed in the animals fed a mixture of these two aglycones (Ohta *et al.*, 2000).

Immunomodulatory properties
Bacillus subtilis (natto), the active culture of natto, activates the production of the inflammatory cytokines IL-6 and IL-8 in epithelial-like human colon carcinoma Caco-2 cells. Moreover, the cytokine secretion induced was suppressed by the tyrosine kinase inhibitors, AG126 and genistein (Hosoi *et al.*, 2003). Pretreatment of human intestinal epithelial cells with soy beverage preparations fermented with pure or mixed cultures of *Streptococcus thermophilus* ST5, *Bifidobacterium longum* R0175, and *Lactobacillus helveticus* R0052 *in vitro* remarkably suppressed TNFα-induced IL-8 production. This indicates that fermentation of soy with selected LAB strains can produce bioactive components with immunomodulatory functions (Wagar *et al.*, 2009). Soymilk kefir has been reported to elevate intestinal IgA levels, and inhibit sarcoma tumor cell growth in an *in vivo* murine model (Liu *et al.*, 2002). A soy-based fermented product prepared with *Aspergillus oryzae* and LAB (*Pediococcus parvulus* and *Enterococcus faecium*) was shown to reduce allergy-associated responses in a murine peanut hypersensitivity model (Zhang *et al.*, 2008). Overall, these findings suggest that soy ferments can also possess immunomodulatory activity, when prepared with appropriate microorganisms and strains.

22.4.4   Aglycone-enriched soy pasta

Fermented soy foods mainly consist of ISF aglycones which have been shown to be more bioavailable in humans than their glycosides. An ISF aglycone-enriched pasta was prepared by addition of ISF aglycones derived from soy germ during the manufacturing process. Hypercholesterolemic adults were given one 80 g serving/day of soy germ pasta containing 33 mg of isoflavones with negligible soy protein. Intake of soy germ pasta significantly reduced total and LDL cholesterol levels by 7.3% and 8.6%, and decreased arterial stiffness and high sensitivity C-reactive protein. However, all the measures returned to baseline when the subjects were switched to conventional pasta (Clerici *et al.*, 2007).

22.4.5   Monascus-fermented soybean extracts (MFSE)

Soybean fermented with a filamentous fungus *Monascus pilosus* contains a significant amount of bioactive ISF aglycones (daidzein, glycitein, genistein; 1.13 mg/g dry weight) and natural statins, mevinolins (2.94 mg/g of dry weight) (Pyo, 2007). Monascus-fermented soybean extracts (MFSE) demonstrated an additive hypolipidemic effect in hyperlipidemic rats than unfermented soybean extracts (UFSE), which have a higher level of glucoside ISF (daidzin, glycitin, and genistin) without mevinolin. The average antioxidant capacities of MFSE were increased by a 5.2 to 7.4-fold compared with those of the UFSE, which are associated with its content of bioactive mevinolins and ISF aglycones produced during Monascus-fermentation. The peptides or proteins with molecular weights of 1 to 3 kDa in the water extracts from Monascus-fermented soybeans showed the highest ACE-inhibitory activity (65.3%), which was remarkably greater (6.5 times) than the control (Pyo and Lee, 2007). Oral intake of MFSE (200 and 400 mg/kg body weight) significantly lowered the serum total cholesterol, triglyceride, and LDL-C levels and elevated high-density lipoprotein cholesterol (HDL-C) levels in hyperlipidemic rats. Dietary MFSE significantly lowered HMG-CoA reductase activity and increased the atherogenic index (ratio of HDL-C/LDL-C) compared with the UFSE group. Moreover, treatment with MFSE significantly reduced the activities of serum aspartate aminotransferase and alanine aminotransferase by averages of 35.6 and 43.2%, respectively compared to the high-fat diet group. The results indicate that MFSE has a more potent hypolipidemic action via improvement of the lipid profiles and suppression of HMG-CoA reductase activity than UFSE in hyperlipidemic rats (Pyo and Seong, 2009).

22.4.6   Soy yogurt or sogurt

Soy yogurts or sogurt are becoming more and more popular because of their low levels of cholesterol and saturated fat, and the fact that they are lactose-free (Drake and Gerard, 2003; Sarkar, 2006). Sogurts prepared with different strains of bacteria may have distinct compositions and functions. For example, a sogurt was developed using LAB (1:1 mixture of *Lactobacillus delbrueckii* subsp. *latis* KFRI 01181 and *Lactobacillus plantarum* KFRI 00144) and MFSE (1.5%, w/v)

(Park and Oh, 2007; Pyo and Song, 2009). It contains high levels of γ-aminobutyric acid (GABA), free amino acids (FAAs), statins, and ISF aglycones compared with the control sogurt (Park and Oh, 2007; Pyo and Song, 2009).

Rabbits with induced hypercholesterolemia were fed soy yogurt or ISF-supplemented soy yogurt fermented with *Enterococcus faecium*, CRL 183 for 60 days. The total cholesterol level (38.1%, and 27.0%, respectively) and the extent of atherosclerosis in the thoracic and abdominal aortas were significantly reduced in both groups, while serum HDL-C concentration was markedly increased. The rise of autoantibodies against oxLDL was prevented. However, when the whole aorta was analysed, animals treated with soy yogurt supplemented with ISF exhibited the greatest reduction in atherosclerotic lesion area. These results suggested that intake of soy yogurt may reduce the risk of CVD by improving the lipid profile and inhibiting the formation of oxLDL autoantibodies, and that supplementation of ISF may enhance the antiatherosleretic effect of soy yogurt (Cavallini *et al.*, 2009). Feeding male Sprague Dawley rats with a diet containing 20% *Lactobacillus*-fermented soy yogurt lowered liver weight, hepatic triglyceride content and plasma cholesterol level compared to the control group fed AIN-93 diet. Furthermore, intake of soy yogurt down-regulated the expression of genes for SREBP-1 and enzymes related to lipogenesis and up-regulated the expression of β-oxidation-related genes in the liver, suggesting that soy yogurt is beneficial in preventing hepatic lipid accumulation (Kitawaki *et al.*, 2009).

Soy yogurt containing bifidobacteria suppressed the proliferation of Ehrlich ascites tumor cells in *in vitro* and *in vivo* studies. Treatment of the tumor cells with soy yogurt containing *Bifidobacterium lactis* Bb-12 or *Bifidobacterium longum* Bb-46 for two hours resulted in 88% and 86% inhibition of their proliferation, respectively. Moreover, dietary supplementation of soy yogurt containing Bb-12 or Bb-46 prolonged the lifespan of the female Swiss albino mice injected intraperitoneally with the tumor cells by 34 and 39%, respectively. The lifespan increase was positively correlated with the number of faeces bifidobacteria (Abd el-Gawad *et al.*, 2004).

22.4.7   Glyceollins-enriched soy yogurt

Phytoalexins are antifungal or antibacterial compounds synthesized in plants under stresses, fungal attack, or elicitor treatment. Glyceollins are a type of isoflavonoid phytoalexins unique to soybeans and synthesized by soy plants under stressed conditions such as fungal infection. Unlike the observed estrogenic effects in other phytochemicals such as genistein and daidzein, glyceollins have potent anti-estrogenic effects on ER signaling and suppresses 17β-estradiol-induced proliferation in MCF-7 cells. The binding affinity of glyceollins to ERα is higher than to ERβ and their antagonistic effect on ERα is greater than on ERβ. This indicates that phytoalexin compounds may be effective in the prevention or treatment of hormone-dependent carcinogenesis (Burow *et al.*, 2001).

Feeding of glyceollin-enriched soy protein in female postmenopausal cynomolgus macaques for three weeks remarkably suppressed estradiol-induced breast proliferation. Furthermore, the estradiol-induced expression of genes for trefoil factor 1 and progesterone receptor, two biomarkers for breast cancer risk, in the breast epithelium was significantly inhibited by dietary addition of glyceollins. This suggests that soybean glyceollins may have potential estrogen-modulating actions in the breast (Wood *et al.*, 2006). The other potential health benefits of phytoalexin-enriched foods may include antioxidant activity, anti-inflammation activity, cholesterol-lowering ability and even anticancer activity.

A glyceollins-enriched soy yogurt developed by Feng S. and co-workers contains 1 mg/g of total glyceollins (Feng *et al.*, 2008). They germinated black soybeans [Glycine max (L.) Merrill] under fungal stress with *Rhizopus oligosporus* for three days. The germinated beans were then homogenized and fermented with LAB containing blended *Streptococcus thermophilus* and *Lactobacillus delbrueckii* subsp. *bulgaricus* FD-DVS YC-X11 to make soy yogurt. Fungal stress led to the generation of glyceollins (Feng *et al.*, 2008).

22.4.8   Okara-based soy foods

Okara is a byproduct of the soy milk production and contains 24.5–37.5% proteins, 9.3–22.3% lipids, 14.5–55.4% crude fibre, and 0.1% isoflavones (Jiménez-Escrig *et al.*, 2008). The crude fibre in okara is mainly composed of cellulose, hemicellulose, and lignin, and is used in enteral nutrition products and some bakery goods such as biscuits and snacks (O'Toole, 1999).

Soy fibre provides important health benefits including improved laxation and cholesterol-lowering ability (Slavin, 1991) and protects gut environment in terms of antioxidant status and prebiotic effect (Jiménez-Escrig *et al.*, 2008). Feeding 10% fibre-rich okara in female Wistar rats significantly reduced body weight gain and blood total cholesterol, and increased antioxidant status and butyrogenic effect in the cecum compared to a control group. In addition, okara-derived soy fibre markedly enhanced calcium absorption and retention (Jiménez-Escrig *et al.*, 2008). In a diet-induced murine obesity model, okara intake (10, 20, 40%) dose-dependently suppressed the body weight gain and development of epididymal white adipose tissue, and prevented increases of plasma total cholesterol, LDL cholesterol, and non-esterified fatty acid as well as steatosis in the liver. Okara intake down-regulated the expression of genes for hepatic fatty acid synthetase, adipose leptin and TNF-α and up-regulated the hepatic cholesterol 7 α-hydroxylase (CYP7A1) gene expression. These results suggest that ingestion of okara-based foods may be effective in preventing obesity (Matsumoto *et al.*, 2007).

22.4.9   Functional soy peptides

Soybeans have been considered as a rich source of good quality of proteins. A variety of peptides can be produced or released during fermentation, *in vitro* hydrolysis, food processing or *in vivo* enzymatic digestion of soy proteins. Many of these peptides are able to modulate different physiological functions, and possess novel properties such as anticarcinogenesis, antihypertensive, antiobesity, hypolipidemic, immunomodulatory and antioxidative actions. It has been shown great potentials for these bioactive peptides to be made into functional beverages and food products.

Anticarcinogenesis peptides

Bowman Birk protease inhibitor (BBI) is an 8 kDa soy protein with 71 amino acids, and can strongly inhibit both trypsin and chymotrypsin. BBI has been shown to be an effective suppressor of carcinogenesis in *in vitro* and *in vivo* models. BBI remains intact and stable after digestion in the simulated intestinal and gastric fluids, and can be internalized into the nucleus of the colonic epithelial cells (Park *et al.*, 2007). The internalized BBI remains active in inhibition of chymotrypsin in intestinal epithelial cells even after digestion. This feature would allow BBI to inhibit critical intracellular proteases and thus suppress malignant transformation (Billings *et al.*, 1991).

Oral administration of BBI suppressed the carcinogenic process induced by various chemical and physical carcinogens in different cells and tissues such as colon, liver, lung, esophagus, cheek pouch of mice, rats and hamsters. About half of an oral dose of BBI can be absorbed into the bloodstream and distributed throughout the body, and excreted via urine. Some of the BBI excreted in urine still remained active (Billings *et al.*, 1992; Yavelow *et al.*, 1983). The calculated half-life of serum BBI is ten hours in both rats and hamsters (Kennedy, 1998). The anticarcinogenic action of BBI is highly efficient. Dietary intake of an amount as low as 0.01% BBI suppressed liver carcinogenesis in mice (St Clair *et al.*, 1990) and colon carcinogenesis in rats (Kennedy, 1998).

Kunitz trypsin inhibitor (KTI) is another potent soybean protease inhibitor. It contains 181 amino acids and is a 20.1 kDa protein. KTI possesses one binding site and has strong inhibition on trypsin and weaker inhibition on chymotrypsin. KTI has been shown to suppress ovarian cancer cell invasion by inhibiting urokinase expression through down-regulation of src-dependent signaling pathways (Inagaki *et al.*, 2005; Kobayashi *et al.*, 2004).

Lunasin is a 43-amino acid peptide derived from 2S soybean albumin. Lunasin inhibited chemically induced carcinogenic transformation in mammalian cells in mice (Lam *et al.*, 2003). *In vitro* study showed that BBI and KTI protect lunasin from digestion of pancreatin. Up to 30% of the lunasin peptide can reach the target tissues and remain intact and bioactive through oral intake. Intraperitoneal injections of lunasin significantly reduced the tumor incidence in a xenograft model of nude mice transplanted with human breast cancer cells (Hsieh *et al.*, 2010). The possible mechanism underlying the anticarcinogenic properties of lunasin might be related to its structural homology to a conserved region of chromatin-binding proteins (Jeong *et al.*, 2003). A motif of lunasin can bind specifically to non-acetylated H3 and H4 histones and prevent their acetylation (de Lumen, 2005).

Hypotensive peptides

Inhibition of angiotension-converting enzyme (ACE) activity is an important parameter used in the screening hypotensive compounds since ACE is a key enzyme involved in the regulation of blood pressure via modulation of rennin-angiotension system. Soy-derived hypotensive peptides have been obtained through enzymatic digestion, fermentation or genetic engineering.

From the peptic digest of soybean proteins, Chen and colleagues isolated 4 hypotensive peptides, Ile-Ala, Tyr-Leu-Ala-Gly-Asn-Gln, Phe-Phe-Leu, and Ile-Tyr-Leu-Leu. Oral intake of these peptides significantly lowered blood pressure in spontaneously hypertensive rats (SHR) (Chen *et al.*, 2003). Kodera and Nio have identified 5 peptides with ACE inhibitory activity from digestion of soybean proteins using protease D3, including Tyr-Val-Val-Phe-Lys, Pro-Asn-Asn-Lys-Pro-Phe-Gln, Asn-Trp-Gly-Pro-Leu-Val, Ile-Pro-Pro-Gly-Val-Pro-Tyr-Trp-Thr, and Thr-Pro-Arg-Val-Phe (Kodera and Nio, 2002). A highly effective anti-hypertensive peptide, RPLKPW, was introduced into the soybean protein subunit using genetic engineering technique. The mutated protein expressed by *E. coli* is highly effective in lowering blood pressure in SHR (Matoba *et al.*, 2001; Onishi *et al.*, 2004). Additionally, many hypotensive peptides can be produced during fermentation of soy foods, such as Val-Ala-His-Ile-Asn-Val-Gly-Lys and Tyr-Val-Trp-Lys from the fermentation with Bacillus natto (Kimura *et al.*, 2000), His-His-Leu from soybean paste (Shin *et al.*, 2001).

Hypocholesterolemic, antiobesity and antioxidant peptides
Soybean-derived peptides with other physiological functions such as lowering blood cholesterol, reducing body fat and weight, and antioxidative activity have also been identified. For example, the α' subunit of the β-conglycinin in the soy has been shown to play a major role in reducing cholesterol level (Manzoni *et al.*, 1998). A glycinin-derived peptide, Leu-Pro-Tyr-Pro-Arg, was also found to have hypocholesterolemic effect in mice after oral intake (Yoshikawa *et al.*, 2000). Leu-Pro-Tyr-Pro-Arg, a glycinin-derived peptide, has been shown to have anorectic effect, and can reduce body fat and weight through decreasing food intake (Takenaka *et al.*, 2000). Matoba demonstrated that enzymatic digestion of soy proteins increased the radical-scavenging activities by three to five times, indicating that the antioxidant peptides may have been released from the intact soybean proteins (Matoba, 2002).

22.5 Safety aspects of soy

Soy foods are generally considered as very healthy foods and are good sources of proteins meeting the physiological needs of humans. Because of the content of estrogen-like ISF and other anti-nutritional factors, concerns on the safety of consuming soy foods/products have been always raised by consumers and health professionals. Especially the potential anti-thyroid and estrogenic or anti-estrogenic effects of soy previously reported in animals and humans still have not been fully understood.

Anti-thyroid actions of soy such as development of goiter or thyroid enlargement were observed in both iodine-deficient rodents (Kimura *et al.*, 1976; McCarrison,

1933; Sharpless *et al.*, 1939; Wilgus *et al.*, 1941) and human infants fed soy diet or soy flour-based formula without iodine fortification (Pinchera *et al.*, 1965; Shepard *et al.*, 1960; Van WYK *et al.*, 1959). Animals fed a soy diet almost doubled the iodine requirement compared to animals fed soy-free diets (Block *et al.*, 1961; Kay *et al.*, 1988; Sharpless *et al.*, 1939). Infants with congenital hypothyroidism who consumed soy formula require about 25% more synthetic hormone than those on soy-free formulas (Chorazy *et al.*, 1995; Jabbar *et al.*, 1997). Additionally, soy components dramatically stimulated the development of thyroid hyperplasia in iodine-deficient rats (Ikeda *et al.*, 2000; Son *et al.*, 2001). Our studies in rats have shown that consumption of 20% alcohol-washed soy protein isolate containing minimal amount of ISF markedly suppressed the binding ability of hepatic thyroid hormone receptor to the thyroid hormone response element of the target genes (Huang *et al.*, 2005; Xiao *et al.*, 2004). These findings suggest that intake of soy may reduce the efficiency of thyroid hormone function, and that soybeans may contain goitrogens that can interfere with the utilization of iodine or functioning of the thyroid gland and cause thyroid problems. However, it appears that consumption of soy could cause goiter or thyroid disorders only in animals or humans consuming diets deficient or marginally adequate in iodine, or who were predisposed to develop goiter (Chang and Doerge, 2000), and in most cases dietary supplementation with adequate iodine can reverse the disorders (Schone *et al.*, 1990). Which component(s) in the soy is responsible for the anti-thyroid effects and the underlying mechanism(s) remain to be identified.

Infants fed soy-based formulas represent one of the groups exposed to high amounts of soy ISF. Blood ISF concentrations in those infants were 13 000–22 000 times higher than plasma estradiol levels in early life, and were 6–11 fold higher on a bodyweight basis than the dose that has hormonal effects in adults consuming soy foods (Setchell *et al.*, 1997). Although studies in rodents showed that oral administration of genistein, one of the major soy ISF, affected reproductive and nonreproductive organs of both sexes (Jefferson *et al.*, 2002, 2009; Montani *et al.*, 2008), the impact of ISF intake from soy foods on early development, endocrine and reproductive functions in humans, particularly the long-term effect, remains to be investigated.

22.6   Future trends

Soybean is a rich source of proteins and bioactive components. Consumption of soy foods has been linked to many beneficial effects such as lower incidences of coronary heart diseases, atherosclerosis, type 2 diabetes and decreased risk of certain types of carcinogenesis as well as better bone health and relief of menopausal symptoms. Research and development of soy functional foods will remain attractive and promising. The future trends include the following.

1 Development of more reliable and specific functional soy foods targeting different subgroups such as patients with diabetes or hypertension, this will

require accurate identification and isolation of bioactive components from soybeans and understanding of the cellular and molecular mechanisms how the effective components exert their functions.

2 Development of functional soy foods with favourable tastes that can be accepted by various groups of consumers, especially for those made by traditional fermentation methods.

3 Development of soybean lines rich in certain bioactive component(s).

4 Standardization of manufacturing procedures and criteria for quality control.

5 Making health claims.

22.7   Sources of further information and advice

Sugano, M (ed.) (2006) *Soy in Health and Disease Prevention*, Taylor & Francis, New York.

Johnson, I and Williamson, G (eds) (2003) *Phytochemical Functional Foods*, Woodhead Publishing Limited, Cambridge.

Gilani, GS and Anderson, JJB (eds) (2002) *Phytoestrogens and Health*, AOCS Press, Champaign, Illinois.

Wilcke, HL, Hopkins, DT and Waggle, DH (eds) (1979) 'Soy protein and human nutrition', Proceedings of a symposium held May 22–23, 1978, in Keystone, Colorado. Academic Press, Inc., New York.

22.8   References

Abd el-Gawad IA, el Sayed EM, Hafez SA, el Zeini HM and Saleh FA (2004), 'Inhibitory effect of yoghurt and soya yoghurt containing bifidobacteria on the proliferation of Ehrlich ascites tumour cells in vitro and in vivo in a mouse tumour model', *Br J Nutr*, **92**, 81–6.

Anthony MS, Clarkson TB, Hughes CL, Morgan TM and Burke GL (1996), 'Soybean isoflavones improve cardiovascular risk factors without affecting the reproductive system of peripubertal rhesus monkeys', *J Nutr*, **126**, 43–50.

Aoki H, Furuya Y, Endo Y and Fujimoto K, (2003a), 'Effect of gamma-aminobutyric acid-enriched tempeh-like fermented soybean (GABA-Tempeh) on the blood pressure of spontaneously hypertensive rats', *Biosci Biotechnol Biochem*, **67**, 1806–8.

Aoki H, Uda I, Tagami K, Furuya Y, Endo Y and Fujimoto K, (2003b), 'The production of a new tempeh-like fermented soybean containing a high level of gamma-aminobutyric acid by anaerobic incubation with Rhizopus', *Biosci Biotechnol Biochem*, **67**, 1018–23.

Billings PC, Brandon DL and Habres JM (1991), 'Internalisation of the Bowman-Birk protease inhibitor by intestinal epithelial cells', *Eur J Cancer*, **27**, 903–8.

Billings PC, St Clair WH, Maki PA and Kennedy AR (1992), 'Distribution of the Bowman Birk protease inhibitor in mice following oral administration', *Cancer Lett*, **62**, 191–7.

Block RJ, Mandl RH, Howard HW, Bauer CD and Anderson DW (1961), 'The curative action of iodine on soybean goiter and the changes in the distribution of iodoamino acids in the serum and in the thyroid gland digests', *Arch Biochem Biophys*, **93**, 15–21.

Brown AW and Shelp BJ (1997), 'The metabolism and functions of gamma-aminobutyric acid (GABA)', *Plant Physiol*, **115**, 1–5.

Burow ME, Boue SM, Collins-Burow BM, Melnik LI, Duong BN, *et al.* (2001), 'Phytochemical glyceollins, isolated from soy, mediate antihormonal effects through estrogen receptor alpha and beta', *J Clin Endocrinol Metab*, **86**, 1750–8.

Cavallini DC, Abdalla DS, Vendramini RC, Bedani R, Bomdespacho LQ, *et al.* (2009), 'Effects of isoflavone-supplemented soy yogurt on lipid parameters and atherosclerosis development in hypercholesterolemic rabbits: a randomized double-blind study', *Lipids Health Dis*, **8**, 40.

Chang HC and Doerge DR (2000), 'Dietary genistein inactivates rat thyroid peroxidase in vivo without an apparent hypothyroid effect', *Toxicol Appl Pharmacol*, **168**, 244–52.

Chen J, Okada T, Muramoto K, Suetsuna K and Yang S (2003), 'Identification of angiotensin I-converting enzyme inhibitory peptides derived from the peptic digest of soybean protein', *J Food Biochem*, **26**, 543–54.

Chien HL, Huang HY and Chou CC (2006), 'Transformation of isoflavone phytoestrogens during the fermentation of soymilk with lactic acid bacteria and bifidobacteria', *Food Microbiol*, **23**, 772–8.

Chorazy PA, Himelhoch S, Hopwood NJ, Greger NG and Postellon DC (1995), 'Persistent hypothyroidism in an infant receiving a soy formula: case report and review of the literature', *Pediatrics*, **96**, 148–50.

Chun J, Kim GM, Lee KW, Choi ID, Kwon GH, *et al.* (2007), 'Conversion of isoflavone glucosides to aglycones in soymilk by fermentation with lactic acid bacteria', *J Food Sci*, **72**, M39–44.

Clerici C, Setchell KD, Battezzati PM, Pirro M, Giuliano V, *et al.* (2007), 'Pasta naturally enriched with isoflavone aglycons from soy germ reduces serum lipids and improves markers of cardiovascular risk', *J Nutr*, **137**, 2270–8.

Coward L, Barnes NC, Setchell KD and Barnes S (1993), 'Genistein, daidzein, and their beta-glycoside conjugates: antitumor isoflaones in soybean foods from American and Asian diets', *J Agric Food Chem*, **41**, 1961–7.

Cushman M, Yanez D, Psaty BM, Fried LP, Heiss G, *et al.* (1996), 'Association of fibrinogen and coagulation factors VII and VIII with cardiovascular risk factors in the elderly: the Cardiovascular Health Study. Cardiovascular Health Study Investigators', *Am J Epidemiol*, **143**, 665–76.

de Lumen BO (2005), 'Lunasin: a cancer-preventive soy peptide', *Nutr Rev*, **63**, 16–21.

Donkor ON and Shah NP (2008), 'Production of beta-glucosidase and hydrolysis of isoflavone phytoestrogens by Lactobacillus acidophilus, Bifidobacterium lactis, and Lactobacillus casei in soymilk', *J Food Sci*, **73**, M15–20.

Drake MA and Gerard PD (2003), 'Consumer attitudes and acceptability of soy-fortified yogurts.', *J Food Sci*, **68**, 1118–22.

Eidelman RS and Hennekens CH (2003), 'Fibrinogen: a predictor of stroke and marker of atherosclerosis', *Eur Heart J*, **24**, 499–500.

Feng S, Saw CL, Lee YK and Huang D (2008), 'Novel process of fermenting black soybean [Glycine max (L.) Merrill] yogurt with dramatically reduced flatulence-causing oligosaccharides but enriched soy phytoalexins', *J Agric Food Chem*, **56**, 10078–84.

Fujita M, Hong K, Ito Y, Fujii R, Kariya K and Nishimuro S (1995), 'Thrombolytic effect of nattokinase on a chemically induced thrombosis model in rat', *Biol Pharm Bull*, **18**, 1387–91.

Fujita M, Hong K, Ito Y, Misawa S, Takeuchi N, *et al.* (1995), 'Transport of nattokinase across the rat intestinal tract', *Biol Pharm Bull*, **18**, 1194–6.

Golbitz P (1995), 'Traditional soyfoods: processing and products', *J Nutr*, **125**, S570–2.

Hachmeister KA and Fung DY (1993), 'Tempeh: a mold-modified indigenous fermented food made from soybeans and/or cereal grains', *Crit Rev Microbiol*, **19**, 137–88.

Hayakawa K, Kimura M and Yamori Y (2005), 'Role of the renal nerves in gamma-aminobutyric acid-induced antihypertensive effect in spontaneously hypertensive rats', *Eur J Pharmacol*, **524**, 120–5.

Hosoi T, Hirose R, Saegusa S, Ametani A, Kiuchi K and Kaminogawa S (2003), 'Cytokine responses of human intestinal epithelial-like Caco-2 cells to the nonpathogenic bacterium Bacillus subtilis (natto)', *Int J Food Microbiol*, **82**, 255–64.

Hsia CH, Shen MC, Lin JS, Wen YK, Hwang KL, *et al.* (2009), 'Nattokinase decreases plasma levels of fibrinogen, factor VII, and factor VIII in human subjects', *Nutr Res*, **29**, 190–6.

Hsieh CC, Hernandez-Ledesma B, Jeong HJ, Park JH and de Lumen BO (2010), 'Complementary roles in cancer prevention: protease inhibitor makes the cancer preventive peptide lunasin bioavailable', *PLoS One*, **5**, e8890.

Hsu RL, Lee KT, Wang JH, Lee LY and Chen RP (2009), 'Amyloid-degrading ability of nattokinase from Bacillus subtilis natto', *J Agric Food Chem*, **57**, 503–8.

Huang W, Wood C, L'Abbe MR, Gilani S, Cockell KA and Xiao CW (2005), 'Soy protein isolate increases hepatic thyroid hormone receptor content and inhibits its binding to the target genes in rats', *J Nutr*, **135**, 1631–5.

Ikeda T, Nishikawa A, Imazawa T, Kimura S and Hirose M (2000), 'Dramatic synergism between excess soybean intake and iodine deficiency on the development of rat thyroid hyperplasia', *Carcinogenesis*, **21**, 707–13.

Ikeda Y, Iki M, Morita A, Kajita E, Kagamimori S, *et al.* (2006), 'Intake of fermented soybeans, natto, is associated with reduced bone loss in postmenopausal women: Japanese Population-Based Osteoporosis (JPOS) Study', *J Nutr*, **136**, 1323–8.

Inagaki K, Kobayashi H, Yoshida R, Kanada Y, Fukuda Y, *et al.* (2005), 'Suppression of urokinase expression and invasion by a soybean Kunitz trypsin inhibitor are mediated through inhibition of Src-dependent signaling pathways', *J Biol Chem*, **280**, 31428–37.

Ishikawa K and Saito S (1978), 'Effect of intraventricular gamma-aminobutyric acid (GABA) on discrimination learning in rats', *Psychopharmacology (Berl)*, **56**, 127–32.

Iwai K, Nakaya N, Kawasaki Y and Matsue H (2002a), 'Inhibitory effect of natto, a kind of fermented soybeans, on LDL oxidation in vitro', *J Agric Food Chem*, **50**, 3592–6.

Iwai K, Nakaya N, Kawasaki Y and Matsue H (2002b), 'Antioxidative functions of natto, a kind of fermented soybeans: effect on LDL oxidation and lipid metabolism in cholesterol-fed rats', *J Agric Food Chem*, **50**, 3597–601.

Jabbar MA, Larrea J and Shaw RA (1997), 'Abnormal thyroid function tests in infants with congenital hypothyroidism: the influence of soy-based formula', *J Am Coll Nutr*, **16**, 280–2.

Jefferson WN, Couse JF, Padilla B, Korach KS and Newbold RR (2002), 'Neonatal exposure to genistein induces estrogen receptor (ER)alpha expression and multioocyte follicles in the maturing mouse ovary: evidence for ERbeta-mediated and nonestrogenic actions', *Biol Reprod*, **67**, 1285–96.

Jefferson WN, Doerge D, Padilla-Banks E, Woodling KA, Kissling GE and Newbold R (2009), 'Oral exposure to genistin, the glycosylated form of genistein, during neonatal life adversely affects the female reproductive system', *Environ Health Perspect*, **117**, 1883–9.

Jeong HJ, Park JH, Lam Y and de Lumen BO (2003), 'Characterization of lunasin isolated from soybean', *J Agric Food Chem*, **51**, 7901–6.

Jiménez-Escrig A, Tenorio MD, Espinosa-Martos I and Ruperez P (2008), 'Health-promoting effects of a dietary fibre concentrate from the soybean byproduct okara in rats', *J Agric Food Chem*, **56**, 7495–501.

Kamao M, Suhara Y, Tsugawa N, Uwano M, Yamaguchi N, *et al.* (2007), 'Vitamin K content of foods and dietary vitamin K intake in Japanese young women', *J Nutr Sci Vitaminol (Tokyo)*, **53**, 464–70.

Kaneki M, Hodges SJ, Hosoi T, Fujiwara S, Lyons A, *et al.* (2001), 'Japanese fermented soybean food as the major determinant of the large geographic difference in circulating levels of vitamin K2: possible implications for hip-fracture risk', *Nutrition*, **17**, 315–21.

Kannel WB (2005), 'Overview of hemostatic factors involved in atherosclerotic cardiovascular disease', *Lipids*, **40**, 1215–20.

Katsuyama H, Ideguchi S, Fukunaga M, Fukunaga T, Saijoh K and Sunami S, (2004), 'Promotion of bone formation by fermented soybean (Natto) intake in premenopausal women', *J Nutr Sci Vitaminol (Tokyo)*, **50**, 114–20.

Kay T, Kimura M, Nishing K and Itokawa Y (1988), 'Soyabean, goitre, and prevention', *J Trop Pediatr*, **34**, 110–13.

Kennedy AR (1998), 'The Bowman-Birk inhibitor from soybeans as an anticarcinogenic agent', *Am J Clin Nutr*, **68**, S1406–12.

Kikuchi-Hayakawa H, Onodera-Masuoka N, Kano M, Matsubara S, Yasuda E and Ishikawa F (2000), 'Effect of soy milk and bifidobacterium-fermented soy milk on plasma and liver lipids in ovariectomized Syrian hamsters', *J Nutr Sci Vitaminol (Tokyo)*, **46**, 105–8.

Kim JY, Gum SN, Paik JK, Lim HH, Kim KC, *et al.* (2008), 'Effects of nattokinase on blood pressure: a randomized, controlled trial', *Hypertens Res*, **31**, 1583–8.

Kim NH, Moon PD, Kim SJ, Choi IY, An HJ, *et al.* (2008), 'Lipid profile lowering effect of Soypro fermented with lactic acid bacteria isolated from Kimchi in high-fat diet-induced obese rats', *Biofactors*, **33**, 49–60.

Kimura A, Takada A, Okada T and Yamada H (2000), 'Microbial manufacture of angiotension I-converting enzyme inhibiting peptides', *Japan: Toyo Hatsuko K K: Jpn Kpkai Tokkyo Koho JP 2000229996 A2 22 Aug 2000 11 p*.

Kimura S, Suwa J, Ito M and Sato H, (1976), 'Development of malignant goiter by defatted soybean with iodine-free diet in rats', *Gann*, **67**, 763–5.

Kitawaki R, Nishimura Y, Takagi N, Iwasaki M, Tsuzuki K and Fukuda M (2009), 'Effects of Lactobacillus fermented soymilk and soy yogurt on hepatic lipid accumulation in rats fed a cholesterol-free diet', *Biosci Biotechnol Biochem*, **73**, 1484–8.

Kobayashi H, Suzuki M, Kanayama N and Terao T (2004), 'A soybean Kunitz trypsin inhibitor suppresses ovarian cancer cell invasion by blocking urokinase upregulation', *Clin Exp Metastasis*, **21**, 159–66.

Kodera T and Nio N (2002), 'Angiotension converting enzyme inhibitors', *PCT Int Appl WO 2002055546 A1 18 43 p Kokai Tokkyo Koho*.

Koenig W (2003), 'Fibrin(ogen) in cardiovascular disease: an update', *Thromb Haemost*, **89**, 601–9.

Kuriyama K, Hirouchi M and Nakayasu H (1993), 'Structure and function of cerebral GABAA and GABAB receptors', *Neurosci Res*, **17**, 91–9.

Lam Y, Galvez A and de Lumen BO (2003), 'Lunasin suppresses E1A-mediated transformation of mammalian cells but does not inhibit growth of immortalized and established cancer cell lines', *Nutr Cancer*, **47**, 88–94.

Lefevre M, Kris-Etherton PM, Zhao G and Tracy RP (2004), 'Dietary fatty acids, hemostasis, and cardiovascular disease risk', *J Am Diet Assoc*, **104**, 410–19.

Liu JR, Wang SY, Lin YY and Lin CW (2002), 'Antitumor activity of milk kefir and soy milk kefir in tumor-bearing mice', *Nutr Cancer*, **44**, 183–7.

Manzoni C, Lovati MR, Gianazza E and Sirtori CR (1998), 'Soybean protein products as regulators of liver low-density lipoprotein receptors. II. a-a' rich commercial soy concentrate and a' deficient mutant differently affect low-density lipoprotein receptor activation', *J Agric Food Chem*, **46**, 2481–4.

Marazza JA, Garro MS and de Giori GS (2009), 'Aglycone production by Lactobacillus rhamnosus CRL981 during soymilk fermentation', *Food Microbiol*, **26**, 333–9.

Matoba N, Doyama N, Yamada Y, Maruyama N, Utsumi S and Yoshikawa M (2001), 'Design and production of genetically modified soybean protein with anti-hypertensive activity by incorporating potent analogue of ovokinin(2–7)', *FEBS Lett*, **497**, 50–4.

Matoba T (2002), 'How does the radical-scavenging activity of soy protein food change during heating', *Daizu Tanpakushitsu Kenkyu*, **5**, 47–50.

Matsumoto K, Watanabe Y and Yokoyama S (2007), 'Okara, soybean residue, prevents obesity in a diet-induced murine obesity model', *Biosci Biotechnol Biochem*, **71**, 720–7.

McCarrison R, (1933), 'The goitrogenic action of soyabean and ground-nut', *Ind J Med Res*, **XXI**, 179–81.

Miniello VL, Moro GE, Tarantino M, Natile M, Granieri L and Armenio L, (2003), 'Soy-based formulas and phyto-oestrogens: a safety profile', *Acta Paediatr Suppl*, **91**, 93–100.

554   Functional foods

Montani C, Penza M, Jeremic M, Biasiotto G, La Sala G, et al. (2008), 'Genistein is an efficient estrogen in the whole-body throughout mouse development', Toxicol Sci, **103**, 57–67.

Morton MS, Arisaka O, Miyake N, Morgan LD and Evans BA (2002), 'Phytoestrogen concentrations in serum from Japanese men and women over forty years of age', J Nutr, **132**, 3168–71.

Nakamura T, Yamagata Y and Ichishima E (1992), 'Nucleotide sequence of the subtilisin NAT gene, aprN, of Bacillus subtilis (natto)', Biosci Biotechnol Biochem, **56**, 1869–71.

Ohta T, Nakatsugi S, Watanabe K, Kawamori T, Ishikawa F, et al. (2000), 'Inhibitory effects of Bifidobacterium-fermented soy milk on 2-amino-1-methyl-6-phenylimidazo[4,5-b] pyridine-induced rat mammary carcinogenesis, with a partial contribution of its component isoflavones', Carcinogenesis, **21**, 937–41.

Okada T, Sugishita T, Murakami T, Murai H, Saikusa T, et al. (2000), 'Effect of the defatted rice germ enriched with GABA for sleeplessness, depression, autonomic disorder by oral administration', Nippon Shokuhin Kagaku Kogaku Kaishi, **47**, 596–603.

Onishi K, Matoba N, Yamada Y, Doyama N, Maruyama N, Utsumi S and Yoshikawa M (2004), 'Optimal designing of beta-conglycinin to genetically incorporate RPLKPW, a potent anti-hypertensive peptide', Peptides, **25**, 37–43.

O'Toole DK (1999), 'Characteristics and use of okara, the soybean residue from soy milk production – a review', J Agric Food Chem, **47**, 363–71.

Pais E, Alexy T, Holsworth RE, Jr. and Meiselman HJ (2006), 'Effects of nattokinase, a pro-fibrinolytic enzyme, on red blood cell aggregation and whole blood viscosity', Clin Hemorheol Microcirc, **35**, 139–42.

Park JH, Jeong HJ and Lumen BO (2007), 'In vitro digestibility of the cancer-preventive soy peptides lunasin and BBI', J Agric Food Chem, **55**, 10703–6.

Park KB and Oh SH (2007), 'Production of yogurt with enhanced levels of gamma-aminobutyric acid and valuable nutrients using lactic acid bacteria and germinated soybean extract', Bioresour Technol, **98**, 1675–9.

Pinchera A, Macgillivray MH, Crawford JD and Freeman AG, (1965), 'Thyroid refractoriness in an athyreotic cretin fed soybean formula', N Engl J Med, **273**, 83–7.

Pyo YH (2007), 'Production of a high value-added soybean containing bioactive mevinolins and isoflavones', J Food Sci Nutr, **12**, 29–34.

Pyo YH and Lee TC (2007), 'The potential antioxidant capacity and angiotensin I-converting enzyme inhibitory activity of Monascus-fermented soybean extracts: evaluation of Monascus-fermented soybean extracts as multifunctional food additives', J Food Sci, **72**, S218–23.

Pyo YH and Seong KS (2009), 'Hypolipidemic effects of Monascus-fermented soybean extracts in rats fed a high-fat and -cholesterol diet', J Agric Food Chem, **57**, 8617–22.

Pyo YH and Song SM (2009), 'Physicochemical and sensory characteristics of a medicinal soy yogurt containing health-benefit ingredients', J Agric Food Chem, **57**, 170–5.

Sarkar S (2006), 'Potential of soyoghurt as a dietetic food', Nutr Food Sci, **36**, 43–9.

Schone F, Jahreis G, Lange R, Seffner W, Groppel B, et al. (1990), 'Effect of varying glucosinolate and iodine intake via rapeseed meal diets on serum thyroid hormone level and total iodine in the thyroid in growing pigs', Endocrinol Exp, **24**, 415–27.

Senbon S. (1940), 'Bacillus natto as the anti-trichophytosis', J Formosan Med Assoc Taipei, **39**, 14–17.

Setchell KD (1998), 'Phytoestrogens: the biochemistry, physiology, and implications for human health of soy isoflavones', Am J Clin Nutr, **68**, S1333–46.

Setchell KD, Zimmer-Nechemias L, Cai J and Heubi JE (1997), 'Exposure of infants to phyto-oestrogens from soy-based infant formula', Lancet, **350**, 23–7.

Sharpless GR, Pearsons J and Prato GS, (1939), 'Production of goiter in rats with raw and with treated soybean flour', J Nutr, **17**, 545–55.

Shepard TH, Pyne GE, Kirschvink JF and McLean CM, (1960), 'Soybean goiter', New Eng J Med, **262**, 1099–103.

Shin ZI, Yu R, Park SA, Chung DK, Ahn CW, Nam HS, Kim KS and Lee HJ (2001), 'His-His-Leu, an angiotensin I converting enzyme inhibitory peptide derived from Korean soybean paste, exerts antihypertensive activity in vivo', *J Agric Food Chem*, **49**, 3004–9.

Slavin J (1991), 'Nutritional benefits of soy protein and soy fibre', *J Am Diet Assoc*, **91**, 816–19.

Son HY, Nishikawa A, Ikeda T, Imazawa T, Kimura S and Hirose M (2001), 'Lack of effect of soy isoflavone on thyroid hyperplasia in rats receiving an iodine-deficient diet', *Jpn J Cancer Res*, **92**, 103–8.

St Clair WH, Billings PC, Carew JA, Keller-McGandy C, Newberne P and Kennedy AR (1990), 'Suppression of dimethylhydrazine-induced carcinogenesis in mice by dietary addition of the Bowman-Birk protease inhibitor', *Cancer Res*, **50**, 580–6.

Sumi H and Ohsugi T (1999), 'Anti-bacterial component dipicolic acid measured in Natto and Natto bacilli', *Nippon Nogei Kagaku Kaishi*, **73**, 1289–91.

Sumi H, Hamada H, Nakanishi K and Hiratani H (1990), 'Enhancement of the fibrinolytic activity in plasma by oral administration of nattokinase', *Acta Haematol*, **84**, 139–43.

Sumi H, Hamada H, Tsushima H, Mihara H and Muraki H (1987), 'A novel fibrinolytic enzyme (nattokinase) in the vegetable cheese Natto; a typical and popular soybean food in the Japanese diet', *Experientia*, **43**, 1110–1.

Suzuki Y, Kondo K, Ichise H, Tsukamoto Y, Urano T and Umemura K (2003b), 'Dietary supplementation with fermented soybeans suppresses intimal thickening', *Nutrition*, **19**, 261–4.

Suzuki Y, Kondo K, Matsumoto Y, Zhao BQ, Otsuguro K, *et al.* (2003a), 'Dietary supplementation of fermented soybean, natto, suppresses intimal thickening and modulates the lysis of mural thrombi after endothelial injury in rat femoral artery', *Life Sci*, **73**, 1289–98.

Takenaka Y, Utsumi S and Yoshikawa M (2000), 'Introduction of enterostatin (VPDPR) and a related sequence into soybean proglycinin A1aB1b subunit by site-directed mutagenesis', *Biosci Biotechnol Biochem*, **64**, 2731–3.

Torres N, Torre-Villalvazo I and Tovar AR (2006), 'Regulation of lipid metabolism by soy protein and its implication in diseases mediated by lipid disorders', *J Nutr Biochem*, **17**, 365–73.

Tsukamoto Y (2004), 'Studies on action of menaquinone-7 in regulation of bone metabolism and its preventive role of osteoporosis', *Biofactors*, **22**, 5–19.

Tsukamoto Y, Ichise H, Kakuda H and Yamaguchi M (2000), 'Intake of fermented soybean (natto) increases circulating vitamin K2 (menaquinone-7) and gamma-carboxylated osteocalcin concentration in normal individuals', *J Bone Miner Metab*, **18**, 216–22.

Udo S (1936), 'Regarding the components of natto: the existence of dipicolinic acid in natto and its effects', *Nippon Nogei Kagaku Kaishi*, **12**, 386–94.

US Food and Drug Administration (1999), 'Food labelling health claims: soy protein and coronary heart disease', *Food and Drug Administration Final rule Fed Register*, **64**, 57699–733.

Van WYK JJ, Arnold MB, Wynn J and Pepper F, (1959), 'The effects of a soybean product on thyroid function in humans', *Pediatrics*, **24**, 752–60.

Wagar LE, Champagne CP, Buckley ND, Raymond Y and Green-Johnson JM (2009), 'Immunomodulatory properties of fermented soy and dairy milks prepared with lactic acid bacteria', *J Food Sci*, **74**, M423–30.

Watanabe N, Fujimoto K and Aoki H (2007), 'Antioxidant activities of the water-soluble fraction in tempeh-like fermented soybean (GABA-tempeh)', *Int J Food Sci Nutr*, **58**, 577–87.

Wilgus HS, Gassner FX, Patton AH and Gustavson RG, (1941), 'The goitrogenicity of soybeans', *J Nutr*, **22**, 43–52.

Wood CE, Clarkson TB, Appt SE, Franke AA, Boue SM, *et al.* (2006), 'Effects of soybean glyceollins and estradiol in postmenopausal female monkeys', *Nutr Cancer*, **56**, 74–81.

Xiao CW (2008), 'Health effects of soy protein and isoflavones in humans', *J Nutr*, **138**, S1244–9.

Xiao CW, L'Abbe MR, Gilani S, Cooke G, Curran I and Papademetriou SA, (2004), 'Dietary soy protein isolate and isoflavones modulate hepatic thyroid hormone receptors in rats', *J Nutr*, **134**, 743–9.

Yamaguchi M and Ma ZJ (2001), 'Inhibitory effect of menaquinone-7 (vitamin K2) on osteoclast-like cell formation and osteoclastic bone resorption in rat bone tissues in vitro', *Mol Cell Biochem*, **228**, 39–47.

Yamaguchi M, Kakuda H, Gao YH and Tsukamoto Y (2000), 'Prolonged intake of fermented soybean (natto) diets containing vitamin K2 (menaquinone-7) prevents bone loss in ovariectomized rats', *J Bone Miner Metab*, **18**, 71–6.

Yamaguchi M, Taguchi H, Gao YH, Igarashi A and Tsukamoto Y (1999), 'Effect of vitamin K2 (menaquinone-7) in fermented soybean (natto) on bone loss in ovariectomized rats', *J Bone Miner Metab*, **17**, 23–9.

Yamaguchi M, Uchiyama S and Tsukamoto Y (2002), 'Stimulatory effect of menaquinone-7 on bone formation in elderly female rat femoral tissues in vitro: prevention of bone deterioration with aging', *Int J Mol Med*, **10**, 729–33.

Yavelow J, Finlay TH, Kennedy AR and Troll W (1983), 'Bowman-Birk soybean protease inhibitor as an anticarcinogen', *Cancer Res*, **43**, s2454–9.

Yoshikawa M, Fujita H, Matoba N, Takenaka Y, Yamamoto T, Yamauchi R, Tsuruki H and Takahata K (2000), 'Bioactive peptides derived from food proteins preventing lifestyle-related diseases', *Biofactors*, **12**, 143–6.

Young VR (1991), 'Soy protein in relation to human protein and amino acid nutrition', *J Am Diet Assoc*, **91**, 828–35.

Zhang T, Pan W, Takebe M, Schofield B, Sampson H and Li XM (2008), 'Therapeutic effects of a fermented soy product on peanut hypersensitivity is associated with modulation of T-helper type 1 and T-helper type 2 responses', *Clin Exp Allergy*, **38**, 1808–18.

23

Functional seafood products

M. Careche and A. J. Borderías, Institute of Food Science, Technology
and Nutrition (ICTAN), Spain, I. Sánchez-Alonso, Institute of the
Structure of Matter (IEM), Spain and E. K. Lund, Institute of Food
Research (IFR), Norwich, UK

Abstract: The development of consumer-oriented functional food products based on
seafood gives an opportunity to enhance its consumption. This chapter describes the main
beneficial health effects of seafood and the potential for development of functional
seafood products, and ends with some examples based on the experience of the authors
on the development of functional seafood products made using restructured fish as the
vehicle matrix and dietary fibres.

Key words: functional seafood products, restructured fish, dietary fibres, antioxidant
dietary fibres.

23.1   Introduction

In general fish is considered to be a healthy part of the diet providing a range of
beneficial nutrients, yet in most European countries and the USA few people
achieve the recommended intake of at least two portions of fish a week, including
oily fish. These recommendations vary between countries and in some an upper
limit of four portions is proposed in response to concerns over accumulation
of toxic substances such as polychlorinated biphenyls (PCB)s and methyl
mercury found in a limited number of species high in the food chain and caught
in particularly polluted waters (Strain *et al.*, 2008; Ginsberg and Toal, 2009).
It is therefore important to provide safe seafood containing key beneficial
compounds.

One way of increasing this consumption is by the development of bespoke
seafood products, with optimal sensory, nutritional, convenience or availability
characteristics. In Europe, beneficial health effects of seafood is actually one of
the drivers for its consumption (Brunso, 2003), but there are certain barriers for

the consumption of fish as such, especially for particular consumer population (Brunso *et al.*, 2008).

Industry is fortifying some foods with components extracted from seafood. Of the various marine ingredients used, omega-3 polyunsaturated fatty acids (PUFA) are the most popular and are included in bread items and other baked goods, dairy products such as milk, cheese, fermented milks, and chocolate milk and infant formulae (Ohr, 2005). They are mainly marketed in US, Europe, Japan and Southeast Asia. This gives an opportunity to increase the daily intake of these compounds through food commodities which are more usual or accepted by consumers. Functional products with seafood as a matrix are mainly found in the canning sector. The claims 'Natural source of omega-3', 'low salt' or 'low fat' are the most commonly attributed to these seafood products, although products enriched in isoflavones, or calcium with casein calcium peptide in order to help calcium absorption, have also been launched to the market.

Many of the nutritional advantages of seafood pose some technological problems in terms of processing or preservation. The highly unsaturated fatty acids make some fish very prone to oxidation, and their proteins may become denatured or aggregated upon storage, leading to shortened storage life. Other nutritional losses derived from the modification or loss of some important nutrients may occur upon improper processing, storage or culinary treatments. Thus, strategies for stabilization of fish matrix components need to be developed alongside other technological innovations and nutritional studies. Species diversity also leads to different nutritional, technological and sensory characteristics of seafood, all of them crucial when developing functional seafood products.

This chapter describes the main beneficial health effects of seafood, the potential for development of functional seafood products and ends with some examples based on the experience of the authors on the development of functional seafood products made by restructured fish as the vehicle matrix.

23.2   Health aspects of seafood

23.2.1   Evidence for health benefits associated with fish consumption

Although consumption of seafoods is generally perceived to be 'healthy' it is unclear whether fish consumption allows us to live longer. However, a diet rich in fish, shell fish and even seaweeds may well provide better health into old age. At a population level, people in countries where fish is a major part of the diet do live longer (Zhang *et al.*, 1999) but when we look at the statistics within countries the data is generally missing or unconvincing for any benefit related to all-cause mortality (Osler *et al.*, 2003; Nakamura *et al.*, 2005). Most of the evidence for benefit has been deduced from population studies. Of these the most convincing are prospective cohort studies in which people who are healthy at the time of asking report on their intake of a wide range of foods as well as other lifestyle factors such as smoking and exercise. Unfortunately the potential benefits of fish have only been relatively recently recognized within the scientific community and so the detail as to types of seafood consumed and how they were cooked is often limited. It is therefore quite difficult to assess intake of specific nutrients associated with fish consumption although plasma omega-3 content does correlate with reported fish consumption (Welch *et al.*, 2006) as does urinary taurine (Wójcik *et al.*, 2010). Beneficial effects found to be associated with fish intake are normally attributed to the omega-3 polyunsaturated fatty acid (PUFA) content of fish oils. However, fish oil intervention studies provide less convincing evidence of protection as regards health outcomes such as cardiovascular disease and cancer (Hooper *et al.*, 2006), but it should be remembered that low detectable responses are a characteristic of intervention studies as they are limited by a number of practicalities affecting length of time of intervention, the choice of target population and whether the intervention is given before or after onset of symptoms. There have been relatively few intervention studies using fish rather than fish oil and these probably suffer even more of the logistic limitations mentioned above. However, a large number of fish oil trials using animal models of various diseases do provide support for a protective effect of fish oils as well as giving insight into potential mechanisms, but a detailed discussion of these is outside the scope of this chapter. Additionally, fish oil studies in human populations have shown protective effects in relation to biomarkers of risk of disease such as beneficial effects on plasma lipoprotein patterns (low-density lipoprotein (LDL), high-density lipoprotein (HDL) cholesterol, etc.) and on cell proliferation and cancer cell death of the epithelial cells lining the intestinal tract. Nevertheless the failure of human intervention studies to show any significant effect on death rates may suggest an effect of fish other than that of omega-3 fatty acids. Such effects could be associated with other nutrients such as selenium and taurine, but the data supporting their health benefits is probably even more limited. For example, the few randomized control diets with taurine have been very small (Wójcik *et al.*, 2010) and data relating to selenium is very mixed.

23.2.2   Evidence in relation to specific diseases

Protective effects of fish consumption have been studied in relation to a wide range of health outcomes including: coronary heart disease, cerebral stroke, various cancers, arthritis, diabetes, cognitive development, cognitive decline, mood disorders and immune function. The evidence suggesting protective effects of seafoods have been recently reviewed in relation to heart disease (Brouwer, 2008), metabolic disorders (Thorsdottir and Ramel, 2008), gastrointestinal disorders (Lund and Kampman, 2008) and cancer (Lund, 2009). Two recent intervention trials have used only fish as an intervention rather than fish plus fish oil capsules, one on gastrointestinal health (Pot *et al.*, 2009a, 2009b, 2010) and the other on a range of markers associated with bone health and weight control (Parra *et al.*, 2007; Thorsdottir *et al.*, 2007; Gunnarsdottir *et al.*, 2008; Ramel *et al.*, 2010) and these show some effects of increased fish intake on systemic health and weight control. Apart from these we must rely on epidemiological studies to assess the effects of fish. Even these are limited, as mentioned above, but those coming from the European Prospective Investigation into Cancer and Nutrition (EPIC) provide good quality data. In this population there was a six- to sevenfold variation in total fish consumption in women and men, between the lowest consumption in Germany and the highest in Spain (Welch *et al.*, 2002). Fish consumption was not associated with any protective effect on breast cancer (Engeset *et al.*, 2006) but it was on colon cancer, even to the extent that high fish consumption appeared to counteract most of the negative effects of a high meat intake (Norat *et al.*, 2005). Reports from this study also show no protective effect on stroke (Myint *et al.*, 2006) although analysis of previous studies had suggested an effect (He *et al.*, 2004a), but a protective effect on diabetes was observed (Patel *et al.*, 2009). Fish consumption is also associated with a lower blood pressure but this effect was mostly explained by a lower body mass index in this group (Appleby *et al.*, 2002). Unfortunately, at present no reports on risk of cardiovascular disease have been published from these studies, but meta-analyses of previous studies suggest a protective effect of fish consumption in this respect (He *et al.*, 2004b; Whelton *et al.*, 2004) with several further individual studies supporting a protective effect having been published in recent years.

23.2.3   Health benefits associated with specific nutrients

Seafoods contain a number of nutrients with potentially beneficial effects. Many of these nutritional factors are known to impact on similar health outcomes but through different mechanisms and thus may act in concert to produce benefit. Probably the best known aspect of seafood consumption in relation to human health is that it is a good source of the omega-3 PUFAs docosahexaenoic acid (DHA) and eicosapentaenoic acid (EPA). EPA and DHA consumption have been linked to reduced risk of cardiovascular disease, colon cancer, cognitive function in both the young and elderly, metal health disorders and a range of chronic inflammatory diseases. The actual quantity of these fatty acids in different seafoods varies between species and depends on the amounts in their diet. For example herring (*Clupea harengus*) and mackerel (*Scomber* spp.) are particularly good sources of omega-3 while lean fish such as cod (*Gadus morhua*) and plaice (*Pleuronectes platessa*), being low in fat, are less so. However, the low fat content of these fish means they provide a low-calorie source of protein and the small amount of fat in their muscle is high in DHA and EPA.

Oily fish is also a considered to be a good source of dietary vitamin D but the UK food tables (Anonymous, 2002) suggest that only cod liver oil and herring, and to a limited extent huss and mackerel, can supply significant amounts of vitamin D, and a very high consumption of even these sources would be required to compensate for lack of sunshine (Ashwell *et al.*, 2010). However, there is an increasing awareness of the possible importance of vitamin D in relation to a wide range of aspects of health such as cancer prevention, heart disease, mental health, inflammatory conditions as well as bone health (Hayes, 2010; Mulligan *et al.*, 2010). As it is frequently suggested that oil-rich fish is eaten to compensate for lack of sunshine in those living closer to the poles, especially those with darker skin colour or who expose little skin or rarely spend time outdoors, it would be desirable to increase the levels of this vitamin in processed seafoods designed for this market. The best known benefit of vitamin D is its role in supporting calcium absorption and bone health. For this effect sufficient calcium must also be available in the diet and so sources of seafood containing high levels calcium such as those in which the bones are included are potentially beneficial. This is normally achieved in canned fish such as salmon (*Salmo salar*), sardines (*Sardina pilchardus*) and anchovies (*Engraulis mordax*). Bombay duck (*Harpadon nehereus*) and dried shrimps are also good sources of calcium but are generally only eaten in small quantities. It should be noted that calcium is not only important in relation to bone health but has also been linked, in combination with vitamin D, to a number of health outcomes including gastrointestinal diseases, diabetes, hypertension and cardiac health.

Seafood is also a potentially good source of selenium as it has been shown to be very bioavailable from fish (Fox *et al.*, 2004). Selenium is required for the proper functioning of key enzymes, most well known of which is the antioxidant enzyme glutathione peroxidise. There are in total 25 such selenoproteins involved in such diverse activities as prevention of lipid peroxidation, thyroid hormone metabolism and inflammatory responses. Optimal selenium intake is believed to be beneficial in relation to cancer prevention, particularly colon and prostate cancers, fertility and overall longevity. The organic forms of selenium are known to be much better absorbed into the body (bioavailable) than inorganic forms. Levels are generally particularly high in a number of shellfish as well as swordfish (*Xiphias gladius*), tuna (*Tunnus* spp.) and salmon but little is known about species-specific differences in bioavailability of selenium. A recent study has identified a novel source of organic selenium, selenoneine, which is present in high quantities in tuna and other fish (Yamashita and Yamashita, 2010). Because of its very recent discovery the bioavailability of this form of selenium remains to be investigated, but this should be a priority as it seems to be the major form of selenium in a number of fish species. We have previously shown that people asked to increase their intake of cod by two portions per week can increase serum selenium levels significantly (Pot *et al.*, 2009b) although not enough to compensate for the generally low levels found in most European populations. Thus selenium enrichment of products is potentially desirable but such developments must take account of the narrow optimal range of intake (30 μg/d–900 μg/d) as excess selenium is recognized to be toxic.

Fish is also traditionally considered to be a good source of readily digestible protein. Although the literature does not fully support the idea that fish protein is any more digestible than other protein sources (Cervantes-Pahm and Stein, 2010; Faber *et al.*, 2010) the balance of amino acids is generally good (Usydus *et al.*, 2009). Furthermore, seafoods, in particular shellfish, are a good source of taurine, which has been suggested to be potentially protective against cardiovascular disease (Wójcik *et al.*, 2010). For example, scallop contains levels in excess of 800 mg/100 g and mussels >600 mg/100 g. In contrast, mammalian meat typically contains less than 50 mg/100 g.

In light of our present still limited knowledge relating to the health benefits of fish we should aim to preserve the known potential beneficial factors associated with fish consumption such as selenium, good PUFA profile, vitamin D and calcium, and low fat and possibly taurine content when producing novel processed seafood products.

23.3   Potential for development of functional seafood products

The increase in functional foods in recent years has occurred as a result of the convergence of several factors, which include the accumulated scientific knowledge of the link between diet, lifestyle, and health; awareness of the consumers of these facts; and the competitive food market (Siro *et al.*, 2008).

Thus, there is an exceptional boom in the functional food and beverage market worldwide, which from 2000 to 2005 increased up to 2.2 times, and has been estimated to increase at the same rate up to 2010, reaching US$ 167 billion (Granato *et al.*, 2010 and references therein). These authors state that the European market for functional foods was estimated to be between 4 and 8 billion US$ in 2003 and this value increased to around 15 billion US$ by 2006, with Germany, France, the United Kingdom and the Netherlands being the most important countries within this market. It varies greatly across regions, with Australasia being clearly dominant, while Eastern Europe and Africa remain very underdeveloped.

Functional seafood can be designed by dietary modulation of farmed fish. Fish can also be seen as a source of functional ingredients to be extracted from, especially, by-products or underutilized species. And, thirdly, fish muscle can be used as a carrier for functional ingredients of marine or other food origins via restructuring technology and several processing technologies. Thus, the potential for the development of functional seafood products has not yet been fully exploited.

23.3.1   Functional seafood products made by dietary modulation

Fatty acids

The PUFA content of fish depends on several factors, for example freshwater fish generally have a low content as compared to saltwater fish. In the case of farmed fish the PUFA content can be tailor-made by the type and source of oil in the feed. It has been shown that dietary supplementation with refined menhaden fish oil markedly increased the n-3 long chain (LC) PUFA content in freshwater species such as Channel catfish (*Ictarus punctatus*) without adversely affecting flavour attributes or storage quality (Morris *et al.*, 2005; Manning *et al.*, 2006). The current inadequate supply of fish meal and fish oil due to the dramatic increase in aquaculture, has led to the development of alternatives from sustainable sources (Naylor *et al.*, 2000). The use of marine algae has been seen as a promising and sustainable alternative source of LC-PUFA.

The use of microalgae thraustochytrid (*Schizochytrium* sp.) to increase the n-3 PUFA content in live feeds such as rotifers and *Artemia nauplii* (Yamasaki *et al.*,

2007) and fairy shrimp (*Streptocephalus dichotomus*) (Velu and Munuswamy, 2004) has been reported in relation to larval fish. The amount of DHA in fish was shown to be effectively increased with inclusion of this microalgae and/or the dinoflagelate *Crypthecodinium cohnii* by feeding larvae (Ganuza *et al.*, 2008) and juvenile in seabream (*Sparus aurata*) (Atalah *et al.*, 2007) and Atlantic salmon (Miller *et al.*, 2007).

Studies conducted with rainbow trout (*Oncorhynchus mykiss*) suggest that the inclusion of more than 3% macroalgae meal (*Macrocystis pyrifera*) in the diet improve the levels of PUFA, specifically EPA and DHA (Dantagnan *et al.*, 2009).

Increasing conjugated linoleic acid (CLA) content in fish is particularly interesting for producing functional fish fillets to enhance their quality for human consumption. CLA includes a group of positional and geometric isomers of linoleic acid containing double bounds. The two main naturally occurring isomers *cis*-9 *trans*-11 and *trans*-10 *cis*-12 are believed to have physiological effects and health benefits (Park and Pariza, 2007; Lock *et al.*, 2009; Tissot-Favre and Waldron, 2009).

CLA isomers have successfully been incorporated into the muscle tissue of freshwater fish, such as channel catfish (*Ictalurus punctatus*) (Manning *et al.*, 2006) and rainbow trout (Bandarra *et al.*, 2006, Valente *et al.*, 2007b) as well as in marine fish such as Atlantic salmon (Berge *et al.*, 2004; Kennedy *et al.*, 2005) or sea bass (*Dicentrarchus labrax*) (Valente *et al.*, 2007a; Makol *et al.*, 2009). Nevertheless different effects on growth performance and metabolic utilization of CLA in fish diets have been described, as they may alter fatty acid metabolism and bone mineralization (Berge *et al.*, 2004; Leaver *et al.*, 2006).

Selenium

Levels of selenium (Se) content in different seafoods have been reported to range from 0.13 mg/kg in species such as halibut (*Hippoglossus hippoglossus*) to 0.73 mg/kg in tuna (*Thunnus thynnus*) (Oehlenschläger, 1997, Souci *et al.*, 2000). Selenium is relatively high in 'niboshi' which is produced by boiling the small Japanese anchovy (*Engraulis japonicus*) for several minutes and then drying (Haratake *et al.*, 2007).

The presence of Se has been reported to increase after supplementation in the form of selenomethionine in salmon (Lorentzen *et al.*, 1994), cutthroat trout (*Oncorhynchus claki bouvieri*) (Hardy *et al.*, 2010), Channel catfish (Wang and Lovell, 1997) and crucian carp (*Carrassius auratus* subsp. *gibelio*) (Zhou *et al.*, 2009).

African catfish (*Clarias goriepinus*) have been fed diets containing γ-glutamyl-selenomethyl-selenocysteine and selenomethyl-selenocysteine enriched garlic over a period of six weeks, and the Se content in the muscle increased linearly with increasing dietary Se levels (Luten and Schram, 2006; Schram *et al.*, 2008). These authors also reported that depuration, a necessary procedure before sacrifice to eliminate off-flavours, has little or no effect on total selenium level in the muscle but changes in flavour due to feed containing garlic disappear as a result of depuration (Luten *et al.*, 2008; Schram *et al.*, 2010).

Taurine
Seafood, especially invertebrates such as molluscs and crustaceans, are high in taurine (300–800 mg per 100 g edible portion) (Dragnes *et al.*, 2009). Marine invertebrates generally have a higher cellular osmolarity than fish and since taurine has an osmoregulatory role, this may explain the higher concentrations. Other factors influencing the taurine concentration *in vivo* of the species are seasonal variations, temperature, salinity and diet (Jones, 1954). There seem to be a direct relation between serum taurine levels and the consumption of seafood (Kim *et al.*, 2003; Brøns *et al.*, 2004; Wójcik *et al.*, 2010).

African catfish fed for six months with fish meals enriched with synthetic taurine at different concentrations (1–18 mg taurine/g wet feed) showed increased levels of this component in muscle in a nonlinear manner (Luten *et al.*, 2008).

23.3.2   Functional components extracted from seafood material

Marine lipids
Major fish species used in the production of fish oil include species such as anchovies, capelin cod, sharks, herring, mackerel, menhaden, salmonids and sardines. In contrast with other fats and oils, marine oils contain high amounts of EPA and DHA (USDA, 2009). Generally, oil is extracted from by-products or from the whole body of certain species. Other sources of PUFA are microalgae and other microorganisms from marine origin that in comparison with fish oils show a less complex fatty acid profile and have strong fish odours.

Marine bioactive peptides
Recently, much attention has been paid to the structural and compositional properties of bioactive peptides from marine proteins that are inactive in the original proteins, but once released by enzymatic hydrolysis have interesting functional properties, at least *in vitro*. Many bioactive peptides have been isolated from undervalued species and marine by-products. Many physiological functions of marine-derived bioactive peptides have been studied, including antihypertensive or angiotensin-I-converting enzyme (ACE) inhibition, antioxidant, anticoagulant, and antimicrobial activities, but these can only be considered suitable for taking to market once bioavailability of these products *in vivo* has been fully assessed. The development of functional marine protein and peptide ingredients has been recently reviewed by Thorkelsson *et al.* (2008). Whereas in recent years a few fermented dairy products with antihypertensive peptides have appeared in both Japanese and European market, they are still not commercially available from marine origin.

Chitin, chitosans and derivates
Chitin occurs naturally, chiefly in the exoskeletons of crustaceans and molluscs, but also in insects and in certain fungi where it is the principal fibrillar polymer of the cell wall. Chitosan is known to possess numerous technological and

physiological properties useful in foods (Shahidi *et al.*, 1999). From a physiological standpoint, its prime function is to reduce intestinal lipid absorption, with reduction of cholesterol and favouring loss of body weight (Ylitalo *et al.*, 2002). It also shows a potential prebiotic effect as a stimulant of selective growth of lactobacilli and bifidobacteria (Lee *et al.*, 2002). Most commercial products are in the form of capsules and tablets. Chitosan is available in a big variety of products with different deacetylation grades and molecular weights or viscosities leading to different properties (Sen, 2005).

In the European market, chitosan is sold in the form of dietary capsules aimed at overweight people while in Japan they are added to commercialized food products such as noodles, potato crisps and biscuits. The US Food and Drug Administration classify chitosan as 'generally recognized as safe (GRAS)'. In the US there are several products in the market that contain chitosan in combination with other nutrients such as lecithin, vitamins, etc., as both supplements and in commercialized juices and chocolates.

Glucosamine, a natural amino sugar found in certain foods such as milk and eggs, which may result from hydrolysis of chitosan, has been developed as a pharmaceutical, as N-acetyl glucosamine, in the treatment of arthritis. It has been added to a range of commercial products and, has been described as an additive in milk (Xu *et al.*, 2004) and milk products in a Chinese patent (Ohr, 2006). An orange juice supplemented with glucosamine has been marketed in the USA, where a commercial glucosamine ingredient has been accorded GRAS status by the US-FDA, which permits the product to be added to a variety of foods and beverages (Anonymous, 2007a).

Fish bones as source of mineral
Tuna bones were in use as a source of calcium in Japan in the mid 1980s in institutional feeding programmes for the elderly and in school meals (Venugopal, 2009). A fish processing company in Japan has successfully processed scales of sardine into an edible food supplement containing calcium and collagen (Anonymous, 2007b). Similarly, canned bite-size chunks of Pacific saury (*Cololabis saira*) rich in calcium, DHA and EPA are commercially available in Japan with added calcium peptide (a milk protein derivate) intended to support calcium absorption. Furthermore, a commercial marine mineral product which also contains sardine bones is available in the USA (Venugopal, 2009). Thus, there is a potential for production of mineral supplements such as calcium from fish bone waste, which can be used for fortifying different foods due to its bioavailability (Shungan, 1996). Other products such as oligopeptides derived from enzymatic degradation of fish bones can be used as a potential calcium-binder (Venugopal, 2009).

Dietary fibre (DF)
Seaweeds are considered a good source of DF and many of the ones currently used for technological purposes are highly soluble (Borderías *et al.*, 2005). Seaweeds contain bioactive compounds with known antioxidant properties, such

as polyphenols, carotenoids and tocopherols (Jiménez-Escrig *et al.*, 2001) associated with the DF. Due to this recently identified antioxidant, a DF concentrate has been developed to be used as a food ingredient (Saura-Calixto and Jiménez-Escrig, 2003).

23.3.3   Restructured fish muscle as a carrier for functional seafood

Restructured seafood products are foods made from minced and/or chopped muscle and which are used, with or without ingredients, to make other products with a new appearance and texture. For some time now there have been products in the market in the form of fish fingers or other shapes intended basically for children as well as seafood products which can mimic other value-added products thus conferring the food a positive image. The reason for restructuring fish muscle has mainly been that the supply of high value seafood products is limited and therefore the need to make the best use of the existing resources. One source of muscle for this technology should be underutilized fish species that otherwise have commercial problems ranging from the size of the fish to their composition, bony structure or unattractive appearance or texture. Additionally, fish by-products from regular processing of more expensive species may be used (Borderías and Pérez-Mateos, 1996).

These restructured products are very good carriers for functional ingredients, since there are fewer technical restrictions compared to inclusion via dietary modulation. However, the method of incorporation may have an impact on bioavailablity. Different types of matrices can be used depending on the integrity of the muscle: from pieces of fillets to minced fish or *surimi*, which is a paste of stabilized myofibrillar proteins with long frozen storage stability and with unique gel-forming abilities. Thus, fish muscle as a food vehicle for bioactive ingredients has a great potential for tailoring foods with the required functional and sensory characteristics. Several ingredients including PUFA, taurine, or soluble DFs have been introduced into restructured fish (Careche *et al.*, 2008).

23.4   Development of functional seafood products with dietary fibres

The development of functional seafood products with each type of matrix has varying degrees of difficulty in terms of technological feasibility, consumer acceptance or functional and nutritional value. A stable environment for the bioactive ingredients, needs to be obtained which has to be compatible with the sensory and techno-functional characteristics of the food. Both issues may call for optimization of the formulations, based on the knowledge of the physical-chemical interactions between the ingredients and the vehicle matrix. Also the bioactive ingredient's health benefit should be maximized and maintained together with the beneficial effects of the matrix itself (IFT, 2005). But the technological developments and the strategies designed to maximize the biological activity of the food component may not be enough to achieve an increase of the consumption of the desired health beneficial compounds or seafood products by the population. Thus this knowledge has to be translated into attractive products for the market, and therefore consumer studies should be integrated from the start of the product development process (Careche *et al.*, 2008).

This section depicts some highlights of the experience of the authors on the development of restructured products enriched with commercial DFs and non-commercial antioxidant DFs. The work was focused on product development assuming the well-known beneficial effect of DFs and PUFA, both of which appear in the positive list of compounds for nutritional claims in the EU regulation (EC, 2006; EU, 2010).

Figure 23.1 describes the roadmap used by the authors for the development of functional seafood products. Initially, the selection and preparation of the ingredients and matrix was performed. Stage 2 covered the studies aiming to find the optimal formulations which included the bioactive compound(s), the seafood matrix and other ingredient(s) needed to achieve the desired product. Here the technological characteristics, the structural features of some selected formulations, the composition analyses, and the sensory properties of the seafood material were explored and the best options were selected for further development. In parallel, consumer studies were conducted, which, together with the input provided by an industrial partner served to prepare some product prototypes. These were tested by consumers in 'Product tests' of some selected products. The final stage led to several seafood product prototypes which differed in the degree of innovation (completely new products *vs* extensions or adaptations of existing ones), consumer targets (selected consumer segments *vs* all consumers), or type of matrix (e.g. mince-based products *vs surimi*) (Careche *et al.*, 2008). The study of *in vitro* antioxidant bioaccessibility of some of the products using antioxidant DFs by

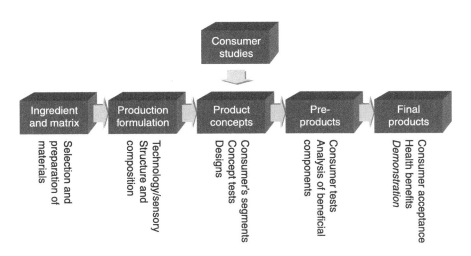

Fig. 23.1 Roadmap for the development of functional seafood products.

intestinal models and the study of water structure and distribution in the seafood matrix and their implications in the reformulation of seafood products were also taken into account.

23.4.1   Selection and preparation of the ingredients and materials

The role of DF in nutrition and health is well established. Knowledge of the beneficial effects of high DF diets has led the development of a large and profitable market of DF-rich products. Most of the DFs used in seafood products are soluble and usually selected for their technological properties, such as high water binding, emulsifying, thickening or gel-forming ability (Park, 2005). There is more limited experience on using insoluble DFs in seafood products (Borderías *et al.*, 2005), and, at the time of the study, none on the use of antioxidant DFs.

The concept of antioxidant DF (ADF) is applied to a vegetable material which contains both DF (>50%) and natural constituents with antioxidant capacity able to inhibit lipid oxidation equivalent to, at least, 200 mg of vitamin E per g of ADF, as well as with a free radical scavenging capacity equivalent to, at least, 50 mg of vitamin E/g. This antioxidant capacity should be an intrinsic property, from natural constituents of the product (Saura-Calixto, 1998). Formulations made with antioxidant DFs (Fig. 23.2), could serve to include DF into the diet

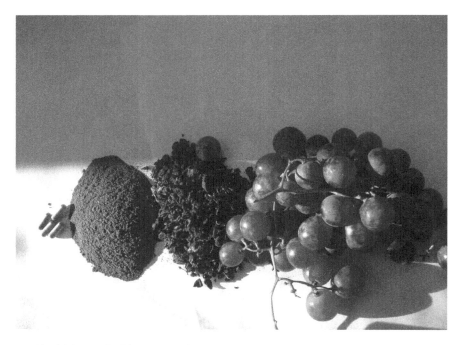

Fig. 23.2   Antioxidant dietary fibres extracted from grapeskin, seeds and pomace.

and to delay lipid oxidation of PUFA contained in fish muscle. Thus the aim was to prove that the inclusion of DF, alone or together with natural antioxidants associated to the DF, led to sensory acceptable restructured products made of fish muscle that fulfil the requirement of 'source of dietary fibre' and/or 'high content of fibre' according to the EU regulation (EC, 2006), which in the case of ADF could act by delaying PUFA oxidation in restructured fish with the subsequent nutritional and sensory advantages associated with these products.

23.4.2 Technological feasibility

The use of different types of restructured fish (*surimi*, minced fish), different underutilized species (horse mackerel (*Trachurus trachurus*) and giant squid (*Dosidicus gigas*)), by-products from regular processing of valued species, as well as regular commercial fish was assessed. Factors such as DF length (wheat DF), particle size of the pomace (red grape), source (white and red grape pomaces, seaweed *fucus*), way of addition of the DF, concentration of fibre/matrix/water, frozen storage, and presence of protective barriers against oxidation, were studied (Sánchez-Alonso *et al.*, 2006, 2007a, 2007b, 2007c, 2008b; Sánchez-Alonso and Borderías, 2008; Careche *et al.*, 2008; Careche and co-workers, 2008; Sánchez-González *et al.*, 2009).

Surimi gel products

Some of the most important technological properties for *surimi* gel products are whiteness, water holding capacity and gel forming ability. In general, wheat DFs confer the products an extra whiteness. Addition of DF needs to be performed by substitution of either water or protein. In the first case, unduly dry gels would be obtained and it is not economically advantageous, therefore, the second option is usually adopted. However, substitution of protein by DF may impair the gelling properties of the mixtures, due to the known effect of lowering protein concentration on this property and the irregular network formed due to the addition of an external, non-gelling compound (Sánchez-Alonso *et al.*, 2006, 2007c). Secondly, it is not necessarily the case that the higher the water holding capacity of the DF the better for the formulation. In fact this can have the effect of dehydrating the protein. This was found to be the case with wheat DF, so that two separate moisture compartments can occur in the matrix, indirectly impairing the gel forming capacity of the muscle protein (Sánchez-González *et al.*, 2009).

Minced fish products

The same technical considerations regarding the way of adding DF apply to minced fish. The main technological advantages of wheat DF was that they effectively bound water, and when the products were battered, they prevent the coating from breaking, also preventing deformation of the cooked portions (Sánchez-Alonso *et al.*, 2007a).

Antioxidant DFs could only be used with minced fish since they dramatically reduced the gel forming ability of *surimi* gels. The chief characteristics of the grape DF concentrates were the high content of total DF (>70%), the relatively high content of soluble DF in comparison with total DF content, and the presence of associated polyphenolic compounds (>5%) (Sánchez-Alonso *et al.*, 2007b, 2008b). Both white and red grape DF was used in proportions of 2 and 4%, and retained the water-holding capacity during frozen storage better than the mixtures without fibre. They also reduced the thaw drip loss and increased the cooking yield. Texture parameters were modified, reducing cohesiveness and hardness (Sánchez-Alonso and Borderías, 2008; Sánchez-Alonso *et al.*, 2008b). The main advantage of these DFs was that they acted as strong antioxidants in frozen stored semi fatty fish minces. Figure 23.3 shows that 2% grape DF was sufficient to delay lipid oxidation in horse mackerel measured by thiobarbituric acid (TBA) values (Sánchez-Alonso and Borderías, 2008). The main drawback was that the colour was very strong and difficult to hide even in horse mackerel or salmon minces.

One of the technological consequences arising from the results of the consumer studies was to use other sources of antioxidant DF, since it was shown that consumers preferred DF of marine origin to their seafood products (Careche *et al.*, 2008). Thus the use of seaweed DF concentrates into restructured fish products was explored. *Fucus* DF acted as antioxidant in a fatty fish species and was suitable technologically, but these DFs conferred the minced fish a dark colour which impaired its potential use (Careche and co-workers, 2008).

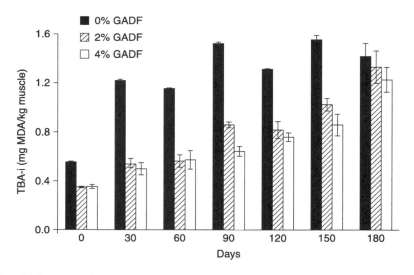

Fig. 23.3 Formation of aldehydes (thiobarbituric acid index (TBA-i) in mg malondialdehyde (MDA)/kg muscle) in samples of minced fish muscle with added grape antioxidant dietary fibre (GADF) during frozen storage at −20 °C.

23.4.3   Product prototypes

Inclusion of dietary fibres into commercial products
In order to test the sensory acceptability of the best formulations tested, as well as the concept of the inclusion of DF into seafood, a product test with 500 consumers was performed with commercial products in association with a company producing restructured fish. Two types of products were chosen, a shredded *surimi* product, suitable as snack food or for inclusion into salads, and a minced fish product, resembling a fillet and suitable as main course. In the first case, wheat DF was used and in the second, both wheat and grape antioxidant DF (Careche *et al.*, 2007; Dopico *et al.*, 2007).

The results showed that products with information about DF and its benefits for health generated positive expectations in the consumers, so that the evaluation prior to tasting was slightly better in the case of products with fibre (Careche *et al.*, 2007, Borderías *et al.*, 2008). Consumers could not detect intrinsic differences between products, except for attributes related to texture. The evaluation of the consumption experience was positive but slightly better for the product without DF. This called for a small optimization step, in order to overcome the dryness and give the product 'smoothness' without compromising the amounts of DF needed for making nutrition claims. The optimization step and scaling up was performed successfully, such that 'high in dietary fibre' claim can be made for commercial products. Furthermore, using triangle tests, no significant differences were obtained between the original formulations and the modified version. Thus the technological feasibility was validated and served to elaborate new products that could be readily commercialized.

Dietary fibres in new product concepts
The product tests also showed that whereas wheat DF enriched products were well received, the grape DF-containing ones were assessed as unsatisfactory due to the strong colour the DF gave to the restructured fish. Additionally, and as mentioned before, consumer survey studies showed that people from certain countries may prefer seaweed DFs in their seafood (Careche *et al.*, 2008). These marine DFs also had a strong greenish colour that may also not be acceptable to the consumers. The combination of technological feasibility and consumer tests narrowed the choice of application of these DFs to already-known products.

Figure 23.4 shows two examples of the range of newly developed products (Sánchez-Alonso *et al.*, 2008a; Borderías *et al.*, 2010). One of these prototypes comprises a cover of *surimi*-based gel enriched with wheat DF stuffed with a mixture of minced fish and freeze-dried seaweed which produces a light green colour. In a limited consumer test with 46 consumers, the cover, the filling and the whole product prior and after tasting was evaluated. Results showed that the colour, rather than a drawback, became an advantage in these new seafood products (Fig. 23.5).

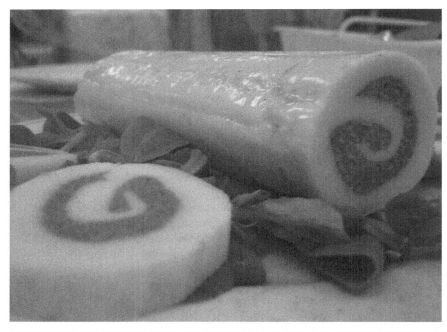

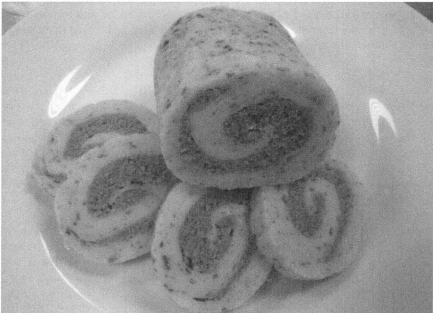

Fig. 23.4   Examples of new restructured products with wheat and antioxidant grapes (top) and seaweed (bottom) dietary fibres which fulfil the nutritional claim 'high in fibre' according to EU legislation.

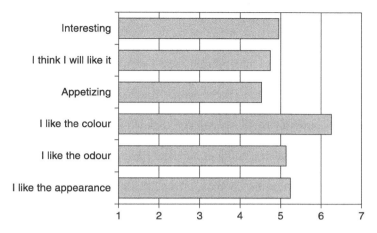

Fig. 23.5 Limited consumer test of the new restructured with wheat and antioxidant seaweed *fucus* dietary fibres. Evaluation prior to consumption. The attribute items were measured on a seven-point agree–disagree scale (1 = totally disagree and 7 = totally agree).

23.4.4 Nutritional and health properties of the developed convenience seafood muscle products with dietary fibres

The aim of the above studies was to develop nutritionally beneficial products from seafood. In preparing these convenience foods we were keen to maintain functionality and preferably to enhance it with the specific aim to be able to make nutritional claims in relation to fibre content (EC, 2006). The prototypes developed, all contained DFs in a sufficient amount to be labeled as a source of DF. The inclusion of *fucus* DF as well as grape DF into seafood muscle products showed additionally to act as antioxidants in fish muscle products thus delaying PUFA oxidation and extending shelf life.

Claims may also be able to be made in relation the PUFA content of these products depending on the marine sources used as ingredients. The developed minced fish products would comply with the requirement of either 'source' or 'high' omega-3 fatty acids (EU, 2010), depending on the type of fish. For example products made of hake spp., the lean fish we used in our experiments, typically 0.55–0.59% fat (Aubourg *et al.*, 2007) and EPA and DHA 10% of total fat (Rubio-Rodriguez *et al.*, 2008), could be additionally labeled as a source of omega-3 fatty acids, since they reach the minimum amounts needed even with the dilution effects at the maximum DF required for nutritional claims. This is more obvious when using semi-fatty (horse mackerel) or fatty (salmon) in the formulations. Other nutrient contents may also be relatively high despite dilution effects.

ADF might also exert an additional beneficial effect due to the antioxidant polyphenols. Pérez-Jiménez *et al.* (2008) observed that antioxidant DFs from grapes may reduce blood pressure and cholesterol levels and reductions appear to be higher than those reported for other fibre sources such as oat fibre or psyllium, possibly due to the combined effects of fibre and antioxidant compounds present in this ADF. According to the authors, a major part of the relatively large amounts of proanthocyanidins reach the colon, where they may provide a high antioxidant status.

With this view, *surimi* and minced type product prototypes and the final restructured product enriched in *fucus* DF were tested for antioxidant capacity by *in vitro* systems which mimic the dynamic processes of the upper and lower gastrointestinal tract. A combination of intestinal models (TIM) was used. Thus, when data become available (Belmann *et al.*, unpublished), a more physiological assessment of the antioxidant capacity of the products during digestion within the gut lumen and the bio-accessibility of different components can be assessed.

If we are to consider the functionality of these products in relation to health it is important to predict how the component ingredients might interact. For example, excessive use of ADF might ameliorate the beneficial effects of PUFAs, some of which are dependent on the pro-oxidant effects of PUFAs within the cell (Latham *et al.*, 2001). Indeed, PUFAs may protect against cancer by specifically inducing apoptosis in cells low in anti-oxidant defences, while in contrast ADF has been shown to reduce apoptosis in the rat colon (López-Oliva *et al.*, 2010). Because intestinal epithelial cells are exposed to much higher concentrations of dietary compounds, especially those that are poorly absorbed, it may be important to check on the bioavailability of the phenolics present in the ADF if given in conjunction with PUFAs as many are not bioavailable without metabolism by the colonic bacteria (Forester and Waterhouse, 2009). Furthermore, this bacterial metabolism may well be modified by the presence of soluble fibre with prebiotic properties.

23.5   Conclusions

The development of consumer-oriented functional food products based on seafood provides an opportunity to enhance the consumption of healthy seafood or bioactive seafood components. This would help achieve weekly recommendations for seafood consumption, both in individuals and low-consuming populations such as are found in Germany and the Netherlands. Alternatively some of their bioactive components can be introduced into other food categories. Altogether it can be considered as an opportunity to make the best use of existing aquatic resources.

The high nutrient density of seafood can be enhanced by dietary modulation of already intrinsic components such as omega-3 fatty acids or selenium, but also other functional ingredients from marine or non-marine origin can be integrated into restructured products. Nutritional claims could already be made in accordance with EU regulation, and thus food technologists and industry have the opportunity for readily applying technology and translating it into new products. This is particularly the case in relation to the integration of DFs into restructured seafood products.

In a next step, to make specific health claims for these products, interactions between compounds with different health benefits in consideration of health functionality of the whole food product should be studied. Therefore, while marine sources can be used to develop new foods which are acceptable to the consumer and about which nutritional claims can be made, more research is required to better understand the health benefits.

23.6   References

Anonymous 2002. *McCance & Widdowson's The Composition of Foods. Integrated Dataset*. http://www.food.gov.uk/science/dietarysurveys/dietsurveys/
Anonymous 2007a. Newsletter, March 14. Institute of Food Technologists, Washington.
Anonymous 2007b. Seafood consumption for stronger bones. *Infofish International*, **3**, 74.
Appleby, P. N., Davey, G. K. and Key, T. J. 2002. Hypertension and blood pressure among meat eaters, fish eaters, vegetarians and vegans in EPIC-Oxford. *Public Health Nutrition*, **5**, 645–54.
Ashwell, M., Stone, E. M., Stolte, H., Cashman, K. D., MacDonald, H., *et al.* 2010. UK Food Standards Agency Workshop Report: an investigation of the relative contributions of diet and sunlight to vitamin D status. *The British Journal of Nutrition*, **104**(4), 603–11.
Atalah, E., Cruz, C. M. H., Izquierdo, M. S., Rosenlund, G., Caballero, M. J., *et al.* 2007. Two microalgae *Crypthecodinium cohnii* and *Phaeodactylum tricornutum* as alternative source of essential fatty acids in starter feeds for seabream (Sparus aurata). *Aquaculture*, **270**, 178–85.
Aubourg, S. P., Lago, H., Sayar, N. and Gonzalez, R. 2007. Lipid damage during frozen storage of Gadiform species captured in different seasons. *European Journal of Lipid Science and Technology*, **109**, 608–16.
Bandarra, N. M., Nunes, M. L., Andrade, A. M., Prates, J. A. M., Pereira, S., *et al.* 2006. Effect of dietary conjugated linoleic acid on muscle, liver and visceral lipid deposition in rainbow trout juveniles (*Oncorhynchus mykiss*). *Aquaculture*, **254**, 496–505.
Berge, G. M., Ruyter, B. and Asgard, T. 2004. Conjugated linoleic acid in diets for juvenile Atlantic salmon (*Salmo salar*); effects on fish performance, proximate composition, fatty acid and mineral content. *Aquaculture*, **237**, 365–80.
Borderías, A. J., Careche, M. and Sánchez-Alonso, I. 2010. *Fish preparation involves rolling layers of fish to form cylindrical roll, where outer layer has white fish muscle salt, white or colored fibre, and optionally added ingredient, and inner layer has chopped fish and vegetable fibre.* Preparado pesquero reestructurado procedimiento de elaboración. Spanish patent (ES2332207-A1).
Borderías, A. J. and Pérez-Mateos, M. 1996. Productos pesqueros reestructurados. *Alimentaria*, **269**, 53–63.
Borderías, A. J., Sánchez-Alonso, I. and Pérez-Mateos, M. 2005. New applications of fibres in foods: Addition to fishery products. *Trends in Food Science & Technology*, **16**, 458–65.
Borderías, J., Sánchez-Alonso, I., Moreno, P., Dopico, D. C., Tudoran, A., *et al.* 2008. Connecting consumer preferences with technical product specifications in wheat dietary fibre enriched seafood restructured products. *In:* Poli, B. M. and Parisi, G. (eds.) *38th Annual WEFTA meeting. Seafood from catch and aquaculture for a sustainable supply: book of abstracts*, Firenze, Italy: Firenze University Press, p. 8.
Brøns, C., Spohr, C., Storgaard, H., Dyerberg, J. and Vaag, A. 2004. Effect of taurine treatment on insulin secretion and action, and on serum lipid levels in overweight men with a genetic predisposition for type II diabetes mellitus. *European Journal of Clinical Nutrition*, **58**, 1239–47.
Brouwer, I. A. 2008. Fish, omega-3 fatty acids and heart disease. *In:* Borresen, T. (ed.) *Improving Seafood Products for the Consumer*. CRC Press-Woodhead Publishing Limited, Cambridge.

Brunso, K. 2003. Consumer research on fish in Europe. *In:* Luten, J. B., Oehlenschlager, J. and Olafsdottir, G. (eds.) *Quality of Fish from Catch to Consumer: Labelling, Monitoring and Traceability.* Wageningen: Wageningen Academic Publishers.

Brunso, K., Hansen, K. B., Scholderer, J., Honkanen, P., Olsen, S. O. and Verbeke, W. 2008. Consumer attitudes and seafood consumption in Europe. *In:* Borresen, T. (ed.) *Improving Seafood Products for the Consumer.* CRC Press-Woodhead Publishing Limited, Cambridge.

Careche, M., Calvo-Dopico, D. and Cañada, J. 2007. Functional food development based on restructured fish and dietary fibre. *In:* SEAFOODplus (ed.) The fourth open SEAFOODplus conference, Bilbao, Spain. *4th SEAFOODplus Conference: Book of Abstracts*, p. 20.

Careche, M. and Co-workers. 2008. The roadmap to consumer driven functional seafood products: an international expedition. *In:* SEAFOODplus (ed.) The fifth open SEAFOODplus conference, Copenhagen. *5th SEAFOODplus Conference: Book of Abstracts*, p. 32.

Careche, M., Saura-Calixto, F., Díaz-Rubio, M. E., Borderías, J., Sánchez-Alonso, I., *et al.* 2008. Developing functional seafood products. *In:* Borresen, T. (ed.) *Improving Seafood Products for the Consumer.* CRC Press-Woodhead Publishing Limited, Cambridge.

Cervantes-Pahm, S. K. and Stein, H. H. 2010. Ileal digestibility of amino acids in conventional, fermented, and enzyme-treated soybean meal and in soy protein isolate, fish meal, and casein fed to weanling pigs. *Journal of Animal Science*, **88**, 2674–83.

Dantagnan, P., Hernandez, A., Borquez, A. and Mansilla, A. 2009. Inclusion of macroalgae meal (*Macrocystis pyrifera*) as feed ingredient for rainbow trout (*Oncorhynchus mykiss*): effect on flesh fatty acid composition. *Aquaculture Research*, **41**, 87–94.

Dopico, D. C., Tudoran, A., Careche, M. and Olsen, S. O. 2007. New functional seafood products: Information, acceptability, health and quality perceptions. *In:* Batista, I., Nunes, M. L., Mendes, R. and Parisi, G. (eds.) 37th Annual WEFTA meeting. Seafood: source of health and well-being, Lisboa, Portugal. National Institute of Biological Resources INRB/IPIMAR, 118.

Dragnes, B. T., Larsen, R., Ernstsen, M. H., Maehre, H. and Elvevoll, E. O. 2009. Impact of processing on the taurine content in processed seafood and their corresponding unprocessed raw materials. *International Journal of Food Sciences and Nutrition*, **60**, 143–52.

EC 2006. Regulation (EC) No 1924/2006 of the European Parliament and of the Council of 20 December 2006 on nutrition and health claims made on foods. *Official Journal of the European Union*, L404.

Engeset, D., Alsaker, E., Lund, E., Welch, A., Khaw, K. T., *et al.* 2006. Fish consumption and breast cancer risk. The European Prospective Investigation into Cancer and Nutrition (EPIC). *International Journal of Cancer*, **119**, 175–82.

EU 2010. Commission Regulation (EU) No 116/2010 of 9 February 2010 amending Regulation (EC) No 1924/2006 of the European Parliament and of the Council with regard to the list of nutrition claims. *Official Journal of the European Union*, L37.

Faber, T. A., Bechtel, P. J., Hernot, D. C., Parsons, C. M., Swanson, K. S., *et al.* 2010. Protein digestibility evaluations of meat and fish substrates using laboratory, avian, and ileally cannulated dog assays. *Journal of Animal Science*, **88**, 1421–32.

Forester, S. C. and Waterhouse, A. L. 2009. Metabolites are key to understanding health effects of wine polyphenolics. *Journal of Nutrition*, **139**, S1824–31.

Fox, T. E., van den Heuvel, E. G., Atherton, C. A., Dainty, J. R., Lewis, D. J., *et al.* 2004. Bioavailability of selenium from fish, yeast and selenate: a comparative study in humans using stable isotopes. *European Journal of Clinical Nutrition*, **58**, 343–9.

Ganuza, E., Benitez-Santana, T., Atalah, E., Vega-Orellana, O., Ganga, R. and Izquierdo, M. S. 2008. Crypthecodinium cohnii and Schizochytrium sp as potential substitutes to fisheries-derived oils from seabream (Sparus aurata) microdiets. *Aquaculture*, **277**, 109–16.

Ginsberg, G. L. and Toal, B. F. 2009. Quantitative approach for incorporating methylmercury risks and omega-3 fatty acid benefits in developing species-specific fish consumption advice. *Environmental Health Perspectives*, **117**, 267–75.

Granato, D., Branco, G. F., Nazzaro, F., Cruz, A. G. and Faria, J. A. F. 2010. Functional foods and nondairy probiotic food development: Trends, Concepts, and Products. *Comprehensive Reviews in Food Science and Food Safety*, **9**, 292–302.

Gunnarsdottir, I., Tomasson, H., Kiely, M., Martinez, J. A., Bandarra, N. M., *et al.* 2008. Inclusion of fish or fish oil in weight-loss diets for young adults: effects on blood lipids. *International Journal of Obesity*, **32**, 1105–12.

Haratake, M., Takahashi, J., Ono, M. and Nakayama, M. 2007. An assessment of Niboshi (a processed Japanese anchovy) as an effective food source of selenium. *Journal of Health Science*, **53**, 457–63.

Hardy, R. W., Oram, L. L. and Moller, G. 2010. Effects of dietary selenomethionine on Cutthroat trout (*Oncorhynchus clarki bouvieri*) growth and reproductive performance over a life cycle. *Archives of Environmental Contamination and Toxicology*, **58**, 237–45.

Hayes, D. P. 2010. Vitamin D and ageing. *Biogerontology*, **11**, 1–16.

He, K., Song, Y., Daviglus, M. L., Liu, K., Van Horn, L., *et al.* 2004a. Fish consumption and incidence of stroke: a meta-analysis of cohort studies. *Stroke*, **35**, 1538–42.

He, K., Song, Y., Daviglus, M. L., Liu, K., Van Horn, L., *et al.* 2004b. Accumulated evidence on fish consumption and coronary heart disease mortality: a meta-analysis of cohort studies. *Circulation*, **109**, 2705–11.

Hooper, L., Thompson, R. L., Harrison, R. A., Summerbell, C. D., Ness, A. R., *et al.* 2006. Risks and benefits of omega 3 fats for mortality, cardiovascular disease, and cancer: systematic review. *British Medical Journal*, **332**, 752–60.

IFT. 2005. *Functional Foods: Opportunities and Challenges. IFT Expert Report* [Online]. Institute of Food Tecnologists. Available: http://www.ift.org/ (accessed July 2010).

Jiménez-Escrig, A., Jiménez-Jimenez, I., Pulido, R. and Saura-Calixto, F. 2001. Antioxidant activity of fresh and processed edible seaweeds. *Journal of the Science of Food and Agriculture*, **81**, 530–34.

Jones, N. R. 1954. Taurine in fresh and iced skeletal muscle of codling (*Gadus-Callarias*). *Biochemical Journal*, **56**, R22–R22.

Kennedy, S. R., Campbell, P. J., Porter, A. and Tocher, D. R. 2005. Influence of dietary conjugated linoleic acid (CLA) on lipid and fatty acid composition in liver and flesh of Atlantic salmon (*Salnio salar*). *Comparative Biochemistry and Physiology B-Biochemistry & Molecular Biology*, **141**, 168–78.

Kim, E. S., Kim, J. S., Yim, M. H., Jeong, Y., Ko, Y. S., *et al.* 2003. Dietary thurine intake and serum thurine levels of women on Jeju Island. *In:* Lombardini, J. B., Schaffer, S. W. and Azuma, J. (eds.) *Taurine 5: Beginning the 21st century*. New York: Kluwer Academic/Plenum Publisher.

Latham, P., Lund, E. K., Brown, J. C. and Johnson, I. T. 2001. Effects of cellular redox balance on induction of apoptosis by eicosapentaenoic acid in HT29 colorectal adenocarcinoma cells and rat colon in vivo. *Gut*, **49**, 97–105.

Leaver, M. J., Tocher, D. R., Obach, A., Jensen, L., Henderson, R. J., *et al.* 2006. Effect of dietary conjugated linoleic acid (CLA) on lipid composition, metabolism and gene expression in Atlantic salmon (*Salmo salar*) tissues. *Comparative Biochemistry and Physiology a-Molecular & Integrative Physiology*, **145**, 258–67.

Lee, H. W., Park, Y. S., Jung, J. S. and Shin, W. S. 2002. Chitosan oligosaccharides, dp 2–8, have prebiotic effect on the Bifidobacterium bifidium and Lactobacillus sp. *Anaerobe*, **8**, 319–24.

Lock, A. L., Kraft, J., Rice, B. H. and Bauman, D. E. 2009. Biosynthesis and biological activity of rumenic acid: a natural CLA isomer. *In:* Destaillats, F., Sébédio, J. L., Dionisi, F. and Chardigny, J. M. (eds.) *Trans Fatty Acids in Human Nutrition*. Bridgewater: The Oily Press.

López-Oliva, M. E., Agis-Torres, A., Goñi, I. and Muñoz-Martínez, E. 2010. Grape antioxidant dietary fibre reduced apoptosis and induced a pro-reducing shift in the glutathione redox state of the rat proximal colonic mucosa. *British Journal of Nutrition*, **103**, 1110–17.

Lorentzen, M., Maage, A. and Julshamn, K. 1994. Effects of dietary selenium or selenomethionine on tissue selenium levels of atlantic salmon (*Salmo salar*). *Aquaculture*, **121**, 359–67.

Lund, E. K. 2009. Fatty acids and cancer prevention. *In:* Knasmüller, S., Demarini, D. M., Johnson, I. T. and Gerhäuser, C. (eds.) *Chemoprevention of Cancer and DNA Damage by Dietary Factors*. Weinheim: Wiley-VCH Verlag GmbH & Co. KGaA.

Lund, E. K. and Kampman, E. 2008. Protective effects of fish consumption in relation to gastrointestinal health. *In:* Borresen, T. (ed.) *Improving Seafood Products for The consumer*. CRC Press-Woodhead Publishing Limited, Cambridge.

Luten, J. B. and Schram, E. 2006. Enrichment of functional selenium in farmed African catfish (*Clarias goriepinus*) by dietary modulation. *In:* Luten, J. B., Jacobsen, C., Bekaert, K., Sæbø, A. and Oehlenschläger, J. (eds.) *Seafood Research from Fish to Dish – Quality, Safety and Processing of Wild and Farmed Seafood*. Wageningen: Wageningen Academic Publishers.

Luten, J. B., Schram, E. and Elvevoll, E. 2008. Tailor-made functional seafood for consumers: dietary modulation of selenium and taurine in farmed fish. *In:* Øyvind Lie, N. (ed.) *Improving Farmed Fish Quality and Safety*. Woodhead Publishing Limited, Cambridge.

Makol, A., Torrecillas, S., Fernandez-Vaquero, A., Robaina, L., Montero, D., et al. 2009. Effect of conjugated linoleic acid on dietary lipids utilization, liver morphology and selected immune parameters in sea bass juveniles (*Dicentrarchus labrax*). *Comparative Biochemistry and Physiology B – Biochemistry & Molecular Biology*, **154**, 179–87.

Manning, B. B., Li, M. H., Robinson, E. H. and Peterson, B. C. 2006. Enrichment of channel catfish (*Ictalurus punctatus*) fillets with conjugated linoleic acid and omega-3 fatty acids by dietary manipulation. *Aquaculture*, **261**, 337–42.

Miller, M. R., Nichols, P. D. and Carter, C. G. 2007. Replacement of fish oil with thraustochytrid Schizochytrium sp L oil in Atlantic salmon parr (*Salmo salar L*) diets. *Comparative Biochemistry and Physiology A – Molecular & Integrative Physiology*, **148**, 382–92.

Morris, M. C., Evans, D. A., Tangney, C. C., Bienias, J. L. and Wilson, R. S. 2005. Fish consumption and cognitive decline with age in a large community study. *Archives of Neurology*, **62**, 1849–53.

Mulligan, M. L., Felton, S. K., Riek, A. E. and Bernal-Mizrachi, C. 2010. Implications of vitamin D deficiency in pregnancy and lactation. *American Journal of Obstetrics and Gynecology*, **202**, 429, 1–9.

Myint, P. K., Welch, A. A., Bingham, S. A., Luben, R. N., Wareham, N. J., et al. 2006. Habitual fish consumption and risk of incident stroke: the European Prospective Investigation into Cancer (EPIC) – Norfolk prospective population study. *Public Health Nutrition*, **9**, 882–8.

Nakamura, Y., Ueshima, H., Okamura, T., Kadowaki, T., Hayakawa, T., et al. 2005. Association between fish consumption and all-cause and cause-specific mortality in Japan: NIPPON DATA80, 1980–99. *American Journal of Medicine*, **118**, 239–45.

Naylor, R. L., Goldburg, R. J., Primavera, J. H., Kautsky, N., Beveridge, M. C. M., et al. 2000. Effect of aquaculture on world fish supplies. *Nature*, **405**, 1017–24.

Norat, T., Bingham, S., Ferrari, P., Slimani, N., Jenab, M., et al. 2005. Meat, fish, and colorectal cancer risk: the European Prospective Investigation into Cancer and Nutrition. *Journal of the National Cancer Institute*, **97**, 906–16.

Oehlenschläger, J. 1997. Marine fish-a source for essential elements?! *In:* Luten, J. B., Borresen, T. and Oehlenschläger, J. (eds.) *Seafood from Producer to Consumer, Integrated Approach to Quality*. Elsevier, The Netherlands.

Ohr, L. M. 2005. Riding the nutraceuticals wave. *Food Technology*, **59**, 95–6.

Ohr, L. M. 2006. Joint health. *Food Technology*, **60**, 57–60.

Osler, M., Andreasen, A. H. and Hoidrup, S. 2003. No inverse association between fish consumption and risk of death from all-causes, and incidence of coronary heart disease in middle-aged, Danish adults. *Journal of Clinical Epidemiology*, **56**, 274–9.

Park, J. W. 2005. Ingredient technology for *surimi* and *surimi* seafood. *In:* Park, J. W. (ed.) *Surimi and Surimi Seafood*, 2nd edition. CRC Press, Taylor and Francis Group.

Park, Y. and Pariza, M. W. 2007. Mechanisms of body fat modulation by conjugated linoleic acid (CLA). *Food Research International*, **40**, 311–23.

Parra, D., Bandarra, N. M., Kiely, M., Thorsdottir, I. and Martinez, J. A. 2007. Impact of fish intake on oxidative stress when included into a moderate energy-restricted program to treat obesity. *European Journal of Nutrition*, **46**, 460–7.

Patel, P. S., Sharp, S. J., Luben, R. N., Khaw, K. T., Bingham, S. A., *et al.* 2009. Association between type of dietary fish and seafood intake and the risk of incident type 2 diabetes: the European Prospective Investigation of Cancer (EPIC) – Norfolk cohort study. *Diabetes Care*, **32**, 1857–63.

Pérez-Jiménez, J., Serrano, J., Tabernero, M., Arranz, S., Diaz-Rubio, M. E., *et al.* 2008. Effects of grape antioxidant dietary fibre in cardiovascular disease risk factors. *Nutrition*, **24**, 646–53.

Pot, G. K., Geelen, A., Majsak-Newman, G., Harvey, L. J., Nagengast, F., *et al.* 2010. Fatty and lean fish consumption reduce serum C-reactive protein levels but not inflammation markers in feces and in colonic biopsies. *Journal of Nutrition*, **140**, 371–6.

Pot, G. K., Habermann, N., Majsak-Newman, G., Harvey, L. J., Geelen, A., *et al.* 2009a. Increasing fish consumption does not affect genotoxicity markers in the colon in an intervention study. *Carcinogenesis*, **31**(6), 1087–91.

Pot, G. K., Majsak-Newman, G., Geelen, A., Harvey, L. J., Nagengast, F. M., *et al.* 2009b. Fish consumption and markers of colorectal cancer risk: a multicenter randomized controlled trial. *American Journal of Clinical Nutrition*, **90**, 354–61.

Ramel, A., Martinez, J. A., Kiely, M., Bandarra, N. M. and Thorsdottir, I. 2010. Moderate consumption of fatty fish reduces diastolic blood pressure in overweight and obese European young adults during energy restriction. *Nutrition*, **26**, 168–74.

Rubio-Rodriguez, N., De Diego, S. M., Beltran, S., Jaime, I., Sanz, M. T. and Rovira, J. 2008. Supercritical fluid extraction of the omega-3 rich oil contained in hake (Merluccius capensis – Merluccius paradoxus) by-products: Study of the influence of process parameters on the extraction yield and oil quality. *Journal of Supercritical Fluids*, **47**, 215–26.

Sánchez-Alonso, I. and Borderías, J. 2008. Technological effect of red grape antioxidant dietary fibre added to minced fish muscle. *International Journal of Food Science and Technology*, **43**, 1009–18.

Sánchez-Alonso, I., Borderias, J. and Careche, M. 2008a. New seafood prototype enriched with coloured dietary fibre. *In:* SEAFOODplus (ed.) The fifth open SEAFOODplus conference, Copenhagen, *5th SEAFOODplus Conference: Book of Abstracts*, p. 53.

Sánchez-Alonso, I., Haji-Maleki, R. and Borderías, A. J. 2006. Effect of wheat fibre in frozen stored fish muscular gels. *European Food Research and Technology*, **223**, 571–6.

Sánchez-Alonso, I., Haji-Maleki, R. and Borderias, J. 2007a. Wheat fibre as a functional ingredient in restructured fish products. *Food Chemistry*, **100**, 1037–43.

Sánchez-Alonso, I., Jiménez-Escrig, A., Saura-Calixto, F. and Borderías, A. J. 2007b. Effect of grape antioxidant dietary fibre on the prevention of lipid oxidation in minced fish: Evaluation by different methodologies. *Food Chemistry*, **101**, 372–8.

Sánchez-Alonso, I., Jiménez-Escrig, A., Saura-Calixto, F. and Borderías, A. J. 2008b. Antioxidant protection of white grape pomace on restructured fish products during frozen storage. *LWT – Food Science and Technology*, **41**, 42–50.

Sánchez-Alonso, I., Solas, M. T. and Borderías, A. J. 2007c. Technological implications of addition of wheat dietary fibre to giant squid (*Dosidicus gigas*) surimi gels. *Journal of Food Engineering*, **81**, 404–11.

Sánchez-González, I., Rodríguez-Casado, A., Careche, M. and Carmona, P. 2009. Raman analysis of surimi gelation by addition of wheat dietary fibre. *Food Chemistry*, **112**, 162–8.

Saura-Calixto, F. 1998. Antioxidant dietary fibre product: A new concept and a potential food ingredient. *Journal of Agricultural and Food Chemistry*, **46**, 4303–6.

Saura-Calixto, F. D. and Jiménez-Escrig, A. 2003. Antioxidant dietary fibre and concentrate of natural antioxidants from Fucus algae and procedures for obtaining them. Spain patent application.

Schram, E., Pedrero, Z., Camara, C., van der Heul, J. W. and Luten, J. B. 2008. Enrichment of African catfish with functional selenium originating from garlic. *Aquaculture Research*, **39**, 850–60.

Schram, E., Schelvis-Smit, R., van der Heul, J. W. and Luten, J. B. 2010. Enrichment of the African catfish *Clarias gariepinus* (Burchell) with functional selenium originating from garlic: effect of enrichment period and depuration on total selenium level and sensory properties. *Aquaculture Research*, **41**, 793–803.

Sen, D. P. 2005. Selected by-products from sea. *In:* Sen, D. P. (ed.) *Advances in Fish Processing Technology*. Allied Publishers, New Delhi, pp. 616–83.

Shahidi, F., Arachchi, J. K. V. and Jeon, Y. J. 1999. Food applications of chitin and chitosans. *Trends in Food Science and Technology*, **10**, 37–51.

Shungan, X. 1996. Calcium powder of freshwater fish bone. *Journal of Shanghai Fishery University*, **5**, 246.

Siro, I., Kapolna, E., Kapolna, B. and Lugasi, A. 2008. Functional food. Product development, marketing and consumer acceptance – A review. *Appetite*, **51**, 456–67.

Souci, S. W., Fachmann, W. and Kraut, H. 2000. *Food Composition and Nutrition Tables*. Medpharm Scientific Publishers, Stuttgart; CRC Press, Boca Raton.

Strain, J. J., Davidson, P. W., Bonham, M. P., Duffy, E. M., Stokes-Riner, A., Thurston, S. W., *et al.* 2008. Associations of maternal long-chain polyunsaturated fatty acids, methyl mercury, and infant development in the Seychelles Child Development Nutrition Study. *Neurotoxicology*, **29**, 776–82.

Thorkelsson, G., Sigurgisladottir, S., Geirsdottir, M., Jóhannsson, R., Guérard, F., *et al.* 2008. Mild processing techniques and development of functional marine protein and peptide ingredients. *In:* Borresen, T. (ed.) *Improving Seafood Products for the Consumer*. CRC Press-Woodhead Publishing Limited, Cambridge.

Thorsdottir, I. and Ramel, A. 2008. Fish consumption and the health of children and young adults. *In:* Borresen, T. (ed.) *Improving Seafood Products for the Consumer*. CRC Press-Woodhead Publishing Limited, Cambridge.

Thorsdottir, I., Tomasson, H., Gunnarsdottir, I., Gisladottir, E., Kiely, M., *et al.* 2007. Randomized trial of weight-loss-diets for young adults varying in fish and fish oil content. *International Journal of Obesity*, **31**, 1560–66.

Tissot-Favre, D. and Waldron, M. 2009. Biosynthesis, synthesis and biological activity of trans-10 cis-12 conjugated linoleic acid (CLA) isomer. *In:* Destaillats, F., Sébédio, J. L., Dionisi, F. and Chardigny, J. M. (eds.) *Trans Fatty Acids in Human Nutrition*. Bridgewater: The Oily Press.

USDA 2009. USDA National Nutrient Database for Standard Reference, Release 22. US Department of Agriculture, Agricultural Research Service.

Usydus, Z., Szlinder-Richert, J. and Adamczyk, M. 2009. Protein quality and amino acid profiles of fish products available in Poland. *Food Chemistry*, **112**, 139–45.

Valente, L. M. P., Bandarra, N. M., Figueiredo-Silva, A. C., Cordeiro, A. R., Simoes, R. M. and Nunes, M. L. 2007a. Influence of conjugated linoleic acid on growth, lipid composition and hepatic lipogenesis in juvenile European sea bass (*Dicentrarchus labrax*). *Aquaculture*, **267**, 225–35.

Valente, L. M. P., Bandarra, N. M., Figueiredo-Silva, A. C., Rema, P., Vaz-Pires, P., *et al.* 2007b. Conjugated linoleic acid in diets for large-size rainbow trout (*Oncorhynchus mykiss*): effects on growth, chemical composition and sensory attributes. *British Journal of Nutrition*, **97**, 289–97.

Velu, C. S. and Munuswamy, N. 2004. Improving the fatty acid profile of fairy shrimp, *Streptocephalus dichotomus*, using a lipid emulsion rich in highly unsaturated fatty acids. *Journal of Agricultural and Food Chemistry*, **52**, 7033–8.

Venugopal, V. 2009. Marine sources of vitamins and minerals. *In:* Venugopal, V. (ed.) *Marine Products for healthcare. Functional and Bioactive Nutraceutical Compounds from the Ocean.* CRC Press, Boca Raton.

Wang, C. and Lovell, R. T. 1997. Organic selenium sources, selenomethionine and selenoyeast, have higher bioavailability than an inorganic selenium source, sodium selenite, in diets for channel catfish (*Ictalurus punctatus*). *Aquaculture,* **152**, 223–34.

Welch, A. A., Bingham, S. A., Ive, J., Friesen, M. D., Wareham, N. J., *et al.* 2006. Dietary fish intake and plasma phospholipid n-3 polyunsaturated fatty acid concentrations in men and women in the European Prospective Investigation into Cancer – Norfolk United Kingdom cohort. *American Journal of Clinical Nutrition,* **84**, 1330–39.

Welch, A. A., Lund, E., Amiano, P., Dorronsoro, M., Brustad, M., 2002. Variability of fish consumption within the 10 European countries participating in the European Investigation into Cancer and Nutrition (EPIC) study. *Public Health Nutrition,* **5**, 1273–85.

Whelton, S. P., He, J., Whelton, P. K. and Muntner, P. 2004. Meta-analysis of observational studies on fish intake and coronary heart disease. *American Journal of Cardiology,* **93**, 1119–23.

Wójcik, O. P., Koenig, K. L., Zeleniuch-Jacquotte, A., Costa, M. and Chen, Y. 2010. The potential protective effects of taurine on coronary heart disease. *Atherosclerosis,* **208**, 19–25.

Xu, Q., Liu, J. and Yuan, Z. 2004. Use of N-acetylglucosamine as additive in milk products of powder or liquid type, applicable in nutriology, food industry, pharmaceutics, healthcare products and medicine. Patent number WO2004093556-A1; CN1533700-A; CN100339014-C.

Yamasaki, T., Aki, T., Mori, Y., Yamamoto, T., Shinozaki, M., *et al.* 2007. Nutritional enrichment of larval fish feed with thraustochytrid producing polyunsaturated fatty acids and xanthophylls. *Journal of Bioscience and Bioengineering,* **104**, 200–206.

Yamashita, Y. and Yamashita, M. 2010. Identification of a novel selenium-containing compound, selenoneine, as the predominant chemical form of organic selenium in the blood of bluefin tuna. *Journal of Biological Chemistry,* **285**, 18134–8.

Ylitalo, R., Lehtinen, S., Wuolijoki, E., Ylitalo, P. and Lehtimaki, T. 2002. Cholesterol-lowering properties and safety of chitosan. *Arzneimittel-Forschung-Drug Research,* **52**, 1–7.

Zhang, J., Sasaki, S., Amano, K. and Kesteloot, H. 1999. Fish consumption and mortality from all causes, ischemic heart disease, and stroke: an ecological study. *Preventive Medicine,* **28**, 520–29.

Zhou, X. X., Wang, Y. B., Gu, Q. and Li, W. F. 2009. Effects of different dietary selenium sources (selenium nanoparticle and selenomethionine) on growth performance, muscle composition and glutathione peroxidase enzyme activity of crucian carp (*Carassius auratus gibelio*). *Aquaculture,* **291**, 78–81.

24

Dietary fibre functional products

F. Guillon, M. Champ, J.-F. Thibault and L. Saulnier, INRA Research Centre, Nantes, France

Abstract: The dietary fibre hypothesis has been based upon pioneering observations of physicians and epidemiologists. They pointed out relationships between diet and chronic diseases such as cardiovascular diseases, diabetes and cancer. Since then, the definition of dietary fibre has been a matter of controversy and today is not fully agreed upon by experts in the field. Most recent definitions encompass all polysaccharides and lignin that resist digestion in the upper gut. Some definitions also include lower molecular weight carbohydrates. Dietary fibres include a wide array of compounds that vary in chemical structures and properties and they might be naturally present in food or incorporated in food to improve nutritional or technological properties. The physicochemical properties of dietary fibre play a key role in the actions on gut function, including fermentation. These properties depend on the source, the processing history of the plant material, as well as the form under which it is ingested. The concept of dietary fibres has stimulated a great deal of research and thrown new insight into the understanding of their metabolic and physiological effects while consumer interest in healthy foods has encouraged technologists in developing enriched food products and new fibre additives as supplements for food. However, there is still a need to bring dietary fibres into more appealing and healthy foods to increase the fibre intake.

Key words: dietary fibre, processing, physicochemical properties, fermentation, systemic responses, colon health, fibre intake.

24.1 Introduction

The term 'dietary fibre' was first coined in 1953 by Hispley to describe plant cell wall components of foods, which he suggested to be protective against toxaemia during pregnancy. However, the dietary fibre hypothesis really emerged in the 1970s from medical workers working on the relationships between diet and incidence of chronic disease, in particular the role of polysaccharides in the diet (Walker 1974, Burkitt and Trowell 1975). For more than three decades, data regarding the beneficial effects of dietary fibre have been accumulating. These materials may participate in the regulation of the gastrointestinal motility, influence glucose and lipid metabolism, promote faecal ouput, slow gastric emptying and affect the secretion of gut hormones, stimulate bacterial metabolic activity, detoxify the colon luminal contents and contribute towards maintaining the equilibrium of the colon ecosystem and integrity of intestinal mucosa (FAO/WHO 1997, Cherbut *et al.* 1995, Guillon *et al.* 1998a, Kritchevsky and Bonfield 1995, Rémésy 1996, Schweizer and Edwards 1992, Southgate *et al.* 1991, Burton-Freeman *et al.* 2002). In this respect, dietary fibre can fit the definition of functional food by the fact that it can affect one or more targeted functions in the body in a positive manner (Diplock *et al.* 1999). The effects of dietary fibre intake on gastrointestinal functions, colorectal cancer, diabetes, cardiovascular health, the immune system, energy balance and weight control have been reviewed recently by Buttriss and Stokes (2008) and Anderson *et al.* (2009) among others.

Despite the tremendous amount of work carried out all over the world, the mechanisms of actions on the functions of the body are not fully understood. A major finding is that it is not only the amount but also the type of dietary fibre that influences physiological response to intake, although emphasis in dietary guidelines remains on increased dietary fibre intake. The physicochemical properties of dietary fibre and their digestive fate have been shown to play a key role in gut function. These properties are related to the source, the processing history of fibre and the form by which it is ingested. Dietary fibre may be present in the diet as plant cell walls or as isolated molecules, endogenous or supplement constituents of food. The chemical structure of dietary constituents and the way the molecules assemble are important in determining their properties. During processing, major changes can occur in the architecture of plant cell walls and in structural features of individual molecules, which can markedly affect fibre properties, food properties and dietary response.

24.2   Defining dietary fibre

The definition of dietary fibre has been a matter of controversy – it took some 16 years for Codex Alimentarius to reach its current global view (Betteridge 2009) – and, today, it is still not fully agreed upon by experts in the field. The debate has focused in particular on whether or not resistant starch and non digestible oligosaccharides should be considered dietary fibres. Over the years, several definitions have been used based on different concepts (Tables 24.1 and 24.2). These definitions can be grouped into three main views. The first relies on a 'botanical' view and regards dietary fibre as mainly plant cell wall constituents. The second group of definitions is based on a chemical view and on related methods used for the measurement of dietary fibre in food. The last view is based on the idea that non-digestibility is the key defining characteristic of dietary fibres. Most recent definitions of dietary fibre fall into this group and consider that dietary

Table 24.1   Different definitions of dietary fibre

Authors	Polymers included in the definition
Trowell, 1972	Cellulose, lignin, hemicelluloses, pectins (skeletal remains of plant cells)
Trowell 1974	Cell-wall polysaccharides + lignin + unavailable associated substances (cutin, suberin, phytic acids)
Trowell *et al.* 1976	Unavailable storage polysaccharides + cell-wall polysaccharides + lignin
Southgate *et al.* 1978	Unavailable polysaccharides + lignin
Southgate *et al.* 1981	Non-starch polysaccharides + lignin
Cummings and Englyst 1987	Non-starch polysaccharides

Source: from Dysseler 1997.

Table 24.2   Suggested definition by organisation or countries

Organisation or countries	Definition and constituents of dietary fibre
CIAA (1992)	Organic constituent non-hydrolysed by human digestive enzymes
CEEREAL (1993)	Indigestible polysaccharides + lignin
Belgium (1993)	Indigestible oligo + indigestible polysaccharides + lignin
Croatia, Germany, Norway and Sweden (1993)	Indigestible polysaccharides + lignin
Scientific Committee for Foods (1994)	Oligosaccharides and polysaccharides and hydrophilic derivatives that are not digested and not absorbed in the upper gut of humans, including lignin.
COST (1994)	Lignin, inositolphosphate, resistant starch, oligosaccharides, plant cell-wall polysaccharides, inulin, polydextrose
FAO/WHO Codex Alimentarius Commission (1995)	The edible plant or animal materials not hydrolysed by the endogenous enzymes of the human digestive tract as determined by the agreed method – AOAC 985.29 and 991.43
Norway (1998)	Material isolated by AOAC Method 985:29 and inulin and oligofructose
AACC (2001)	The edible parts of plants or analogous carbohydrates that are resistant to digestion and absorption in the human small intestine with complete or partial fermentation in the large intestine. These include polysaccharides, oligosaccharides, lignin, and associated plant substances. Dietary fibres promote beneficial physiological effects including laxation, and/or blood cholesterol attenuation, and/or blood glucose attenuation
The Food Nutrition Board (FNB) of the Institute of Medicine of the National Academies, USA (2001)	Dietary fibre consists of non-digestible carbohydrates and lignin that are intrinsic and intact in plants. Added fibre consists of isolated, non-digestible carbohydrates that have beneficial physiological effects in humans. Total fibre is the sum of dietary fibre and added fibre

Organisation or countries	Definition and constituents of dietary fibre
EU (2007)	Carbohydrate polymers with three or more monomeric units, which are neither digested nor absorbed in the human small intestine and belong to the following categories:
	• edible carbohydrate polymers naturally occurring in the food as consumed
	• edible carbohydrate polymers which have been obtained from food raw material by physical, enzymatic, or chemical means and which have a beneficial physiological effect demonstrated by generally accepted scientific evidence
	• edible synthetic carbohydrate polymers which have a beneficial physiological effect demonstrated by generally accepted scientific evidence
	Lignin and other minor non-carbohydrates are not considered fibre when separated from the carbohydrate polymers and added to a food
FAO/WHO Codex Alimentarius Commission (2009)	Dietary fibre means carbohydrate polymers[1] with ten or more monomeric units[2] which are not hydrolysed by the endogenous enzymes in the small intestine of humans and belong to the following categories:
	• edible carbohydrate polymers naturally occurring in the food as consumed
	• carbohydrate polymers, which have been obtained from food raw material by physical, enzymatic or chemical means and which have been shown to have a physiological effect of benefit to health as demonstrated by generally accepted scientific evidence to competent authorities
	• synthetic carbohydrate polymers which have been shown to have a physiological effect of benefit to health as demonstrated by generally accepted scientific evidence to competent authorities

Source: from Dysseler 1997, Guo 2009 and McCleary 2010.

Notes:
[1] When derived from a plant origin, dietary fibre may include fractions of lignin and/or other compounds associated with polysaccharides in the plant cell walls. These compounds also may be measured by certain analytical method(s) for dietary fibre. However, such compounds are not included in the definition of dietary fibre if extracted and re-introduced into a food.
[2] Decision on whether to include carbohydrates from three to nine monomeric units should be left to national authorities.

fibre encompasses all polysaccharides (not just non-starch polysaccharides) and lignin that resist digestion in the upper gastrointestinal tract. They typically include a wide array of compounds (Table 24.3) that vary in chemical structure and properties: non-starch polysaccharides from plant cell walls, lignin, gums, microbial polysaccharides, inulin and resistant starch.

Some definitions of this type also include lower molecular weight carbohydrates, such as oligosaccharides not digested in the small intestine, but a consensus has

Table 24.3 Classification and chemical characteristics of the main dietary fibres

Class	Components	Structure (bonds backbone) in	Main sources
Polysaccharides of cell walls in higher plants	Cellulose	beta-D-glucan (4 linked)	No fractionated plant material
	Hemicelluloses	Xyloglucans (4-linked–D-glucans with attached side chains)	Dicotyledons
		Xylans (beta-D-4 linked)	Dicotyledons
		Arabinoxylans-glucuronoarabinoxylans	Monocotyledons
		Mixed linkage beta-D-glucan (3 and 4 linked)	Monocotyledons, more abundant in barley, oat grains
	Pectic susbtances	Galacturonans and rhamnogalacturonans	Dicotyledons
		Arabinan (alpha-L-5 linked, with attached side chains)	
		Arabinogalactan 1(beta-D-4 linked galactan with attached side chains)	
Other molecules	Lignin	Complex polyphenolic polymer	Mature plants
Hydrocolloids from seaweed extracts	Carrageenans	Sulfated polymers composed of galactose and anhydrogalactose	Red seaweeds, mainly *Chondrus crispus*
	Alginates	Polymers of D-mannuronic and L-guluronic acids, monomers occur in blocks	Brown seaweeds; mainly *Laminaria digitata*, stipes of *Laminaria hyperborea, Ascophyllum nodosum Fucus serratus*
Microbial sources	Xanthan gum	Backbone identical to cellulose with trisaccharide side-chains composed of alpha-D-mannose, beta-D-glucuronic acid and a terminal beta-D-mannose	*Xanthomonas campestris*
	Gellan gum	Linear backbone composed of 1,3-beta-D-glucose, 1,4-beta-D-glucuronic acid, 1,4 beta-D-glucose and 1,4 alpha-D-rhamnose	*Pseudomonas elodea*

Category	Name	Structure	Source
Plant exudates	Gum arabic	Structure close to arabinogalactan of type II with more complex side chains	From different species of acacia
	Gum Karaya	Structure close to pectins; side chains containing glucuronic acid	*Sterculia*
	Gum tragacanth	Pectic and arabinogalactan II structures	*Astragalus gummifer*
Seeds extracts	Guar gum	Galactomannan, ratio D-galactose to D-mannose: 1:2	Endosperm of leguminosae seeds *Cyamopsis teragonolobus*
	Locust bean (carob) gum	Galactomannan, ratio D-galactose to D-mannose: 1:4	*Cerotona siliqua*
	Psyllium	Polysaccharide composed of arabinose, xylose and galacturonic acid	*Plantago ovata*
Roots extracts	Konjac	Acetylated glucomannan	Amorphophallus *konjac*
Modified cellulose and pectins	Modified cellulose	Carboxymethyl cellulose Methyl cellulose Hydroxypropylmethyl cellulose	
	Pectins	Low and high methyl esterified amidated pectins	Apple pomace, citrus peel
Resistant starches	Physical trapped starches	Alpha1-4,1-6 linked glucose units	Whole grains, legume seeds and cereals
	Resistant starch granules	Native starches having a B-type X ray diffraction pattern	Raw potato, green banana; high amylose starches High amylose starches, any kind of starch
	Retrograded amylose		
Oligosaccharides	Fructo-oligosaccharides	Oligosaccharides mainly composed of fructose (glucosyl (fructosyl)$_n$ fructose)	Extracted from Chicory roots (Raftilose® or enzymatically synthesised from sucrose (Actilight®, Neosugar)
	α-Galactosides (raffinose, stachyose, verbascose)	Sucrose – (galactose)$_n$ = from 1 to 3	Pulse (beans, lentils, peas)

Source: adapted from Lineback 1999 and Dreher 1999.

not been reached on this point. The definitions adopted by AACC International in 2001 (Anon 2001) and the EU in 2007 (EC Directive 2008/100/EC Annex II) include oligosaccharides, whereas the definition agreed on at the 2009 meeting of the Codex Alimentarius' Codex Committee on Nutrition and Foods for Special Dietary Uses (CCNFSDU) leaves the decision on whether or not to include carbohydrates from 3 to 9 monomeric units up to national authorities (ALINORM 10/33/26). The CCNFSDU definition can be found in Table 24.2. For a more extensive discussion of the evolution of definitions of dietary fibre, and the CCNFSDU definition in particular, see Betteridge (2009).

It should also be mentioned that for a considerable period, different types of dietary fibres were divided into two groups – soluble or insoluble fibre – depending on whether they resisted fermentation in the large bowel (insoluble) or not (soluble). However, this categorisation is now understood to be misleading, as some so-called insoluble fibres are actually fermented in the large bowel. The solubility in water of a fibre also does not always correlate with its physiological effects (Buttriss and Stokes 2008).

Resistant starch (RS), included in more recent definitions of dietary fibre, has been defined, relying on a physiological concept, as the sum of starch and the products of starch degradation not absorbed in the small intestine of healthy individuals (Asp *et al.* 1992, 1996). As a matter of fact there are many reasons why starch may be incompletely digested and absorbed during passage through the digestive tract. These can be divided into extrinsic or intrinsic factors. Extrinsic factors are related to the environment of starch in food, for example enclosure in intact cells. Intrinsic factors refer to the characteristics of the starch, resistant native starch granules, chemically modified starches, and retrograded starch occurring in processed foods. Older methods for determination of total dietary fibre (TDF) (e.g. AOAC 1995) used to lead to an underestimation of resistant starch. The 'gold standard' for resistant starch measurement is *in vivo* quantification of the amount of undigested starch in the illeal effluent (a direct measure of starch in the digesta that passes from the small intestine to the large intestine, but this is impractical for routine analysis (Birkett and Brown 2008). Alternative analytical methods have been proposed to predict the ileal digestibility of starch in healthy subjects. They have been validated on the basis of *in vivo* data (Champ *et al.* 1999) or ileostomates (Asp *et al.* 1996). These methods are not exempt from criticism and none of them presently available has been shown to measure all RS. The new AACC International approved method for TDF (32-45.01) (also accepted as AOAC method 2009.01) aims to give a measurement of RS in line with *in vivo* results (McCleary, 2010).

Non-digestible oligosaccharides, also referred to as resistant oligosaccharides, are defined based on physiological (they resist hydrolysis by acid and enzymes in the upper gut due the nature of their glycosidic linkages) and chemical criteria (degree of polymerisation). The precise boundary between oligosaccharides and polysaccharides is arbitrary but generally oligosaccharides are defined as saccharides containing from 3 to 10 monosaccharides (< Ø10: FAO/WHO 1997, 10: Asp *et al.* 1992, Cho *et al.* 1999b, Voragen 1998). This definition includes oligosaccharides with prebiotic properties with a degree of polymerisation in the range 3–10. Some of the most important oligosaccharides are fructo-oligosaccharides and alpha galactosides. Previously, the predominant methods used for the determination of total dietary fibre did not measure oligosaccharides because of their ethanol/water solubility. Specific enzymatic or HPLC methods have been employed to measure oligosaccharides directly in foods (Coussement 1999). Adaptations of the AOAC method have been applied with success to determine oligofructosaccharides in foods (Dysseler *et al.* 1999). AACC International method 32-45.01 aims to recover non-digestible oligosaccharides intact so that they can subsequently be measured (McCleary 2010).

24.3   Sources of dietary fibre

Within food systems, dietary fibre is found in two main forms: as intrinsic constituents of various plant foods or as additions as a supplement. As supplements, they can be used as ingredients (> 5%) or additives (< 5%).

24.3.1   Endogenous

Cereals and cereal products, roots, tubers, vegetables, nuts and fruits are all sources of dietary fibre. When considering dietary fibre in these foods, it is mainly the role of cell walls that is being considered. The cell wall is a dynamic complex structure surrounding the plant cells, exterior to the plasmalemma. The composition and the properties are constantly adapted to growth, differentiation and variations in the environment of the cell. Schematically, cell walls can be divided into two classes: primary cell walls are those deposited by growing plant cells; they are thin and hydrated. The primary cell wall of most flowering plants is a composite polymeric structure in which crystalline cellulose interlocked with xyloglucans is embedded in a matrix of pectic polysaccharides, with a small amount of the structural proteins intercalated in the matrix (Carpita and Gibeaut 1993; Carpita and McCann 2000; Cosgrove 1997, 2005; Selvendran and Robertson 1990).

The individual macromolecules are held together by covalent, ionic, hydrogen bonds and van der Waals forces. Physical enmeshment may also be involved. Cellulose plays a major role in determining the strength of the cell wall; xyloglucans may bind tightly to the surface of cellulose and act as a lubricating agent to prevent cellulose aggregation. Pectins are thought to determine the porosity of the cell walls and thus limit the diffusion of molecules through the walls; they may control the charge environment of microdomains in the cell walls; they may be involved in the defence response of the plant against invading organisms. Primary cell walls can vary in composition, thickness and morphology, depending on the source and physiological stage of the plant. This type of wall is found in parenchymatous tissue, which is the major tissue of the pulp of fruits and vegetables. In grasses, the branched arabinoxylans and mixed linked beta glucans are thought to play the role that xyloglucans play in dicotyledons (Carpita and Gibeaut 1993, Carpita and McCann 2000).

As primary cell walls cease growth, the walls become thicker by deposition of more layers of matrix polysaccharides and cellulose. They can be impregnated with lignin to form stiff and uncompressible walls. The cells with thickened walls have specialised functions, providing rigidity, transporting water and nutrients or protecting the plant from desiccation or predators. They are part of the epidermis, collenchyma, sclerenchyma and vascular conducting tissues. These tissues generally may contribute a small amount of the plant material ingested but may also play a major role in the physical effects of fibre.

Some substances such as cutin, suberin, complex internal ester of hydroxy aliphatic acids may be deposited at the epidermal or subepidermal surface of organs (stems, leaves or roots, tubers). They prevent water loss and impede microbial digestion of the external walls.

Physically inaccessible starch found in partly milled grains and seeds and starchy foods cooked and cooled can be regarded as a natural source of RS. Fructans such as inulin and fructo-oligosaccharides occur as photosynthetic products of storage in a number of plants such as Jerusalem artichokes, onions, asparagus, chicory, leek, garlic. In Jerusalem artichokes and onions, they may account for up to 60–70% of the dry matter.

Another example of naturally occurring oligosaccharides are the alpha galactosides (Voragen 1998). Alpha galactosides derived from sucrose (raffinose, stachyose, verbascose) are mainly in leguminous seeds. They account for 2–8% of the dry matter. Another group of alpha galactosides in legumes are glucose galactosides (melibiose and mannitriose) and inositol galactosides (galactinol, galactopinitol, ciceritol). Ciceritol has been reported as the major alpha galctosides in chickpeas (Quemener and Brillouet 1983, Bernabé et al. 1993). In seeds, the exact role(s) of alpha galactosides is not clearly established. It has been suggested that they may be storage molecules as they disappear at the onset of sprouting. They can also participate in the protection of seed against desiccation and freezing. There are some differences between flatulence-inducing potential alpha galactosides. Ciceritol may be less flatogenic than sucrose galactosides (Fleming 1981).

We consume different organs of the plant, and each contain a range of different tissues and cell types (Table 24.4). These different levels of organisation must be taken into account to further understand the behaviour of fibre under processing and their physiological implications.

24.3.2   Supplements

Concentrates
Fibre concentrates arise mainly from the processing of fruit, vegetable, legume or cereal sources (Guillon and Thibault 1996). Fibre concentrates are, by definition, fibre enriched. Concentrated sources of dietary fibre from fruits and vegetables can be obtained through dehydration processes. These concentrates potentially can be used as ingredients for high fibre products. The appearance of the ingredient

Table 24.4   Structure of plant foods

Plant foods		Main tissues present
Cereal foods	Flours, product derived from flours	Thin walls structures from the endosperm, extensively broken
	Whole grains	Grains almost intact; the cellular structure is retained
	Brans	Thicker, more lignified walls (pericarp, seed coat, nucellar layer) with small amounts of endospermal walls (aleurone, layer, some amount of the starch endosperm)
Fruits		For the most part undifferentiated parenchymatous tissues with small amount of lignified vascular tissues. Outer skin cutinised
Leafy vegetables	Leaves, petioles, stems and associated structures such as flowers	Parenchymatous tissues and variable amounts of vascular and support tissues. Outer tissues cutinised and may be suberinised
Seed legumes		Thick, not lignified seed coats which are cutinised. Cotyledons (or endospermal tissues) with rather thick wall compared to those encountered in the cereal endosperm
Tubers		Suberinised skin; thin wall undifferentiated cells with storage polysaccharides. Vascular lignified tissues in small amount
Roots		Outer tissues often suberinised; most of the time undifferentiated tissues except in mature roots where vascular lignified tissues may be significantly developed

Source: adapted from Southgate, 1995.

and its functionality will depend on the fibre matrix and changes induced by the treatments. Heated force air dehydration can lead to some collapses of the cell walls while freeze drying, or instant controlled depression can better preserve the walls and thus the appearance and texture of the product.

Concentrates can also be co-products of agricultural and food by-products. They result from mechanical treatment aiming at separating different tissues in plant material or from extraction processes for isolating particular components such as pectins, starch, proteins or juice.

Bran from cereals is the coarse outer layer of the kernel and is generally separated from cleaned and scoured grains during milling. In parboiled rice, the harvested rice is subjected to soaking and steaming before being dried and milled. Oat bran is probably the most popular bran product. It has been introduced, with success, into reduced-calorie breads, baked goods, beverages and meat substitutes.

Rice bran may be as effective as oat bran in lowering blood cholesterol and this has stimulated interest for the product. It can be added to baked goods, breads, snacks and extruded foodstuffs.

New fractionation processes are developed in order to separate the interesting parts of the wheat bran from the undesirable ones (Hemery *et al.* 2007). Most fractionation processes comprise two steps, fragmentation process and the separation step. Innotative separation involving electrostatic separation of particles has been introduced (Bohm *et al.* 2003, Bohm and and Kratzer, 2005). This sorting process makes it possible to obtain practically pure aleurone powder that contains about 90% of aleurone layer (Buri *et al.* 2004). This layer has been shown to have great nutritional interest, and to concentrate most of the minerals and vitamins of wheat grain (Pomeranz, 1988). In particular, it contains interesting proportion of β-glucans, phenolic compounds and other phytochemicals (Buri *et al.* 2004) and exhibit anti-oxydant capacity (Zhou *et al.* 2004, MateoAnson *et al.* 2008).

Seed legumes are also a source of fibre concentrate, obtained from milled or dehulled seeds fractionated to obtain starch and protein concentrates. Two types of fibre with distinct characteristics are generated: from the hulls and the residual cotyledons.

Sugar fibre can derive from sugar beet pulp, co-product from the sugar beet industry or directly produced from the beet root as starting material. In both cases, the roots are first washed to eliminate the bulk of sand and process to extract sucrose. In the latter case, the process is adapted to minimise or avoid colour and odour formation during processing. In the former case, the beet pulp is further treated to remove taste, colour and odour. Then the fibre is dried. Several processes have been patented and sugar beet fibre is now available on the market under various trade names.

The precursors of fruit fibre concentrates correspond mostly to the tissues produced upon expression of fruit juice. The pulp is generally extensively washed to remove residual sugars and then dried. Generally they exhibit unique flavour and taste.

The composition and properties of these fibres depend on the major constitutive tissues, and preservation of the cell integrity on the processing (Table 24.5) they are going through. Concentrates are generally incorporated into foods to increase the dietary fibre content of food. Fibre ingredients that exhibit high water retention capacity can be used as bulking agents or fat replacers. Depending on their end use, many of the fibre ingredients are undergoing further processing to improve their functionality and, therefore, extend their use.

Isolates
Isolates are obtained either by extraction in liquid medium, purification and recovery of one type of polysaccharides (pectins, alginates, carrageenans, beta glucans inulin, alpha galactosides), by drying and grinding of native exsudates (arabic, ghatti gums) or by organic synthesis (polydextrose). The extraction conditions differ according to the polysaccharides extracted. Guar and carob

Table 24.5 Chemical composition of some fibre concentrates

Fibre	TDF	Rha-Fuc	Ara	Xyl	Man	Gal	Glc*	Uronic acid	Lignin	Starch	Proteins	Ashes
Wheat bran[1]	50.4	nd	9.6	16.5	1.3	1.2	11.0 (98%)	6.6	2.6	18.6	15.8	4.0
Oat bran[2]	86.2	nd	4.1	26.3	0.1	1.2	45.2 (83%)	nd	14.9	nd	4.5	5.6
Maize bran[2]	71.9	nd	4.5	8.6	0.1	1.2	56.4 (94%)	nd	1.2	nd	8.8	2.1
Barley bran[2]	72.6	nd	6.3	21.7	0.1	0.7	33.5 (84%)	nd	10.4	nd	9.4	6.9
Apple fibre[3]	83.3	1.1	6.8	4.9	1.3	4.0	22.2	20.6	nd	7.0	6.2	1.2
Citrus fibre[3]	76.0	1.3	8.0	2.7	2.0	6.0	20.6	30.0	nd	traces	7.0	5.1
Soy fibre (cotyledon)[4]	79.8	3.6	12.9	4.7	1.2	27.0	12.4	15.8	nd	nd	nd	nd
Soy fibre (hull)[4]	75.6	1.3	5.7	9.4	5.4	2.8	39.9	10.2	nd	nd	nd	nd
Sugar beet[3]	76.8	1.0	19.5	1.4	1.4	4.1	18.0	19.0	1.8	traces	9.6	4.7
Pea fibre (hull)[5]	91.5	0.9	4.2	14.6	1.0	1.2	45.1	12.7	nd	0.0	3.8	1.7

Sources: 1 Ralet et al. 1990; 2 Schimberni et al. 1982; 3 Cloutour 1995; 4 Lo 1989; 5 Ralet et al. 1993.
Notes:* non-starch glucose; () percentage of cellulosic glucose; nd: not determined.

gums flours are prepared from milled cotyledons. Beta glucan preparations (oat gum) can be obtained by wet milling of oat grain. Many of the isolated polysaccharides find industrial applications as techno-functional ingredients (thickening agents or emulsion stabilisers). In this context, they are used at set concentrations (usually 0.5–2.0%). The incorporation in high amounts of polysaccharides with texturing properties, apart from necessitating adaptation of the formulation and technology, may have detrimental effects on the organoleptic properties of the end products.

The major products sold as cellulose fibre preparation are derived from woody plants through pulping and bleaching process. The bleached cellulose pulp is a white product, which may then be dried and mechanically sized (Ang and Miller 1991). The manufacturing processes likely differ between manufacturers resulting in final product with distinct chemical or physical properties. Variations of the final product also may be ascribed to differences in the starting material. Powdered cellulose can be promoted for reducing calories in foods, while maintaining the texture, structure and mouth feel of the product. Cellulose can be chemically modified to produce water-soluble cellulose gums. The chemically modified celluloses include carboxymethyl cellulose, methyl cellulose and hydroxypropylmethyl cellulose. They are generally used as additives and can improve stability in baked goods and sauces. Because of filming properties, some cellulose derivatives are used as binders in food matrices and may serve as oil barrier for fried products.

Several patents have been filed over the last few years for the production of RS (Wursch 1999). Generally, starch is heated in water more than 100 °C to hydrate and gelatinise and then cooled for a sufficient time to retrograde and form RS. The yield of RS mainly depends on the amylose content, and amylose-rich starches (amylomaize, high amylose pea or barley starches) are generally preferred as starting materials. The yield of RS can be increased by playing on various processing steps (debranching of the gelatinised starch and fractionation, extrusion cooking after high temperature gelatinisation) and conditions (concentration, temperature, storage time). Yield can be finally improved by subsequent hydrolysis of the unretrograded starch with enzymes. The final product is a bland white powder with no flavour or taste. RS can be incorporated into foods as bulking agent, dietary fibre or fat mimetic.

Polydextrose is prepared by vacuum thermal polymerisation of glucose using sorbitol as a plasticiser and citric acid as catalyst (Craig et al. 1999). The average degree of polymerisation is about 12. It can be used in foods as functional ingredients (sugar and partial fat replacer, humectant, cryoprotectant, freezing point depression) or as dietary fibre.

Fructo-oligosaccharides are prepared enzymatically from inulin (enzymatic hydrolysis) or sucrose (transglycosylation) (De Leenheer 1996, Coussement 1999). They are mainly used as dietary fibres (prebiotic effects). As a technological agent, they can help to reduce sucrose and fat content while maintaining texture and mouth feel of the product (dairy products, ice cream, sorbet). Enzymatic hydrolysis processes can also be applied to produce oligosaccharides from plant cell wall polysaccharides (Voragen 1998, Vasquez *et al.* 2000; Drakoularakou *et al.* 2004). Very recently, a new beta-glucan, obtained by partial hydrolysis of barley beta-glucan and arabinoxylo-oligosaccharides (AXOS) produced by hydrolysis of arabinoxylan rich cereal products were also added to the list of prebiotics (Grootaert *et al.* 2007, Swennen 2006).

24.3.3 Amounts of dietary fibre in some foods

Data on the amount of dietary fibre in foods varies according to the definition of dietary fibre chosen and the measurement method used. There can be considerable variation between different methods to measure 'total' dietary fibre content in some foods (Lunn and Buttriss 2007). Until recently, mainly two types of methods have been used for the measurement of dietary fibre in foods, namely enzymatic gravimetric methods whereby the fibre is isolated and weighed (AOAC methods) and component analysis methods in which individual dietary fibre saccharides are determined more or less specifically (Englyst *et al.* 1994). In the Englyst methods, lignin and RS are excluded. With the AOAC method, lignin (+ cutins, tannins, Maillard products) and part of the RS are included (Table 24.6). Oligosaccharides are not recovered. Lunn and Buttriss (2007) review different methods for the measurement of dietary fibres in more detail. As the definition of dietary fibre has evolved, new methods to measure total dietary fibre have been developed, such as AOAC 2009.01 Total Dietary Fiber (CODEX Definition) by Enzymatic-Gravimetric Method and Liquid Chromatography. In contrast to earlier AOAC methods to measure total dietary fibre, this incorporates an enzyme digest protocol that is more consistent with the human digestive system and uses liquid chromatography to quantify non-digestible oligosaccharides (McCleary 2010).

Table 24.6 Dietary fibre content of some foods (g/100 g edible portion)

Food	Moisture	Dietary fibre content	
		Non-starch polysaccharides[1]	Total fibre[2]
Banana	75.1	1.1	1.6
French beans	13.3	4.7	nd
Beans, green	11.3	17.0	40.0
Lentils, green	10.8	8.9	nd
Potatoes	79.0	1.3	1.8
Wheat	14.0	9.0	12.6
Maize	12.0	nd	11.0
Rice	11.8	2.0	3.5
Oat	8.9	6.8	10.3

Source: FAO–WHO 1997.
Notes: [1] Non-starch polysaccharides (Englyst *et al.* 1994); [2] Total dietary fibre (AOAC 1995).

Table 24.7 presents some values of dietary fibre amount in foods. These foods are natural sources of dietary fibre as there are no available data for industrial foods where fibre preparations are added for their functional properties. The analytical values were obtained by the AOAC method (1995).

Table 24.7 shows that foods generally regarded as good sources of fibre, fresh vegetables and fruits, are in fact low-fibre foods. These foods contain large amounts of water and even if rich on a dry weight basis, their contribution to fibre intake is relatively low. Expressed on a dry weight basis the most fibre-concentrated foods are brans (mainly breakfast cereals), vegetables, fresh and dried fruits, legume seeds, muesli and wholemeal breads.

Table 24.7   Dietary fibre content of some foods (g/100 g edible portion*)

	Moisture	Dietary fibre content		
		Total	Insoluble	Soluble
'French' bread	29.2	2.7	1.9	0.8
White surdough bread	37.1	1.9	1.3	0.6
Wholewheat surdough bread	39.7	8.1	7.0	1.1
Cookies: brownies	12.8	2.5	1.7	0.8
Cookies: butter	4.7	2.4	1.6	0.8
Croissants	20.4	2.3	1.4	0.9
Cornflakes: plain	2.8	2.0	1.7	0.3
Puffed rice	6.5	1.4	1.0	0.4
Muesli	5.0	12.0		
Wheat bran (breakfast cereals)	2.9	35.3	32.8	2.5
Wheat flakes	2.4	11.4	9.6	1.8
Barley bran	3.5	70	67.0	3.0
Parboiled rice: cooked	77	0.5		
Rice: cooked	77.5	0.7	0.7	0
Brown rice: cooked	73.1	1.7		
Pasta: macaroni	69.6	2.0	1.7	0.3
Boiled potatoes	79.5	1.3	1.0	0.3
French fried potatoes	48.6	3.0	1.5	1.5
Peas, green canned	80.7	4.5	3.6	0.9
Peas, green boiled	76.9	6.7	5.0	1.7
Peas frozen, boiled	81.6	4.4	3.2	1.2
Beans, green, canned		2.1	1.4	0.7
Beans, green, boiled		2.5	1.5	1.0
Carrots, raw	88.5	2.4	1.1	1.3
Carrots, cooked	90.5	2.7	1.2	1.5
Lettuce	96.0	0.7	0.5	0.2
Tomatoes, raw	94.5	1.2	0.8	0.4
Apple	84.6	1.5	1.3	0.2
Bananas	75.7	1.7	1.2	0.5
Kiwi	83.0	3.4		
Punes, dried	26.2	7.3	31	4.2

Source: Dreher 1999.
* Mainly analysed by the AOAC (1995).

24.4   Processing dietary fibre ingredients

Many fibre supplements are age-old familiar and have been modified in some way to improve their functionality (all the parameters that make food acceptable for processing and to the consumer) while still providing an enhanced level of dietary fibre. For example, gums, algal polysaccharides and pectins have been used for years to thicken – to impart viscosity to aqueous phase in food systems. They provide texture and mouth feel. They can stabilise suspensions, emulsions, foams, impart freeze/thaw stability and control syneresis. Because of their impact on the texture and sensory property of the end products, they are generally used in low amounts. Insoluble fibre or composite (mixture of soluble and insoluble) preparations are mainly used as texturing and/or bulking agents.

The physicochemical properties of fibre preparation play a key role in their functionality: fibre dimensions, hydration/rheological properties and fat binding/retention properties. The colour and flavour are also of importance.

A second generation of fibres with optimised properties for targeted applications has been emerging. Our purpose here is to examine the impact of some processes on the properties of some fibre preparations.

24.4.1   Grinding

Most of the fibre concentrates are available at different particle sizes. Partitioning may be done and fractions with different chemical compositions obtained, depending on the origin and history of the cell wall material (Auffret *et al.* 1994). Brans, which contain different tissues, are particularly affected (Heller *et al.* 1977). For example, glucan-enriched fraction from oat can be easily obtained by mechanical separation because the beta glucans are concentrated in the outermost endosperm layer (the subaleurone). This is not the case with barley as the beta glucans are more or less evenly distributed throughout the whole kernel.

Grinding can also affect the physical characteristics of fibre. The milling process used can be of importance (Sidiras *et al.* 1990). Ball milling not only reduces particle size but can also severely disrupt the crystalline order of cellulose. The effect is proportional to the time of ball milling. Hammer mill has no effect on cellulose crystallinity.

Grinding may affect hydration characteristics of the fibres as well as texture (Table 24.8). However, the most marked changes concern the kinetics of water uptake; the ground fibre is instantaneously hydrated compared to the raw fibre (Auffret *et al.* 1994). However, extensive milling can lead to a decrease in the specific surface area. Atmospheric humidity can provoke agglomeration of particles and collapse of some cellular structures, thus decreasing porosity (Fan *et al.* 1980, Gharpuray *et al.* 1983). Grinding can also affect the binding properties of the fibre (Ryden and Robertson 1995). These effects are mainly related to changes in the physical structure of the fibre and in particular to increased specific surface area.

Table 24.8 Hydration characteristics of some fibre concentrates

Source of fibre	Particle size (μm)	Swelling (ml/g)	Water retention (g water/g dry pellet)	Water absorption (ml water/g dry fibre)	Reference
Sugar beet fibre	500–200 μm	11.5	26.5		1
		19.3	32.9		2
	390	14.7	19.7		3
	385	21.4	22.6	8.8	4
	205	15.9	19.2	7.3	4
	540	11.0	26.6		5
	660	13.5	7.2		6
Citrus fibre		15.7	11.2	5.2	7
	540	15.7	10.4	7.0	4
	235	13.3	8.6	7.0	4
	420	14.7	10.4		6
	139	10.4	10.7	4.6	8
Apple fibre	540	9.6	6.9	3.8	6
	250	8.6	5.5	4.6	6
	133	7.4	5.4		8
Pea hull	500	6.0	7.1	2.4	9
	80	5.6	7.1	2.7	9
	950	9.9	4.3	1.9	4
	300	7.8	6.2	2.8	4
	560	6.2	4.2	2.7	6
	100	6.5	3.9	3.3	6
	67	6.6	3.8	3.7	8
Wheat bran	500–250		6.4	2.7	10
	900	11.9	6.8	1.0	4
	320	5.9	3.0	0.9	4
	1000–500	7.0	7.0		5
	Coarse	7.4	5.6		11
	Ground	6.4	6.6		11
Maize bran		5.7	2.4		12
Oat bran		5.53	3.5		12
Resistant starch	40	5.6	3.5	3.0	8
	84	7.4	3.1	3.9	

Sources: 1 Bertin *et al.* 1988; 2 Ralet *et al.* 1991; 3 Auffret *et al.* 1993; 4 Auffret *et al.* 1994; 5 Renard *et al.* 1994; 6 Cloutour 1995; 7 Thibault *et al.* 1988; 8 Robertson *et al.* 2000; 9 Ralet *et al.* 1993; 10 Ralet *et al.* 1990; 11 Ponne *et al.* 1997, 1998.

24.4.2   Heat treatments

As previously mentioned, fibre concentrates are generally supplied in a dry form. It improves the fibre shelf life without the addition of chemicals and reduces package size. Different drying methods are used in the food industry: convection, under vacuum, freeze drying, etc. The characteristics of the fibre products must be taken into account to design the procedure that minimises adverse effects. For example, agglomeration, deformation or darkening of the products must be avoided or at least minimised. It is also important to maintain or improve hydration properties of the fibre if they are to be used as texturing and bulking agents. Drying, most of the time depresses swelling and water retention capacities of the sample (Table 24.9) (Larrauri 1999, Femenia et al. 1999). Moreover, a partial modification of some dietary fibre components may also occur. This can be

Table 24.9   Effect of processing on the hydration properties of some dietary fibres

Dietary fibre	Treatment	Swelling (ml/g)	Water retention capacity (g water/g)	Reference
Sugar beet fibre	Native	10.8	6.1	1
	Depectinated – soft drying	22.8	13.1	1
	Depectinated – drastic drying	27.6	14	1
	Native	19.3	32.9	2
	Extruded	14.4	28.2	2
Cauliflower-based fibre supplements	Native (fresh)	22.9	19.9	3
	Freeze dried	19.4	8.318.7	3
	Boiled	27.4	24.6	3
	Dried 40 °C	16.9	12.8	3
	Dried 75 °C	4.2	5.7	3
Apple fibre	Dried 50 °C	32.0	13.9	4
	Dried under vacuum (80 °C, 13 mbar)	54.4	22.2	4
	Freeze-dried	50.6	20.5	4
	High rate freezing + dried under vacuum	56.7	17.9	4
	CID + dried under vacuum	46.8	18.6	4
Pea hull	Native	6.2	4.2	5
	Mercerised + freeze-drying	8.6	6.0	5
	Depectinated + freeze –drying	11.7	7.2	5
	Depectinated + mercerised + freeze drying	9.7	6.8	5
	Native	6.0	7.1	2
	extruded	5.2	4.3	2
Wheat bran	Native	7.0	7	6
	Delignified	11.0	10.4	6
	Native	nd	6.4	7
	Extruded	nd	6.0	7

Sources: 1 Guillon et al. 1998; 2 Thibault et al. 1988; 3 Femenia et al. 1999; 4 Guillon, personal communication; 5 Cloutour 1995; 6 Renard et al. 1994; 7 Ralet et al. 1990.

observed with a sample exposed to variable periods of temperature treatments while at a relatively high moisture. Femenia *et al.* (1999) found no changes in solubility of non-starch polysaccharides for fresh, freeze-dried and 40 °C dried fibre from cauliflower but a decrease in sample dried at 75 °C. The lowest swelling and water retention capacities were also obtained with samples dried at 75 °C. Close association between polysaccharides within the cell walls in dehydrated samples could reduce pore volume and restrict the extent of rehydration. Similar results have been observed with sugar beet and submitted to pectin extraction prior to drying. Freeze-drying led to a maintenance or increase of swelling and water retention capacity while drastic drying at high temperature resulted in a decrease of these properties (Guillon *et al.* 1998b, Cloutour 1995).

The wall is a strong mechanical component of living cells. It allows high turgor pressure and gives the cell its shape. However, when stress overpasses mechanical resistance of the wall, an irreversible deformation of the cell is obtained. This type of deformation occurs in most drying processes, except in the case of freeze-drying. Blanching prior to drying contributes towards increasing the permeability of the cell walls and induces an increase of the deformation. The drying conditions have a strong impact on shrinking. Products rapidly dried generally contain more void volumes and show a lower density than products slowly dried.

Drying can also affect certain bioactive compounds in fruit and vegetable products (Larrauri 1999). A decrease of polyphenol contents of red grape pomace peels was observed on drying at a temperature above 100 °C. Carotenoids seem sensitive to high temperature and losses occur during dehydration of carrots at 60 °C.

24.4.3   Thermo-mechanical treatment

Fibre-rich preparation may be extrusion cooked to modify its functionality. The results on different fibres show that extrusion cooking has a moderate effect on the hydration properties of pea hull brans, sugar beet or lemon fibre (Table 24.9). In contrast, extrusion cooking can influence solubility of the fibres. Wheat bran and other cereals need a high amount of energy, and about 15% of soluble material is obtained (Ralet *et al.* 1990). Less energy is required for the hulls and a similar amount of material is solubilised (Ralet *et al.* 1993). Ferulylated heteroxylans and glucans are solubilised from wheat bran, and arabinans, heteroxylans and pectins from pea hull. Extrusion of oat bran cereals in which the beta-glucan has a range of molecular weights cause loss of the integrity of the cell walls and dispersion of the beta-glucan dispersed throughout the cereal. Differences in the hardness and density of the extruded cereals are also evident as the molecular weight was reduced (Tosh *et al.* 2010).

The main effect of extrusion cooking of sugar beet pulp, lemon and apple fibre is to increase by up to 40% the water solubility of pectins in cold water (Thibault *et al.* 1995). The soluble pectins can have high molecular weight and high degree of methylation. They can form gel as other high methoxy (HM) pectins (Ralet *et al.* 1994).

A new process has been developed to fit the industrial demand for products with preserved nutritional quality and improved functionality. This process is named 'instant controlled depression' and associates texturation and drying processes (Louka and Allaf 1998). It consists of submitting the material to thermal processing at high pressure for a short time and then flash expansion. The operation interpolated after the pre-drying stage permits expansion of the dried products, by self-vaporisation of the residual water. As a result, the product recovers its original shape. Its organoleptic properties are close to those of freeze-dried products. The colour is preserved and its ability to rehydrate safeguarded. The quality of the end product depends on the operating conditions and on the characteristics of the raw material. The energy cost compared to freeze-drying is low. This process has been applied with success to small cubes of fruits and vegetables.

24.4.4 Chemical treatments

Hydration properties of fibre can be altered substantially by treating them with solvents, oxidants, acid or alkaline. The action of these chemicals is mainly to extract more or less selectively compounds such as pectins, hemicelluloses and lignins. The extent of extraction depends on the concentration of the chemical and on the temperature conditions.

At the laboratory scale, it has been demonstrated that substantial removal of pectins by relatively mild chemical treatment leads to an increase of the pore volume of sugar beet fibre, and thus of the water hydration properties (Table 24.9) (Auffret *et al.* 1993, Guillon *et al.* 1998b). Similar results have been obtained with pea hull (Weightman *et al.* 1994). However, if the chemical treated fibre undergoes harsh drying, its hydration properties become limited, probably because of structural collapse of the fibre matrix (Table 24.9).

Removal of compounds is not necessarily a prerequesite to increase the hydration properties. The swelling action of water on cellulosic material is enhanced by the breakdown of intra- and interchain bonds by alkaline agent or phosphoric acid (Sinitsyn *et al.* 1991).

Bleaching can be used to lighten fibre material. For this purpose, hydroxide peroxide treatment has been applied (Gould *et al.* 1989). Phenolic compounds and other phytochemicals may be lost. Peroxide can induce the release of carbohydrates bound to phenolic compounds. This treatment can increase the fibre's ability to absorb water, soften and swell when hydrated. For example, treated wheat straw can be used as high substitute for a portion of flour in cakes without introducing undesirable sensory characteristics or causing deterioration of the baking performance (Jasberg *et al.* 1989).

24.4.5 Enzymatic treatment

Endogenous phytase activity in wheat grain can be used to reduce phytate levels but exogenous enzyme can also make a significant contribution (Jayarajah *et al.* 1997). The endogenous phytase activity results in destruction of phytate without accumulation of inositol phosphate intermediates, and at low moisture levels, without modification of the fibre components through polysaccharidase activities which may be present in bran.

Enzymatic treatments can be applied to improve the functionality of fibre preparations. The properties mainly concerned are the hydration properties and solution viscosity. Oat beta-glucans and guar gum may be hydrolysed to provide grades developing different viscosity in solution. The treatment results in a decrease of molecular weight and yield products with generally improved resistance to thermal, pH, and shear degradation when compared to the high molecular weight parents.

Treatment of pea hull and apple fibres with pectinolytic and cellulolytic enzymes has been found to increase the proportion of water-soluble fibre and confer the matrix with a softer texture, making easier its incorporation into foods (Caprez *et al.* 1987).

Xylanase preparations find widespread use in the baking industry to improve handling characteristics of the dough, loaf volume and crumb structure of the bread, especially bread containing high amount of dietary fibre (Poutanen 1997). The enzymes degrade *in situ* the water-insoluble arabinoxylans present in discrete endosperm cell wall particles, thus causing a substantial enrichment in the water-soluble arabinoxylans with corresponding increase in viscosity of the aqueous phase (Poutanen *et al.* 1998). The improving action of pentosanases on the volume of bread may be compared to those reported when high molecular weight soluble pentosans or guar gum are added to flour ingredients. Of course when added in excess, enzymes induce an extensive depolymerisation of the water-soluble arabinoxylans, thus causing a decrease in viscosity and a deterioration of the dough quality.

24.5   Processing foods containing dietary fibre

Most foods are processed for consumer convenience in the food industry or at home. Industrial processing is applied to prolong shelf life of the products or to produce foods ready to eat or easy to prepare while preserving their quality, i.e. texture, colour, flavour, palatability and nutritional quality. Industrial processing mainly includes heat treatments, thermo-mechanical and non-thermal treatments.

24.5.1   Heat treatment
Wet heat treatment mainly includes blanching, boiling, canning, steaming and microwaving. The major consequences of processing are release of cell contents and the solubilisation of labile dietary fibre components, i.e. pectins, beta glucans, arabinoxylans, oligosaccharides. The extent of solubilisation of the cell wall polysaccharides depends on the chemical nature of the polysaccharide and its association with other macromolecules within cell walls, and on the processing parameters (temperature, duration, etc). During cooking and processing, there can

be extensive breakdown of pectic polysaccharides through a beta-eliminative degradation. This results in significant reduction of the molecular weight and thus increases solubilisation (Anderson and Clydesdale 1980, Varo *et al.* 1984, Stolle-Smits *et al.* 1995, Svanberg *et al.* 1997). The viscosity of the water-soluble dietary fibre decreases following intense heat treatment, in accordance with a shift towards a lower molecular weight (Svanberg 1997). As a result of partial solubilisation of cell wall components, the insoluble fibre matrix can exhibit higher swelling because of a looser and more porous network. Depending on the pore size distribution, the water retention capacity may be increased or decreased. For leafy vegetables, the tissues become softer. In seed legumes, pectins cementing the cells are solubilised, leading to separation of cotyledon cells. Blanching applied to inactive enzymes, although it can also cause some solubilisation. For example, blanching carrots leads to a deesterification of pectic polysaccharides (Plat *et al.* 1991), and the change has been mainly ascribed to enzyme activity rather than beta elimination. Pectin methyl esterase is known to remain active at increased temperatures (Lopez *et al.* 1997), and activity can be affected by intracellular cations release during cell metabolism or disruption (Alonso *et al.* 1997). It can influence the texture or tissue firmness in vegetables (Wu and Chang 1990). Microwave cooking is generally considered as a mild form of heat treatment. Applied to green beans, microwaving slightly affected the total dietary fibre content but a shift toward lower molecular weight of the water-soluble fibre was observed (Svanberg 1997). Only severe microwaving (repeated treatment) decreased the total fibre content (Svanberg 1997). The polysaccharides in cereal fibres are not susceptible to beta elimination during cooking or processing. Moreover, the presence of phenolic compounds may limit the extractability of arabinoxylans.

Dry heat treatment such as baking or roasting, does not significantly alter the dietary fibre composition. In extreme conditions, a significant increase in the lignin content and a decrease in water hydration properties can be observed (Camire 1999). This could be ascribed to the formation of Maillard products. Maillard products arise from the reaction of sugars and proteins, often leading to browning and development of flavour. They are not digested by endogenous enzymes in the small intestine and therefore can contribute towards increased amount of total dietary fibre.

Heat treatment followed by a cooling period can induce the formation of RS in starchy foods. The amount will depend on the botanical source, the ratio of amylose to amylopectin, processing parameters (temperature, amount of water, cooling) and storage conditions. The RS content of common food cereals food like breads, breakfast cereals, pasta and rice is generally below 3%, potato 4–5%, potato flakes 3% (Asp *et al.* 1996). In the case of cooked cereal products (rice, pasta, bread), RS does not seem to increase during storage or freezing (Wursch 1999). In contrast, deep-fat frying or storing cooked potato in the cold increases by up to about 12% the starch into RS. Repeated heating and cooling can lead to an accumulation of RS but the increase in absolute is relatively small compared to amount generated on the first heating/cooling cycle. Starch lipid and starch protein complexes can also be formed during cooking and these are more resistant to alpha amylase (Holm *et al.* 1983).

24.5.2   Thermo-mechanical treatment

Extrusion cooking is nowadays currently used by the food industry for various types of snacks, ready-to-eat cereal products, etc. In a typical twin extruder, the product is fed in and transported by rotation of the screws. Here, the product is submitted to heat and shear. At the end of extruder, the product is forced to pass through a die, and then water can be vaporised leading to an expanding product.

Extrusion of wheat or rye flour under normal conditions does not induce the formation of high amount of RS (Bjorck *et al.* 1984, Lue *et al.* 1990). No changes in these conditions are observed in the total amount of dietary fibre and a slight increase in the amount of soluble fibre at the expense of the insoluble fraction is reported (Varo *et al.* 1983, Bjorck *et al.* 1984). While under drastic conditions, an increase in the amount of total fibre and a significant conversion of insoluble to soluble fractions has been found (Bjorck *et al.* 1984). This increase in total dietary fibre is not ascribed to an increase of RS. Popping and flaking only slightly change the composition of cereals. Soluble carbohydrates fractions are generally only a little enhanced by the treatments. The treatments bring disorganisation of the endosperm of grains, but the outer layers (aleurone and adjacent layer) are generally preserved. Popping of maize grains causes heterogeneous reactions within the grain (Farber and Gallant 1976). In the unpopped peripheral zones, starch granules are partly swollen while the inner part of the endosperm shows an alveolar structure where starch is completely gelatinised and pushed against the remnant cell walls. Steam flaking, especially with maize, generally produces a disorganisation of the cell structure: the cell walls are broken, and content of the cell more or less dispersed. Starch granules appear slightly deformed, partly gelatinised and fissured. Intensive mechanical/thermal treatments generally increase the accessibility and digestibility of starch.

In the case of legumes, flaking compared to cooking results in a lower amount of resistant starch. In the case of beans, 9–11% of total starch was resistant in flake beans (Schweizer *et al.* 1990) against 16.5% in cooked beans (Noah *et al.* 1998).

24.5.3   Freezing

Enzyme activities and, in particular, pectinolytic activities are only slowed at freezer temperature. This means that in long storage periods, pectin solubilisation and degradation may occur. Starch can retrograde in frozen foods, leading to the formation of RS. Freezing can be accompanied by ice crystal formation, which can lead to disruption of the cell walls. This phenomenon can increase the release of cell content and the solubilisation of cell wall polysaccharides on cooking (Rahman *et al.* 1971). The formation and size of ice crystals depends on the temperature and rate of freezing. Preservation of the quality of products requires rapid freezing.

24.5.4   Fermentation

Fermented legumes are an integral and significant part of the diet in developing countries. It has been suggested as an economical method of processing and preserving foods. Fermentation has been shown to enhance the nutritive value of legumes, reduces some anti-nutritional endogenous compounds and improves consumer acceptability. It increases vitamins, removes some anti-nutritional factors such as trypsin inhibitors and eliminates alpha galactosides, compounds related to flatus production.

24.5.5   Germination

Malting is a well-established process used to produce cereal substrates for fermented beverages. Malted cereals may be used to formulate nutritious products, including infant and weaning foods. Grain germination is associated with water uptake. Subsequently, an activation process signalled by hormones arising from the embryonic axis results in synthesis and secretion of hydrolytic and other enzymes. These enzymes depolymerise cell polysaccharides, and the protein and starch reserves of the endosperm. Thus, germination induces chemical and biochemical changes in the seed. It can decrease the amount of alpha galactosides, lectins, trypsin inhibitors and phytate. Substantial solubilisation and degradation of some cell wall polysaccharides by endogenous enzymes may occur. For example, during malting endogenous beta glucanase is synthesised, which results in the depolymerisation of beta barley glucans, thus decreasing their capacity to increase viscosity of aqueous solution (Fincher and Stone 1986). Extensive degradation of cell arabinoxylans, the other major components of cereal endosperm cell walls, also occurs in germinating wheat grain (Fincher and Stone 1986). Germination can lead to the synthesis of new compounds, some of which have high bioactivity and can increase the nutritional value and stability of the grains. For example, the germination of rye for six days at 15–25 °C increase the content of folate and methanol soluble phenolic compounds by 2–3.5 fold (Liukonnen *et al.* 2003).

Combination of fermentation and germination has been shown to increase the bioactive potential of wholemeal rye (Katina *et al.* 2007) Thus, although the amount of dietary fibre may be quantitatively equivalent in cooked/processed to that in raw material, their properties may be altered.

24.6   The physiological effects of dietary fibre

While the amount and source of fibre may be important for dietary responses, it is equally important to describe properties of fibre used if mechanisms responsible for fibre activity(ies) are to be understood. Physical and chemical properties will determine local responses (direct effects as the result of the presence of dietary fibre in the digestive tract) and associated systemic responses which may be expected with ingestion of a particular fibre. These properties include viscosity for soluble fibre, water retention, binding/adsorption properties, particle size. The fermentation of dietary fibre through the products and residues of fermentation and impact on the microflora also play a key role in the effects ascribed to dietary fibre.

24.6.1   Physicochemical properties involved in the physiological effects of dietary fibre

Water-soluble polysaccharides and viscosity
Some water-soluble polysaccharides such as pectins, gums, arabinoxylans and the (1–3,1–4)-beta-D-glucans may form viscous solutions. Inclusion of these polysaccharides in a meal can increase the volume and viscosity of digesta in the upper gut. They can delay gastric emptying in the stomach, which can promote satiety. This can also reduce emulsification of dietary lipids in the acid medium of the stomach and subsequently lower the extent of lipid assimilation. In the lumen of the small intestine, viscosity can resist the effects of gastrointestinal motility. It can impede the diffusion of digestive enzymes towards their substrates, which slows down digestion. It can also slow down the release and transit of the products of hydrolysis towards the absorptive surface of the mucosa. The direct systemic response is a steady rate of nutrient delivery in the circulation resulting in lower post-prandial level.

Viscosity is imparted by the chemical structure of the polysaccharides (amount of space occupied by the macromolecules generally characterised by intrinsic viscosity) and also by the cross-linkages between the macromolecules (Morris 1990, Dikeman and Fahey 2006, Cui and Wang 2009, Wood 2010). Concentration temperature, ionic concentration, pH, association with proteins, and shear forces are all involved.

Treatments that induce hydrolysis of pectins, beta glucans, arabinoxylan or various gums into lower molecular weight molecules will contribute towards reduced capacity of these molecules to increase the viscosity of digesta. In contrast, some treatments such as extrusion cooking can increase the amount of water-soluble molecules without extensively splitting them. Thus, it is important to consider the property of fibre in food as it is eaten.

Moreover, although not digested by endogenous enzymes in the upper gut, macromolecules can undergo significant degradation. For example, pectins can be solubilised through disruption of calcium bridges under acidic conditions (in the stomach) or through beta elimination at a near neutral pH (e.g. in the small intestine). The extent and location of this degradation could have a nutritional impact. Changes in ionic environment and pH throughout the gastrointestinal tract can also influence the solubility and viscosity of polysaccharides. This is generally observed with polyelectrolytes (pectins, alginates). For example, at a high concentration alginate can form a gel in the stomach and may be soluble in the small intestine. The concentration in the lumen may be different from that in ingested food. In particular, the total volume of digesta may adapt in response to ingestion of viscous solution, partly offsetting the difference in initial viscosity.

As a consequence, the viscosity of fluid digesta may vary within the gut. This means that the measured viscosity of a fibre source may bear little relationship to the viscosity in the digestive segments of interest. At least the concentration, structure and molecular weight of the polymer (degree of space occupancy by the polymer) must be documented in the segment of the digestive tract under consideration for interpreting the data. Because most of the polysaccharides exhibit shear thinning, only one value at a single shear rate has no meaning. Morris (1990, 1992) recommends measuring the viscosity at a few shear rates and then derive the maximum viscosity (η_0) and the shear rate ($\gamma_{1/2}$) required to reduce viscosity to $\eta_{0/2}$.

Adsorption/binding ions and bile acids
The ability of certain fibre to adsorb or entrap bile acids and phospholipids has been suggested as a potential mechanism by which dietary fibre, containing uronic acids or phenolic acids, may increase faecal excretion of bile acids. An increased bile acid excretion results in higher cholesterol turnover from the body. The exact mechanisms by which fibre sequesters bile acids are unclear; hydrophobic (fibre-containing phenolics) and ionic interactions (fibre-containing uronic acids) have been suggested (Thibault *et al.* 1992). *In vivo*, some fibre preparations (Wolever 1995) increase ileal and faecal excretions of sterols and lipids, but which help adsorption or increase of the fluid digesta viscosity account for this effect is still questionable.

Fibre consisting of lignified or coarse tissues such as rice straw are identified as neutraceuticals with binding properties (Robertson 1998). Insoluble dietary fibres and dietary fibre-rich preparations with more or less intact cell wall structures, such as cereal products (bread, brans), linseed and psyllium seeds, alcohol-insoluble substances from fruits and vegetables are able *in vitro* to bind bile acids. Strongest interactions occurr with chenodeoxycholic acid, deoxycholic acid, hyodeoxycholic acid, and lithocholic acid (Dongowski, 2009). Milling, relieving the constraint on accessibility to the binding surface and allowing a greater partitioning of compounds from fibre, can increase the affinity for some toxic heterocyclic amines in foods (Robertson 1998).

Adsorption has often been measured by methods similar to those used for water retention capacity, and both absorption and entrapment in the cell wall matrix can account for the retention. The prevailing chemical environment and characteristics of the fibre fractions in the small intestine must be taken into account for physiogically reliable measurements of the binding capacity.

Water absorption/retention properties
Insoluble fibre can absorb, swell and entrap water within its porous matrix. Water retention properties contribute towards the bulking effect of fibre in the colon. They can take part in the dilution of cytotoxic substances in the large intestine, thus reducing harmful potency.

The hydration properties depend on the chemistry of the individual components of fibres, the way they are assembled in the cell walls, the anatomy and the particle size of the fibres. Fibre mainly composed of primary cell walls exhibits general higher values than fibre with secondary cell walls (Table 24.8) (Thibault *et al.* 1992, 1994).

Environmental conditions such as pH, ionic strength and nature of the ions can influence the hydration values of fibres containing polyelectrolytes (charged groups such as carboxyl in fibre rich in pectins, carboxyl and sulfate groups in fibres from algae) (Thibault *et al.* 1992, 1994).

Processes, such as grinding, drying, heating or extrusion cooking for example, provided that they modify the composition and the physical properties of the fibre matrix, will strongly affect the hydration properties (Thibault *et al.* 1992). Fibres with high values for hydration properties are generally well fermented, probably because bacteria and their secreted enzymes can rapidly diffuse and reach their substrates (Auffret *et al.* 1993, Cloutour 1995, Guillon *et al.* 1998b). In the colon, the most effective stool bulkers are low fermented fibres, because they retain a proportion of their matrix and thus are still able to bind water. Wheat bran and ispaghula are the reference fibres for this effect.

Different aspects of fibre hydration can be distinguished and a need was identified for a clear definition. In particular there should be a distinction between absorption, uptake, holding and binding. The definition of hydration properties arising from the European PROFIBRE project are:

Swelling: 'the volume occupied by a known weight of fibre under the condition used'.

Water retention capacity: 'the amount of water retained by a known weight of fibre under the condition used' – it is preferred to either water-holding capacity or water-binding capacity.

Water absorption: 'the kinetics of water movement under defined conditions'.

Swelling and water retention capacity provide a general view of fibre hydration and can provide information useful for fibre-supplemented foods. Water absorption can provide more information on the fibre, in particular its substrate pore volume, and will help our understanding of the behaviour of fibre in foods or during gut transit.

For each parameter, several methods have been proposed for their measurement but not always with a clear picture of what is being measured. Generally, swelling is measured as settled bed volume and water retention capacity as the amount of water retained after centrifugation by the insoluble substrate (pellet). Water absorption is measured using a Baumann apparatus or using osmotic pressure/dialysis techniques. When assessing the behaviour of fibre in food and in the digestive tract from the hydration properties, the physical fibre matrix properties as well as the physicochemical conditions prevailing in their environment in food or gut lumen should be taken into account. Hydration properties of the fibre matrix before ingestion may bear little relationship to the fibre in the colon as the result of fibre fermentation.

Disruptibility of the cell walls

In food with intact cells, the release of nutrients can be related to resistance of cell walls to disruption. Nutrients entrapped within the cellular structure cannot be digested until the cell walls have been damaged. In the case of starchy foods, the amount of starch escaping digestion and reaching the large intestine is increased in foods with intact cell walls.

Factors that influence cell wall disruptibility are structure, lignification and mechanical and thermo-mechanical treatments. Secondary cell walls are generally more resistant to mechanical stress. This means, for example, that the outer layer of cereal kernel or legume seeds will be more preserved than cell walls of the starchy endosperms. The physical structure of food can also be significantly disrupted in the mouth, due to chewing. The extent of disruption, depends on the food rheological properties. The physical degradation of food results in an increase of the available surface to enzymes. Thus, it can significantly affect the overall process of digestion and postprandial blood response.

Light microscopy can be used to examine the physical structure of food. Again, the main difficulty is to evaluate damages occurring within the digestive tract. In this respect, more *in vivo* data are required.

Particle size

Particle size can play a role in controlling a number of events occurring in the digestive tract (e.g. transit time, fermentation and faecal excretion). The rate of fermentation is proportional to the external surface area in contact with the bacteria for fibres with a low porosity such hulls and brans. Coarse wheat bran is more effective in regulating transit time than fine bran. Particles can induce an increased excitation of colonic mechanoreceptors, stimulating contractile activity in favour of a higher propulsion of digesta (Cherbut 1995, Edwards 1995). The decrease of intestinal transit time associated with these fibres protects the colon from prolonged exposure to cytotoxic substances which may also be carcinogenic.

Particle size is related to the processing history of the fibre product. Mechanical treatment such as grinding but also chewing decreases the particle size. Wet heat treatments that release a large amount of pectins through weakening the middle lamella can induce a concomitant loss of intercellular adhesion. Degradation of the fibre matrix by colonic bacteria can lead to an almost complete disintegration of the particles.

Particle size distribution can be measured by different methods, like sieving, or methods based on the change in resistivity of a conducting medium, or optical methods (laser diffraction, microscopy and image analysis computer) (Allen 1988). All of these methods are based on different principles. They will give different values for the same material but classification for a range of materials will be preserved. All have some drawbacks and limitations. The form of the fibre, wet or dry, is of importance as some fibres may swell in solution and as a consequence, their particle size increases. The measurement of particle size in a wet form of residue of fermentation may be more relevant when assessing the bulking effects of fibre in the large intestine. In any case, when giving particle size values, the methods used and the form of the fibre must be clear.

24.6.2 Fermentation patterns

Dietary fibre makes a substantial contribution as a substrate for fermentation. It has been found in the ileostomy model that the mean excretion of dry weight and energy were 50 g/d and 800 kJ/d, respectively on a low fibre diet, and 88 g/d and 1700 kJ/d on a high fibre diet (Langkilde and Andersson 1998). Effects of dietary fibre on bowel function like faecal mass, stool frequency, regulation of colonic pH and salvage of energy from non-digestible foods are directly related to their fermentation pattern (Cherbut 1995, Edwards 1995, Wong *et al.* 2006). Poorly fermented fibres contribute towards increased bulk in the large intestine, thereby reducing the risk for constipation and possibly also colonic cancer. Highly fermentable fibres, through the products of metabolism, are involved in physiological effects on the colon mucosa (Bingham 1990, Cummings 1995, Higginson 1995, McIntyre *et al.* 1993, Sakata 1995) and colon function (Edwards 1995) as well as post-absorptive actions on the liver and other tissues (Wolever 1995, Darcy-Vrillon and Duée 1995, Demigné *et al.* 1995, Topping and Pant 1995). They contribute towards maintaining the ecosystem equilibrium (Salminen *et al.* 1998). In addition, some fibre sources such as fructo-oligosaccharides can selectively stimulate the growth of health-promoting bacteria, including bifidobacteria and lactobacilli (Salminen *et al.* 1998, Van Loo *et al.* 1999). They may be the main genera responsible for the protective barrier function and for stimulating healthy immune response in adults. Recently the group of N. Delzenne and P. Cani in Belgium suggested that some fibres and mainly prebiotics could have a beneficial effect on metabolic syndrome and in overweighed and obese individuals (Cani *et al.* 2009). Fructans promote *Bifidobacterium* spp. in humans (Roberfroid 2007) and animal models (Cani *et al.* 2007). This prebiotic, when administrated to mice fed a high-fat diet, decreases plasma lipopolysaccharides (LPS), improves glucose tolerance and glucose-induced insulin secretion, and normalised plasma and adipose tissue proinflammatory cytokines (Cani *et al.* 2007).

All dietary fibres are not fermented to the same extent or at the same rate (Table 24.10). Factors controlling fermentation are related to the substrates available for fermentation, the microflora and its activity, and the host.

Microbial degradation requires the contribution of a different group of bacteria linked in a trophic chain. Polysaccharide-degrading bacteria hydrolyse polymers into smaller fragments that can be used by saccharolytic species. The rate and extent of fermentation depends on the physical structure of the fibre matrix (access of bacteria to their substrates) and on the chemical structure of the individual polysaccharides (Guillon *et al.* 1996). Fibre products rich in secondary tissues (bran, hull) are poorly fermented compared to fibre mainly composed of parenchyma tissue (fruits, vegetables). Soluble polysaccharides are fermented at a higher rate than equivalent polysaccharides within cell walls. Highly and randomly branched polysaccharides are generally fermented at a lower extent than blocked branched polysaccharides. Some polysaccharides such as carrageenans and ulvan are not degraded by colonic bacteria while their constitutive monomers or dimers are (Bobin-Dubigeon *et al.* 1997, Mathers *et al.* 1998). It has been suggested that bacteria do not possess the enzymatic equipment necessary for their breakdown. Polysaccharidase synthesis is generally induced by exposure to the substrates and repressed by the products of reaction (Macfarlane

Table 24.10 Factors affecting the fermentation pattern of dietary fibre (percentage of sugar disappearance after *in vitro* batch incubation)

Sources	Treatment	Particle size (µm)	WRC (g H_2O/g dry pellet)	Apparent sugar disappearance, 4 h*–6 h**	Apparent sugar disappearance, 24 h	Reference
Beet fibre	Commercial fibre	660	7.2	14 ± 0**	70 ± 1	1
Citrus fibre	Commercial fibre	420	10.4	44 ± 2**	81 ± 1	1
Pea fibre (hull)	Commercial fibre	1950	4.8	6 ± 1**	22 ± 7	1
Pea fibre	Grinded	560	4.2	3 ± 1**	22 ± 2.0	1
Pea fibre	Grinded	115	3.3	10 ± 1**	41 ± 2	1
	Treated with pectinolytic enzymes + cellulase	30	nd	1 ± 3**	10 ± 3	1
	Mercerised	520	6.0	5 ± 0**	10 ± 2	1
	Partial removal of pectins	950	7.2	17 ± 2**	26 ± 0	1
	Extensive removal of pectins	650	6.8	29 ± 1**	29 ± 2	1
Apple fibre	Commercial fibre	540	6.9	13 ± 2**	51 ± 4	1
	Grinded	250	5.5	31 ± 4**	67 ± 2	1
	Partial removal of pectins	264	8.5	40 ± 1**	73 ± 2	1
Carrageenans				6 ± 6**	29 ± 4	2
Alginates				31 ± 1**	83 ± 1	2
Acacia gum					49 ± 12	3
Actilight					74 ± 11	3
Novelose (RS: 61.4, type B)	Removal of digestible starch			5*	87	4
Hylon®7(RS: 27.4, type B)	Removal of digestible starch			8*	57	4

Source: 1 Cloutour 1995; 2 Bobin-Dubigeon 1996; 3 Michel *et al.*, 1998; 4 Martin *et al.*, 1998.

and Degnan 1996). In addition, the course of fermentation depends on the microflora composition, which varies from one individual to another, and intra-individually in the cell population densities of the principal taxonomic groups (Macfarlane and Macfarlane 1993). The main bacteria reported to be able to hydrolyse polysaccharides are *Bacteroides*, *Bifidobacterium*, *Ruminococcus* and some species of *Eubacterium* and *Clostridium*. *Bacteroides* is the bacterial genus presenting the highest degree of metabolic versality and is predominant in the microflora.

Some substrates (e.g. fructo-oligosaccharides, inulin), known as prebiotics, can promote selectively the growth and/or the activity of one or a limited number of bacteria in the colon.

End products of fermentation include short chain fatty acids (SCFA), mainly acetate, propionate and butyrate and gases (H_2, CO_2 and in some cases CH_4). The amount and molar ratios of the three main SCFAs vary substantially, depending on the substrate type (Table 24.11). The nature of the monomers seems not to play a major role in the determination of SCFA profiles. Acetic acid is the major SCFA produced, whatever the substrate. The highest proportion is seen with pectin-type material. Starch is generally associated with a large proportion of butyrate while the highest proportion of propionic acid is observed with arabinogalactan, guar gum and galacto-oligosaccharides. Botham *et al.* (1998) showed that different glucans yielded different SCFA profiles; fermentation of cellulose produced mainly acetate while pea starch generated less acetate (47%) but more butyrate (36%) and more propionate (15%). Fermentation of arabinoxylan has been associated with a proliferation of the bifidobacteria, lactobacilli and eubacteria groups and a high proportion of butyric acid in the SCFA produced (Hughes *et al.* 2007, Pastell *et al.* 2009, Knudsen and Laerke 2010).

SCFAs are mainly absorbed and stimulate salt and water absorption. They are metabolised by the colon epithelium, liver and muscle (Wong *et al.* 2006). Acetic

Table 24.11   Short chain fatty acid profile of some dietary fibre

Substrates rich in:	Example	Short fatty acid profiles
Cellulose		High amount of acetate
Beta-glucans	Oat bran	High amount of buyrate and relatively low amount of acetate*
Resistant starch	Retrograded or native Eurylon®, Hylon®, Crystalean®	High amount of butyrate and relatively low amount of acetate
Wheat bran		High amount of butyrate
Fructo-oligosaccharides	Actilight	High amount of butyrate and relatively amount of acetate
Inulin		High amount of propionate and acetate*
Pectins		High amount of acetate
Galactomannans		High amount of propionate

* Excerpted from Botham *et al.* 1998.

acid is the only SCFA that can be detected in peripheral blood. Propionic acid is mainly metabolised in the liver and is mainly discussed in relation to effects on carbohydrate and cholesterol metabolisms.

Among short chain fatty acids produced during colonic fermentation of dietary fibre, butyrate has a specific interest. It is the preferential fuel of colonocytes. Butyrate has anticancer properties, since it modulates several key intestinal epithelial cell functions, such as proliferation, differentiation, inflammation and apoptosis (Segain *et al.* 2000, Thibault *et al.* 2007, Hamer *et al.* 2008).

While the amount of fibre may be important for dietary response it is equally important to describe its source and properties if mechanisms responsible for fibre activity(s) are to be understood. Numerous mechanisms of action have been identified which are related to physicochemical properties and fermentation patterns in the large intestine. The fact that fibre sources differ in their susceptibility to undergo modification during cooking and processing must be considered. The physicochemical environment prevailing in different areas of the digestive tract as the changes occurring within the fibre matrix during passage must also be taken into account. More in vivo data are still required. Moreover, methods for measurement of the physicochemical properties that are relevant from a physiological point of view are still needed.

The relationships between target function of the body and improved state of health and/or reduced risk of disease remain to establish. Moreover, most of our knowledge is derived from studies where model fibres were used at doses that were not always realistic. More data are needed with food as eaten, and as part of a complex diet to confirm attributes of fibres.

24.7   Recommended intakes of dietary fibre

The document entitled 'Dietary fibre intakes in Europe' and published in 1993 by the European Community within the framework of COST 92 provides a record of fibre intake in the different member states of the European Union. The range value is from 21 to 25.3 g/day. It is obvious that the data are obtained by different methods of intake calculation but also of food analysis, which makes comparison difficult. The contribution of food containing added fibre for technological or functional purposes is not taken into account. Cereals, followed by vegetables, including pulses and potato, are the main food group contributors to dietary fibre intake. Of course, there are variations between countries. For example, consumption of cereals is highest in North Europe and lowest in South Europe. For comparison, dietary fibre intake in the United States of America is said to average 12–14 g per day (Miller Jones 2008).

Nutritional recommendations about fibre intake in the different countries relies on the same analytical basis (Cho *et al.* 1999a). In agreement with a proposal from Organisation Mondiale de la Santé (World Health Organization), Dupin and co-workers (1992) suggest in France a daily intake of 30–40 g dietary fibre. Several other countries, such as Denmark and Sweden, suggest a lower intake, namely 25–30 g dietary fibre/day. The Netherlands and USA express their recommendation as g fibre/MJ or 2000 Kcal. Recommendations are based on what hitherto has been known about fibre. Most of the time, the guidelines are qualitative. They emphasise the need to eat more fruit and vegetables, and to avoid fat. Dietary diversity is encouraged more than precise nutritional guidelines.

24.8   Conclusions and future trends

Dietary fibre has been accepted in the prevention and management of disease in Western society. Dietary fibre exerts its direct physiological effect throughout the gastrointestinal tract in addition to metabolic activities.

The food industry has the opportunity to improve the health of customers and/ or to reduce their risk of disease through foods with added activities. One difficulty for food companies when dealing with dietary fibre is to meet both nutritional and technological requirements; and most often, a compromise must be found. In the last few years, ingredient suppliers have been engaged in research aimed at further improving the quality of fibre, which in part determines how much fibre can be added to foods and contribute towards their quality and nutritional attributes. It is important to further understand the effects of cooking and processing on fibre functionality and to take major notice of them. Novel generations of fibre (modified or mixtures of fibres with complementary properties) with optimised properties for specific application of final products have been developed. However, food companies still need to establish and develop innovative ways to bring dietary fibre into more products. Fibre supplementation of foods remains a largely empirical process. Predictive models for the mechanisms involved in successful incorporation of fibre in foods must be developed.

Well-validated relevant biomarkers to physiological functions and health end points are crucial to demonstrate accurately that food is truly effective. If appealing and believable, fibre-rich products will contribute significantly to dietary guidelines.

The success of foods for cholesterol reduction and for well-balanced intestinal flora are examples of possible success with this approach. Modern research on dietary fibre has been ongoing for almost 30 years. There is no doubt that further development regarding effects of dietary fibre and associated substances will be important for the development of nutritious foods and for improved public health.

24.9   References

Allen, T. (1998) 'Granulométrie', Technique de l'Ingénieur, 1040–66.
Alonso, J., Howell, N. and Canet, W. (1997) 'Purification and characterisation of two pectinmethylesterase from persimmon (Diospyros kaki)', *J Sci Food Agric*, **75**, 352–8.
Anderson, N.E. and Clydesdale, F.M. (1980) 'Effects of processing on the dietary fibre content of wheat bran, pureed green beans, and carrots', *J Sci*, **45**, 1533–7.
Anderson, J.W., Baird, P., Davis, R.H., Ferreri, S., Knudtson, M., *et al.* (2009) 'Health benefits of dietary fiber', *Nutr Rev*, **67**(4), 188–205.

Ang, J.F. and Miller, W.B. (1991) 'Multiple functions of powdered cellulose as a food ingredient', *Amer Assoc Cereal Chem*, **36**(7), 558–64.

Anonymous (1999) 'Ingrédients "santé": une forme pétillante, RIA, Spécial FIE 99, HS juillet-aout, 97–108.

Anonymous (2001) 'The definition of dietary fiber', *Cereal Foods World*, **46**(3), 112–29.

AOAC International (1995) 'Total, soluble and insoluble dietary fiber in foods. AOAC official method 991.43', *Official Methods of Analysis*, 16th edn.

Asp, N.G., Van Amelsvoort, J.M.M. and Hautvast, J.G.A.J. (1996) 'Nutritional implication of resistant starch', *Nutr Res Rev*, **9**, 1–31.

Asp, N.G., Schweizer, T.F., Southgate, D.A.T. and Theander, O. (1992) 'Dietary fibre analysis'. In: T.F. Schweizer and C.A. Edwards (eds), *Dietary Fibre: A Component of Food*, pp. 57–101, ILSI Human Nutrition Reviews, London, Springer-Verlag.

Auffret, A., Barry, J.-L. and Thibault, J.-F. (1993) 'Effect of chemical treatments of sugar beet fibre on their physico-chemical properties and on their in vitro fermentation', *J Sci Food Agric*, **61**, 195–203.

Auffret, A., Ralet, M.-C., Guillon, F., Barry, J.-L. and Thibault, J.-F. (1994) 'Effect of grinding and experimental conditions on the measurement of hydration properties of dietary fibres', *Lebensm Wiss U Technol*, **27**, 166–72.

Bernabe, M., Fenwick, R., Frias, J., Jimenez-Barbero, J., Price, K., *et al.* (1993) 'Determination by NMR spectroscopy of the structure of ciceritol, a pseudotrisaccharide isolated from lentils', *J Agri Food Chem*, **41**, 870–2.

Bertin, C., Rouau, X. and Thibault, J.-F. (1988) 'Structure and properties of sugar beet fibres', *J Sci Food Agric*, **44**, 15–29.

Betteridge, V. (2009) 'Dietary fibre: an evolving definition', *Nutr Bull*, **34**(2), 122–5.

Bingham, S.A. (1990) 'Mechanisms and experimental and epidemiological evidence relating dietary fibre (non-starch polysaccharides) and starch to protection against large bowel cancer', *Proc Nutr Soc*, **49**, 153–71.

Birkett, A.M. and Brown, I.L. (2008) 'Resistant starch and health'. In B.R. Hamaker (ed), *Technology of Functional Cereal Products*, pp. 63–85, Woodhead Publishing, Cambridge.

Bjorck, I., Nylan, M. and Asp, N.G. (1984) 'Extrusion cooking and dietary fiber: effects on dietary fiber content and on degradation in the rat intestinal tract', *Cereal Chem*, **61**, 174–9.

Bobin-Dubigeon, C. (1996) 'Caractérisation chimique, physico-chimique et fermentaire de produits alimentaires à base d'algues', thèse de doctorat, Université de Nantes, 194.

Bobin-Dubigeon, C., Lahaye, M., Guillon, F., Barry, J.-L. and Gallant, D.J. (1997) 'Factors limiting the biodegradation of Ulva sp cell wall polysaccharides', *J Sci Food Agric*, **75**, 341–51.

Bohm, A., Bogoni, C., Behrens, R. and Otto, T. (2003) 'Method for the extraction aleurone from bran.' US Patent Application Publication US 2003/0175384 A1 Applicant Buhler A.G.

Bohm, A. and Kratzer, A. (2005) 'Method for isolating aleurone particles.' US Patent Application Publication US 2005/0103907 A1 Applicant Buhler A.G.

Botham, R.L., Ryden, P., Robertson, J.A. and Ring, S.G. (1998) 'Structural features of polysaccharides and their influence on fermentation behaviour'. In F. Guillon *et al.* (eds), *Functional Properties of Non-digestible Carbohydrates*, pp. 46–51, Nantes, INRA.

Burkitt, D.O. and Trowell, H.C. (1975) *Refined Carbohydrates Foods and Disease: Implication of Dietary Fiber*, London, Academic Press.

Burton-Freeman B., Davis, P.A. and Schneeman, B.O. (2002) 'Plasma cholecystokinin is associated with subjective measures of satiety in women', *Am J Clin Nutr*, **76**(3), 659–67.

Buri, R.C., Von Reding, W. and Gavin, M.H. (2004) 'Description and characterization of wheat aleurone', *Cereal Foods World*, **49**, 247–82.

Buttriss, J.L. and Stokes, C.S. (2008) 'Dietary fibre and health: an overview', *Nutrition Bulletin*, **33**(3), 186–200.

Camire, M.E. (1999) 'Chemical and physical modification of dietary fibre'. In S.S. Cho, L. Prosky and M. Dreher (eds), *Complex Carbohydrates in Foods*, pp. 373–84, New York, Marcel Dekker.

Cani, P.D., Neyrinck, A.M., Fava, F., Knauf, C., Burcelin, R.G., *et al.* (2007) 'Selective increases of bifidobacteria in gut microflora improve high fat-diet-induced diabetes in mice through a mechanism associated with endotoxaemia', *Diabetologia*, **50**, 2374–83.

Cani, P.D., Possemiers, S., de Van, W.T., Guiot, Y., Everard, A., Rottier, O., *et al.* (2009) 'Changes in gut microbiota control inflammation in obese mice through a mechanism involving GLP-2-driven improvement of gut permeability', *Gut*, **58**, 1091–1103.

Caprez, A., Arrigoni, E., Neukom, H. and Amadó, R. (1987) 'Improvement of the sensory properties of two different dietary fibre sources through enzymatic modification', *Lebens Wiss Technol*, **20**, 245–50.

Carpita, N.C. and Gibeaut, D.M. (1993) 'Structural models of the primary walls of flowering plant', *Plant J*, **3**, 1–30.

Carpita, N.C. and McCann, M.C. (2000) 'The cell wall.' In W. Buchanan, W. Gruissem and R. Jones (eds), *Biochemistry and Molecular Biology of Plants*, pp. 52–108, Washington DC, American Society of Biologists.

Champ, M., Martin, L., Noah, L. and Gratas, M. (1999) 'Analytical methods for resistant starch'. In S.S. Cho, L. Prosky and M. Dreher (eds), *Complex Carbohydrates in Foods*, pp. 169–87, New York, Marcel Dekker.

Cherbut, C. (1995) 'Fermentation et fonction digestive colique', *Cah Nutr Diét*, **30**, 143–7.

Cherbut, C., Barry, J.-L., Lairon, D. and Durand, M. (1995) *Dietary Fibre: Mechanisms of Action in Human Physiology and Metabolism*, Paris, John Libbey Eurotex.

Cho, S.S., O'Sullivan, K. and Rickard, S. (1999a) 'Worldwide dietary fiber intake: recommendations and actual consumption patterns'. In S.S. Cho, L. Prosky and M. Dreher (eds), *Complex Carbohydrates in Foods*, pp. 411–29, New York, Marcel Dekker.

Cho, S.S., Prosky, L. and Dreher, M. (1999b) *Complex Carbohydrates in Foods*, New York, Marcel Dekker.

Cloutour, F. (1995) 'Caractéristiques des fibres alimentaires: influence sur leur fermentation in vitro par la flore digestive de l'homme', thèse de doctorat, Université de Nantes, 130.

Cosgrove, D.J. (1997) 'Assembly and enlargement of the primary cell wall in plants', *Annu Rev Cell Dev Biol*, **13**, 171–201.

Cosgrove, D.J. (2005) 'Growth of the plant cell wall', *Nature Reviews Molecular Cell Biology*, **6**, 850–61.

Coussement, P. (1999) 'Inulin and oligofructose as dietary fiber: analytical, nutritional and legal aspects'. In S.S. Cho, L. Prosky and M. Dreher (eds), *Complex Carbohydrates in Foods*, pp. 203–11, New York, Marcel Dekker.

Craig, S.A.S., Holden, J.F., Troup, J.P., Auerbach, M.H. and Frier, H. (1999) 'Polydextrose as soluble fiber and complex carbohydrate'. In S.S. Cho, L. Prosky and M. Dreher (eds), *Complex Carbohydrates in Foods*, pp. 229–48, New York, Marcel Dekker.

Cummings, J.H. (1995) 'Short chain fatty acids'. In G.R. Gibson and G.T. Macfarlane (eds) *Human Colonic Bacteria: Role in Nutrition, Physiology and Pathlogy*. pp. 101–130, Boca Raton, FL, CRC Press.

Cummings, J.H. and Englyst, H. (1987) 'Fermentation in the human large intestine and the available substrate', *Am J Clin Nutr*, **45**, 1243–55.

Cui, S.W. and Wang, Q. (2009) 'Cell wall polysaccharides in cereal: chemical structure and functional properties', *Structural Chem*, **20**, 291–7.

Darcy-Vrillon, B. and Duée, P.H. (1995) 'Fibre effect on nutrient metabolism in splanchnic and peripheral tissues'. In C. Cherbut, J.-L. Barry, D. Lairon and M. Durand (eds), *Dietary Fibre: Mechanisms of Action in Human Physiology and Metabolism*, pp. 83–94, Paris, John Libbey Eurotex.

De Leenheer, L. (1996) 'Production and use of inulin: industrial reality with a promising future'. In H. van Bekkum, H. Ròper and F. Voragen (eds), *Carbohydrates as Organic Raw Materials III*, pp. 67–92, NL-2509JC The Hague, CRF Cabohydrate Research Foundation.

Demigné, C., Morand, C., Levrat, A.-M., Besson, C., Moundras, C. and Remesy, C. (1995) 'Effect of propionate on fatty acid and cholesterol synthesis and on acetate metabolism in isolated rat hepatocytes', *Br J Nutr*, **74**, 209–19.

Dikeman, C.L. and Fahey, G.C. (2006) 'Viscosity related to dietary fiber: a review', *Crit Rev Food Sci Nutr*, **46**, 649–63.

Diplock, A.T., Agget, P.J., Ashwell, M., Bornet, F., Fern, E.B. and Roberfroid, R. (1999) 'Functional food science in Europe', Foreword, *Br J Nutr*, **81**, S1–27.

Dongowski, G. (2009) 'Determination of interactions in vitro between dietary fibre-rich products and bile acids', *Ernahrung*, **33**, 298–313.

Drakoularakou, D., McCartney, A., Rastall, R. and Gibson, G.R. (2004) 'Established and emerging prebiotics and their effects on the gut microflora', *Agro Food Indust Hi Tech*, **15**, 18–20.

Dreher, M. (1999) 'Food sources and uses of dietary fiber'. In S.S. Cho, L. Prosky and M. Dreher (eds), *Complex Carbohydrates in Foods*, pp. 327–71, New York, Marcel Dekker.

Dupin, H., Abraham, J. and Giachetti, I. (1992) 'Apports nutritionnels conseillés pour la population française', Paris, Editions Lavoisier Technique et Documentation.

Dysseler, P. (1997) 'Fibres alimentaires: définition et sources de fibres alimentaires'. Conference: Propriétés et utilisation: intérêts fonctionnels et nutritionnels', Fibres Alimentaires, Ingrédients Fonctionnels et Nutritionnels. Résultats de trois programmes européens, Rennes, 14 March 1997.

Dysseler, P., Hoffem, D., Fockedey, J., Quemener, B., Thibault, J.-F. and Coussement, P. (1999) 'Determination of inulin and oligofructose in food products (modified AOAC dietary fibre method)'. In S.S. Cho, L. Prosky and M. Dreher (eds), *Complex Carbohydrates in Foods*, pp. 213–27, New York, Marcel Dekker.

European Commission Directive 2008/100/EC Annex II.

Edwards, C. (1995) 'Dietary fibre, fermentation and the colon'. In C. Cherbut, J.-L. Barry, D. Lairon and M. Durand (eds), *Dietary Fibre: Mechanisms of Action in Human Physiology and Metabolism*, pp. 51–60, Paris, John Libbey Eurotex.

Englyst, H., Quigley, M.E. and Hudson, G.J. (1994) 'Determination of dietary fibre as non-starch polysaccharides with gas-liquid chromatographic, high-performance liquid chromatographic measurement of constituent sugars', *Analyst*, **119**, 1497–1509.

Fan, L.T., Lee, Y.H. and Beardmore, D.H. (1980) 'Mechanism of enzymatic hydrolysis of cellulose: effects of major structural features of cellulose on enzymatic hydrolysis', *Biotechnol Bioeng*, **22**, 177–9.

FAO/WHO, (1997) 'Carbohydrates in human nutrition', FAO Food and Nutrition Paper 66. Report of a Joint FAO/WHO Expert Consultation, Rome, April 1997.

Farber, B. and Gallant, D.J. (1976) 'Evaluation de divers traitements technologiques des céréales', *Ann Zootech*, **25**, 13–30.

Femenia, A., Selvendran, R.R., Ring, S.G. and Robertson, J.A. (1999) 'Effect of heat treatment and dehydration on properties of cauliflower fiber', *J Agric Food Chem*, **47**, 728–732.

Fincher, G.B. and Stone, B.A. (1986) 'Cell walls and their components in cereal grain technology'. In *Advances in Cereal Science and Technology*, vol. VIII, pp. 207–295, St Paul, MN, American Association of Cereal Chemists.

Fleming, S.E. (1981) 'A study of relationships between flatus potential and carbohydrate distribution in legume seeds', *J Food Sci*, **46**, 794–803.

Gharpuray, M.M., Lee, Y.-H. and Fan, L.T. (1983) 'Structural modification of lignocellulosics by pretreatments to enhance enzymatic hydrolysis', *Biotechnol Bioeng*, **25**, 157–72.

Gould, J.M., Jasberg, B.K. and Cote, G.C. (1989) 'Structure–function relationship of alkaline peroxide treated lignocellulose', *Cereal Chem*, **66**, 213–17.

Grootaert, C., Delcour, J.A., Courtin, C.M., Broekaert, W.F., Verstraete, W. and Van de Wiele, T. (2007) 'Microbial metabolism and prebiotic potency of arabinoxylan oligosaccharides in the human intestine', *Trends Food Sci Tech*, **18**, 64–71.

Guillon, F., Amadó, R., Amara-Collaço, M.T., Andersson, H., Asp, N.G., *et al.* (1998a) *Functional Properties of Non-digestible Carbohydrates*, Nantes, INRA.

Guillon, F., Auffret, A., Robertson, J.A., Thibault, J.-F. and Barry, J.L. (1998b) 'Relationships between physical characteristics of sugar-beet fibre and its fermentability by human faecal flora', *Carbohydrate Polymers*, **37**, 185–97.

Guillon, F., Cloutour, F. and Barry, J.-L. (1996) 'Dietary fibre: relationships between intrinsic characteristics and fermentation pattern'. In Y. Málki and J.H. Cummings (eds), *Proceedings of COST Action 92, Espoo, Finland, Dietary Fibre and Fermentation in the Colon*, pp. 117–29, Brussels, European Commission.

Guillon, F. and Thibault, J.-F. (1996) 'Les fibres alimentaires, additifs ou ingrédients alimentaires?' *Actualités en diététique*, **22**, 897–903.

Guo, M. (2009) 'Dietary fiber and dietary fiber rich foods'. In M. Guo, *Functional Foods: Principles and Technology*, pp 63–111, Cambridge, Woodhead Publishing.

Hamer, H.M., Jonkers, D., Venema, K., Vanhoutvin S., Troost, F.J. and Brummer, R.J. (2008) 'Review article: the role of butyrate on colonic function', *Aliment Pharmacol Ther*, **27**, 104–19.

Heller, S.N., Rivers, J.M. and Hackler, L.R. (1977) 'Dietary fibre: the effect of particle size and pH on its measurement', *J Food Sci*, **42**, 436–9.

Hemery, Y., Rouau, X., Lullien Pellerin, V., Barron, C. and Abecassis, J. (2007) 'Dry processes to develop wheat fractions and products with enhanced nutritional quality' *J Cereal Sci*, **46**, 327–47.

Higginson, J.M.D. (1995) 'Fiber and cancer: historical perspectives'. In D. Kritchevsky and C. Bonfield (eds), *Dietary Fiber in Health and Disease*, pp. 174–190, St Paul, MN, Eagan Press.

Hispley, E.H. (1953) 'Dietary fibre and pregnancy toxaemia', *Brit Med J*, **2**, 420–22.

Holm, J., Bjorck, I., Ostrouska, S., Eliasson, A.-C., Asp, N.-G., *et al.* (1983) 'Digestibility of amylose-lipid complexes in vitro and in vivo', *Starch*, **35**, 294–8.

Hughes, A., Shewry, P.R., Li, L., Gibson, G.R., Sanz, M.L. and Rastall, R.A. (2007) 'In vitro fermentation by human fecal microflora of wheat arabinoxylans', *J Agric Food Chem*, **55**, 4589–95.

Jasberg, B.K., Gould, J.M. and Warner, K. (1989) 'High fiber, noncaloric flour subtitute for baked foods: alkaline peroxide-treated lignocellulose in chocolate cake', *Cereal Chem*, **66**, 209–13.

Jayarajah, C.N., Trang, H.-R., Robertson, J.A. and Selvendran, R.R. (1997) 'Dephytinisation of wheat bran and the consequences for fibre matrix non-starch polysaccharides', *Food Chem*, **58**, 5–12.

Katina, K., Liukonnen, K.H., Kaukovirta-Norja, H., Adlercreutz, H., Heinonen, S.M., *et al.* (2007) 'Fermentation-induced changes in the nutritional value of native or germinated rye', *J Cereal Sci*, **46**, 348–55.

Knudsen, K.E.B. and Laerke, H.N. (2010) 'Rye arabinoxylans: molecular structure, physicochemical properties and physiological effects in the gastrointestinal Tract', *Cereal Chem*, **87**, 353–62.

Kritchevsky, D. and Bonfield, C. (1995) *Dietary Fiber in Health and Disease*, St Paul, MN, Eagan Press.

Langkilde, A.M. and Andersson, H. (1998) 'Amount and composition of substrate entering the colon'. In F. Guillon *et al.* (eds), *Functional Properties of Non-digestible Carbohydrates*, pp. 140–142, Nantes, INRA.

Larrauri, J.A. (1999) 'New approaches in the preparation of high dietary fibre powders from fruit by-products', *Trends in Food Sci and Technol*, **10**, 3–8.

Lineback, D. (1999) 'The chemistry of complex carbohydrates'. In S.S. Cho, L. Prosky and M. Dreher (eds), *Complex Carbohydrates in Foods*, pp. 115–129, New York, Marcel Dekker.

Liukonnen, K.H., Katina, K., Wilhelmsson, A., Myllymaki, O., Lampi, A.M., *et al.* (2003) 'Process-induced changes on bioactive compounds in whole grain rye', *Proceeding of Nutrition Society*, **62**, 117–22.

Lo, G.S. (1989) 'Nutritional and physical properties of dietary fiber from soybeans', *Cereal Foods World*, **34**, 530–4.

Lopez, P., Sanchez, A.C., Vercet, A. and Burgos, J. (1997) 'Thermal resistance of tomato polygalacturonase and pectinmethyl esterase at physiological pH', *Food Res Technol*, **204**, 146–50.

Louka, N. and Allaf, K. (1998) 'Improvement of the quality of dried vegetable product by controlled instantaneous decompression'. In F. Guillon *et al.* (eds) *Functional Properties of Non-digestible Carbohydrates*, pp. 81–2, Nantes, INRA.

Lue, S., Hsieh, F., Peng, I.C. and Huff, H.E. (1990) 'Expansion of corn extrudates containing dietary fiber: a microstructure study', *Lebensm Wiss u Technol*, **23**, 165–73.

Lunn J. and Buttriss J.L. (2007) 'Carbohydrates and dietary fibre', *Nutr Butt*, **32**(1), 21–64.

Macfarlane, G.T. and Degnan, B.A. (1996) 'Catabolite regulatory mechanisms in relation to polysaccharide breakdown and carbohydrate utilization'. In Y. Málki and J.H. Cummings (eds), *Proceedings of COST Action 92, Dietary Fibre and Fermentation in the Colon*, pp. 117–129, Brussels, European Commission.

Macfarlane, G.T. and Macfarlane, S. (1993) 'Factors affecting fermentation reactions in the large bowel', *Nutr Soc Proc*, **52**, 367–73.

McIntyre, A., Gibson, P.R. and Young, G.P. (1993) 'Butyrate production from dietary fibre and protection against large bowel cancer in a rat model', *Gut*, **34**, 386–91.

Martin, L.J.M., Dumon, H.J.W. and Champ, M.M.J. (1998) 'Production of short chain fatty acids from resistant starch in a pig model', *J Sci Food Agric*, **77**, 71–80.

Mateo Anson, N., Van den Berg, R., Havenaar, R., Bast, A., and Haenen, G., (2008) 'Ferulic acid from aleurone determines the antioxidant potency of wheat grain (Triticum aestivum L.),' *J Agric Food Chem*, **56**, 5589–94.

Mathers, J.C., Roper, C.S., Cherbut, C., Hoebler, C., Darcy-Vrillon, B. and Vaudelade, P. (1998) 'Physiological responses to polysaccharides: are rats and pigs good models for humans?' In F. Guillon *et al.* (eds) *Functional Properties of Non-digestible Carbohydrates*, pp. 110–12, Nantes, INRA.

McCleary, B. (2010) 'Development of an integrated total dietary fiber method consistent with the Codex Alimentarius definition', *Cereal Foods World*, **55**(1), 24–8.

Michel, C., Kravtchenko, T.P., David, A., Gueneau, S., Kozlowski, F. and Cherbut, C. (1998) 'In vitro prebiotic effects of Acacia gums onto the human intestinal microbiota depends on the botanical origin and environment pH', *Anaerobe*, **4**, 257–66.

Miller Jones, J. (2008) 'Fiber, whole grains and disease prevention'. In B.R. Hamaker (ed.), *Technology of Functional Cereal Products*, pp. 46–62, Cambridge, Woodhead Publishing.

Morris, E.R. (1990) 'Shear thinning of random coil polysaccharides: characterisation by two parameters from a simple linear plot', *Carbohydr Polym*, **13**, 85–96.

Morris, E.R. (1992) 'Physico-chemical properties of food polysaccharides'. In T.F. Schweizer and C. Edwards (eds), *Dietary Fibre, A Component of Food: Nutritional Function in Health and Disease*, pp 41–56, ILSI Europe, Berlin, Springer-Verlag.

Noah, L., Guillon, F., Bouchet, B., Buleon, A., Molis, C., Gratas, *et al.* (1998) 'Digestion of carbohydrate from white beans (*Phaseolus vulgaris* L.) in healthy humans', *J Nutr*, **128**, 977–85.

Pastell, H., Westerman, P., Meyer, N.S., Tuomainen, P. (2009) '*In vitro* fermentation of arabinoxylan-derived carbohydrates by bifidobacteria and mixed fecal microbiota', *J Agric Food Chem*, **57**(18), 8598–8606.

Plat, D., Ben-Halom, N., Levi, A., Reid, D. and Goldschmidt, E. (1991) 'Changes in pectic susbtances in carrots during hydration with and without blanching', *Food Chem*, **39**, 1–12.

Pomeranz, Y. (1988) 'Chemical composition and kernel structures'. In Y. Pomeranz (ed.), *Wheat: Chemistry and Technology*, pp 97–158, St Paul, MN, AACC.

Ponne, C.T., Armstrong, D.R. and Luyten, H. (1997) 'Food fibres as technological agents in foods'. In F. Guillon *et al.* (eds) *Plant Polysaccharides in Human Nutrition: Structure, Function, Digestive Fate and Metabolic Effects*, pp. 6–12, Nantes, INRA.

Ponne, C.T., Armstrong, D.R. and Luyten, H. (1998) 'Influence of dietary fibres on textural properties of food'. In F. Guillon *et al.* (eds) *Functional Properties of Non-digestible Carbohydrates*, pp. 61–5, Nantes, INRA.

Poutanen, K. (1997) 'Enzymes, an important tool in the improvement of the quality of cereal foods', *Trends Food Sci Techn*, **8**, 300–6.

Poutanen, K., Suirtti, T., Aura, A-M., Liukonnen, K. and Autio, K. (1998) 'Influence of processing on the ceral dietary fibre complex: what do we know?' In F. Guillon *et al.* (eds), *Functional Properties of Non-digestible Carbohydrates*, pp. 66–70, Nantes, INRA.

Quemener, B. and Brillouet, J.-M. (1983) 'Ciceritol, a pinitol digalactoside from seeds of chickpea lentil and white lupin', *Phytochem*, **22**, 1745–51.

Rahman, A.R., Henning, W.L. and Westcoot, D.E. (1971) 'Histological and physical changes in carrots as affected by blanching, cooking, freezing, freeze-drying and compression', *J Food Sci*, **36**, 500–2.

Ralet, M.-C., Thibault, J.-F. and Della Valle, G. (1991) 'Solubilization of sugar-beet pulp cell wall polysaccharides by extrusion cooking', *Lebensm Wiss u Technologie*, **24**, 107–12.

Ralet, M.-C., Axelos, M. and Thibault, J.-F. (1994) 'Gelation properties of extruded lemon cell walls and their water soluble pectins', *Carbohydr Res*, **260**, 271–82.

Ralet, M.-C., Della Valle, G. and Thibault, J.-F. (1993) 'Raw and extruded fibre from pea hulls. Part I: composition and physico-chemical properties', 17–23; 'Part II: structural study of the water-soluble polysaccharides', 25–34, *Carbohydrate Polymers*, **20**, 17–34.

Ralet, M.-C., Thibault, J.-F. and Della Valle, G. (1990) 'Influence of extrusion cooking on the physico-chemical properties of wheat bran', *J Cereal Sci*, **11**, 249–59.

Remesy, C. (1996) 'Intérêt nutritionnel des fibres et des micronutriments apportés par les fruits et légumes', *Actualités en diététique*, **22**, 883–95.

Renard, C.M.G.C., Crepeau, M.-J. and Thibault, J.-F. (1994) 'Influence of ionic strength, pH and dielectric constant on hydration properties of native and modified fibres from sugar-beet and wheat bran', *Indus Crops Prod*, **3**, 75–84.

Roberfroid, M. (2007) 'Prebiotics: the concept revisited', *J Nutr*, **137**, S830–7.

Robertson, J.A. (1998) 'Application of plant-based byproducts as fiber supplements in processed foods', *Recent Res Devel in Agric Food Chem*, **2**, 705–17.

Robertson, J.A., De Monredon, J.-F., Dysseler, P., Guillon, F., Amado, R. and Thibault, J.-F. (2000) 'Hydration properties of dietary fibre and resistant starch: a European collaborative study', *Lebensm Wiss u Technologie*, **33**, 72–9.

Ryden, P. and Robertson, J.A. (1995) 'The effect of fibre source and fermentation on the apparent hydrophobic binding properties of wheat bran in preparations for the mutagen 2-amino-3, 8-dimethylimidazol 4, 5-F quinoxaline (MEIQX)', *Carcinogenesis*, **16**, 209–16.

Sakata, T. (1995) 'Effects of short chain fatty acids on gastrointestinal epithelial cells'. In C. Cherbut, J.-L. Barry, D. Lairon and M. Durand (eds), *Dietary Fibre: Mechanisms of Action in Human Physiology and Metabolism*, pp. 61–68, Paris, John Libbey Eurotex.

Salminen, S., Bouley, C., Boutron-Ruault, M.-C., Cummings, J.H., Franck, A., *et al.* (1998) 'Functional food science and gastrointestinal physiology and function', *British J Nutr*, **80** (Supp. 1), S147–71.

Schimberni, M., Cardinali, F., Sodini, G. and Canela, M. (1982) 'Chemical and functional characteristics of corn bran, oat hull and barley hull flour', *Lebensm Wiss u Technol*, **15**, 337–9.

Schweizer, T.F., Andersson, H., Langkilde, A.M., Reimann, S. and Torsdottir, I. (1990) 'Nutrients excreted in ileostomy effluents after consumption of mixed diets with beans and potatoes. II. Starch, dietary fibre and sugars', *Eur J Cli Nutr*, **44**, 567–75.

Schweizer, T.F. and Edwards, C.A. (1992) *Dietary Fiber: A Component of Food*, London, Springer-Verlag, pp. 41–45.

Segain, J.-P., Raingeard de la Blétière, D., Bourreille, A., Leray, V., Gervois, N., *et al.* (2000) 'Butyrate inhibits inflammatory responses through NFkappaB inhibition: implications for Crohn's disease'. *Gut*, **47**, 397–403.

Selvendran, R.R. and Robertson, J.A. (1990) 'The chemistry of dietary fibre: an holistic view of the cell wall matrix'. In D.A.T. Southgate, K. Waldron, I.T. Johnson and G.R. Fenwick (eds), *Dietary Fibre: Chemical and Biological Aspects*, RSC Special Publication No. 83, Cambridge. Royal Society of Chemistry.

Sidiras, D.K., Koulas, D.P., Vgenpoulos, A.G. and Koukios, E.G. (1990) 'Cellulose crystallinity as affected by various technical processes', *Cellulose Chem Technol*, **24**, 309–17.

Sinitsyn, A.P., Gusakov, A.V. and Vlasenko, A.E.Y. (1991) 'Effect of structural and physicochemical features of cellulosic substrates on the efficiency of enzymatic hydrolysis', *Appl Biochem Biotechnol*, **30**, 43–59.

Southgate, D.A.T. (1995) 'The structure of dietary fiber'. In D. Kritchevsky and C. Bonfield (eds), *Dietary Fiber in Health and Disease*, pp. 26–36, St Paul MN, Eagan Press.

Southgate, D.A.T., Hudson, G.J., and Englyst, H. (1978) 'The analysis of dietary fibre: the choice for the analyst', *J Sci Food Agric*, **29**, 979–98.

Southgate, D.A.T. (1981) 'What is the dietary fibre', *Food Technol Austr*, **33**, 24–5.

Southgate, D.A.T., Waldron, K., Johnson, I.T. and Fenwick, G.R. (1991) *Dietary Fibre: Chemical and Biological Aspects*, RSC Special Publication No. 83, Cambridge, Royal Society of Chemistry.

Stolle-Smits, T., Beekhuizen, J.G., Van Dijk, C., Voragen, A.G.J. and Recourt, K. (1995) 'Cell wall dissolution during industrial processing of green beans (Phaseolus vulgaris L.)', *J Agri Food Chem*, **43**, 2480–6.

Svanberg, M. (1997) 'Effects of processing on dietary fibre in vegetables', thesis, Department of Applied Nutrition and Food Chemistry, Lund Institute of Technology, Lund University, Lund, Sweden, p. 138.

Svanberg, M., Suortti, T. and Nyman, M. (1997) 'Effects of processing on physicochemical properties of dietary fibre in carrots'. In F. Guillon *et al.* (eds), *Plant Polysaccharides in Human Nutrition: Structure, Function, Digestive Fate and Metabolic Effects*, pp. 13–19, Nantes, INRA.

Swennen, K., Courtin, C.M., Lindemans, G.C.J.E. and Delcour, J.A. (2006) 'Large scale production and characterisation of wheat bran arabinoxylooligosaccharides', *J Sci Food Agric*, **86**, 1722–31.

Thibault, R., Blachier, F., Darcy-Vrillon, B., De Coppet, P., Bourreille, A, and Segain, J.P. (2007) 'Butyrate utilization by the colonic mucosa in inflammatory bowel diseases: a transport deficiency', *Inflamm Bowel Dis*, **16**(4), 684–95.

Thibault, J.-F., Della Valle, G. and Ralet, M.-C. (1998) 'Produits riches en parois végétales et fraction hydrosoluble accrue, leur obtention, leur utilisation et compositions les contenant', Brevet français no 88-11601, 5 September 1988.

Thibault, J.-F., Lahaye, M. and Guillon, F. (1992) 'Physicochemical properties of food plant cell walls'. In T.F. Schweizer and C. Edwards (eds), *Dietary Fibre, A Component of Food. Nutritional Function in Health and Disease*, pp. 21–39, ILSI Europe, Berlin: Springer-Verlag.

Thibault, J.-F., Ralet, M.-C., Axelos, M.A.V. and Della Valle, G. (1995) 'Effects of extrusion-cooking of pectin rich materials', Pectins and Pectinases, Wageningen (Pays-Bas), 3–7 December 1995.

Thibault, J.-F., Renard, M.G.C. and Guillon, F. (1994) 'Physical and chemical analysis of dietary fibres in sugar-beet and vegetable'. In J.F. Jackson and H.F. Linskens (eds), *Modern Methods of Plant Analysis, vol. 16, Vegetable and Vegetable Products*, pp. 23–55, Heidelberg, Springer-Verlag.

Topping, D.L. and Pant, I. (1995) 'Short-chain fatty acids and hepatic lipid metabolism: experimental studies'. In J.H. Cummings, J.C. Rombeau and T. Sakata (eds), *Physiological and Clinical Aspects of Short-chain Fatty Acids*, pp. 495–508, Cambridge, Cambridge University Press.

Tosh, S.M., Brummer, Y., Miller, S.S., Regand, A., Defelice, C., *et al.* (2010) 'Processing affects the physicochemical properties of beta-glucan in oat bran cereal' *J Agric Food Chem*, **58**, 7723–30.

Trowell, H. (1972) 'Dietary fibre and coronary heart disease', *Revue Européenne d'Etudes Cliniques et Biologiques*, **17**(4), 345–9.

Trowell, H. (1974) 'Definition of fiber', *Lancet*, **1**, 503–8.

Trowell, H., Southgate, D.A.T., Wolever, T.M.S., Leeds, A.R., Gassul, M.A., and Jenkins, D.J.A. (1976) 'Dietary fiber redefined', Lancet, **1**, 967.

Van Loo, J., Cummings, J.H., Delzenne, N., Englyst, H., Frank, A., *et al.* (1999) 'Functional food properties of non digestible oligosaccharides: a consensus report from the ENDO project' (DG XII AIRII-CT94-1095), *Br J Nutr*, **81**, 121–32.

Varo, P., Laine, R. and Koivistoinen, P. (1983) 'Effect of heat treatment on dietary fiber: interlaboratory study', *J Assoc Off Anal Chem*, **66**, 933–8.

Varo, P., Veijalainen, K. and Koivistoinen, P. (1984) 'Effect of heat treatment on the dietary fibre contents of potato and tomato', *J Food Technol*, **19**, 485–92.

Vásquez, M.J., Alonso, J.L., Domínguez, H. and Parajó, J.C. (2000) 'Xylooligosaccharides: manufacture and applications'. *Trends Food Sci Tech*, **11**, 387–93.

Voragen, A.G.J. (1998) 'Technological aspects of functional food-related carbohydrates', *Trends in Foods Science and Technology*, **9**, 328–35.

Walker, A.R.P. (1974) 'Dietary fibre and the pattern disease', *Ann Intern Med*, **80**, 663–4.

Weightman, R.M., Renard, M.G.C., Gallant, D.J. and Thibault, J.-F. (1994) 'Structure and properties of the polysaccharides from pea hulls. Part II: Modification of the composition and physico-chemical properties of commercial pea hulls by chemical extraction of the constituent polysaccharides', *Cabohyd Polym*, **24**, 139–48.

Wolever, T.M.S. (1995) 'Short chain fatty acids and carbohydrate metabolism'. In H.J. Binder, J.H. Cummings and K.H. Soergel (eds), *Short Chain Fatty Acids*, pp. 251–259, Falk Symposium 73, 8–10 September, 1995, Dordrecht, Kluwer Academic.

Wong, J.M., De Souza, R., Kendall, C.W., Emam, A. and Jenkins, D.J. (2006) 'Colonic health: fermentation and short chain fatty acids', *J Clin Gastroenterol*, **40**, 235–43.

Wood, P.J. (2010) 'Oat and rye beta glucan: properties and function', *Cereal Chemistry*, **87**, 315–30.

Wu, A. and Chang, W.H. (1990) 'Influence of precooking on the firmness and pectic substances of three stem vegetables', *Int J Food Sci Technol*, **25**, 558–63.

Wursch, P. (1999) 'Production of resistant starch'. In S.S. Cho, L. Prosky and M. Dreher (eds), *Complex Carbohydrates in Foods*, pp. 71–111, New York, Marcel Dekker.

Zhou, K., Laux, J.J. and Yu, L. (2004) 'Comparison of swiss red wheat grain and fractions for their antioxidant properties', *J Agric Food Chem*, **52**, 1118–23.

Index

Lightning Source UK Ltd.
Milton Keynes UK
UKOW07n0214101114

241140UK00009B/124/P

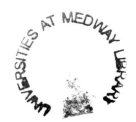

9 781845 696900